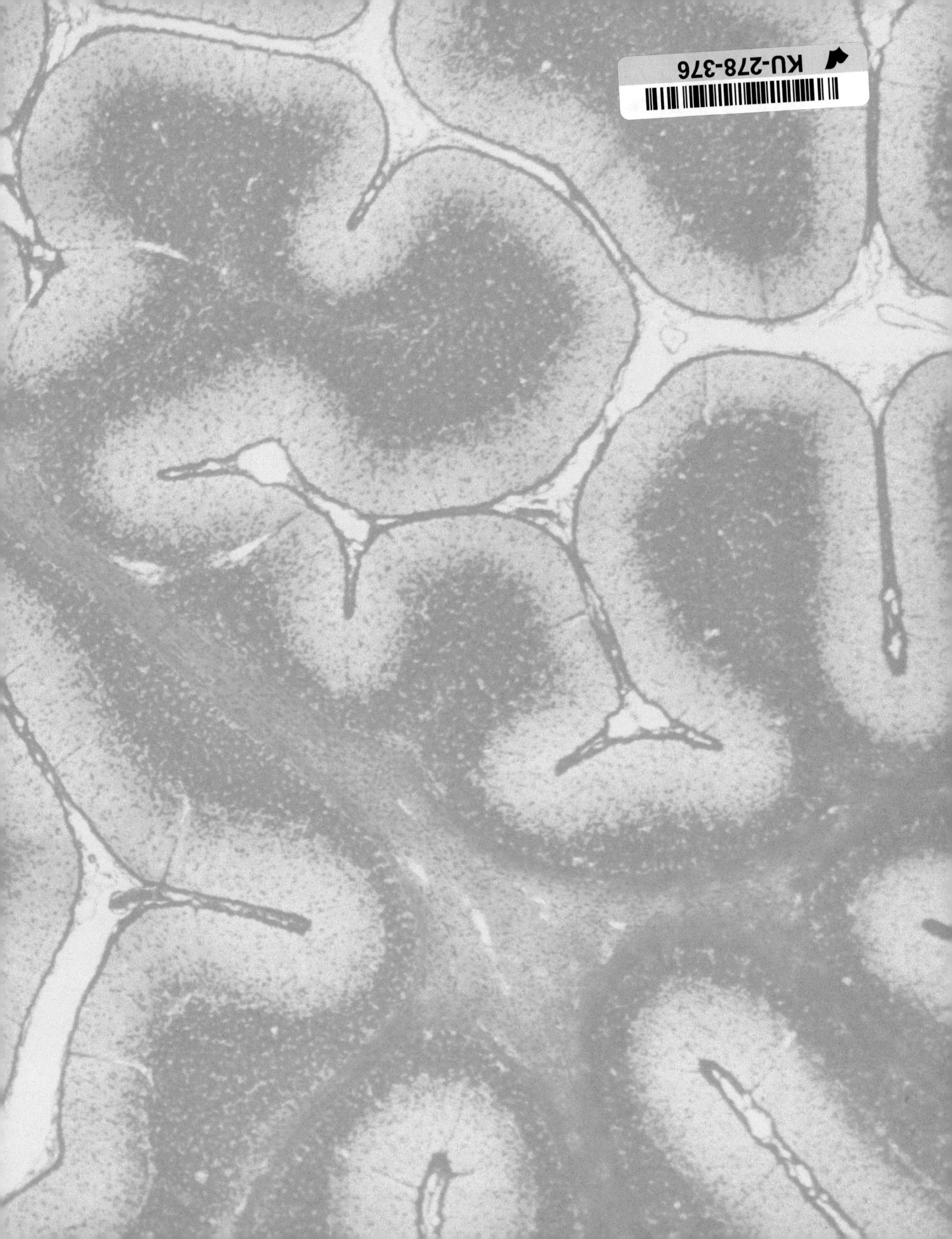

THE BRAIN BOOK

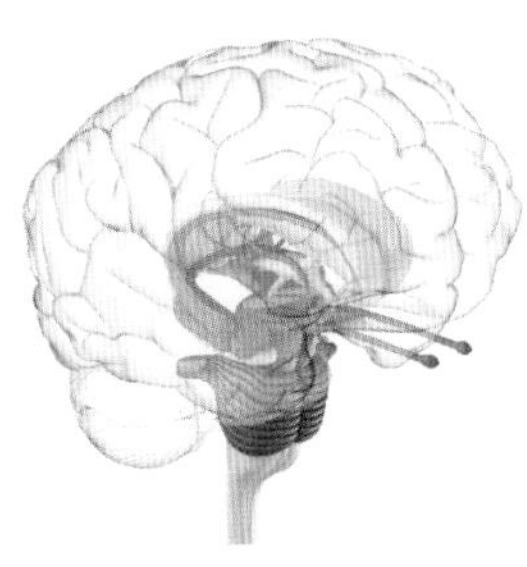
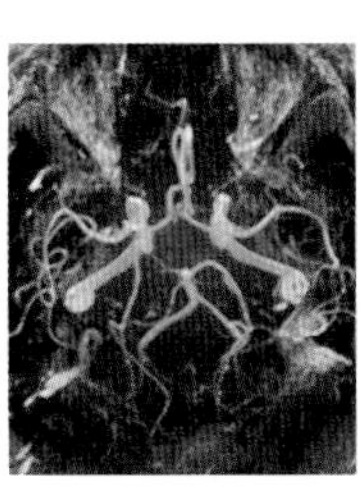
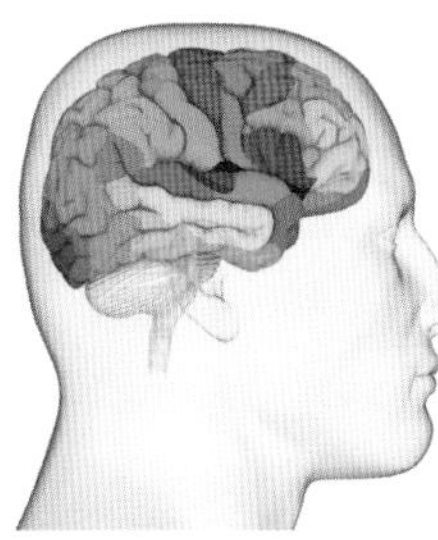
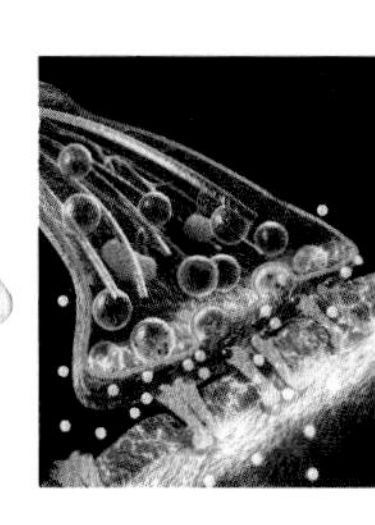
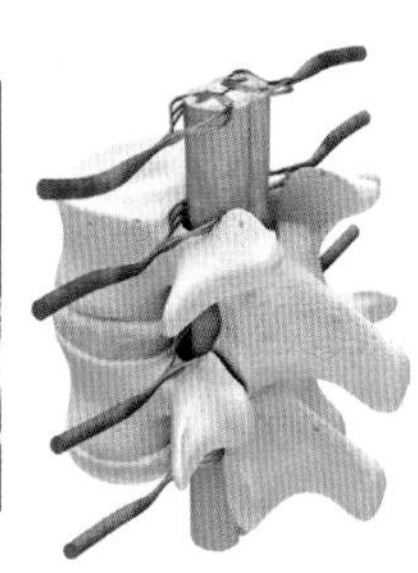

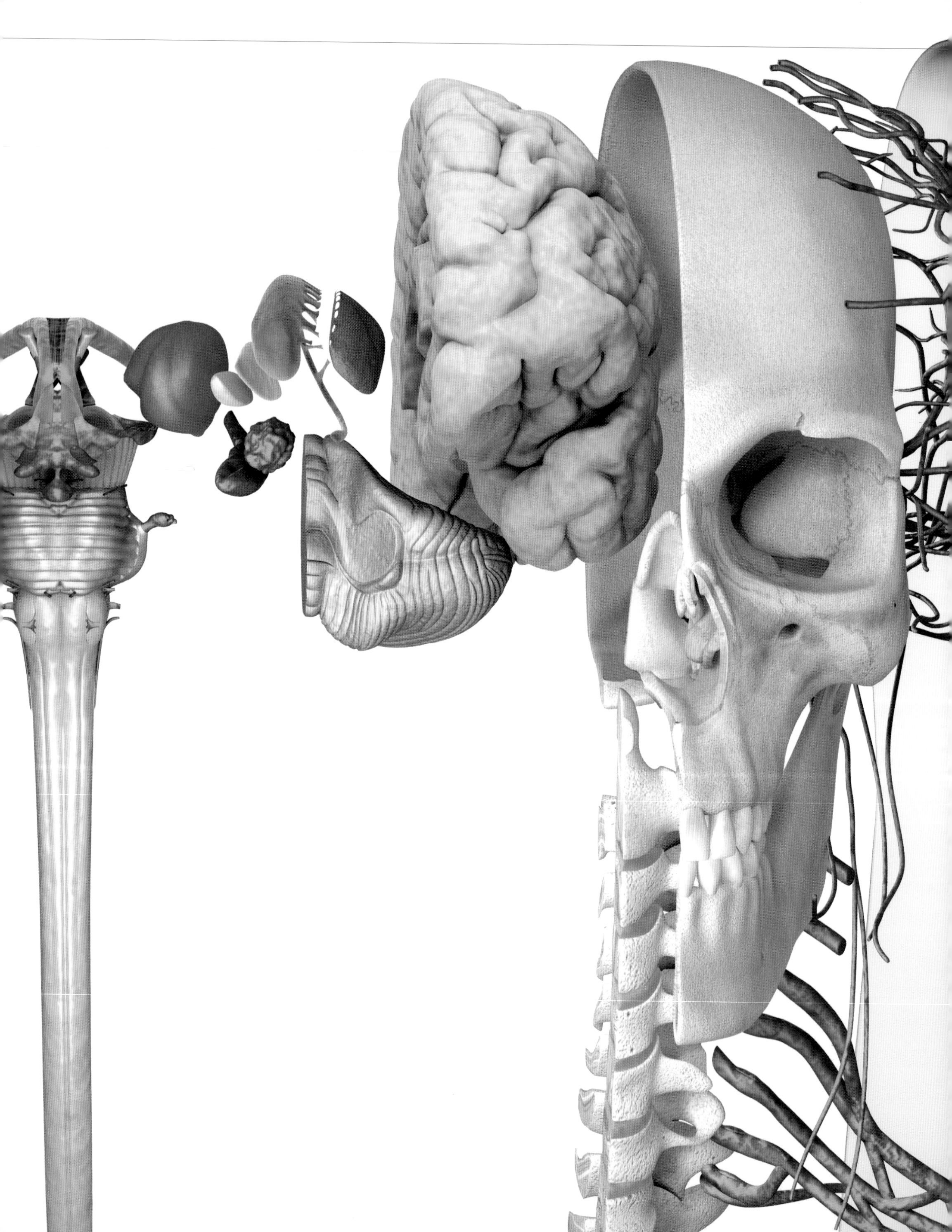

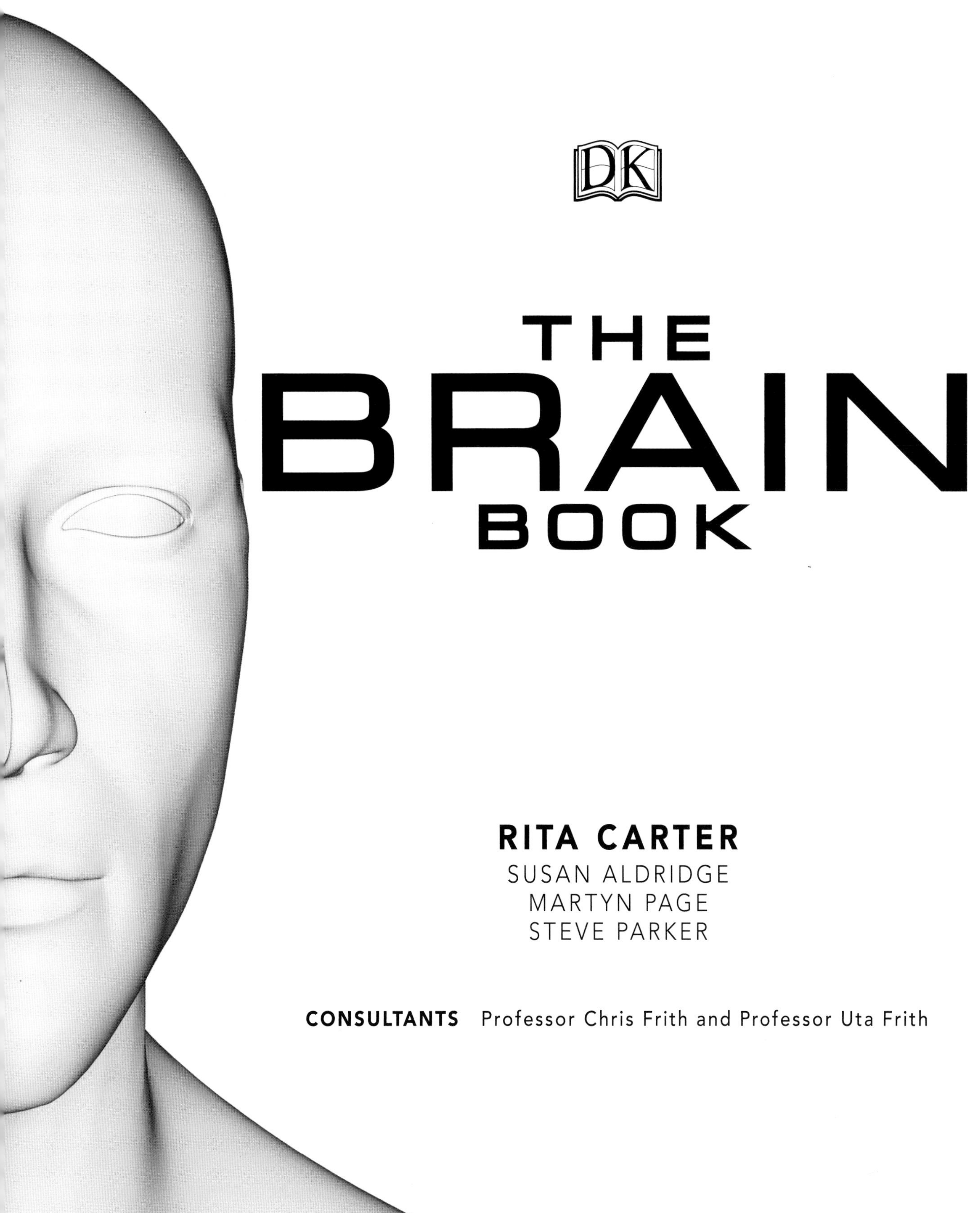

DK

THE BRAIN BOOK

RITA CARTER
SUSAN ALDRIDGE
MARTYN PAGE
STEVE PARKER

CONSULTANTS Professor Chris Frith and Professor Uta Frith

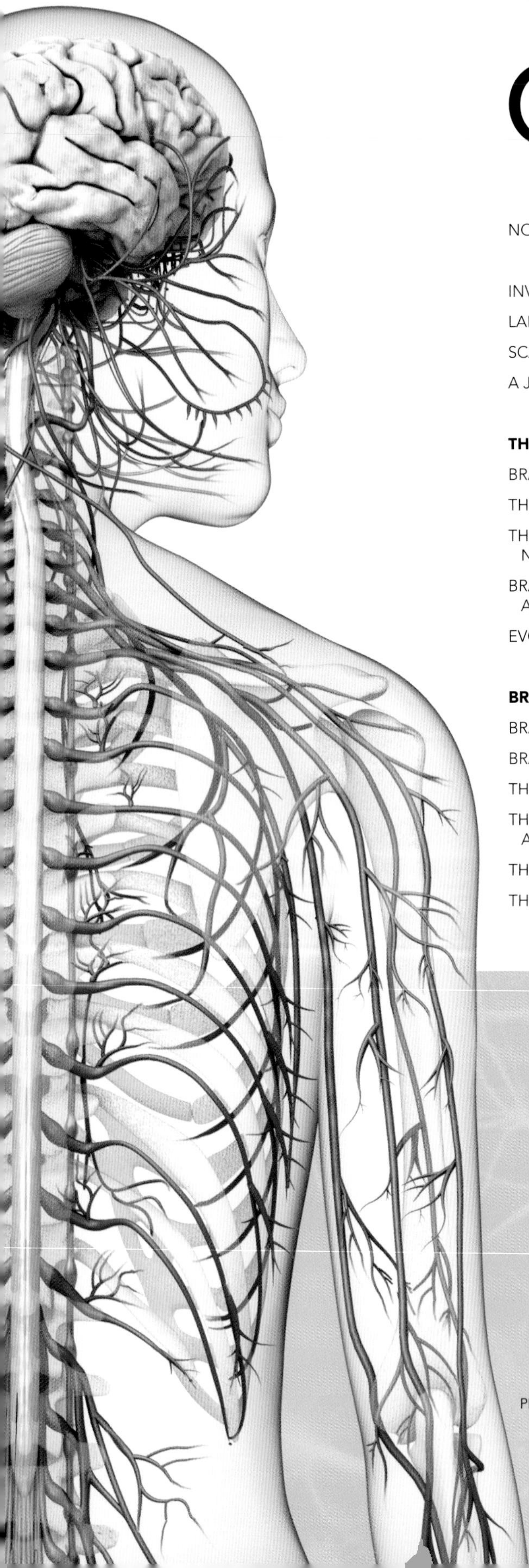

CONTENTS

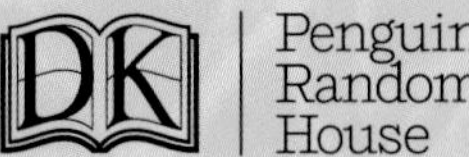

THIRD EDITION

DK DELHI

SENIOR EDITOR Rupa Rao
ART EDITOR Sonakshi Singh
MANAGING EDITOR Rohan Sinha
MANAGING ART EDITOR Sudakshina Basu
DTP DESIGNER Bimlesh Tiwary
PICTURE RESEARCHER Sumedha Chopra
PICTURE RESEARCH MANAGER Taiyaba Khatoon
PRE-PRODUCTION MANAGER Balwant Singh
PRODUCTION MANAGER Pankaj Sharma

DK LONDON

SENIOR EDITOR Peter Frances
PROJECT EDITOR Ruth O'Rourke-Jones
PROJECT ART EDITOR Francis Wong
MANAGING EDITOR Angeles Gavira Guerrero
MANAGING ART EDITOR Michael Duffy
JACKET DESIGN DEVELOPMENT MANAGER Sophia MTT
PRODUCER, PRE-PRODUCTION Gillian Reid
SENIOR PRODUCER Meskerem Berhane
ASSOCIATE PUBLISHER Liz Wheeler
ART DIRECTOR Karen Self
DESIGN DIRECTOR Phil Ormerod
PUBLISHING DIRECTOR Jonathan Metcalf

FIRST EDITION

SENIOR EDITOR Peter Frances
SENIOR ART EDITOR Maxine Lea
PROJECT EDITORS Nathan Joyce, Ruth O'Rourke, Miezan van Zyl
EDITORS Salima Hirani, Katie John, Rebecca Warren
PROJECT ART EDITORS Alison Gardner, Siân Thomas, Francis Wong
DESIGNER Riccie Janus
EDITORIAL ASSISTANT Elizabeth Munsey
INDEXER Hilary Bird
PROOFREADER Polly Boyd
PICTURE RESEARCHER Liz Moore
JACKET DESIGNER Duncan Turner
SENIOR PRODUCTION CONTROLLER Inderjit Bhullar
PRODUCTION EDITOR Tony Phipps

CREATIVE TECHNICAL SUPPORT Adam Brackenbury, John Goldsmid
MANAGING EDITOR Sarah Larter
SENIOR MANAGING ART EDITOR Phil Ormerod
PUBLISHING MANAGER Liz Wheeler
REFERENCE PUBLISHER Jonathan Metcalf
ART DIRECTOR Bryn Walls
ILLUSTRATORS Medi-Mation, Peter Bull Art Studio

This edition published in 2019
First published in Great Britain in 2009 by
Dorling Kindersley Limited
80 Strand, London, WC2R 0RL

A Penguin Random House Company
20 10 9 8 7 6 5 4 3
004–306003–Jan/2019

The Brain Book provides information on a wide range of medical topics, and every effort has been made to ensure that the information in this book is accurate. The book is not a substitute for medical advice, however, and you are advised always to consult a doctor or other health professional on personal health matters.

A CIP catalogue record for this book is available from the British Library

ISBN 978-0-2413-0225-5

Printed in China

A WORLD OF IDEAS:
SEE ALL THERE IS TO KNOW

www.dk.com

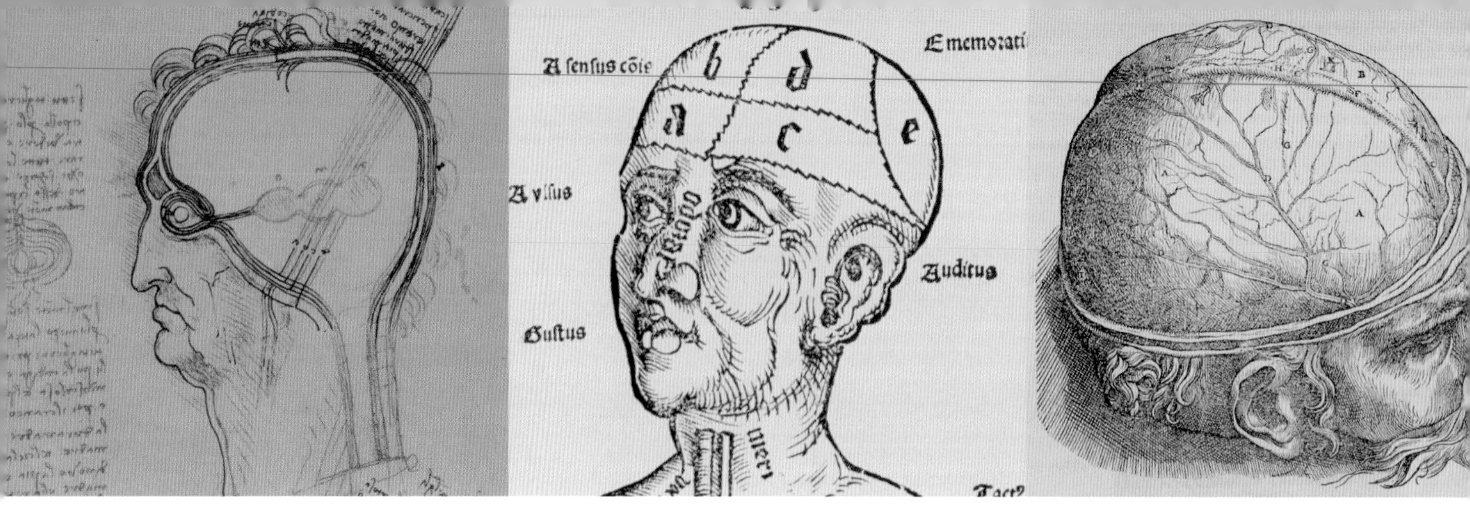

NO ORDINARY ORGAN

The human brain is like nothing else. As organs go, it is not especially prepossessing – 1.4kg (3lb) or so of rounded, corrugated flesh with a consistency somewhere between jelly and cold butter. It doesn't expand and shrink like the lungs, pump like the heart, or secrete visible material like the bladder. If you sliced off the top of someone's head and peered in you wouldn't see much happening at all.

SEAT OF CONSCIOUSNESS

Given this, it is perhaps not surprising that for centuries the contents of our skulls were regarded as relatively unimportant. When they mummified their dead, the ancient Egyptians scooped out the brains and threw them away, yet carefully preserved the heart. The Ancient Greek philospher, Aristotle, thought the brain was a radiator for cooling the blood. René Descartes, the French scientist, gave it a little more respect, concluding that it was a sort of antenna by which the spirit might commune with the body. It is only now that the full wonder of the brain is being realized.

The most basic function of the brain is to keep the rest of the body alive. Among your brain's 100 billion neurons, there are those that regulate your breathing, heartbeat, and blood pressure; and others that control your hunger, thirst, sex drive, and sleep cycle. On top of this the brain generates the emotions, perceptions, and thoughts that guide your behaviour. Then it directs and executes your actions. Finally, it is responsible for the conscious awareness of the mind itself.

THE DYNAMIC BRAIN

Until about 100 years ago, the only evidence that brain and mind were connected derived from "natural experiments" – accidents in which head injuries created aberrations in their victims' behaviour. Dedicated physicians mapped out areas of the cerebral landscape by observing the subjects of such experiments while they were alive – then matching their deficits to the damaged areas of their brains. It was slow work because the scientists had to wait for their subjects to die before they could look at the physiological evidence. As a result, until the early twentieth century, all that was known about the physical basis of mind could have been contained in a single volume.

Since then, scientific and technological advances have fuelled a neuroscientific revolution. Powerful microscopes made it possible to look in detail at the brain's intricate anatomy. A growing understanding of electricity allowed the dynamics of the brain to be recognized and then, with the advent of electroencephalography (EEG), to be

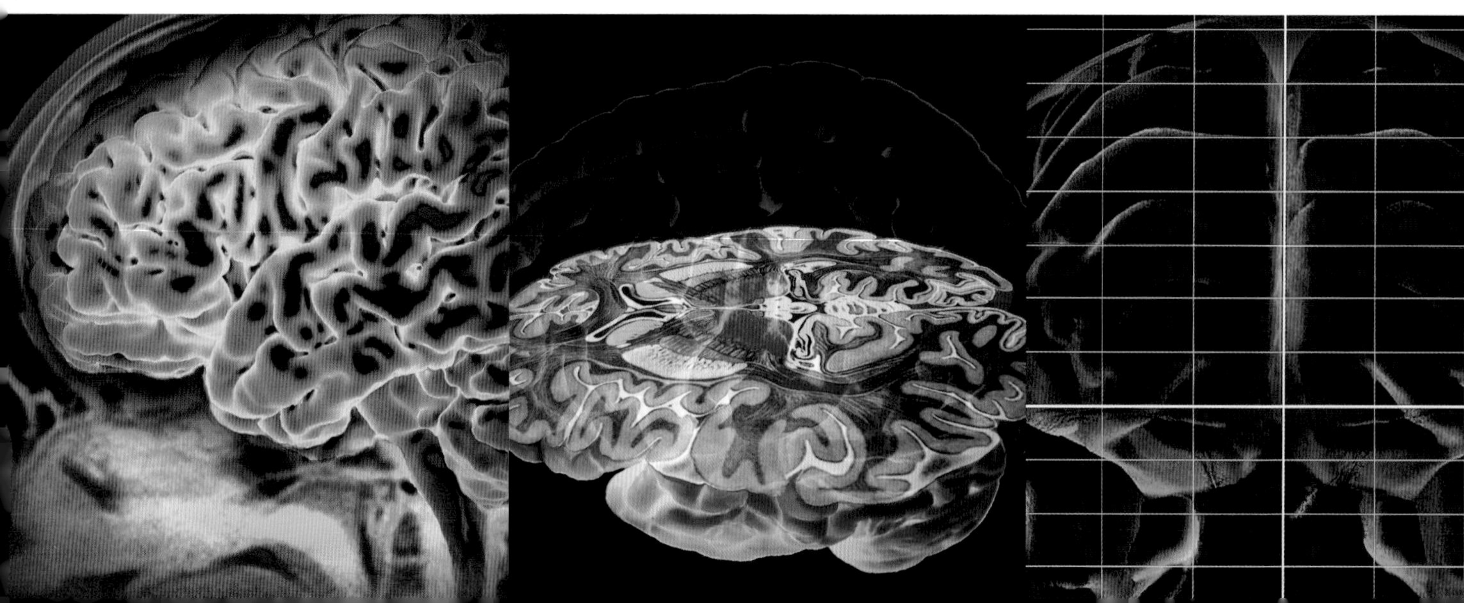

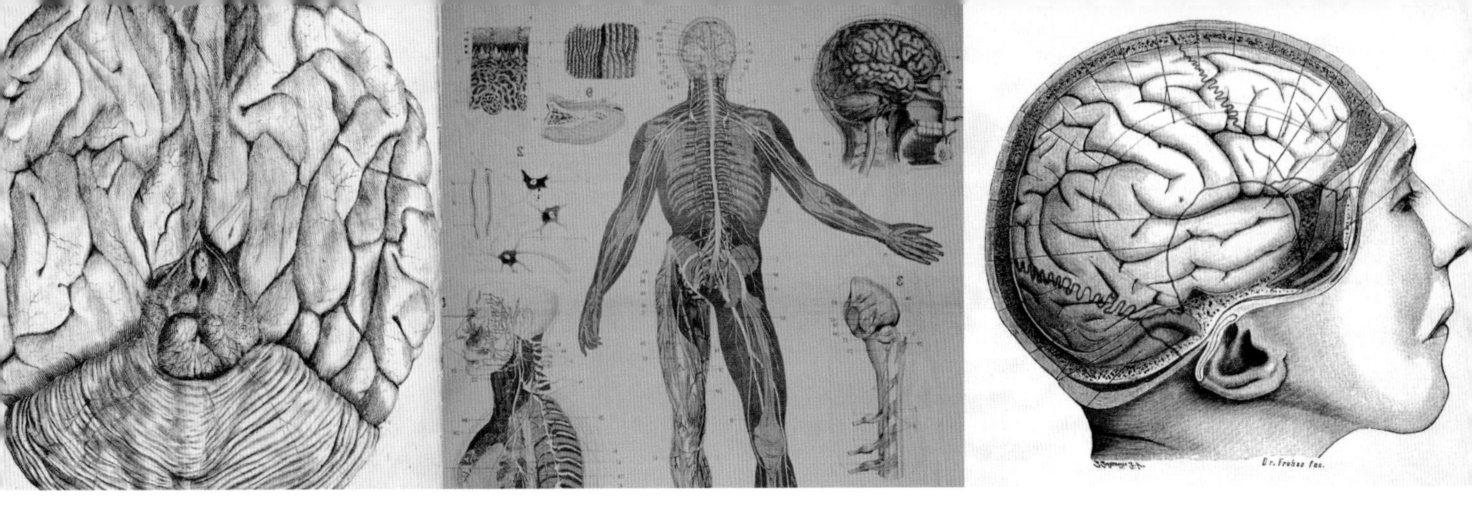

observed and measured. Finally, the arrival of functional brain imaging machines allowed scientists to look inside the living brain and see its mechanisms at work. In the last 20 years, positron emission tomography (PET), functional magnetic resonance imaging (fMRI), and, most recently, magnetic encephalography (MEG) have between them produced an ever more detailed map of the brain's functions.

LIMITLESS LANDSCAPE

Today we can point to the circuitry that keeps our vital processes going, the cells that produce our neurotransmitters, the synapses where signals leap from cell to cell, and the nerve fibres that convey pain or move our limbs. We know how our sense organs turn light rays and sounds waves into electrical signals, and we can trace the routes they follow to the specialized areas of cortex that respond to them. We know that such stimuli are weighed, valued, and turned into emotions by the amygdala – a tiny nugget of tissue punching way above its weight. We can see the hippocampus retrieve a memory, or watch the prefrontal cortex make a moral judgement. We can recognize the nerve patterns associated with amusement, empathy, – even the thrill of *schadenfreude* at the sight of an adversary suffering defeat. Rather than just a map, the picture emerging from imaging studies reveals the brain to be an astonishingly complex, sensitive system in which each part affects almost every other. "High level" cognition performed by the frontal lobes, for instance, feeds back to affect sensory experience – so what we see when we look at an object is shaped by expectation, as well as by the effect of light hitting the retina. Conversely, the brain's most sophisticated products can depend on its lowliest mechanisms. Intellectual judgements, for example, are driven by the bodily reactions that we feel as emotions, and consciousness can be snuffed out by damage to the humble brainstem. To confuse things further, the system doesn't stop at the neck but extends to the tips of your toes. Some would argue it goes beyond – to encompass other minds with which it interacts.

Neuroscientific investigation of the brain is very much a work in progress and no-one knows what the finished picture will look like. It may be that the brain is so complicated that it can never understand itself entirely. So this book cannot be taken as a full description of the brain. It is a single view, from bottom to top, of the human brain as we know it today – in all its beauty and complexity. Be amazed.

Rita Carter

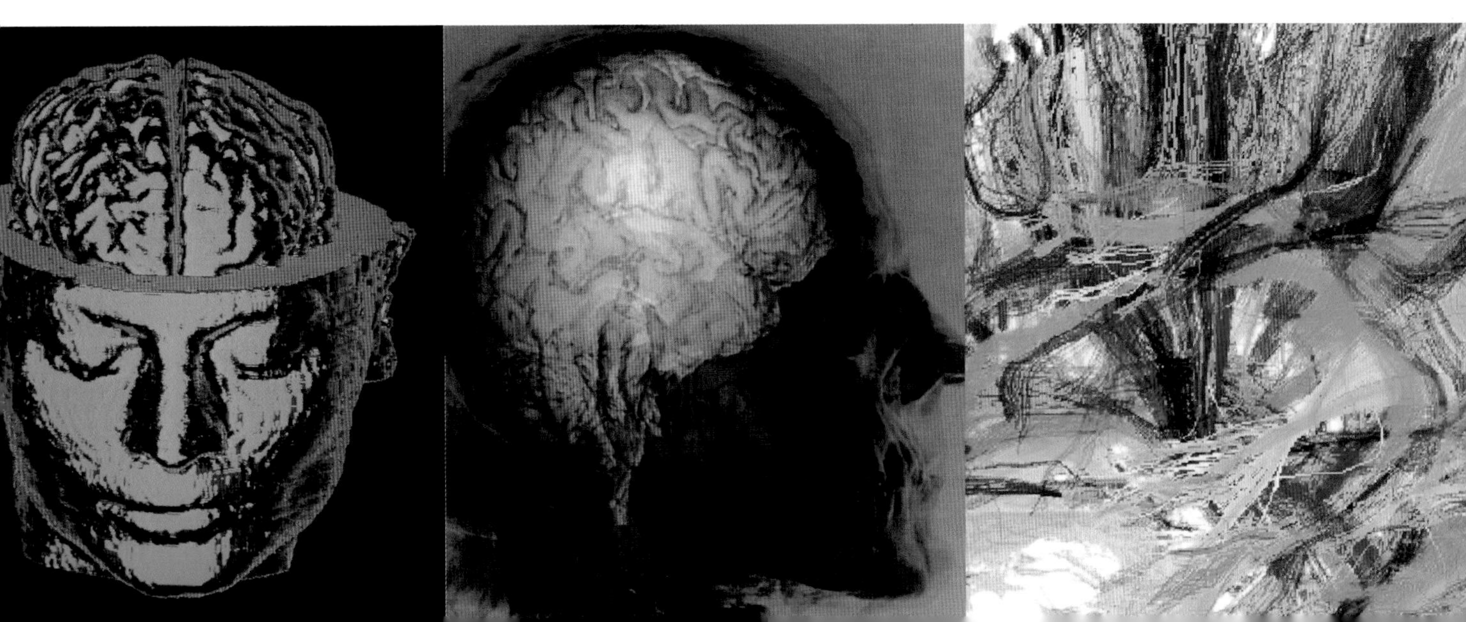

INVESTIGATING THE BRAIN

THE BRAIN IS THE LAST OF THE HUMAN ORGANS TO GIVE UP ITS SECRETS. FOR A LONG TIME, PEOPLE WERE NOT EVEN ABLE TO UNDERSTAND WHAT THE BRAIN IS FOR. THE DISCOVERY OF ITS ANATOMY, FUNCTIONS, AND PROCESSES HAS BEEN A LONG AND SLOW JOURNEY ACROSS THE MILLENNIA, AS HUMAN KNOWLEDGE ABOUT THIS MYSTERIOUS ORGAN HAS DEVELOPED AND ACCUMULATED.

EXPLORING THE BRAIN

The brain is particularly difficult to investigate because its structures are minute and its processes cannot be seen with the naked eye. The problem is compounded by the fact that its most interesting product – consciousness – does not feel like a physical process, so there was no obvious reason for our distant ancestors to associate it with the brain. Nevertheless, over the centuries, philosophers and physicians built up an understanding of the brain and, in the last 25 years, with the advent of brain-imaging techniques, neuroscientists have created a detailed map of what was once an entirely mysterious territory.

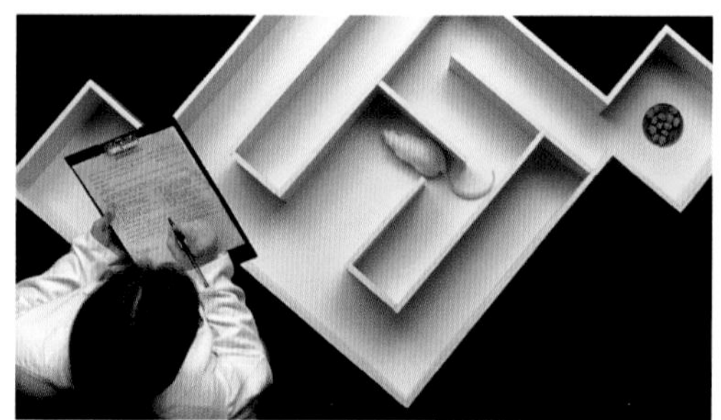

USING RATS
The brains of rats are very similar to human brains. Until imaging techniques were developed, the only way scientists were able to look directly at brain tissue was by using the brains of rats and other non-human animals.

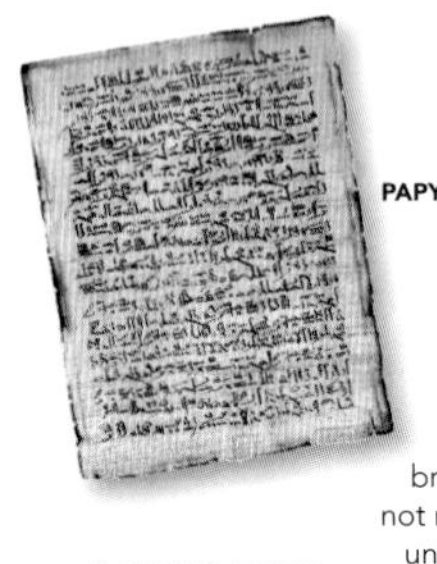

PAPYRUS

4000 BCE
Early Sumerian writing notes the euphoric effect of poppy seeds.

2500 BCE
Trepanation (boring holes into the skull) is a common surgical procedure across many cultures, possibly used for relieving brain disorders such as epilepsy, or for ritual or spiritual reasons.

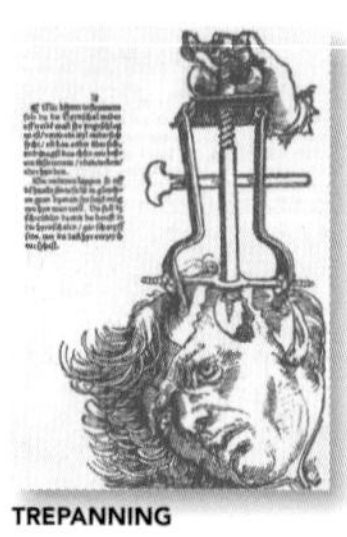

TREPANNING

1700 BCE
Egyptian papyrus gives a careful description of the brain, but Egyptians do not rate this organ highly; unlike other organs, it is removed and discarded before mummification, suggesting that it was not considered to be of any use in future incarnations.

450 BCE
Early Greeks begin to recognize the brain as the seat of human sensation.

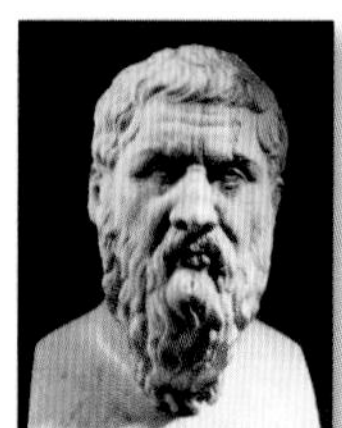

PLATO

387 BCE
The Greek philosopher Plato teaches at Athens; he believes the brain is the seat of mental processes.

335 BCE
Greek philosopher Aristotle restates the ancient belief that the heart is the superior organ; the brain, he claims, is a radiator to stop the body overheating.

ARISTOTLE

170 BCE
Roman physician Galen theorizes that human moods and dispositions are due to the four "humours" (liquids that are held in the brain's ventricles). The idea persists for more than 1,000 years. Galen's anatomical descriptions, used by generations of physicians, were based mainly on work on monkeys and pigs.

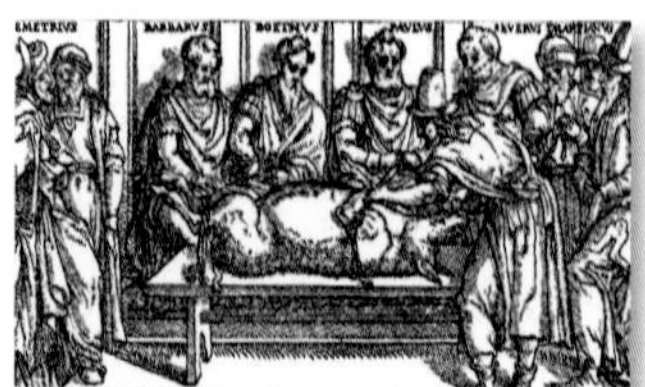

GALEN AT WORK

4000 BCE | 3000 BCE | 2000 BCE | 1000 BCE | 1500 | 1600 | 1700 | 1800

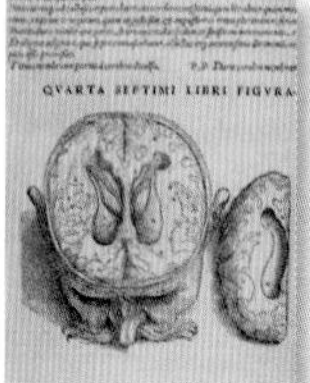

DRAWING THE BRAIN

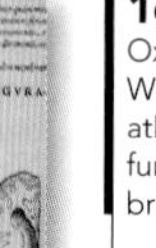

1543
Andreas Vesalius, a European physician, publishes the first "modern" anatomy, with detailed drawings of the human brain.

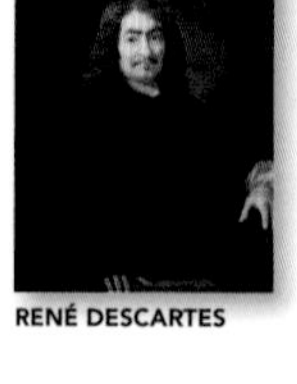

RENÉ DESCARTES

1649
French philosopher René Descartes describes the brain as a hydraulic system that controls behaviour. "Higher" mental functions are generated by a spiritual entity, however, which interacts with the body via the pineal gland.

1664
Oxford physiologist Thomas Willis publishes the first brain atlas, locating various functions in separate brain "modules".

BRAIN ATLAS

1774
German physician Franz Anton Mesmer introduces "animal magnetism", later called hypnosis.

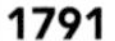

1791
Luigi Galvani, an Italian physicist, discovers the electrical basis of nervous activity by making frogs' legs twitch.

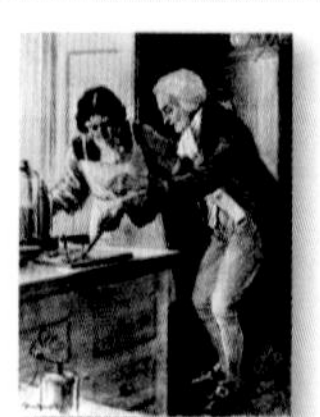

LUIGI GALVANI

1848
Phineas Gage has his brain pierced by an iron rod (see p.141).

1849
German physicist Hermann von Helmholtz measures the speed of nerve conduction and subsequently develops the idea that perception depends upon "unconscious inferences".

THE ADVENT OF IMAGING TECHNIQUES

Scientists were unable to find out much about the workings of the brain until relatively recently. The only way they were able to match functions such as sight, emotion, or speech to the locations in the brain in which they are controlled was to find a person in whom a faculty was disturbed due to injury, and then wait until they were dead in order to look at the location and extent of the brain damage. Otherwise, scientists could only guess at what was happening to the brain by observing people's behaviour. Today, modern imaging techniques such as functional MRI and EEG (see p.12) allow neuroscientists to see the electrical activity in the brain as a person carries out various tasks or thought processes. This allows them to link types of actions, emotions, and so on, to specific types of activity in the brain. The freedom to observe the brain that imaging techniques have afforded has allowed for an explosion of knowledge within neuroscience, and has deepened our understanding of the brain and how it works.

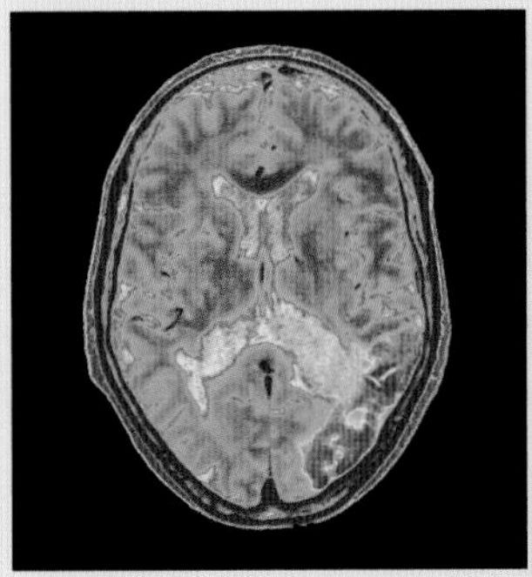

MAGNETIC RESONANCE IMAGING
Brain scans can reveal damaged tissue – the red area in the MRI scan above indicates damage caused by a stroke.

Electrode "cap"

ELECTRODES
Neural activity can be measured by attaching electrodes to the scalp. These pick up electrical activity in the brain and transform it into a digital record.

1850
Franz Joseph Gall founds phrenology (see p.10), which attributes different personality traits to specific areas of the head.

1859
Charles Darwin publishes *On the Origin of Species.*

1862–74
Broca and Wernicke (see p.10) discover the two main language areas of the brain.

1873
Italian scientist Camillo Golgi publishes the silver nitrate method, making it possible to see nerves in their entirety. He wins the Nobel Prize in 1906.

NERVE CELLS

1874
Carl Wernicke publishes on aphasia (language disorders after brain damage).

1889
Santiago Ramón y Cajal proposes that nerve cells are independent elements and the basic units of the brain in *The Neuron Doctrine.* He wins the Nobel Prize in 1906.

Circa 1900
Sigmund Freud abandons an early career in neurology to study psychodynamics. The success of Freudian psychoanalysis eclipsed physiological psychiatry for half a century.

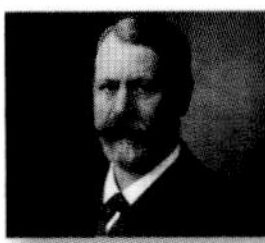

SIGMUND FREUD

1906
Santiago Ramón y Cajal describes how nerve cells communicate.

NERVE CELLS IN RODENT HIPPOCAMPUS

1906
Alois Alzheimer describes presenile degeneration (see p.231).

1909
Korbinian Brodmann describes 52 discrete cortical areas based on neural structure. These areas are still used today (see p.67).

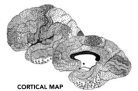

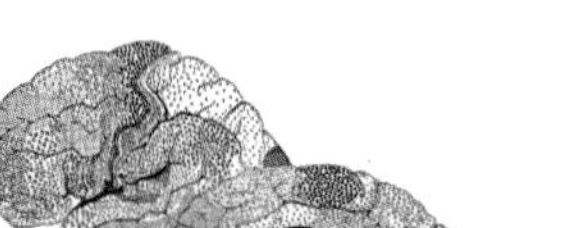

CORTICAL MAP

1914
British physiologist Henry Hallett Dale isolates acetylcholine, the first of the neuro-transmitters (see p.73) to be discovered. He wins the Nobel Prize in 1936.

1919
Irish neurologist Gordon Morgan Holmes localizes vision to the striate cortex (the primary visual cortex).

1924
The first electroencephalograms are produced by Hans Berger.

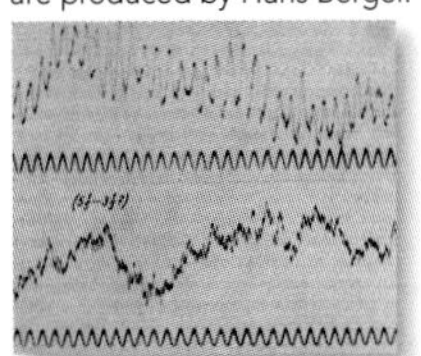

ELECTROENCEPHALOGRAPHY

1934
Portuguese neurologist Egas Moniz carries out the first leucotomy operations (later known as lobotomies, see p.11). He also invented angiography, one of the first techniques that allowed scientists to make images of the brain.

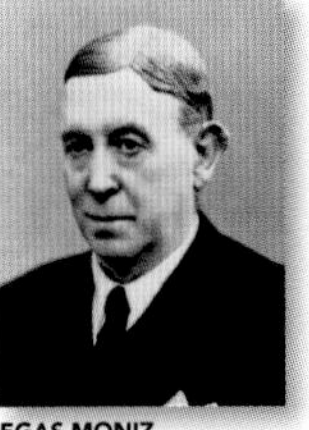

EGAS MONIZ

1953
Brenda Milner describes patient HM (see p.159), who suffers memory loss after hippocampal surgery.

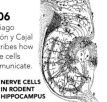

1957
W. Penfield and T. Rasmussen devise a motor and sensory homunculus (see pp.10 and 103).

1970–80
Brain scanning is developed: PET, SPECT, MRI, and MEG all emerge during this decade.

1973
Timothy Bliss and Terje Lomo describe long-term potentiation (see p.156).

1981
Roger Wolcott Sperry is awarded the Nobel Prize for his work on the different functions of the two brain hemispheres (see pp.11 and 205).

1983
Benjamin Libet writes on the timing of conscious volition (see p.11).

1991
Mirror neurons are discovered by Giacomo Rizzolatti in Parma (see pp.11 and 122–23).

2013
The European Union and United States start human brain simulation projects. The Connectome, a global co-operative endeavour, delivers its first charts of the connections between neurons.

1900

2000

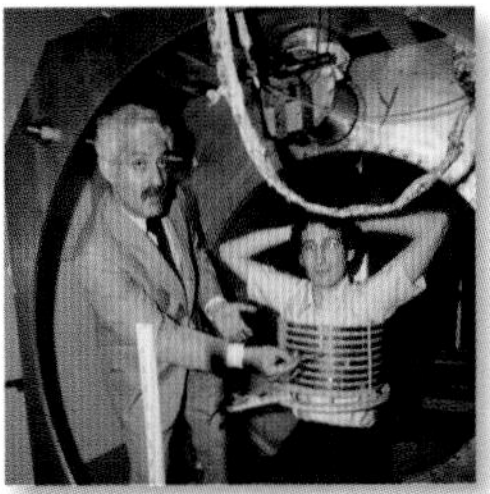

EARLY MAGNETIC IMAGING

LANDMARKS IN NEUROSCIENCE

MOST OF THE KNOWLEDGE WE HAVE ABOUT THE BRAIN HAS BEEN GATHERED BY SLOW, PAINSTAKING RESEARCH INVOLVING LARGE TEAMS OF PEOPLE. HOWEVER, OCCASIONALLY THE HISTORY OF NEUROSCIENCE HAS BEEN PUNCTUATED BY DRAMATIC DISCOVERIES OR IDEAS, OFTEN ARISING FROM THE WORK OF A SINGLE SCIENTIST. SOME OF THESE SUBSEQUENTLY PROVED TO BE VALUABLE BREAKTHROUGHS WHILE OTHERS, THOUGH INFLUENTIAL, PROVED TO BE DEAD ENDS.

PHRENOLOGY
Franz Joseph Gall

Gall thought that personality could be read by feeling the contours of the skull. He theorized that various faculties were localized in the brain and that the strongest were correspondingly large, making the skull bulge measurably. It was hugely popular in nineteenth-century America and Europe – nearly every town had a phrenology institute. Although nonsense, Gall's idea that brain functions are localized has turned out to be largely true. Imaging research aimed at locating brain functions is often called "modern phrenology".

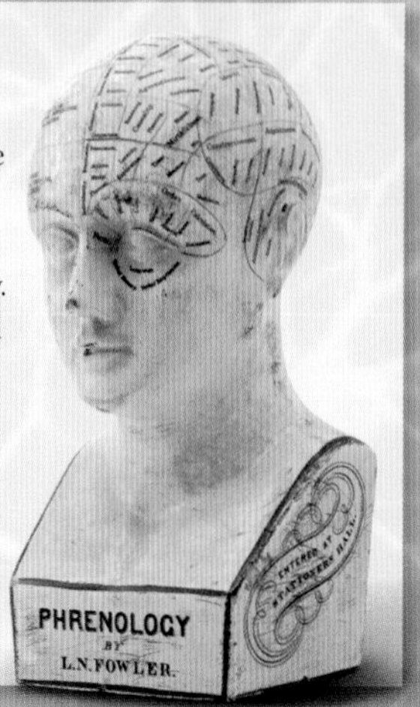

PHRENOLOGY HEAD
Models such as this claimed to show the bulges on the skull that revealed a person's character. Categories included "blandness" or "benevolence".

THE MAN WHO LOST HIMSELF
Phineas Gage

This polite, well-liked American railroad foreman changed dramatically, becoming "grossly profane", after an accident destroyed part of his brain (see p.141). His case was the first to show that faculties such as social and moral judgement can be localized to the frontal lobes.

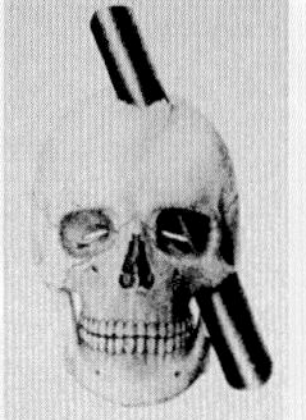

FATEFUL INJURY
This reconstruction of Phineas Gage's skull shows how an iron rod damaged the frontal lobes of his brain.

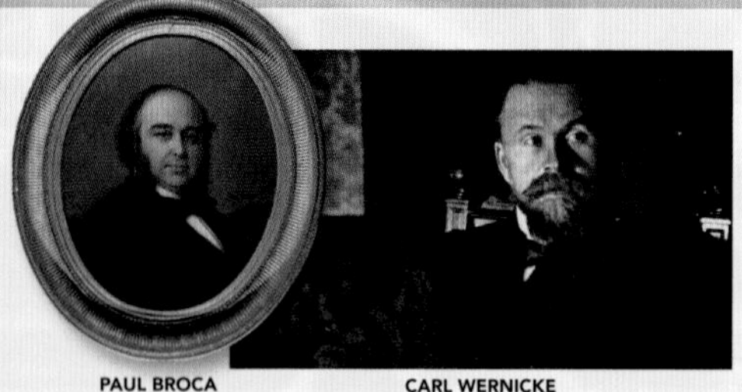

PAUL BROCA   CARL WERNICKE

LANGUAGE AREAS
Broca and Wernicke

In 1861, French physician Paul Broca described a patient who he named "Tan", as it was the only word "Tan" could say. When Tan died, Broca examined his brain and found damage to part of the left frontal cortex. This part of the brain became "Broca's Area" (see p.148). In 1876, German neurologist Carl Wernicke found that damage to a different part of the brain (which became known as "Wernicke's Area") also caused language problems. These two scientists were the first to clearly define functional areas of the brain.

EARLY BRAIN IMPLANT
José Delgado

Spanish neurologist Dr José Delgado invented a brain implant that could be remotely controlled by radio waves. He found that animal and human behaviour could be controlled by pressing a button. In a famous experiment, conducted in 1964, Delgado faced a charging bull, bringing it to a halt at his feet by activating the implant in its brain. In another, he put a device in the brain of a chimp that was bullying its mate. He put the control in the cage where the victim chimp used it to "turn off" the bully's bad behaviour.

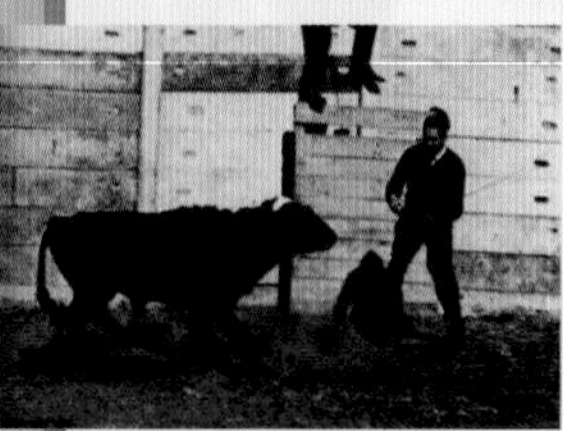

DELGADO AND THE BULL

MAPPING THE BRAIN
Wilder Penfield

The first detailed maps of human brain function were made by Canadian brain surgeon Wilder Penfield. He worked with patients undergoing surgery to control epilepsy. While the brain was exposed, and the patient conscious, Penfield probed the cortex with an electrode and noted the responses of the patient as he touched each part. Penfield's work was the first to reveal the role of the temporal lobe in recall and map the areas of the cortex that control movement and provide bodily sensations.

CANADIAN STAMP

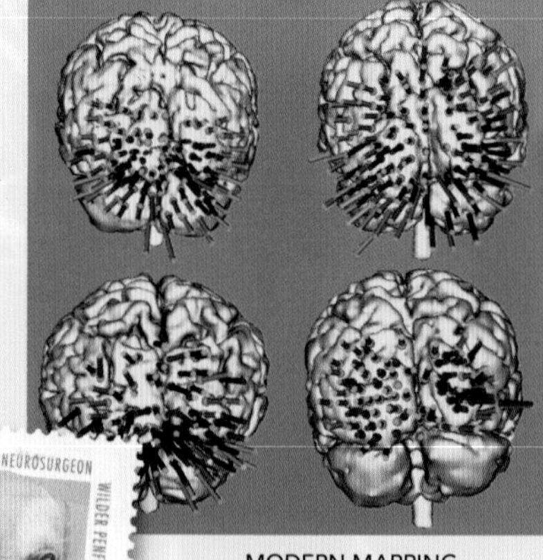

MODERN MAPPING
Today advanced imaging (see above) allows neural activity to be matched to mental tasks. However, much of the basic map was established by Penfield half a century earlier.

LOBOTOMY

The first lobotomies were performed in the 1890s, but they only took off in the 1930s when the Portuguese neurosurgeon Egas Moniz found that cutting the nerves that run from the frontal cortex to the thalamus relieved psychotic symptoms in some of his patients. Moniz's work was picked up by US surgeon Walter Freeman, who invented the "ice pick lobotomy". From 1936 until the 1950s, he advocated lobotomy as a cure for a range of problems, and between 40,000 and 50,000 patients were lobotomized. The operation was overused and is now thought abhorrent. However, in many cases it eased suffering: a follow-up of patients in the UK found 41 per cent were "recovered" or "greatly improved", 28 per cent were "minimally improved", 25 per cent had "no change", 4 per cent had died, and 2 per cent were worse off.

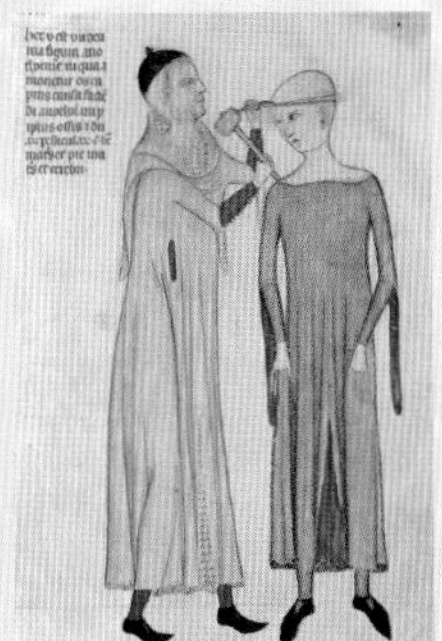

TREPANATION
The practice of drilling holes in the head has been used since prehistoric times as a treatment for a vast array of illnesses. The modern equivalent, craniotomy, is carried out to relieve pressure within the skull.

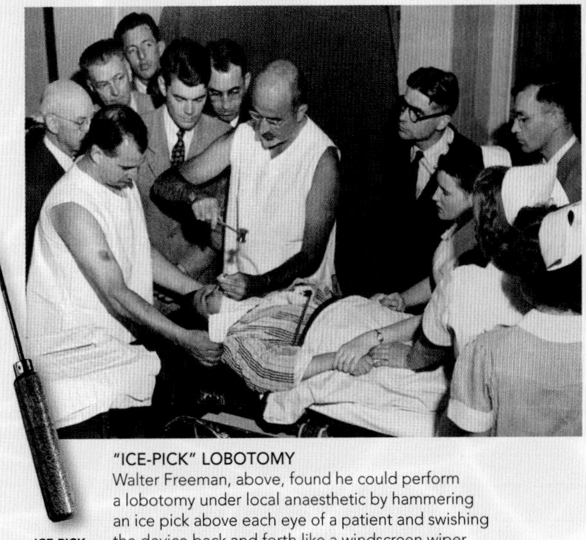

ICE PICK

"ICE-PICK" LOBOTOMY
Walter Freeman, above, found he could perform a lobotomy under local anaesthetic by hammering an ice pick above each eye of a patient and swishing the device back and forth like a windscreen wiper.

MAKING MEMORIES
Henry G. Molaison

In 1953, aged 27, "HM" underwent an operation in the USA, to stem severe epilepsy. The surgeons, then unaware of the functions of the hippocampus, took out a large area of that part of his brain (see p.159). When he came round, he was unable to lay down new memories and remained so for the rest of his life. The tragic accident demonstrated the crucial role of the hippocampus in recall.

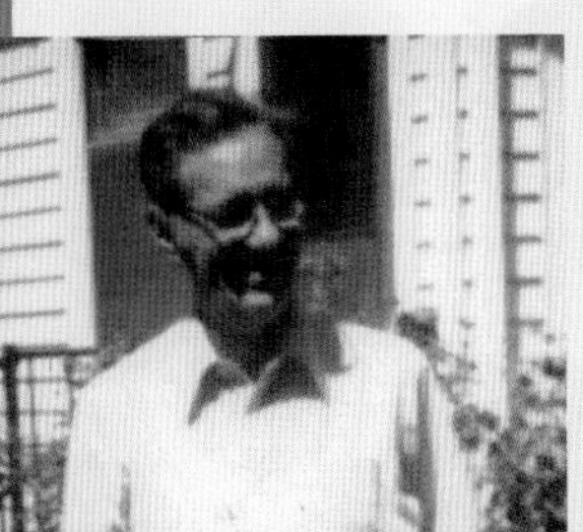

FROZEN IN TIME
Henry G. Molaison – generally known only as "HM" – was one of the most studied patients in the history of modern medicine.

CONSCIOUS DECISIONS
Benjamin Libet

A series of ingenious experiments by US neuroscientist Benjamin Libet (see p.191) in the early 1980s demonstrated that what we think are conscious "decisions" to act are actually just recognition of what the unconscious brain is already doing. Libet's experiments have profound philosophical implications because, on the face of it, the results suggest that we do not have a conscious choice about what we do, and therefore cannot consider ourselves to have free will.

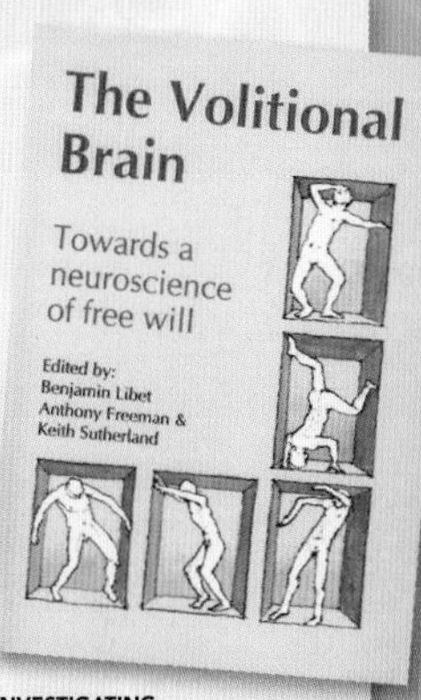

INVESTIGATING FREE WILL

SPLIT-BRAIN EXPERIMENTS
Roger Sperry

Neurobiologist Roger Sperry conducted the split-brain experiments (see p.204) on people whose brain hemispheres were surgically separated in the course of treatment for epilepsy. They showed that, under certain conditions, each hemisphere could hold different thoughts and intentions. This raised the profound question of whether a person has a single "self".

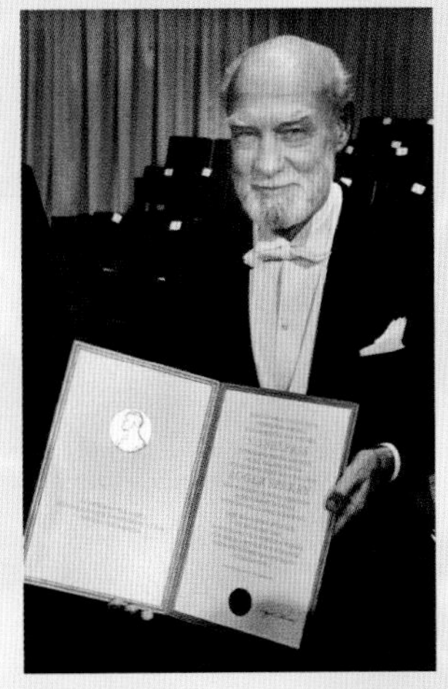

ROGER SPERRY RECEIVES THE NOBEL PRIZE IN 1981

MIRROR NEURONS

Mirror neurons (see pp.122–23) were discovered in 1991 – by accident. A group of researchers in Italy, led by Giacomo Rizzolatti, were monitoring neural activity in the brains of monkeys as they made reaching movements. One day a researcher inadvertently mimicked the monkey's movement while it was watching, and found that the neural activity in the monkey's brain that sparked up in response to the sight was identical to the activity that occurred when the monkey made the action itself. Mirror neurons are thought by some to be the basis of theory of mind, mimicry, and empathy.

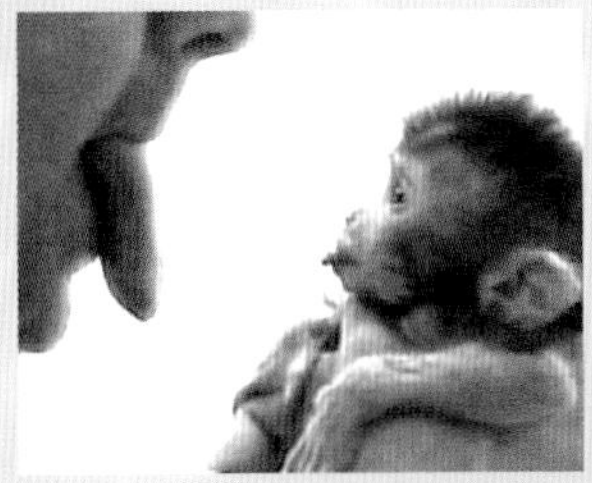

MIMICKING MACAQUE
Mirror neurons produce automatic mimicry by producing a similar state in an observer's brain to the state of the person they are watching.

SCANNING THE BRAIN

BRAIN IMAGING TECHNIQUES CAN BE DIVIDED INTO TWO DIFFERENT TYPES: ANATOMICAL IMAGING, WHICH GIVES INFORMATION ABOUT THE STRUCTURE OF THE BRAIN, AND FUNCTIONAL SCANNING, WHICH ALLOWS RESEARCHERS TO SEE HOW THE BRAIN WORKS. USED TOGETHER, THESE TECHNIQUES HAVE REVOLUTIONIZED NEUROSCIENCE.

A WINDOW ON THE BRAIN

The structure of the brain is well known, but until recently the way it created thoughts, emotions, and perceptions could only be guessed at. Imaging technology has now made it possible to look inside a living brain and see it at work. The brain works by generating tiny electrical charges. Functional imaging reveals which areas are most active. This may be done by measuring electrical activity directly (EEG), picking up magnetic fields created by electrical activity (MEG), or measuring metabolic side-effects such as alterations in glucose absorption (PET) and blood flow (fMRI).

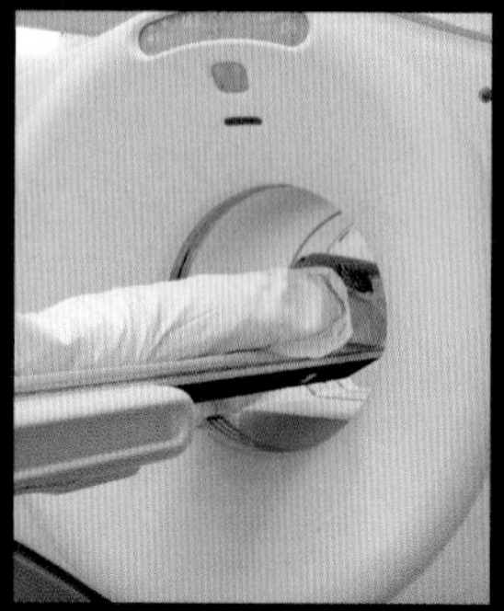

PET SCANNER
Positron emission tomography (PET) scanners detect signals from radioactive markers in tissues to show activity in the brain.

FUNCTION

The brain is composed of modules that are specialized to do specific things. Functional brain imaging is largely about identifying which ones are most concerned with doing what. This has allowed neuroscientists to build a detailed map of brain functions. We now know where perceptions, language, memory, emotion, and movement occur. By showing how various functions work together, imaging also gives us a glimpse into some of the most sophisticated aspects of human psychology. For example, observing a person's brain making a decision, we see that apparently rational decisions are driven by the emotional brain. Imaging the brains of master chess players shows why expertise depends on practice. Watching the brain of a person seeing a frightened face shows that emotion is contagious.

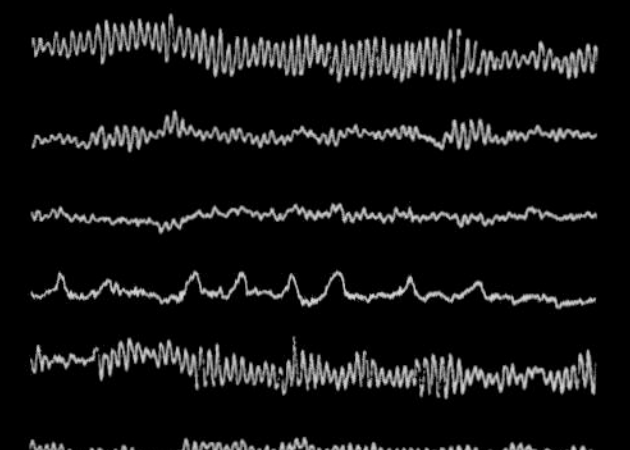

BRAIN WAVES
Electroencephalographs (EEGs) show electrical activity caused by nerve cells firing. They record distinct "brain waves", which reflect the speed of firing in different states of mind.

PET SCANS
These scans involve injecting a volunteer with a radioactive marker that attaches to glucose in the brain. Areas of high activity (red) attract glucose for fuel. The marker dye shows which parts of the brain are firing.

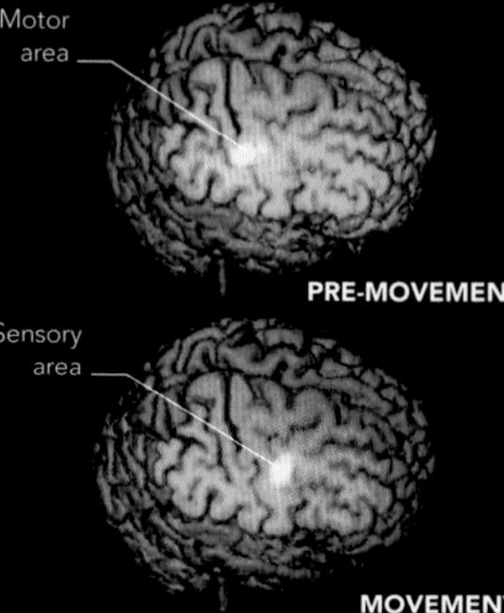

REAL-TIME ACTIVITY
Magnetoencephalography (MEG) picks up magnetic traces of brain activity. It is poor at showing where activity occurs, but good at pinpointing timing. Here, a brain plans a finger movement, then 40 milliseconds later its activity shifts as the movement is made.

ANATOMY

The brain looks very different according to how you view it. Computed tomography (CT) imaging combines the use of a computer and fine X-rays to produce multiple "slices" of the body. It allows you to see normally obscured body tissues, such as the inside of the brain, from any angle or level, with the delicate inner structures thrown into clear relief. Artificial colouring of the areas further distinguishes one part from another. CT scans are purely structural – they show the form of the organ but not how it works. They are very good at showing contrast between soft tissues and bone, and are therefore useful in diagnosing tumours and blood clots.

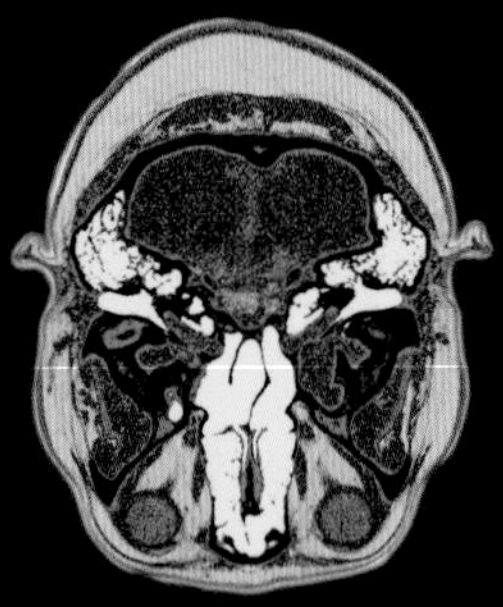

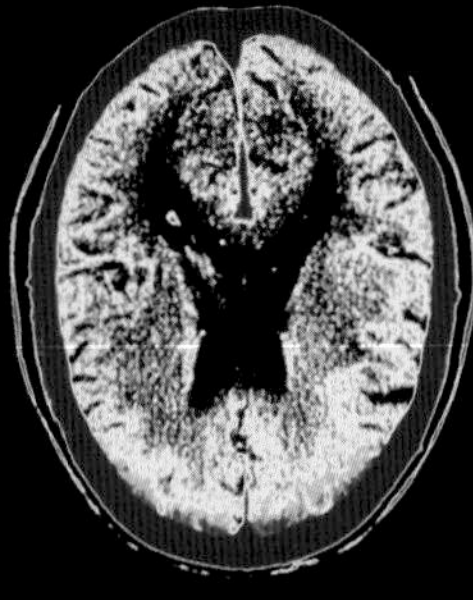

STRUCTURAL DETAILS
These CT images show different tissues in detail. The image on the left shows the cerebellum and eyeballs in red, the bones in blue and green, and the sinuses and ear cavities are bright yellow. The image on the right shows a healthy brain (front at bottom). The black areas are the fluid-filled ventricles.

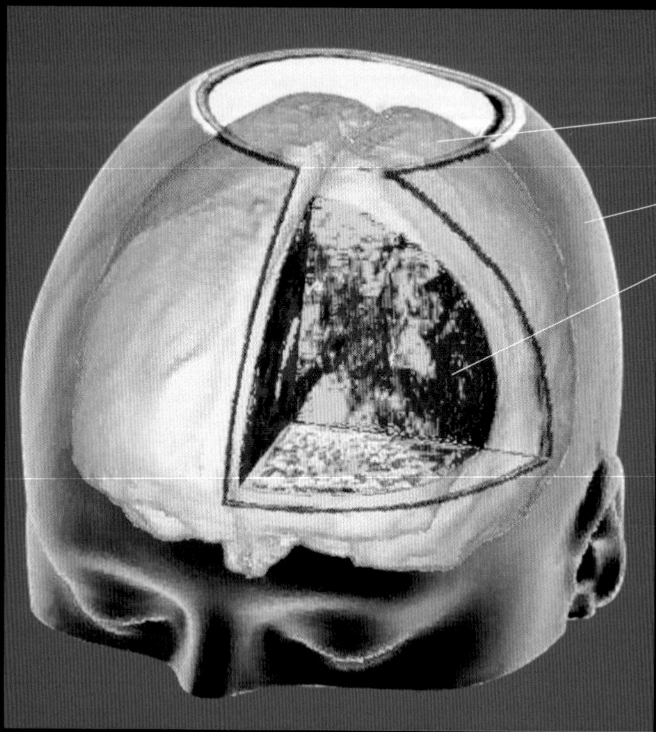

3-D BRAIN
CT allows pictures of brains to be displayed in three dimensions, and "sliced" to reveal the inner workings. Here, the front right quarter of the brain's coverings and surface are cut away to reveal the tissues beneath.

MAGNETIC RESONANCE IMAGING

Magnetic resonance imaging (MRI) provides a better contrast between tissue types than CT. Instead of using X-rays, it uses a powerful magnetic field, which causes hydrogen atoms in the body to realign. The nuclei of the atoms produce a magnetic field that is "read" by the scanner and turned into a three-dimensional computerized image. The brain is scanned at a rapid rate (typically once every 2–3 seconds) to produce "slices" similar to those in CT scans. Increases in neural activity cause changes in the blood flow, which alter the amount of oxygen in the area, producing a change in the magnetic signal. Functional MRI (fMRI) involves showing differing levels of electrical activity in the brain, overlaid on the anatomical details.

NERVE PATHWAYS IN THE BRAIN
A refinement of MRI called diffusion tensor imaging picks up the passage of water along nerve fibres. Here, the blue fibres run from top to bottom, the green from front to back, and the red between the two hemispheres.

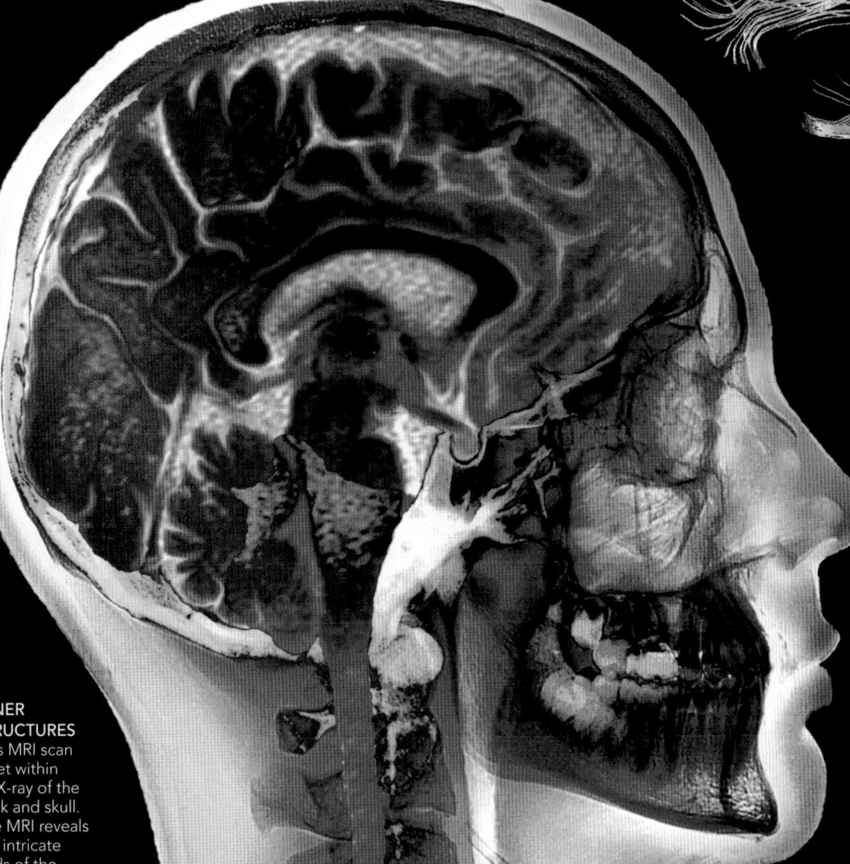

INNER STRUCTURES
This MRI scan is set within an X-ray of the neck and skull. The MRI reveals the intricate folds of the brain tissue.

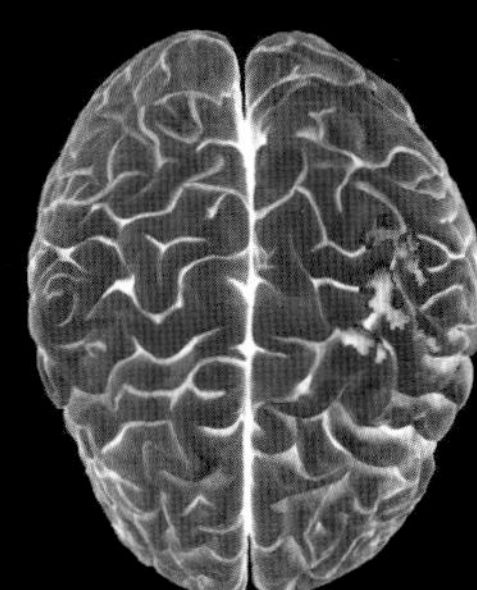

MOVEMENT
FMRI is very good at localizing brain activity. In this image (front of brain at bottom), the red area shows activity in the part responsible for moving the right hand. Each side of the body is controlled by the opposite hemisphere of the brain.

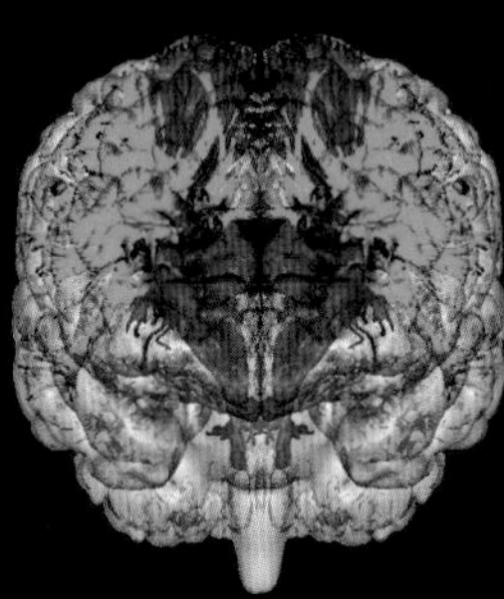

FIBRE DETAIL
This diffusion tensor image shows another view of the nerve fibres. The green fibres link the various parts of the limbic system. The blue fibres run from the cerebellum, which joins on to the spine. The red fibres connect the two hemispheres.

COMBINED IMAGING

Each type of imaging has its advantages. MRI is good on detail, for example, but is too slow to chart fast-moving events. EEG and MEG are fast but are not so good at pinpointing location. To get scans that show both fast processes *and* location, researchers use two or more methods to produce a combined image. Here (right), for example, high-resolution MRI, taking about 15 minutes to acquire is combined with a low-resolution fMRI, which takes seconds to produce and shows the location of activity in the brain areas used in hearing language. The areas shift during a task like this, because it involves many aspects, and they have to work fast and in concert. The areas used in a task vary from person to person, so studies often combine data from volunteers to give an average.

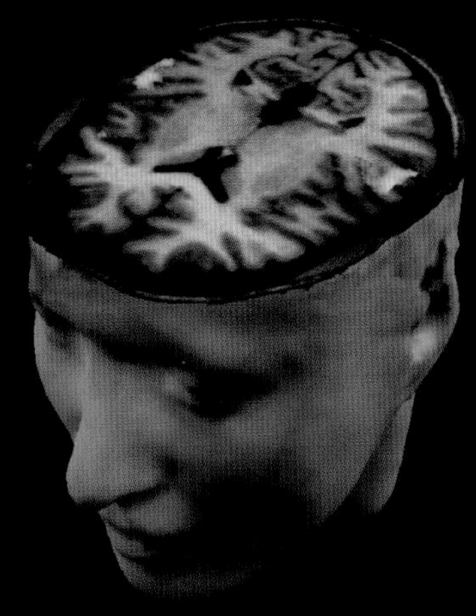

STUDYING LANGUAGE
In most people, the main language areas of the brain are located in the left hemisphere, so this area shows greater activity when a person listens to spoken words. The right hemisphere is also required for complete hearing, and for distinguishing tone and rhythm.

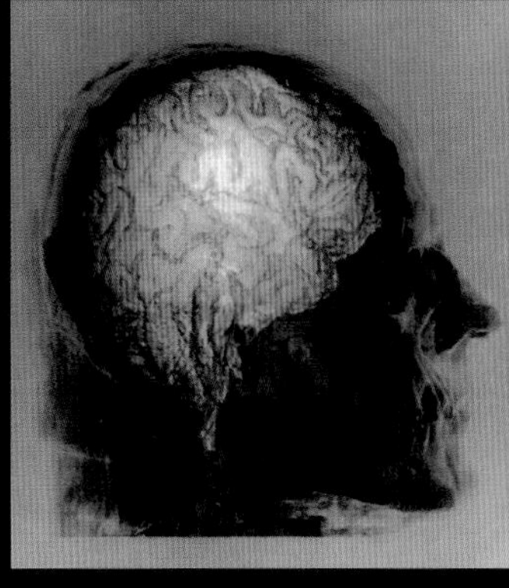

SLICED TOGETHER
Here, a combined CT and MRI scan shows the surface folds of the brain. It also reveals the skull bones and the top vertebrae.

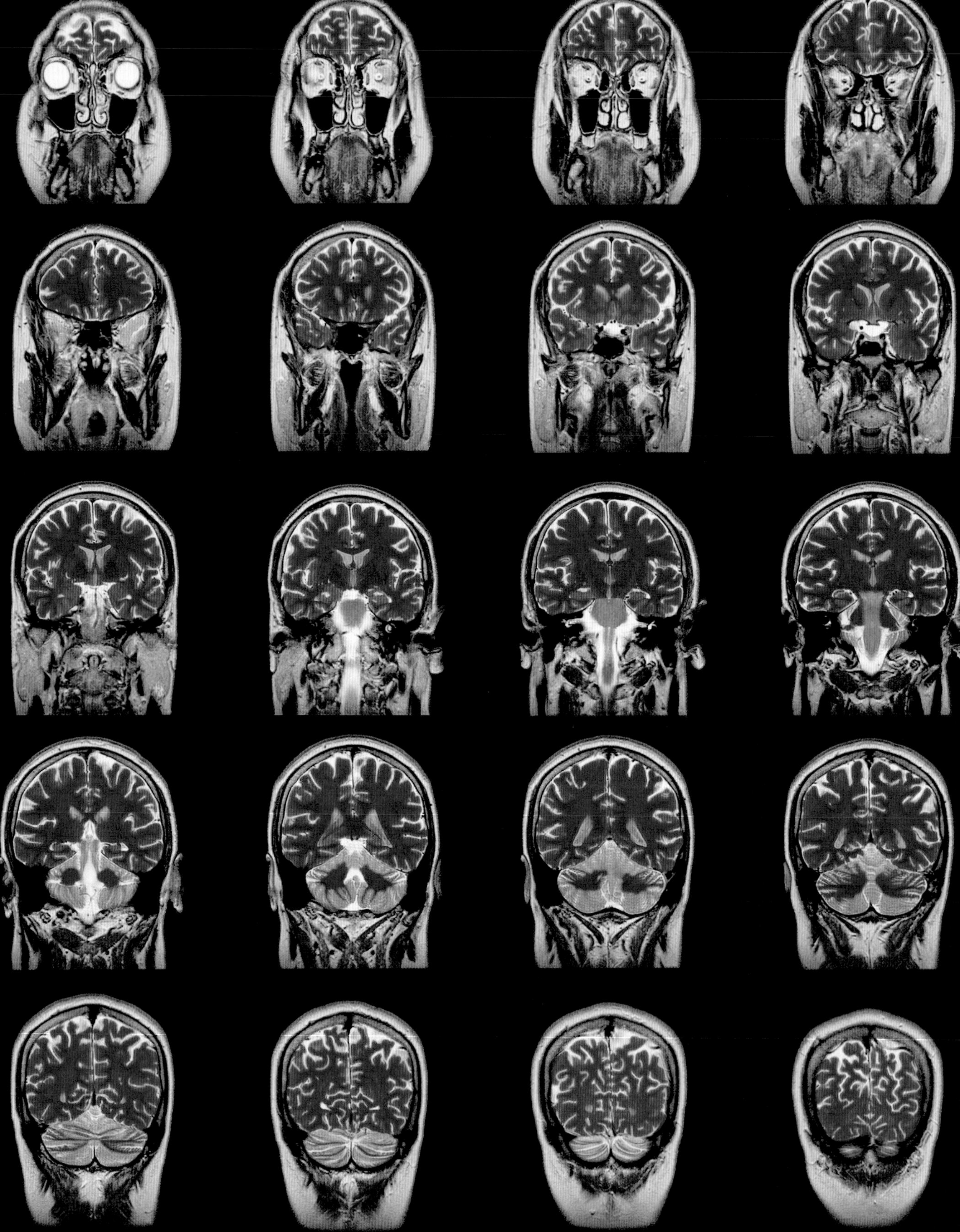

A JOURNEY THROUGH THE BRAIN

THE BRAIN IS THE MOST COMPLEX ORGAN IN THE BODY AND IS PROBABLY THE MOST COMPLEX SYSTEM KNOWN TO HUMANKIND. OUR BRAIN CONTAINS BILLIONS OF NEURONS THAT ARE CONSTANTLY SENDING SIGNALS TO EACH OTHER, AND IT IS THIS SIGNALLING THAT CREATES OUR MINDS. WITH THE HELP OF MODERN SCANNING TECHNOLOGY, WE NOW KNOW ABOUT BRAIN STRUCTURE IN GREAT DETAIL.

In the nineteenth century, much was learned about the structure of the brain by removing it from the body after death. Knowledge of the workings of the living human brain could only be gained by studying people with damaged brains, for example Phineas Gage (see p.141), but the precise location of this damage could not be known while the patient was still alive. Everything changed with the invention of brain scanners at the end of the twentieth century. In the following pages, we shall undertake a journey through the brain of a healthy, 55-year-old man revealed by magnetic resonance imaging (MRI). In these images, we can see the many components of the brain. We are starting to understand the function of some of these, but we are only at the very beginning of this journey of understanding.

The captions that accompany the scans indicate the most likely function of various brain regions. But these regions often have many functions, and these functions depend upon interactions with other brain regions. Most structures in the brain are paired, with identical counterparts in the left and right hemispheres, so structures identified in one hemisphere are mirrored in the opposite one. The scans themselves have been coloured, so that the cerebrum appears in red, the cerebellum in light blue, and the brainstem in green.

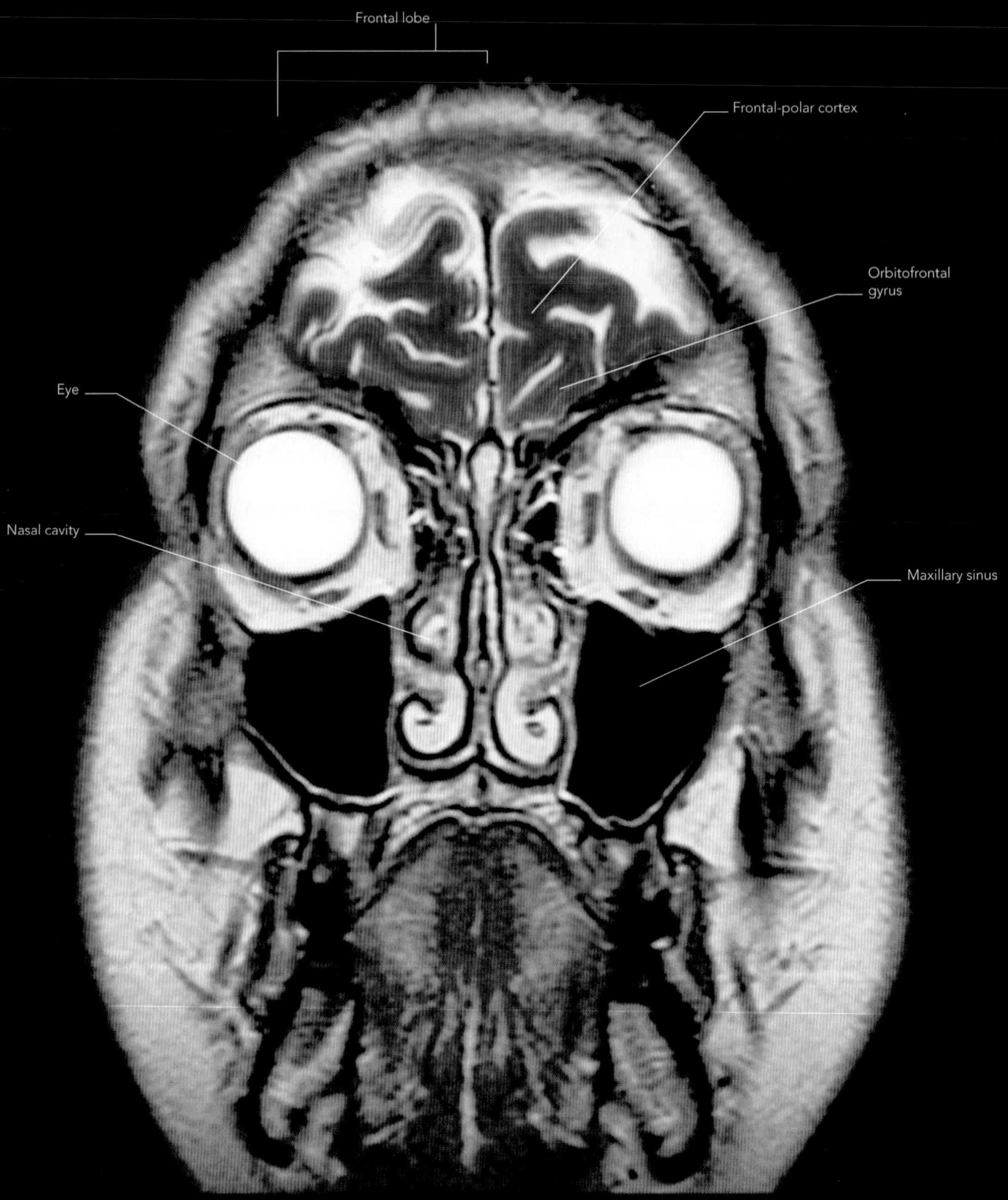

Frontal lobe

Frontal-polar cortex

Orbitofrontal gyrus

Eye

Nasal cavity

Maxillary sinus

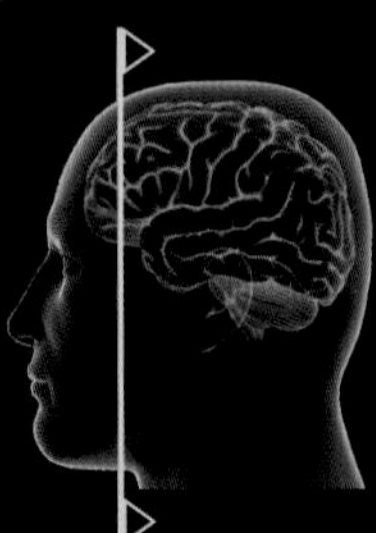

1 THE FRONTAL-POLAR CORTEX
The frontal-polar cortex is the most recently evolved part of the prefrontal cortex in the frontal lobe and is concerned with forward planning and the control of other brain regions. This slice, right at the front of the brain, also reveals other features of the skull, including the eyes, nasal cavity, maxillary sinus, and tongue.

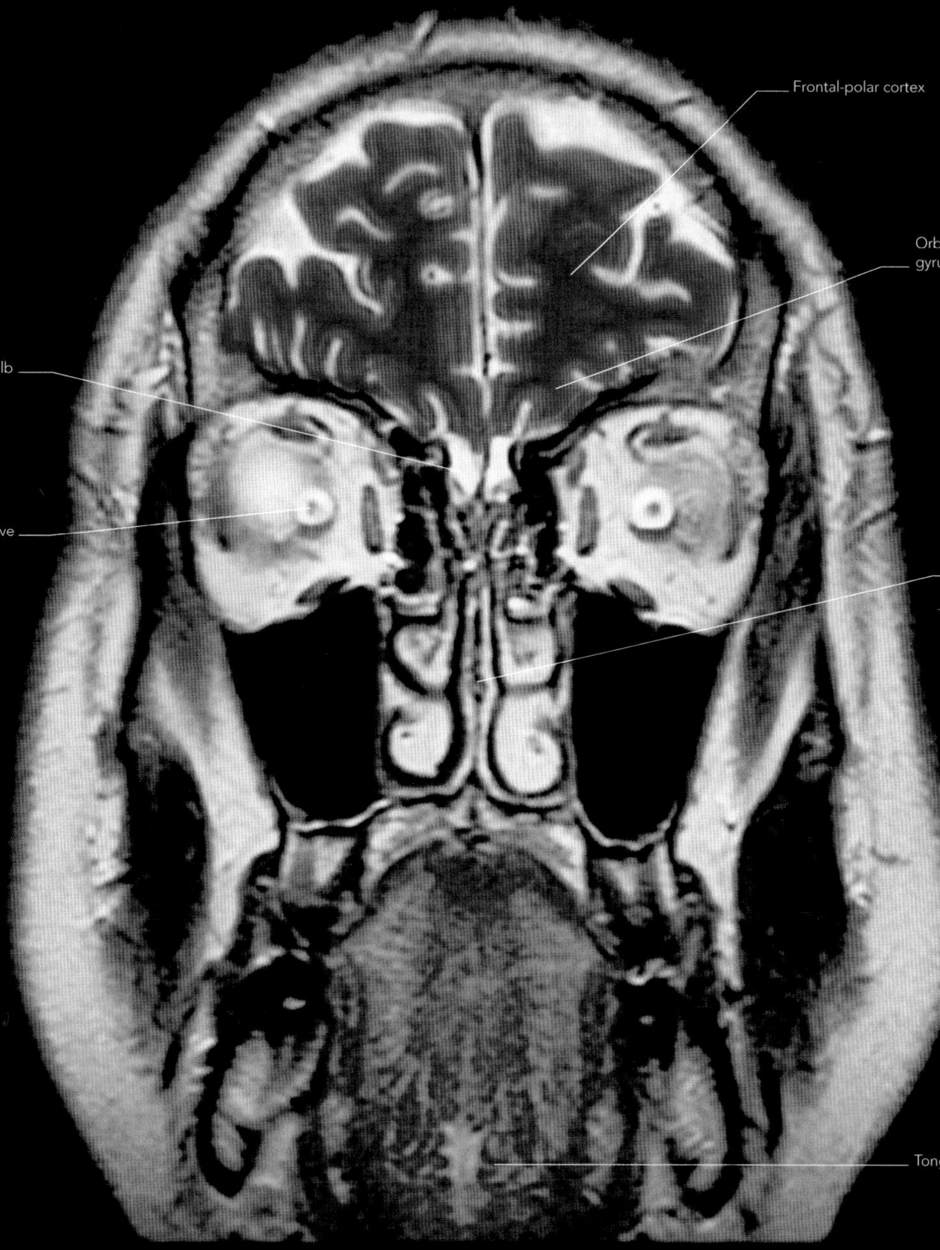

Frontal-polar cortex

Orbitofrontal gyrus

Olfactory bulb

Optic nerve

Nasal septum

Tongue

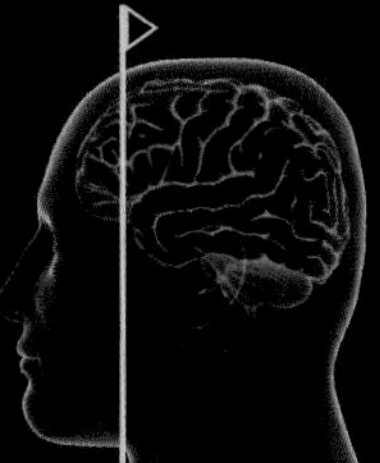

2 THE FRONTAL LOBE

The frontal lobe, of which the prefrontal cortex is the front part, is the largest of the brain's lobes and the latest to evolve. The frontal lobe is devoted to the control of action – precise control of muscles at the back, high-level planning at the front. In this slice, the optic nerve can also be seen carrying visual information from the eye to the brain.

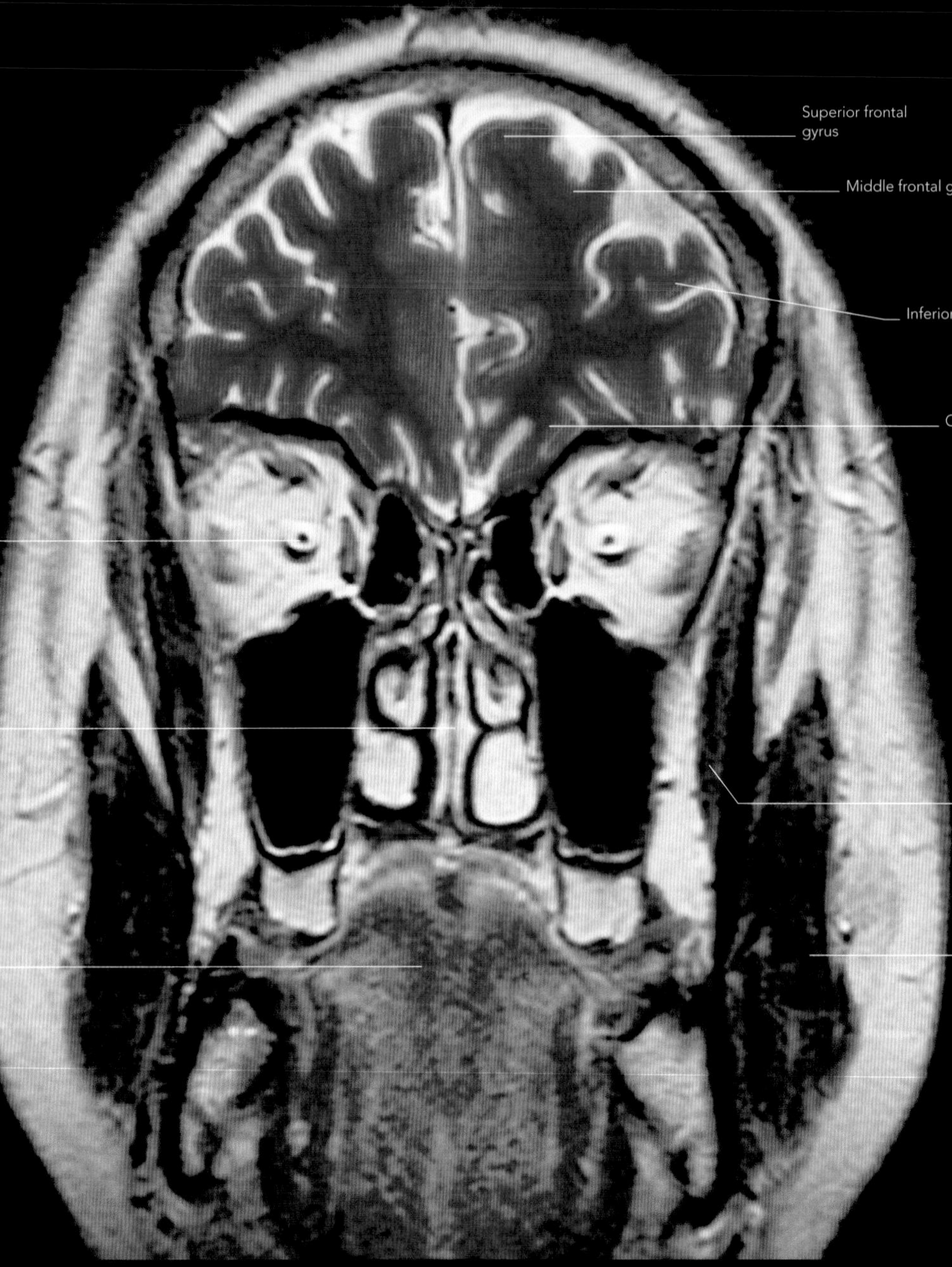

Superior frontal gyrus

Middle frontal gyrus

Inferior frontal gyrus

Orbitofrontal gyrus

Optic nerve

Nasal septum

Temporalis muscle

Tongue

Masseter muscle

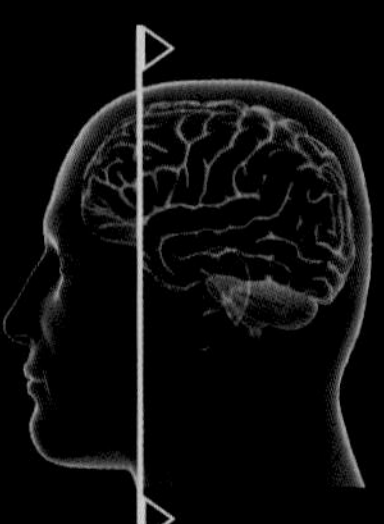

3 THE CORTEX
The cortex, which appears on these scans as yellow lines, is heavily folded, creating a large surface area. The major ingoing folds (sulci, singular sulcus) are used as landmarks to define brain regions. The bulges between the ingoing folds are known as gyri (singular, gyrus). The major components of the frontal lobe are the superior, middle, and inferior frontal gyri.

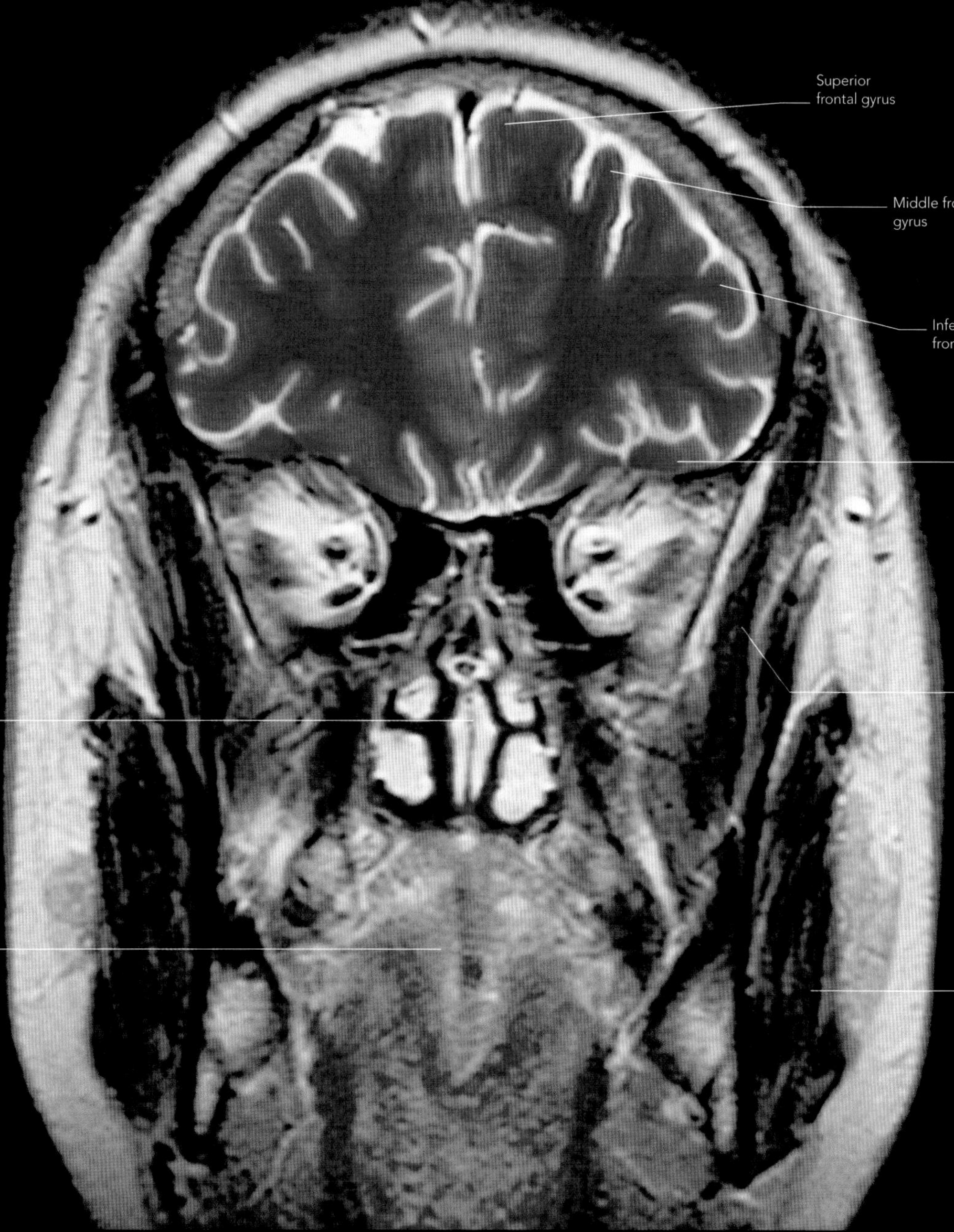

Superior frontal gyrus

Middle frontal gyrus

Inferior frontal gyrus

Orbitofrontal gyrus

Temporalis muscle

Nasal septum

Tongue

Masseter muscle

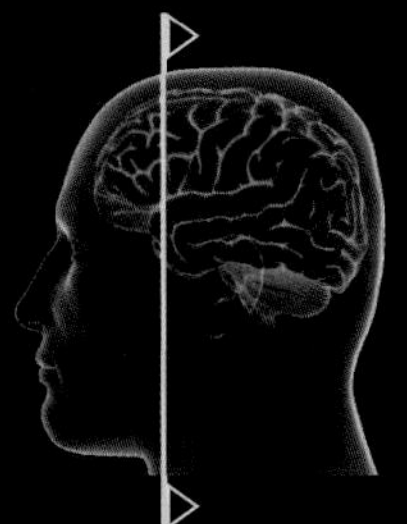

4 THE ORBITOFRONTAL GYRI

The orbitofrontal gyri, located at the bottom of the brain, receive signals about smell and taste. Like the rest of the prefrontal cortex, this area is concerned with predicting the future, but specializes in predictions about rewards and punishments and therefore emotions. This area is connected with the amygdala (see slice 9, p.24).

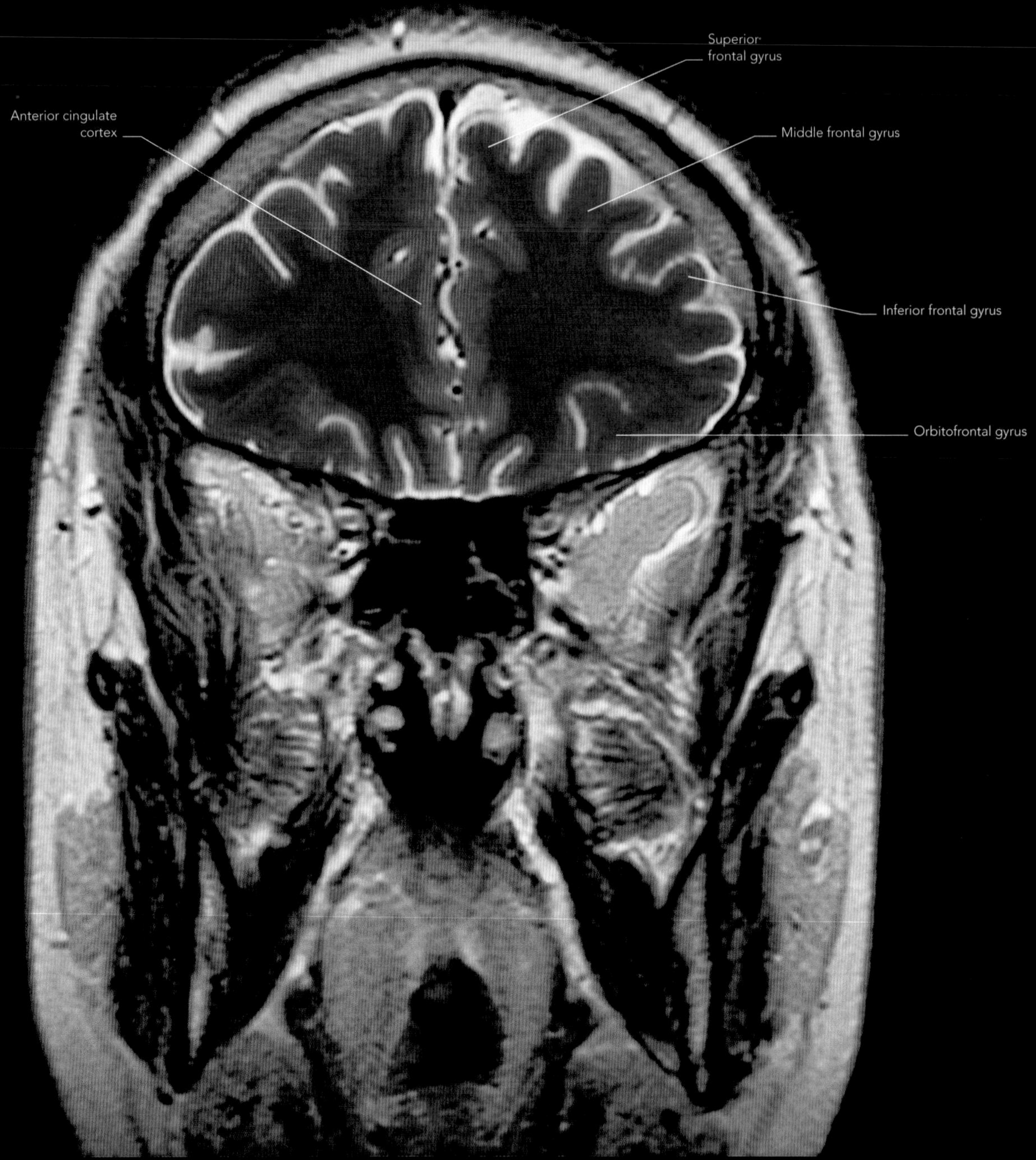

Superior frontal gyrus

Anterior cingulate cortex

Middle frontal gyrus

Inferior frontal gyrus

Orbitofrontal gyrus

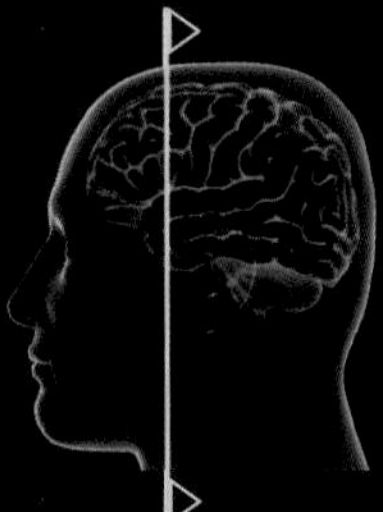

5 THE ANTERIOR CINGULATE CORTEX
Here we see the beginning of the anterior cingulate cortex, which lies between the two hemispheres. This sits alongside the limbic system. It is involved in linking emotions to actions and predicting the consequences of actions. The back part of the anterior cingulate cortex has direct connections with the motor system.

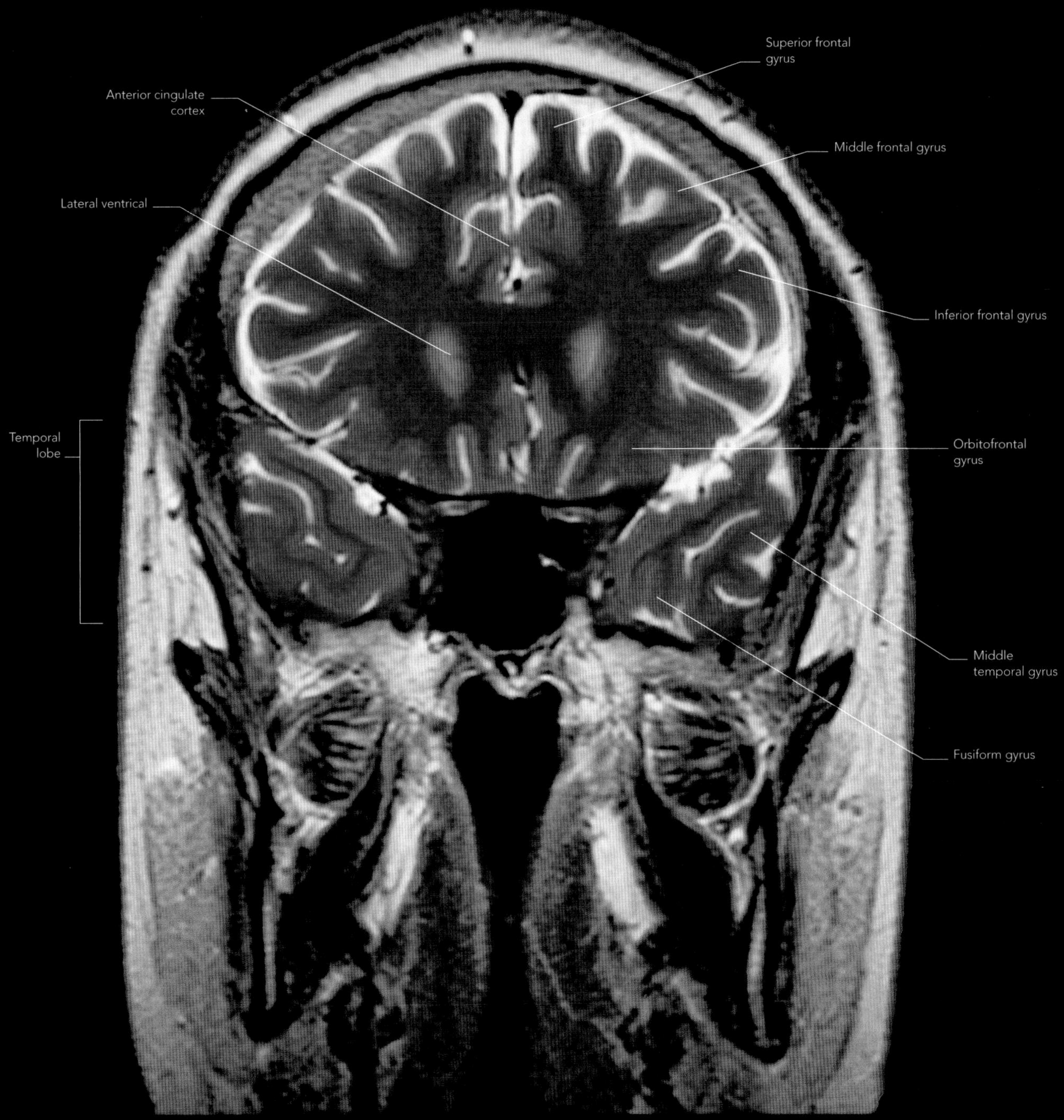

Superior frontal gyrus
Anterior cingulate cortex
Middle frontal gyrus
Lateral ventrical
Inferior frontal gyrus
Temporal lobe
Orbitofrontal gyrus
Middle temporal gyrus
Fusiform gyrus

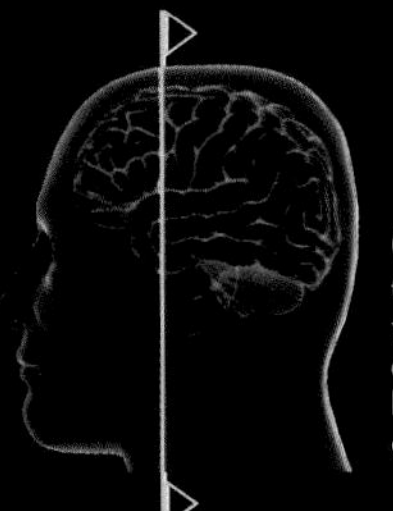

6 THE TEMPORAL LOBES
In this slice, the temporal lobes come into view for the first time. At the very front of the temporal lobes (the temporal poles), knowledge acquired from all the senses is combined, along with emotional tone. We can also see the lateral ventricles in the middle of the slice. These are parts of a system of fluid-filled spaces in the middle of the brain.

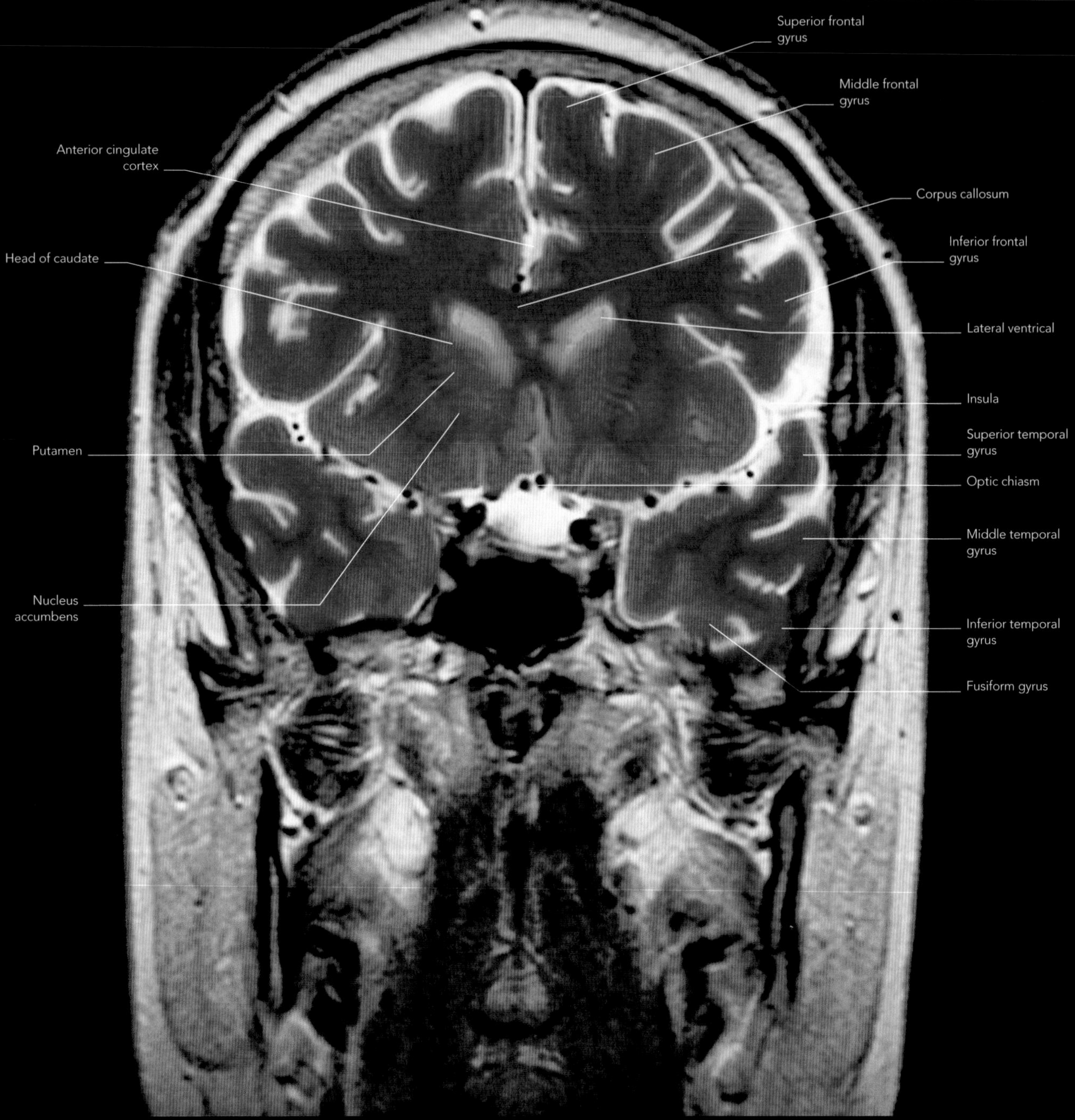

Superior frontal gyrus

Middle frontal gyrus

Anterior cingulate cortex

Corpus callosum

Inferior frontal gyrus

Head of caudate

Lateral ventrical

Insula

Superior temporal gyrus

Putamen

Optic chiasm

Middle temporal gyrus

Nucleus accumbens

Inferior temporal gyrus

Fusiform gyrus

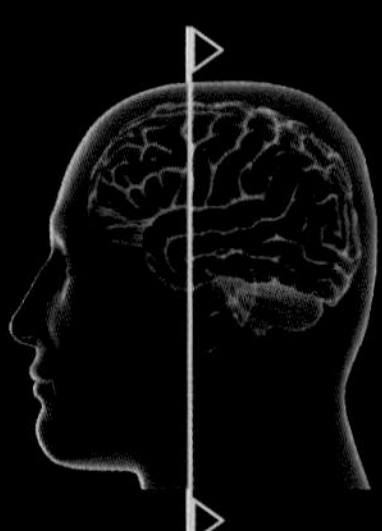

7 THE INSULA

The insula is a fold of cortex hidden deep in the brain between the frontal and the temporal lobes. Signals about the internal state of the body – such as heart rate, temperature, and pain – are received here. Also visible in this slice is the corpus callosum, the band of nerve fibres that joins the brain's left and right hemispheres.

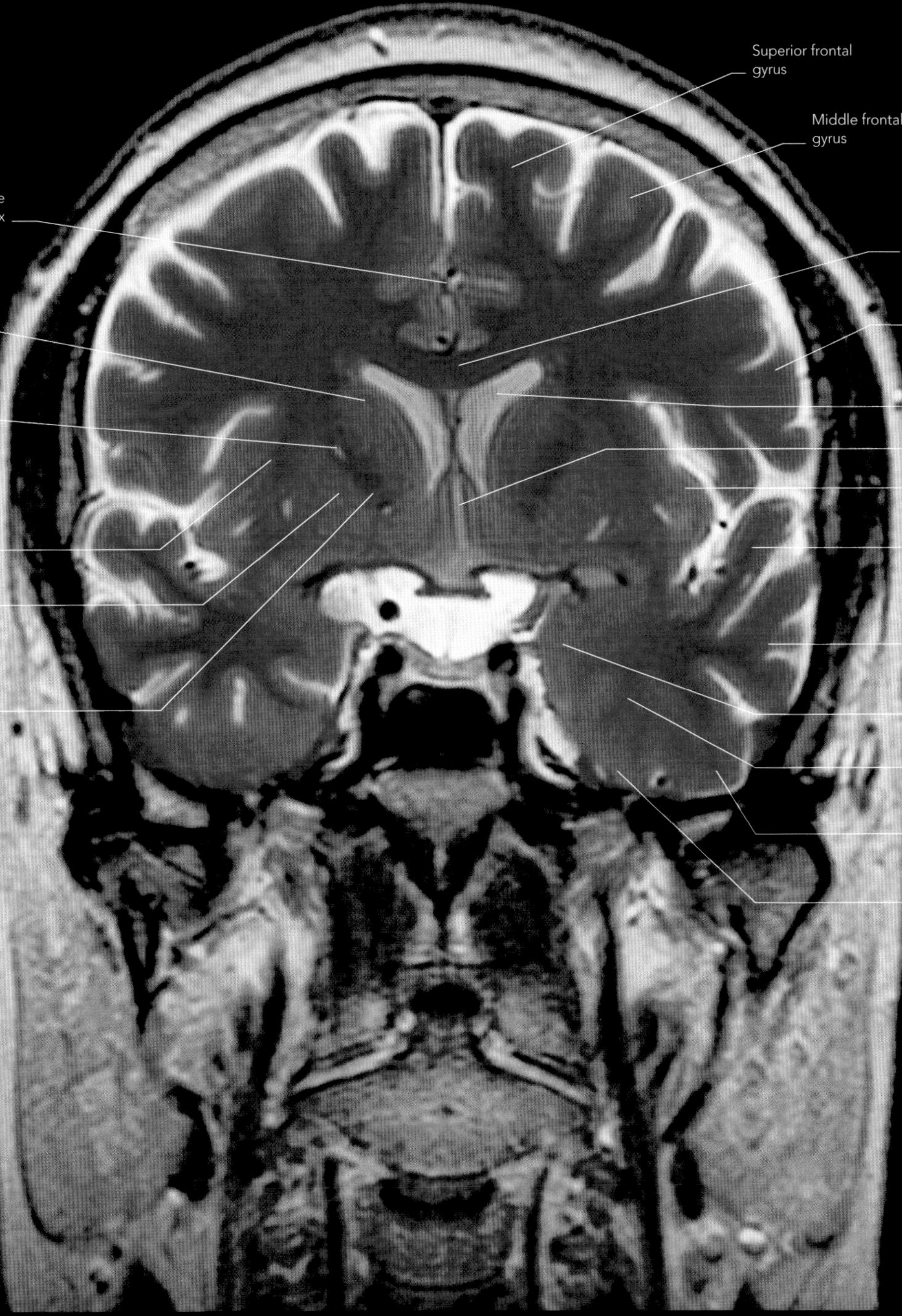

Superior frontal gyrus
Middle frontal gyrus
Anterior cingulate cortex
Corpus callosum
Inferior frontal gyrus
Head of caudate
Lateral ventrical
Internal capsule
Third ventrical
Insula
Putamen
Superior temporal gyrus
External globus pallidus
Middle temporal gyrus
Internal globus pallidus
Amygdala
Hippocampus
Inferior temporal gyrus
Fusiform gyrus

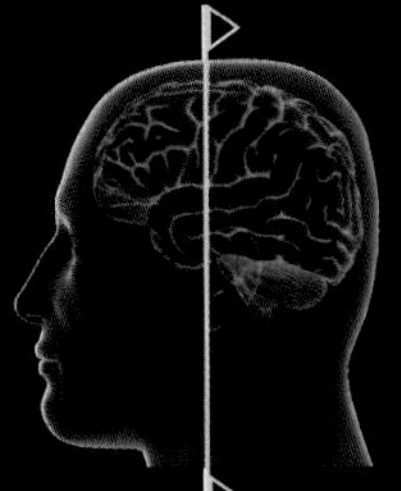

8 THE BASAL GANGLIA Located in the middle of the brain, the basal ganglia include the caudate, putamen, and globus pallidus. Also known as nuclei, ganglia are clumps of grey matter (or nerve-cell bodies) surrounded by white matter. The basal ganglia are linked to the cortex, the thalamus, and the brainstem and are concerned with motor control and decision making.

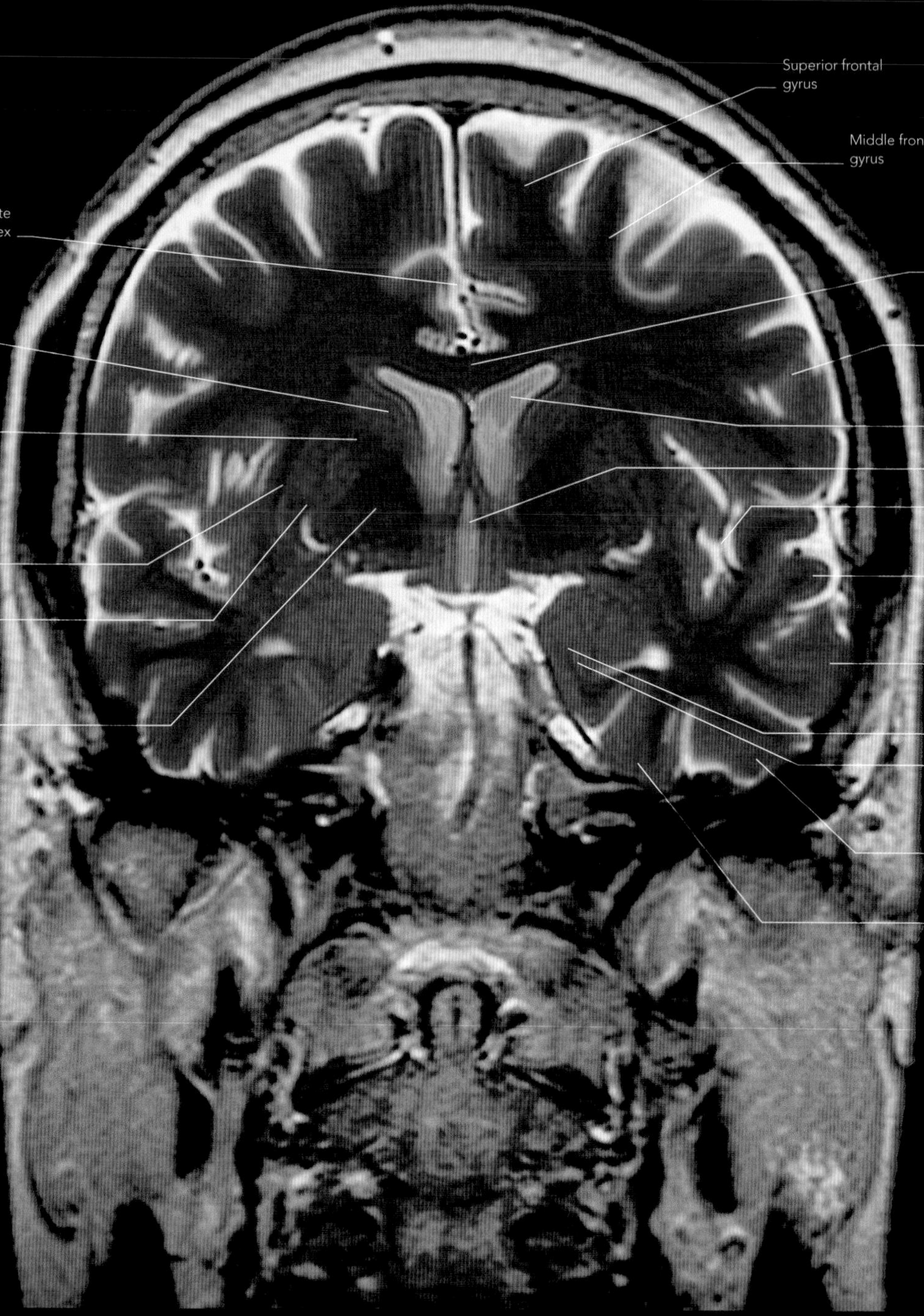

Superior frontal gyrus
Middle frontal gyrus
Anterior cingulate cortex
Corpus callosum
Inferior frontal gyrus
Head of caudate
Lateral ventrical
Internal capsule
Third ventrical
Insula
Putamen
Superior temporal gyrus
External globus pallidus
Middle temporal gyrus
Internal globus pallidus
Amygdala
Hippocampus
Inferior temporal gyrus
Fusiform gyrus

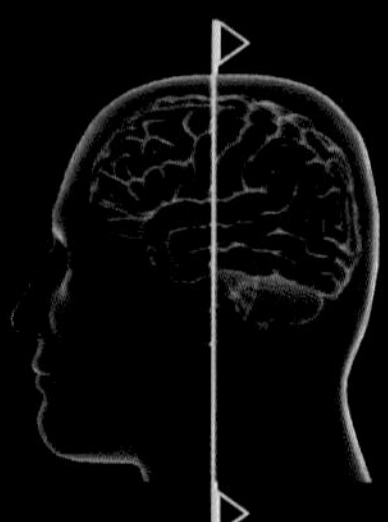

9 THE AMYGDALA AND HIPPOCAMPUS
This slice includes the amygdala and the front part of the hippocampus. Both structures lie in the inner part of the temporal lobe. The amygdala is involved in learning to approach or avoid things and hence with emotion. The hippocampus has a critical role in spatial navigation and memory of past experiences, including routes between places.

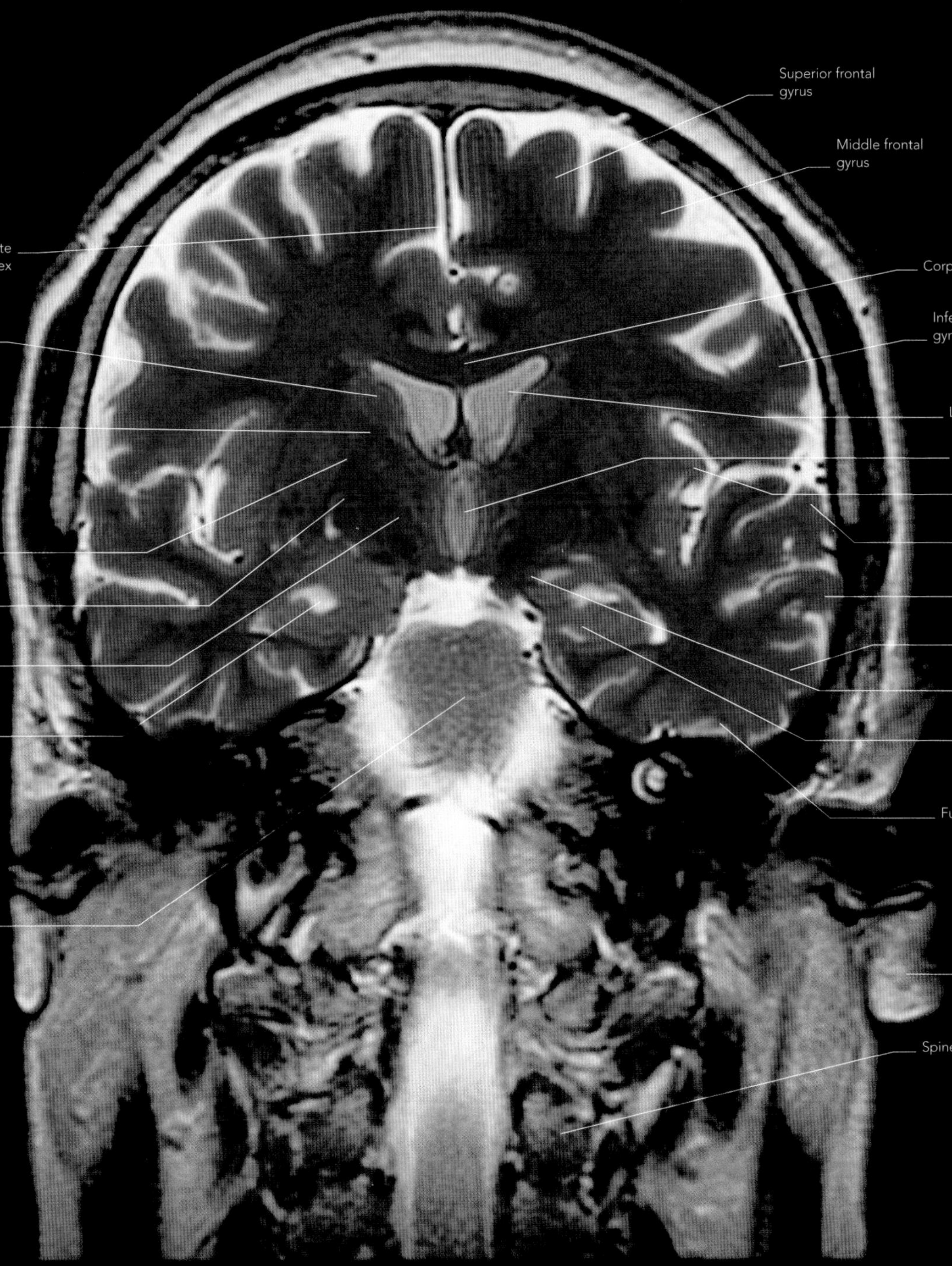

Superior frontal gyrus

Middle frontal gyrus

Anterior cingulate cortex

Corpus callosum

Inferior frontal gyrus

Head of caudate

Lateral ventrical

Internal capsule

Third ventrical

Insula

Superior temporal gyrus

Putamen

Middle temporal gyrus

External globus pallidus

Inferior temporal gyrus

Internal globus pallidus

Amygdala

Temporal horn of lateral ventrical

Hippocampus

Fusiform gyrus

Pons

Ear

Spine

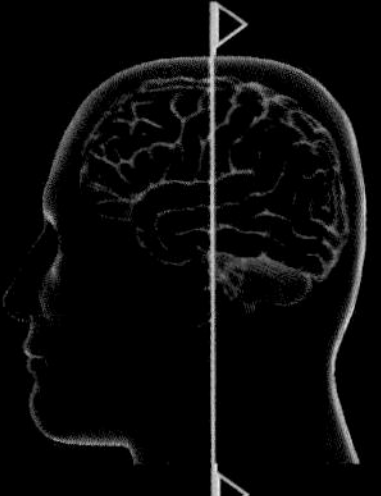

10 BROCA'S AREA

Here we approach the back of the frontal lobe. The bottom of the inferior frontal gyrus in the left hemisphere, just above the insula, contains Broca's area, which has a critical role in speech and language. At the bottom of the slice, we see the front of the brainstem, the pons, which joins the brain to the spinal cord.

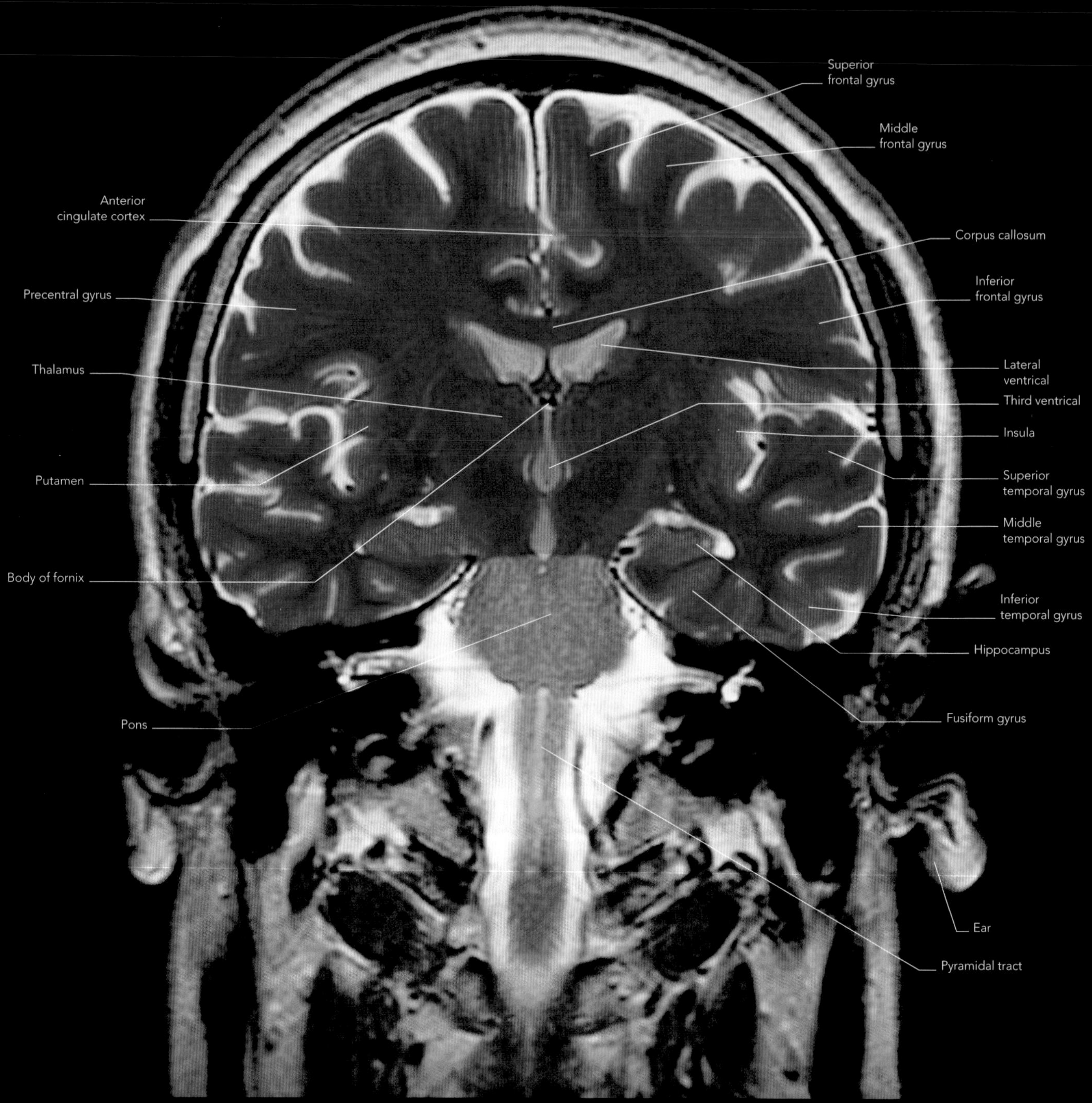

Superior frontal gyrus
Middle frontal gyrus
Anterior cingulate cortex
Corpus callosum
Precentral gyrus
Inferior frontal gyrus
Thalamus
Lateral ventrical
Third ventrical
Insula
Putamen
Superior temporal gyrus
Middle temporal gyrus
Body of fornix
Inferior temporal gyrus
Hippocampus
Pons
Fusiform gyrus
Ear
Pyramidal tract

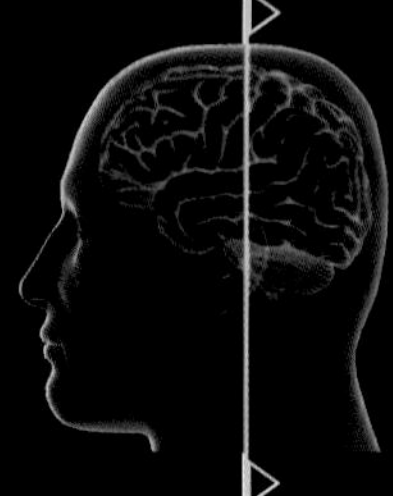

11 THE THALAMUS

This slice includes the thalamus, which lies between the cerebrum and the brainstem. A complex structure, it is made up of more than 20 nuclei (see p.60). The thalamus acts in a similar way to a relay station, taking in information from all the senses (except smell) and sending them on to different parts of the cerebral cortex.

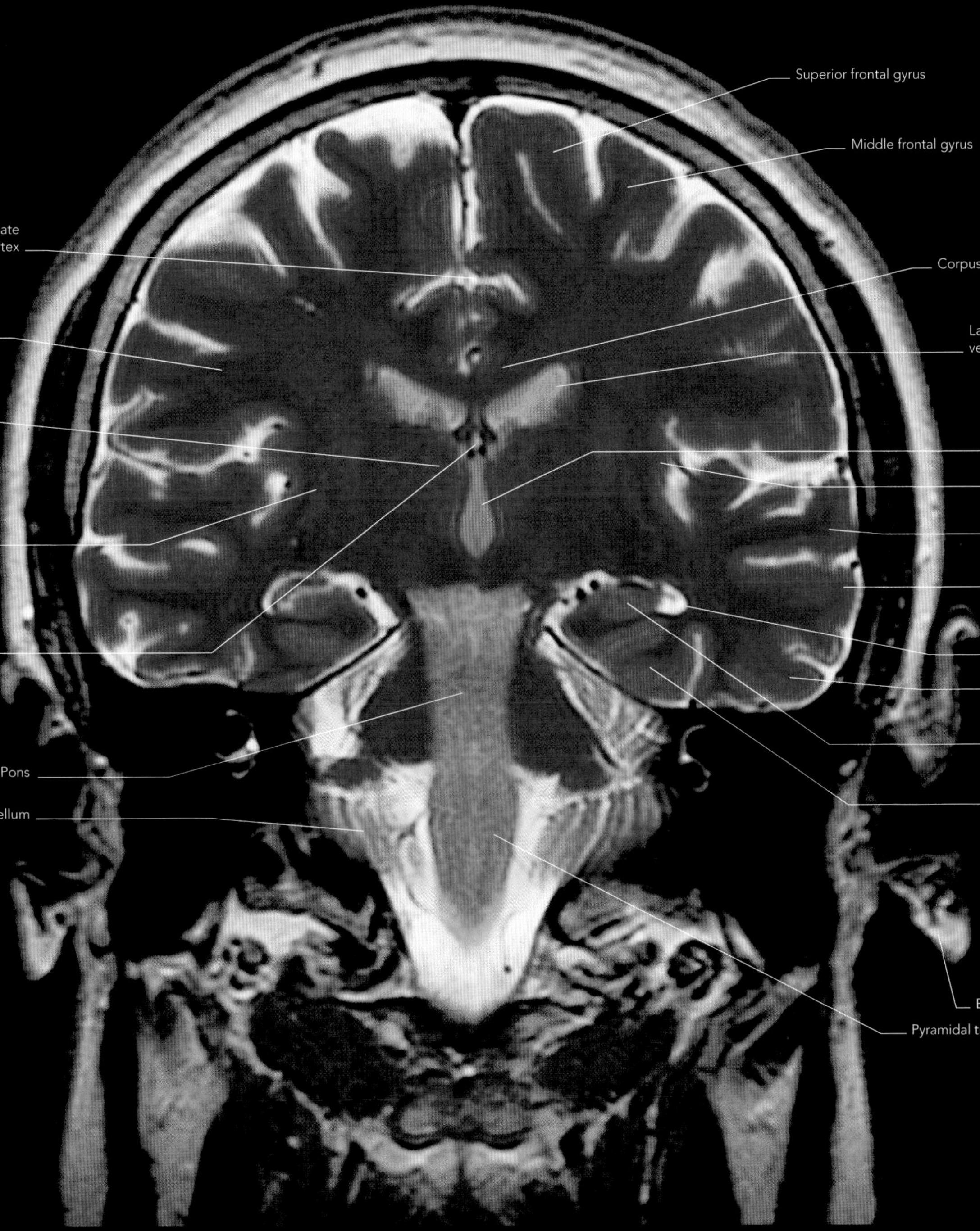

Anterior cingulate cortex
Precentral gyrus
Thalamus
Putamen
Body of fornix
Pons
Cerebellum
Superior frontal gyrus
Middle frontal gyrus
Corpus callosum
Lateral ventrical
Third ventrical
Insula
Superior temporal gyrus
Middle temporal gyrus
Temporal horn of lateral ventrical
Inferior temporal gyrus
Hippocampus
Fusiform gyrus
Ear
Pyramidal tract

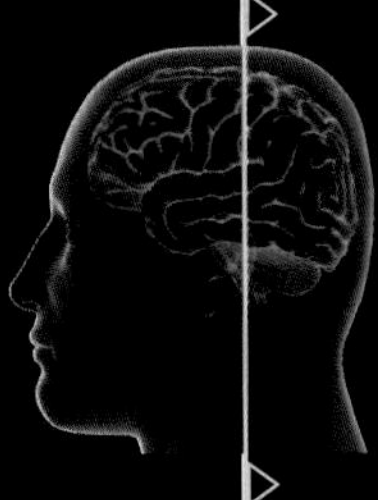

12 THE BRAINSTEM

The brainstem (in green) joins the brain to the spinal cord and contains a number of structures such as the pons. The brainstem has a special role in the control of basic bodily functions, including the control of heart rate and breathing. It also relays signals from the brain to the muscles and from senses in all parts of the body to the brain.

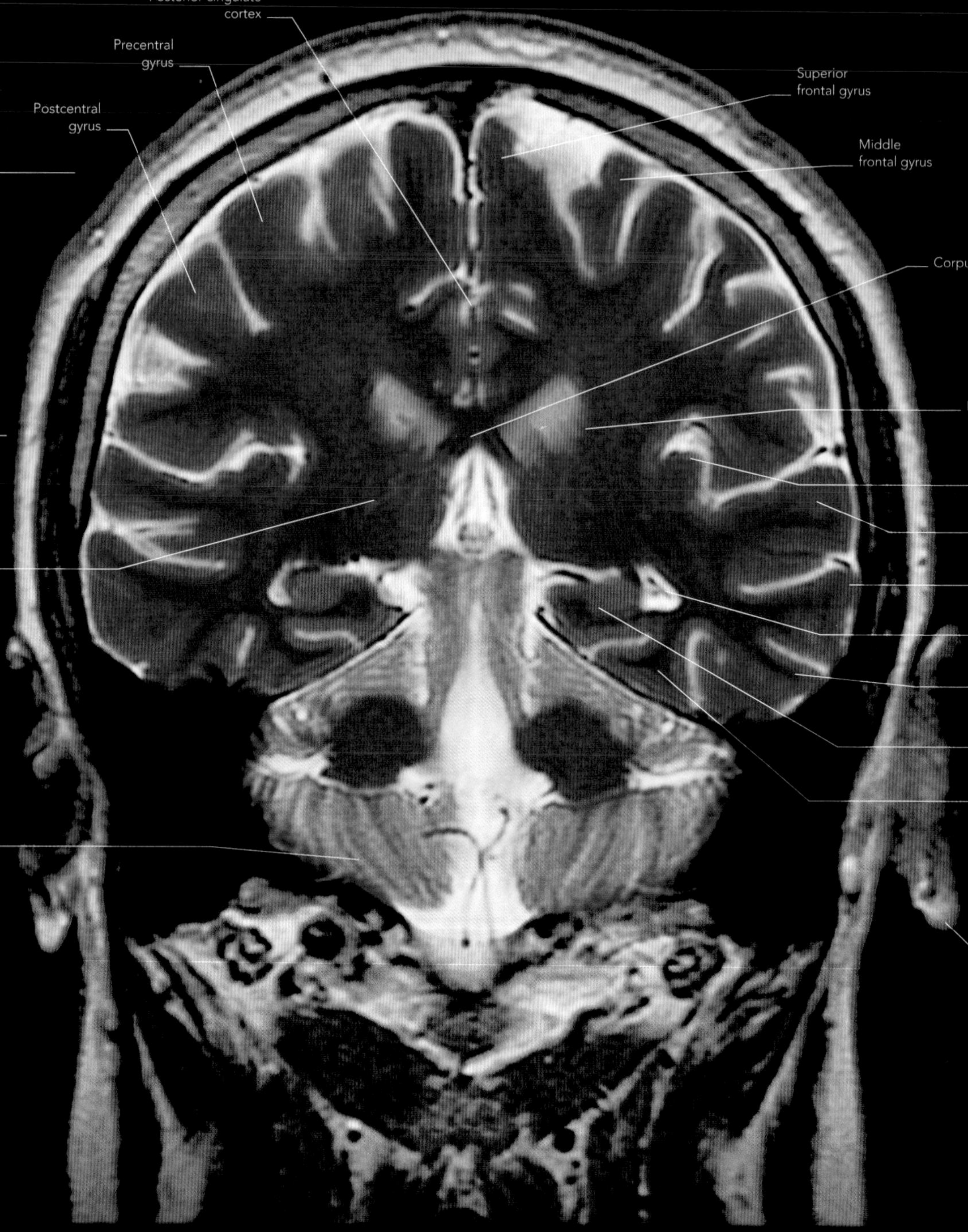

Posterior cingulate cortex
Precentral gyrus
Postcentral gyrus
Parietal lobe
Superior frontal gyrus
Middle frontal gyrus
Corpus callosum
Lateral ventrical
Insula
Superior temporal gyrus
Pulvinar of the thalamus
Middle temporal gyrus
Temporal ho
lateral ventric
Inferior temporal gyrus
Entorhinal corte
Fusiform gyr
Cerebellum
Ear

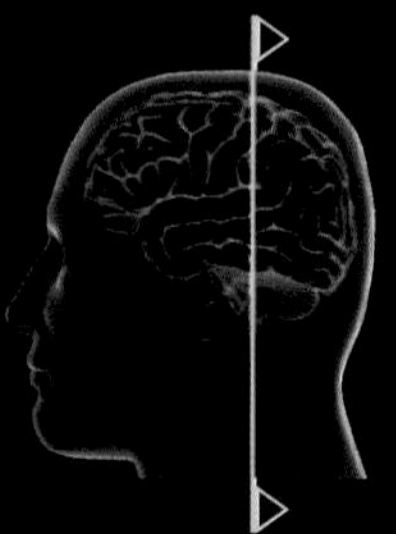

13 THE PARIETAL LOBE

The parietal lobe includes the supramarginal gyrus and the angular gyrus (see slices 14–20, pp.29–35). The parietal lobe integrates signals from many of the senses (including visual information that arrives via the dorsal route, see pp.82–83) to estimate the position of the body and the limbs in space. This information is critical when we reach for and grasp objects.

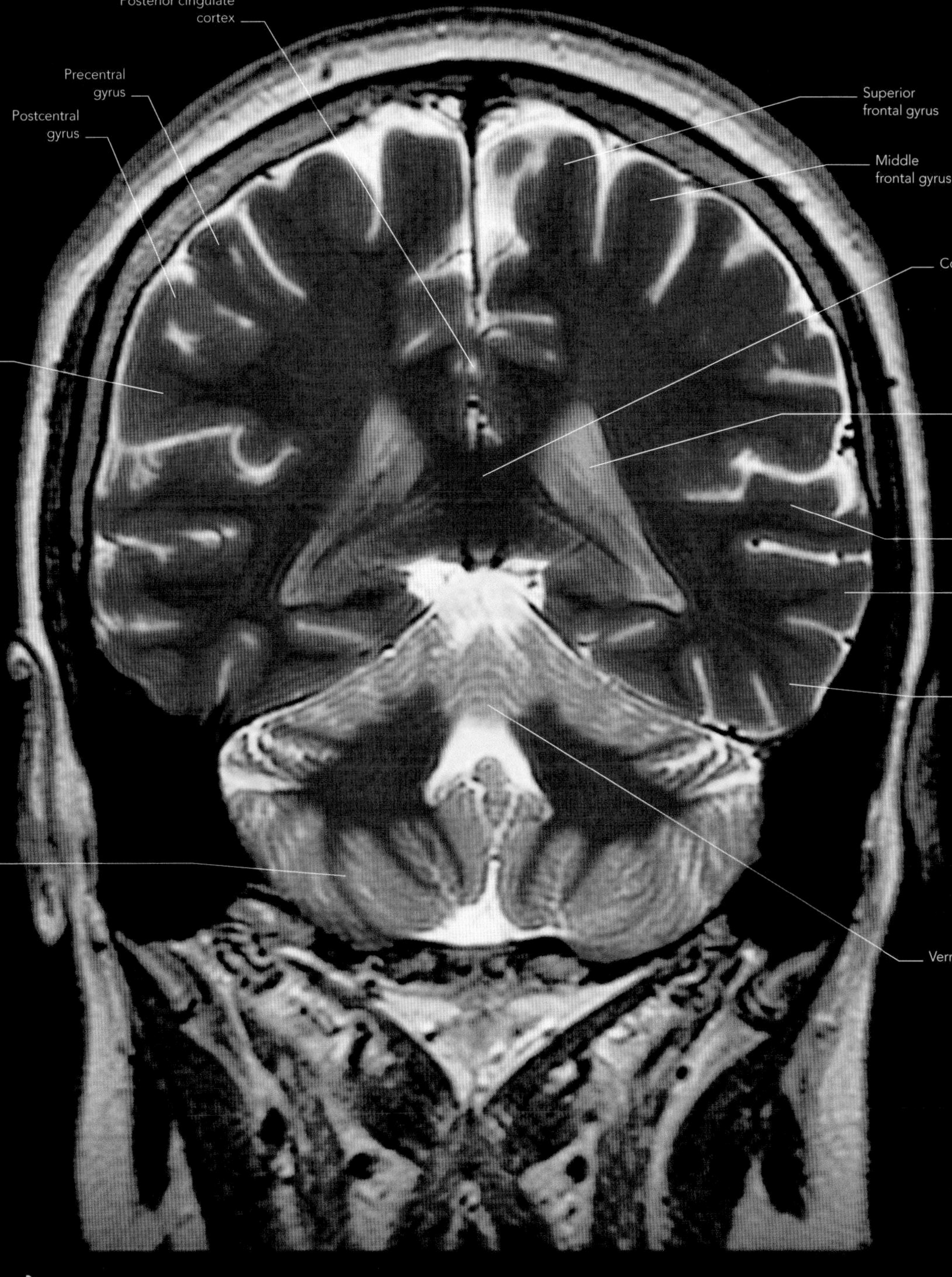

Posterior cingulate cortex
Precentral gyrus
Postcentral gyrus
Superior frontal gyrus
Middle frontal gyrus
Corpus callosum
Supramarginal gyrus
Lateral ventrical
Superior temporal gyrus
Middle temporal gyrus
Inferior temporal gyrus
Cerebellum
Vermis

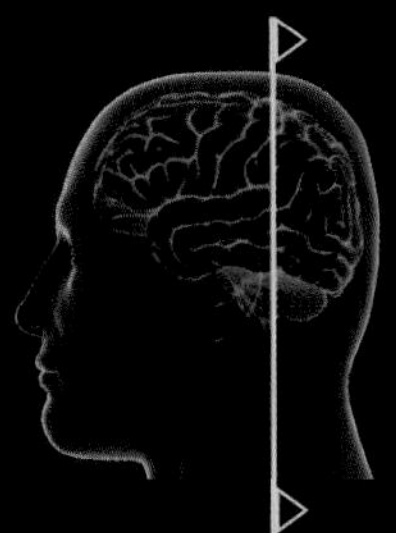

14 THE PRECENTRAL AND POSTCENTRAL GYRUS The last part of the frontal cortex is the precentral gyrus.This contains the motor strip, where different regions send signals to control different parts of the body. The immediately adjacent part of the parietal cortex (the postcentral gyrus) has a corresponding sensory strip, where sensory signals are received from different parts of the body.

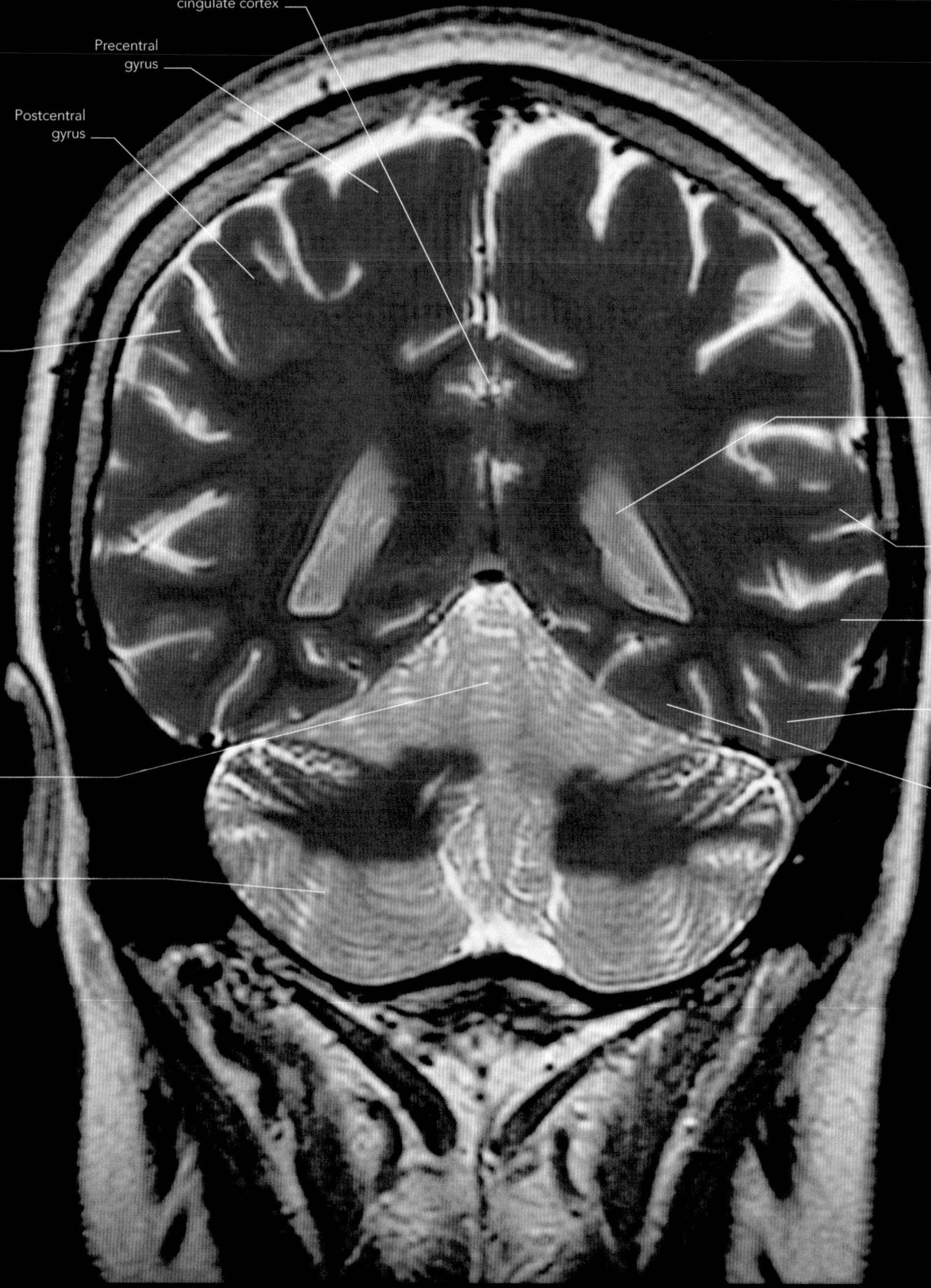

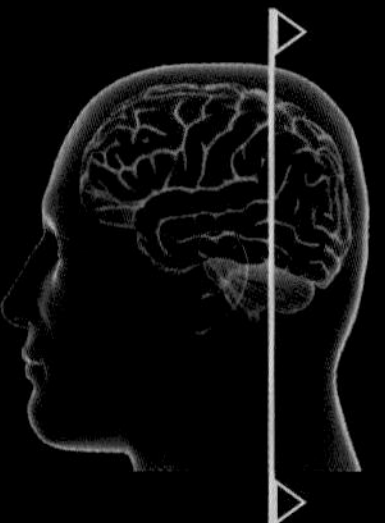

15 THE PRIMARY AUDITORY CORTEX
The primary auditory cortex, where signals from the ears reach the cortex via the thalamus, lies along the very top of the superior temporal gyrus, in the fissure between the temporal lobe and the parietal lobe. Adjacent to the primary auditory cortex is Wernicke's area, where incoming sounds are turned into words.

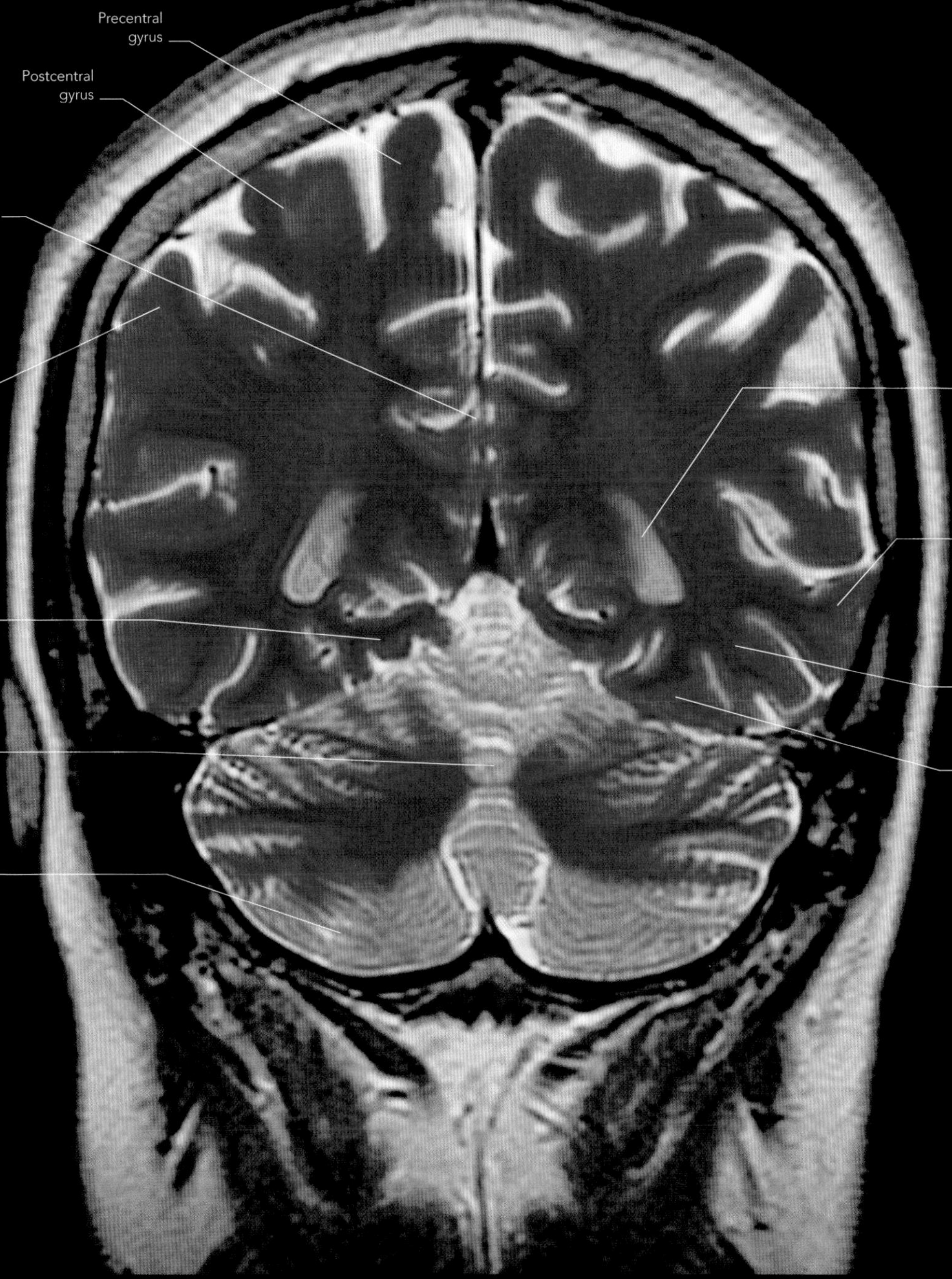

Precentral gyrus

Postcentral gyrus

Posterior cingulate cortex

Supramarginal gyrus

Occipital gyrus

Vermis

Cerebellum

Lateral ventrical

Middle temporal gyrus

Inferior temporal gyrus

Fusiform gyrus

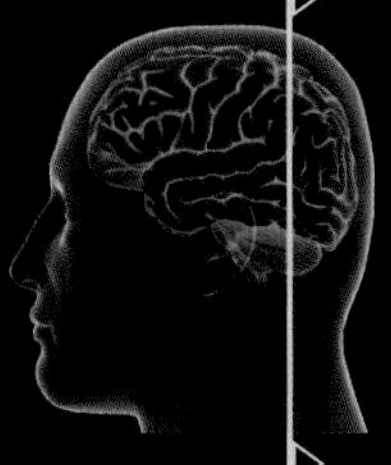

16 THE FUSIFORM GYRUS
The inferior temporal gyrus and the fusiform gyrus at the bottom of the temporal lobe are two areas concerned with recognition of objects. Part of the fusiform gyrus, known as the face-recognition area, is specialized for recognizing faces. It not only identifies facial features but also scrutinizes them for meaning, and so plays an important part in social interaction.

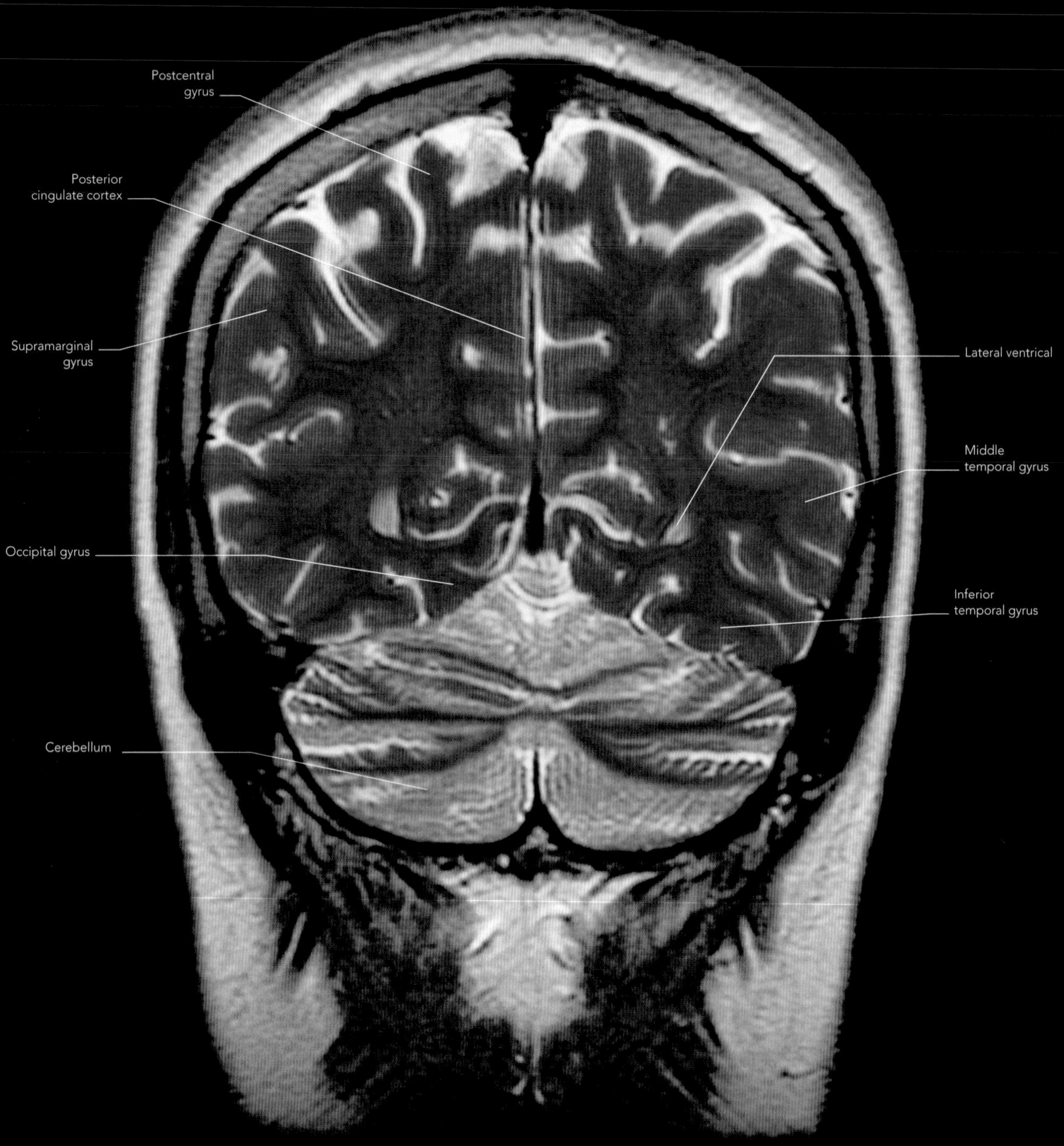

Postcentral gyrus

Posterior cingulate cortex

Supramarginal gyrus

Lateral ventrical

Middle temporal gyrus

Occipital gyrus

Inferior temporal gyrus

Cerebellum

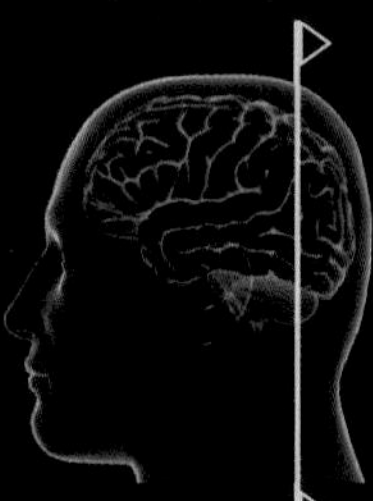

17 THE CEREBELLUM

The cerebellum (coloured light blue) is the highly convoluted "little brain" that sits at the back and below the main brain (also known as the cerebrum). The cerebellum is concerned with fine motor control and the timing of movements. There are many connections between the cerebellum and the motor cortex.

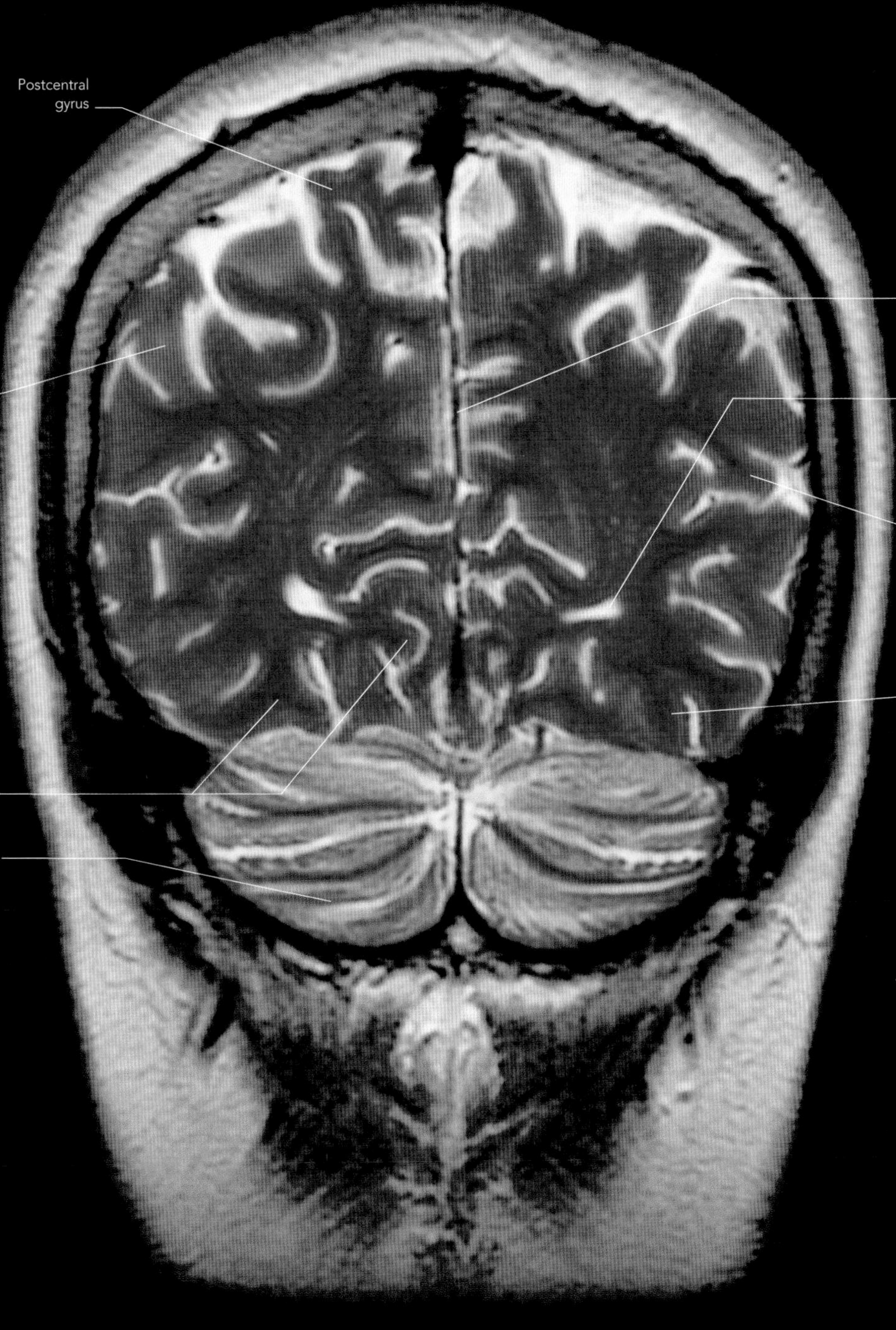

Postcentral gyrus

Precuneus

Supramarginal gyrus

Lateral ventrical

Angular gyrus

Occipital lobe

Inferior temporal gyrus

Occipital gyrus

Cerebellum

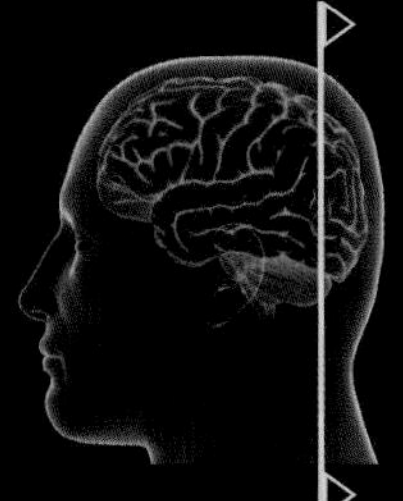

18 THE OCCIPITAL LOBE

The occipital lobe is concerned with vision. In the forward-most areas, signals from the primary visual cortex (see slice 20, p.35) are analysed in terms of features such as shape and colour. This information is then sent forwards to the inferior temporal cortex (see slice 16, p.31), along a pathway called the ventral route, and used for object recognition.

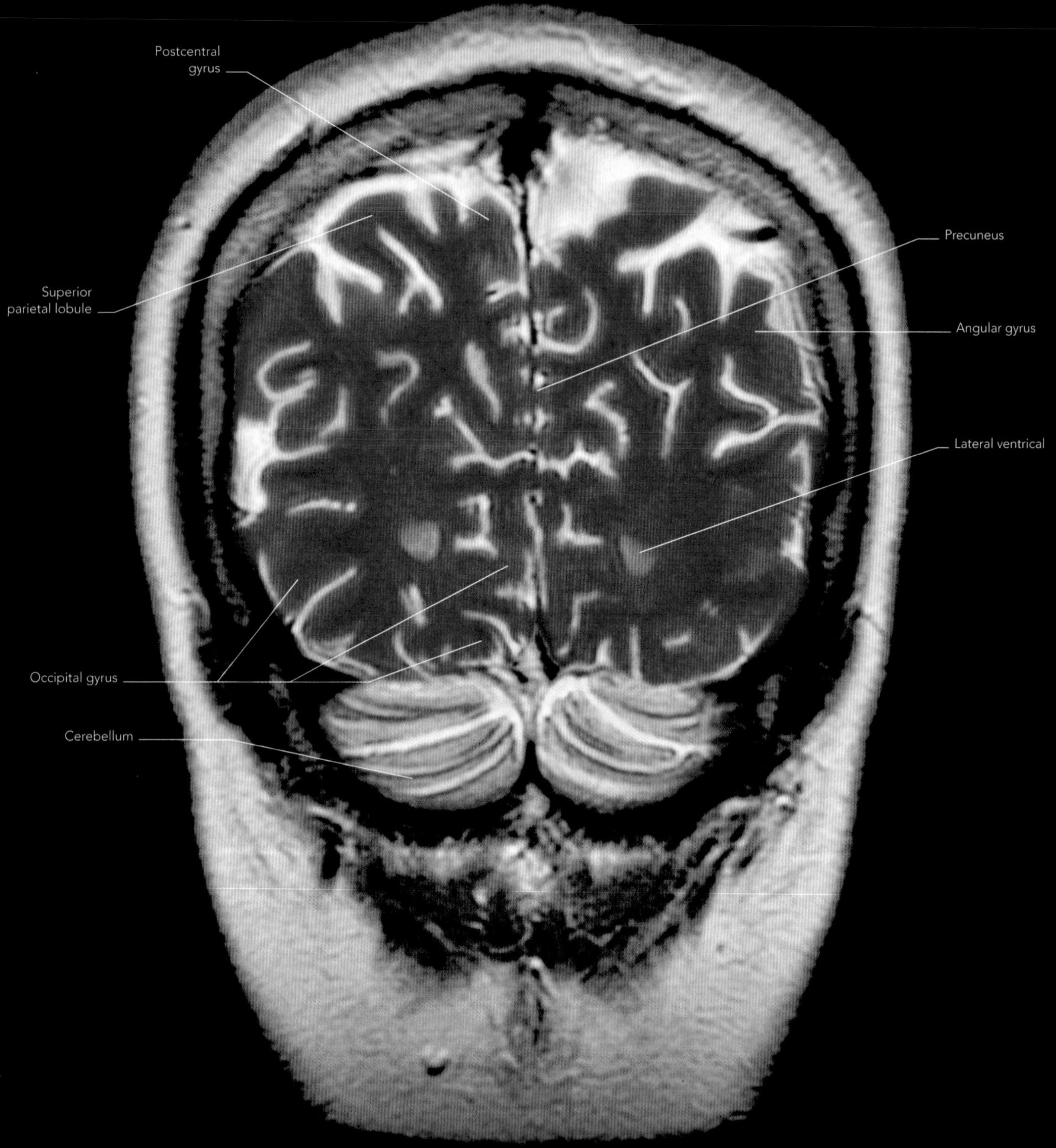

Postcentral gyrus

Superior parietal lobule

Precuneus

Angular gyrus

Lateral ventrical

Occipital gyrus

Cerebellum

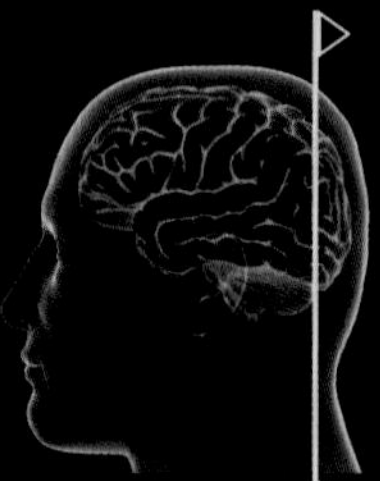

19 THE PRECUNEUS AND THE POSTERIOR CINGULATE CORTEX

The precuneus in the back part of the parietal lobe and posterior cingulate cortex (see slice 17, p.32) lie between the two hemispheres. These remain some of the more mysterious regions of the brain. They probably have a role in memory, especially memories about the self.

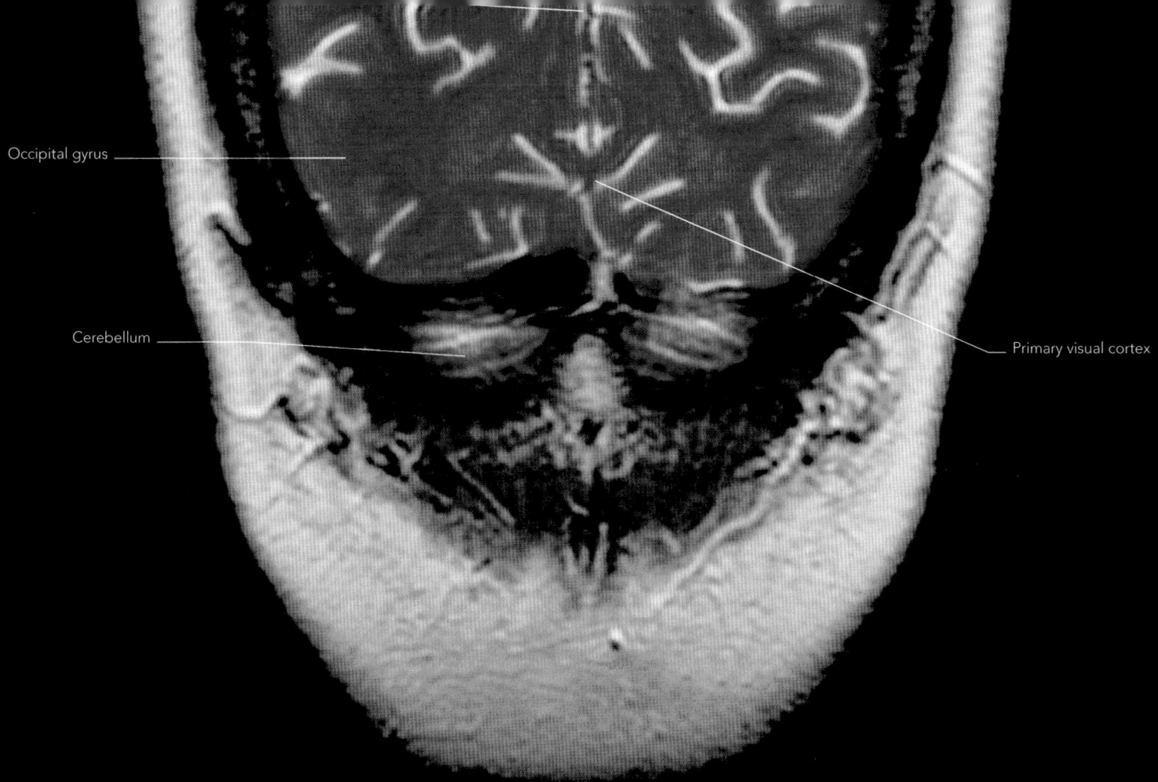

Occipital gyrus

Cerebellum

Primary visual cortex

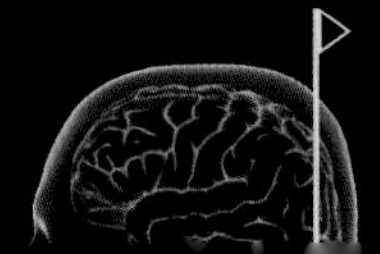

20 THE PRIMARY VISUAL CORTEX

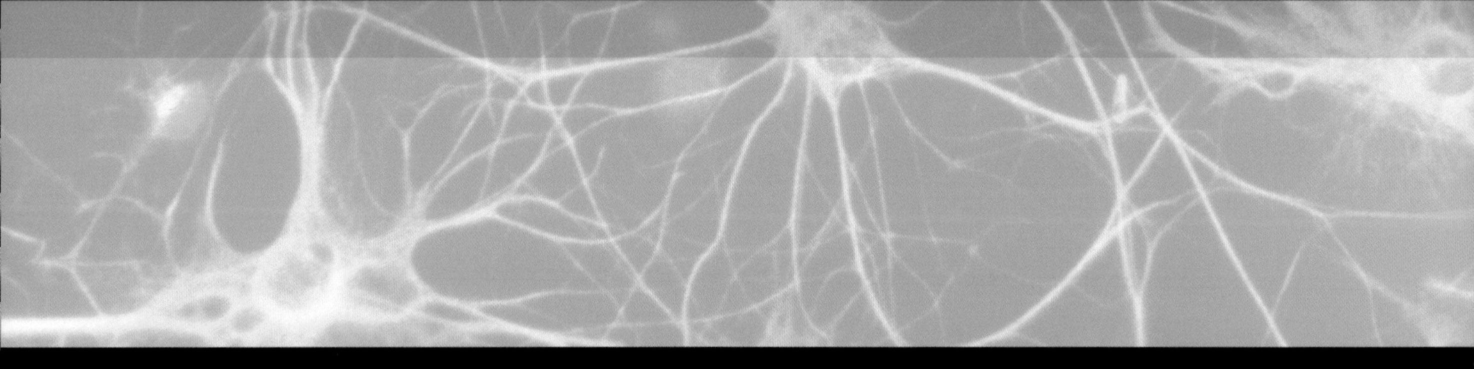

THE HUMAN BRAIN KEEPS US PRIMED TO RESPOND TO THE WORLD AROUND US. IT IS AT THE HUB OF A VAST AND COMPLEX COMMUNICATIONS NETWORK THAT CONSTANTLY SEEKS AND COLLECTS INFORMATION FROM THE REST OF THE BODY AND THE OUTSIDE WORLD. AS THE BRAIN INTERPRETS THIS INFORMATION, IT GENERATES EXPERIENCES: SIGHTS AND SOUNDS, EMOTIONS AND THOUGHTS. BUT ITS PRIMARY FUNCTION IS TO PRODUCE CHANGES IN THE BODY. THESE INCLUDE LIFE-SUSTAINING BASICS SUCH AS THE REGULAR CONTRACTIONS OF THE HEART THROUGH TO THE COMPLEX ACTIONS THAT CONSTITUTE BEHAVIOUR.

THE BRAIN AND THE BODY

BRAIN FUNCTIONS

THE PRIMARY TASK OF THE BRAIN IS TO HELP MAINTAIN THE WHOLE BODY IN AN OPTIMAL STATE RELATIVE TO THE ENVIRONMENT, IN ORDER TO MAXIMIZE THE CHANCES OF SURVIVAL. THE BRAIN DOES THIS BY REGISTERING STIMULI AND THEN RESPONDING BY GENERATING ACTIONS. IN THE PROCESS, IT ALSO GENERATES SUBJECTIVE EXPERIENCE.

WHAT THE BRAIN DOES

The brain receives a constant stream of information as electrical impulses from neurons in the sense organs. The first thing it does is determine whether the information warrants attention. If it is irrelevant or just confirmation that everything is staying the same, it is allowed to fade away and we are not conscious of it. But if it is novel or important, the brain amplifies the signals, causing them to be represented in various regions. If this activity is sustained for long enough, it will result in a conscious experience. In some cases, thoughts are taken one step further, and the brain instructs the body to act on them, by sending signals to the muscles to make them contract.

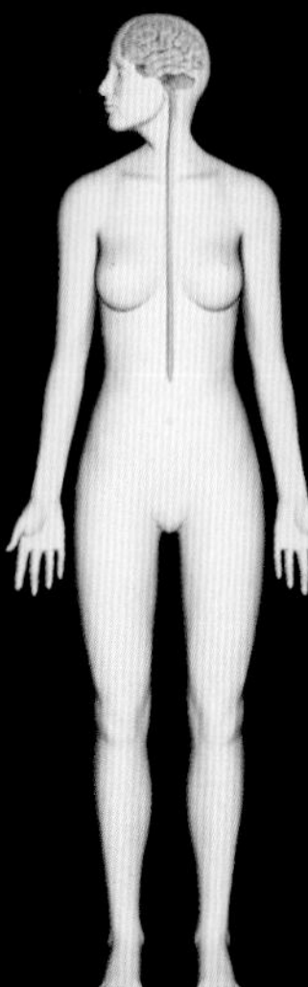

THE BRAIN AND BODY
The brain and spinal cord constitute the central nervous system, which is the body's main control centre, responsible for co-ordinating all of the processes and movement in the body.

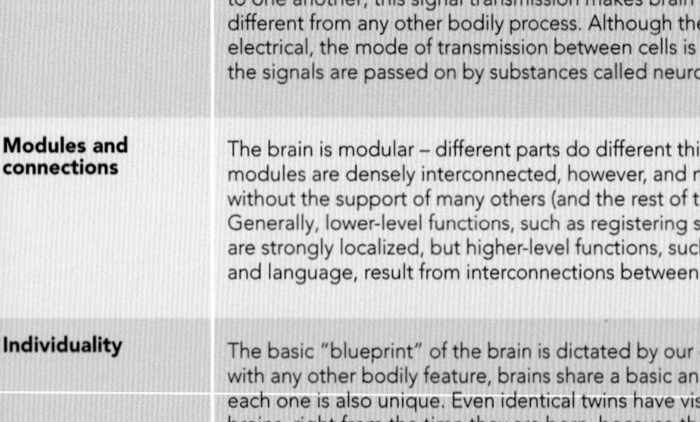

KEY FEATURES OF THE BRAIN

FEATURE	DESCRIPTION
Processing information	The brain registers a vast amount of information. However, only a very small amount of this is actually selected for processing to the point at which it enters our consciousness and can be reported. Experience that cannot be reported is not conscious. Unconscious brain processing nevertheless guides and sometimes initiates actions (see p.116 and p.191).
Sending signals	The brain consists of about 1000 billon cells. Roughly 10 per cent are specialized electrical cells called neurons, which send signals to one another; this signal transmission makes brain function different from any other bodily process. Although the signals are electrical, the mode of transmission between cells is chemical – the signals are passed on by substances called neurotransmitters.
Modules and connections	The brain is modular – different parts do different things. The modules are densely interconnected, however, and none works without the support of many others (and the rest of the body). Generally, lower-level functions, such as registering sensations, are strongly localized, but higher-level functions, such as memory and language, result from interconnections between brain areas.
Individuality	The basic "blueprint" of the brain is dictated by our genes. As with any other bodily feature, brains share a basic anatomy, but each one is also unique. Even identical twins have visibly different brains, right from the time they are born, because the brain is exquisitely sensitive to its environment. The differences between individual brains result in each person having a unique personality.
Plasticity	Brain tissue can be "strengthened" and built up like a muscle, according to how much it is exercised. So, if a person learns and practises a skill, such as playing a musical instrument or doing mathematics, the part of their brain concerned with that task will grow physically bigger. It also becomes more efficient and enables the person to perform the task more skilfully.

HOW THE BRAIN DOES IT

No-one knows exactly how electrical activity turns into experience. That remains a famously hard problem, which has yet to be cracked (see p.179). However, much is now known about the brain processes that turn incoming information into the various components of subjective experience, such as thoughts or emotions. Much depends on where the information comes from. Each sense organ is specialized to deal with a different type of stimulus – the eyes are sensitive to light, the ears to sound waves, and so on. The sense organs respond to these stimuli in much the same way – they generate electrical signals, which are sent on for further processing. But the information from each organ is sent to a different part of the brain, and then processed along a different neural pathway. Where information is processed therefore determines what sort of experience it will generate.

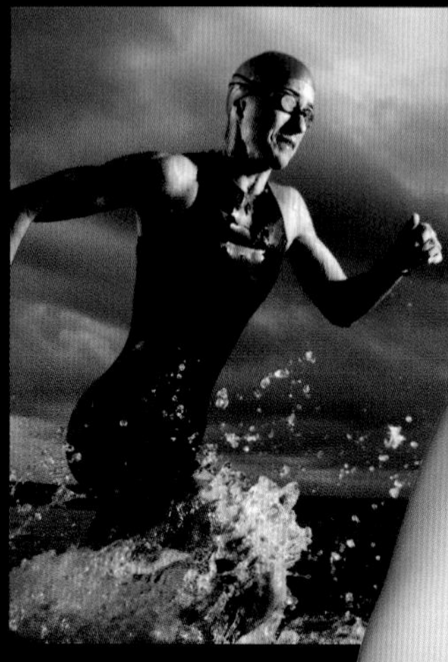

ACTIONS
Certain brain areas are specialized to produce bodily movement. Brainstem modules control automatic internal actions, such as the lung and chest movements needed for breathing, the beating of the heart, and the constriction or dilation of blood vessels to control blood pressure. In conscious activities, the primary motor cortex sends messages (via the cerebellum and basal ganglia) to the muscles of the limbs, trunk, and head to create gross movements.

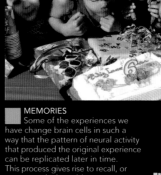

MEMORIES
Some of the experiences we have change brain cells in such a way that the pattern of neural activity that produced the original experience can be replicated later in time. This process gives rise to recall, or memory, which enables us to use past experiences as a guide to how to behave in the present.

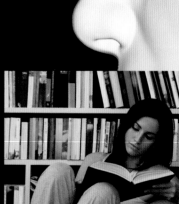

LANGUAGE
Language involves both producing speech and analysing what others say to understand the meaning. It depends on the brain's ability to link objects with abstract symbols and then to convey the symbols – and thus the ideas they represent – to others via words. As well as facilitating communication between people, language enables individuals to reflect on their own ideas.

EMOTIONS

Certain stimuli (including some thoughts and imaginings) cause changes in the body by activating areas in the limbic system, especially the amygdala. Conscious "feelings" occur when signals from the limbic system are sent on to "association areas" in the prefrontal cortex that support consciousness. During adolescence, the amygdala is relied heavily upon for processing emotional information, as the prefrontal cortex only matures when a person reaches their late 20s.

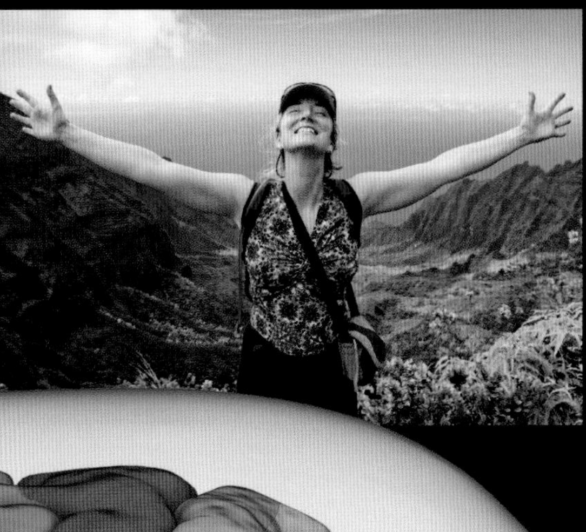

BRAIN FACTS	
FEATURE	**FACT**
Structure	The brain is highly compact. If you smoothed out all the wrinkles in the cortex, the brain would cover an area of about 2,300 square cm (2 ½ square ft).
Connectivity	The brain has around 100 billion neurons. There are more potential connections between the neurons than there are atoms in the universe.
Growth	A fetus grows neurons at the rate of 250,000 a minute. A person is born with nearly all the neurons they will ever have, but the neural networks are not mature yet.
Signalling speed	Information travels at different speeds within different types of neurons. Transmission speeds range from 1 to over 100 metres/sec (3 to 330 feet/sec).
Utilizing the whole brain	The claim that we only use 10 per cent of our brains is false – we use all of it. Some complex functions, such as memory, involve many areas at once.
Regeneration	You do not "lose" brain cells as you age, although some functions may decline. You can maintain the networks or even form new ones by exercising your brain.
Pain-free zone	Brain tissue has no pain receptors, so despite the fact it registers pain from all parts of the body, it does not actually feel pain itself.

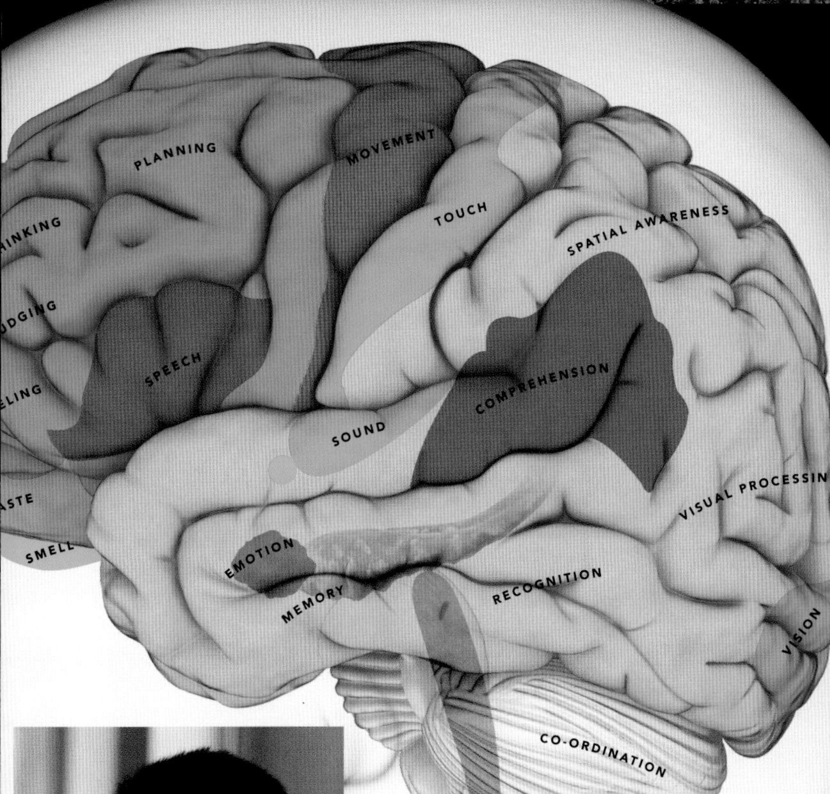

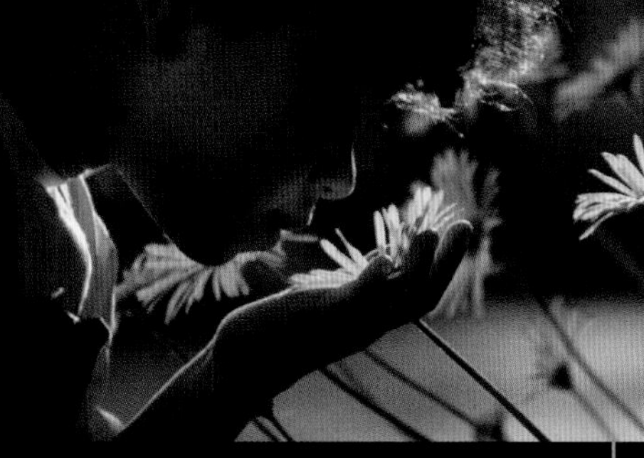

SENSATIONS

Information from the environment enters the brain via the different sense organs and is transmitted to specific areas of the cerebral cortex called the primary sensory areas. This information includes some input from the body itself. In the absence of external stimuli, the sensory areas continue to be active and are thought to generate the experiences that we know as dreams, hallucinations, and imagination.

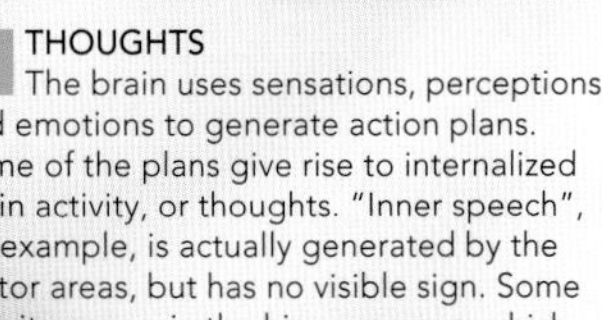

THOUGHTS

The brain uses sensations, perceptions, and emotions to generate action plans. Some of the plans give rise to internalized brain activity, or thoughts. "Inner speech", for example, is actually generated by the motor areas, but has no visible sign. Some activity occurs in the hippocampus, which we experience as recollection.

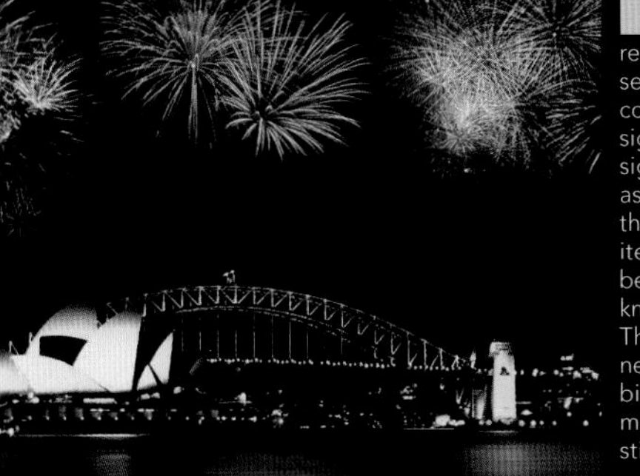

PERCEPTIONS

Most of the time we are receiving information from many sensory areas at once, as with the combination of auditory and visual signals at a fireworks display. These signals may be communicated to association areas, which bind all of this information together. If these items of "bound" information become conscious, they form what is known as a multi-sensory perception. There is a great deal of current neuroscientific research on how the binding process forms a unified, multi-sensory perception, as it is still not fully understood.

THE NERVOUS SYSTEM

THE NERVOUS SYSTEM IS THE BODY'S MAJOR COMMUNICATION AND CONTROL NETWORK. DATA, IN THE FORM OF ELECTRICAL SIGNALS, IS RELAYED CONSTANTLY FROM THE SENSE ORGANS TO AND FROM THE BRAIN, THROUGH COMPLEX NETWORKS OF NEURONS AND ON A TIMESCALE MEASURED IN MILLISECONDS.

Although it is a single, unified communications network, the nervous system consists of three anatomical and functional subdivisions. The central nervous system (CNS) is the co-ordinating system for the body. It comprises the brain and spinal cord, which are surrounded and protected by the skull and vertebral column respectively. The peripheral nervous system (PNS) is a complex network of nerves extending across the body, branching out from 12 pairs of cranial nerves originating in the brain and 31 pairs of spinal nerves emanating from the spinal cord. It relays information between the body and the brain in the form of nerve impulses. It has an afferent division (through which messages are sent to the brain) and an efferent division (which carries messages from the brain to the body). Finally, there is the autonomic nervous system (ANS), which shares some nerve structures with both the CNS and PNS. It functions "automatically" without conscious awareness, controlling basic functions, such as body temperature, blood pressure, and heart rate.

Sensory input travels quickly from receptor points throughout the body via the afferent network of the PNS to the brain, which processes, co-ordinates, and interprets the data in just fractions of a second. The brain makes an executive decision that is conveyed via the efferent division of the PNS to muscles, which take the action needed to respond to environmental change rapidly.

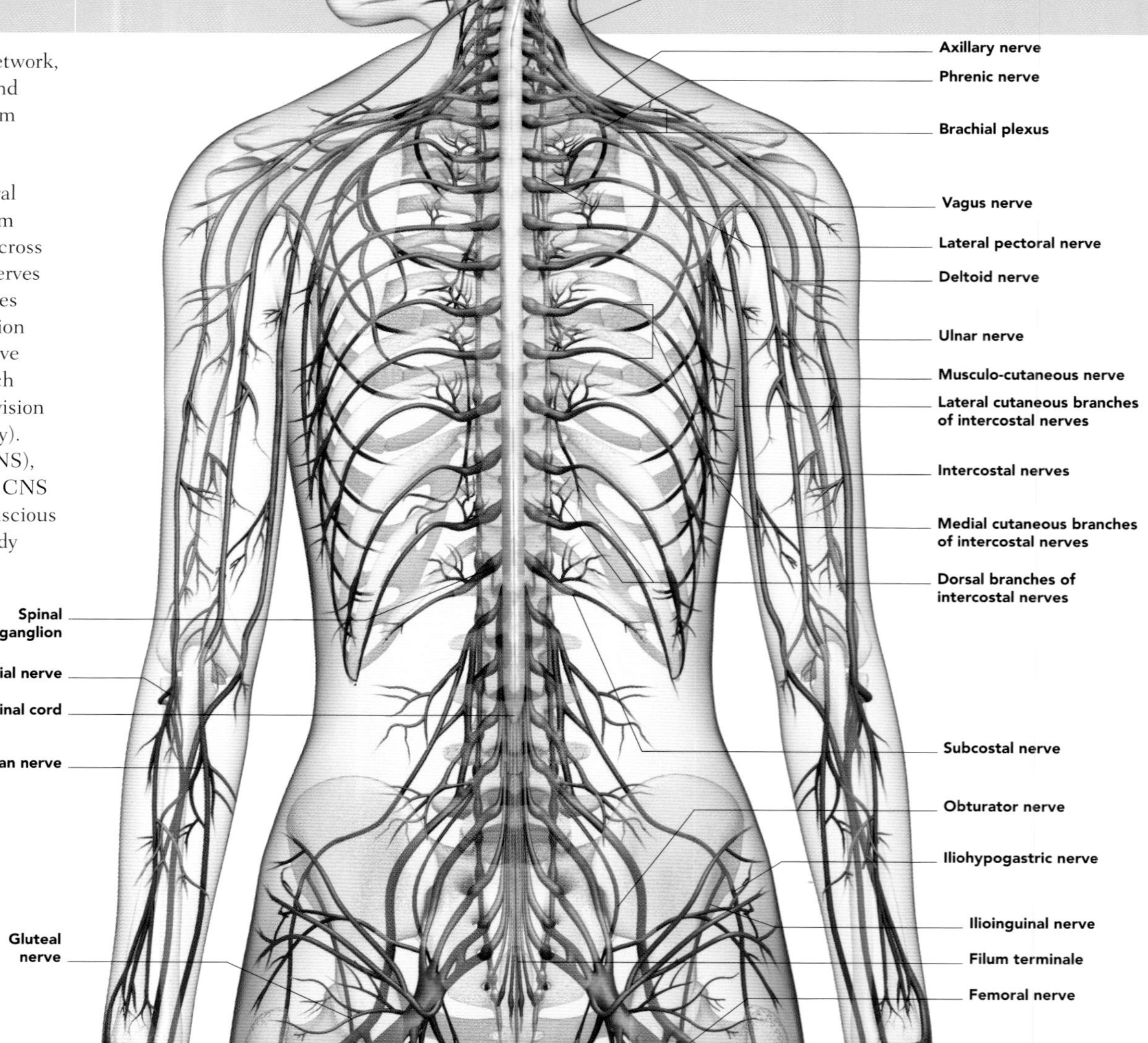

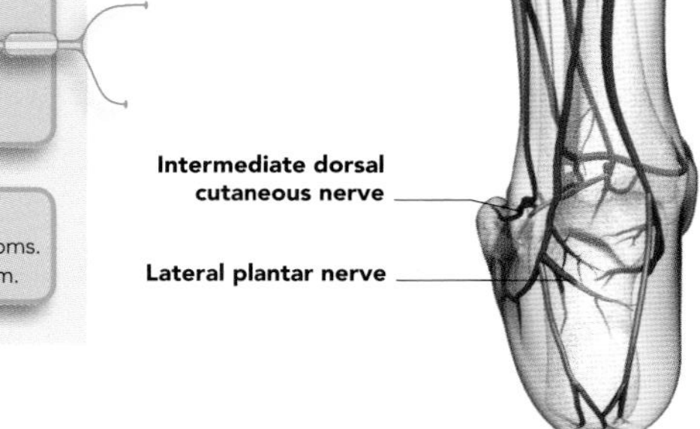

THE BRAIN AND THE BODY

Increasingly, the interaction between brain and body is being understood in much finer detail. The organisation of the nervous system (and for that matter all the other systems of the body, such as the cardiovascular and endocrine systems) can be considered at various different functional levels, from the entire system down to individual cells, the basic unit of all living things. The chart below shows six of these levels and their features. While it is possible to view organs with the naked eye, tissues, networks, cells, and molecules all have to be viewed with the aid of a microscope.

SYSTEM – THE CENTRAL NERVOUS SYSTEM
The brain and the spinal cord together make up the CNS.

ORGAN – THE BRAIN
The central organ of the CNS, the brain is a complex, integrated collection of tissues that controls the functions of the human body.

TISSUES – NUCLEI
These are groups of neurons (nuclei) that work together to perform specialized functions.

NETWORKS
Neural networks consist of thousands of neurons and the connections between them (synapses).

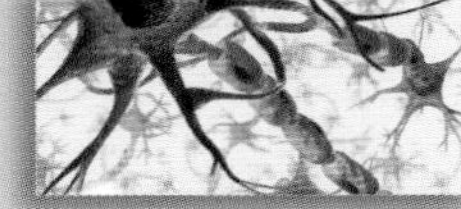

CELLS – NEURONS
Neurons are the basic units of the CNS. They transmit electrical signals, process the data, and communicate with each other via synapses.

MOLECULES
These are the smallest recognized unit, comprising two or more atoms. All the body's cells contain working parts made of millions of them.

THE BRAIN AND THE NERVOUS SYSTEM

THE BRAIN SITS AT THE TOP OF THE BODY, DIRECTING AND CO-ORDINATING ALL ACTION AND ACTIVITY THROUGHOUT ITS ENTIRETY. IT DOES SO VIA THE SPINAL CORD AND THE NERVES THAT STEM FROM IT AT VARIOUS POINTS ALONG ITS LENGTH, BRANCHING OUT INTO A NETWORK THAT SPANS THE WHOLE BODY.

cortex
brainstem

EXTENT OF THE SPINAL CORD
The spinal cord extends from the brainstem down to the first lumbar vertebra, where it forms a filament, known as the filum terminale, which extends to the coccyx.

spinal cord
filum terminale
coccyx
lumbar region

THE SPINAL CORD

The spinal cord carries information to and from the brain and all parts of the body except the head, which is served by the cranial nerves. The signals that travel along the spinal cord are known as nerve impulses. The cord itself comprises a bundle of nerve fibres, which are the long projections of nerve cells. They extend from the base of the brain to the lower region of the spine. The cord is roughly the width of a pencil, tapering at its base to a narrow bunch of fibres. Data from the sensory organs in different parts of the body is collected via the spinal nerves and transmitted along the spinal cord to the brain. The spinal cord also sends motor information, such as movement commands, from the brain out to the body, which is again transmitted via the spinal nerve network.

SPINAL CORD ANATOMY
The core of the spinal cord is grey matter, which is composed of nerve cells (neurons). The outer layer of white matter insulates the long fibres (axons) that extend from the nerve cells.

Nerve fibres
Bundles of nerve fibres carry signals to and from spinal cord and specific areas of the brain

White matter

Grey matter

Central canal
Filled with cerebrospinal fluid, which provides nourishment

Spinal nerve
Carries both sensory and motor information between brain and body

Anterior fissure
Deep groove along front of spinal cord

Motor nerve rootlet
Individual nerve fibre that emerges from front of spinal cord; carries signals to muscles

Sensory root ganglion
Cluster of nerve cell bodies on each spinal nerve; partially processes incoming signals

Sensory nerve root
Nerve splits into rootlets that enter spinal cord at rear, carrying incoming signals about touch sensations to brain

Subarachnoid space

Pia mater

Arachnoid

Dura mater

Meninges
Three layers of connective tissues that protect spinal cord; cerebrospinal fluid fills space under middle layer

FRONT OF BODY

Spinal nerve root
Spinal nerve
Spinal cord
Vertebra
REAR OF BODY

HOW SPINAL NERVES ATTACH
There are gaps in the vertebrae of the backbone through which spinal nerves enter the spinal cord. The nerves divide into spinal nerve roots, each made up of tiny rootlets that enter the back and front parts of the cord.

SPINAL NERVES

There are 31 pairs of spinal nerves. These branch out from the spinal cord, dividing and subdividing to form a network connecting the spinal cord to every part of the body. The spinal nerves carry information from receptors around the body to the spinal cord. From here the information passes to the brain for processing. Spinal nerves also transmit motor information from the brain to the body's muscles and glands, so the brain's instructions can be carried out swiftly.

SPINAL REGIONS
Each of the 31 pairs of nerves belong to one of four spinal regions – cervical, thoracic, lumbar, or sacral.

Cervical region
Eight pairs of cervical nerves serve chest, head, neck, shoulders, arms, and hands

Thoracic region
12 pairs of thoracic nerves connect to back and abdominal muscles and intercostal muscles

Lumbar region
Five pairs of lumbar nerves form network to serve lower abdomen, thighs, and legs

Sacral region
Six pairs of sacral nerves connect to legs, feet, and anal and genital areas

DERMATOMES

Spinal nerves contain a special fibre, the dorsal root, that sends sensory information from the skin to the brain. Each pair of spinal nerves (bar one pair) serves a specific area of the body, or dermatome. Nerve fibres in contact with skin receptors join up along the network of fibres in one dermatome to form the relevant dorsal root, which enters the spinal cord and conveys sensory impulses from that dermatome to the brain.

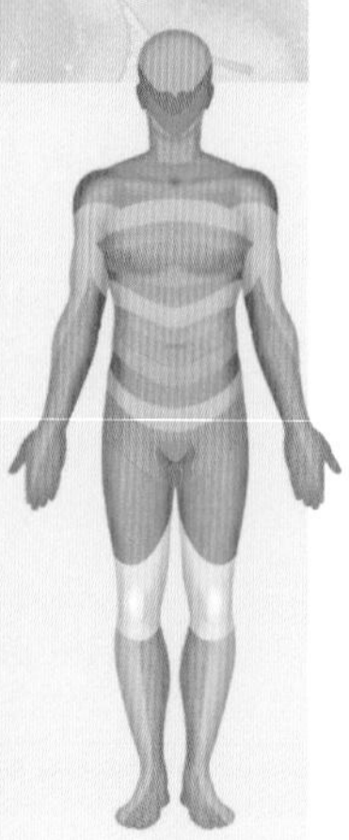

MAP OF DERMATOMES
This map shows the 30 dermatomes of the body. Each zone is served by a corresponding pair of spinal nerves.

CRANIAL NERVES

There are 12 pairs of cranial nerves that are linked directly to the brain, without entering the spinal cord. They allow sensory information to pass from the organs of the head, such as the eyes and ears, to the brain and also convey motor information from the brain to these organs – for example, directions such as moving the mouth and lips in speech. The cranial nerves are named after the body part they serve, such as the optic nerve for the eyes, and are also assigned Roman numerals, following anatomical convention.

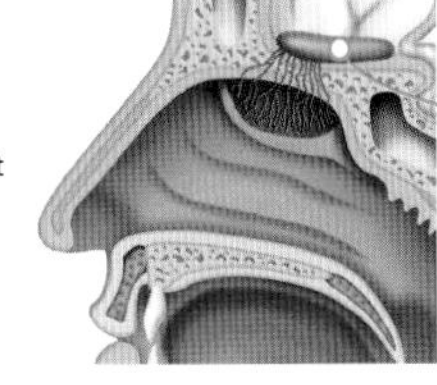

Olfactory nerve (I, sensory)
Smell molecules in nasal cavity trigger nerve impulses that pass along this nerve to olfactory bulb, then on to limbic areas (see pp.64–65) of brain

Optic nerve (II, sensory)
Visual information from retina is conveyed to brain by optic nerve at back of eye; optic nerves from both eyes meet at point known as optic chiasm, then signals from both visual fields are sent to opposite sides of brain

Oculomotor, trochlear, and abducens nerves (III, IV, VI, motor)
Three nerves regulating voluntary movements of eye muscles, allowing movement of eyeball and eyelids; oculomotor nerve also allows for pupil constriction

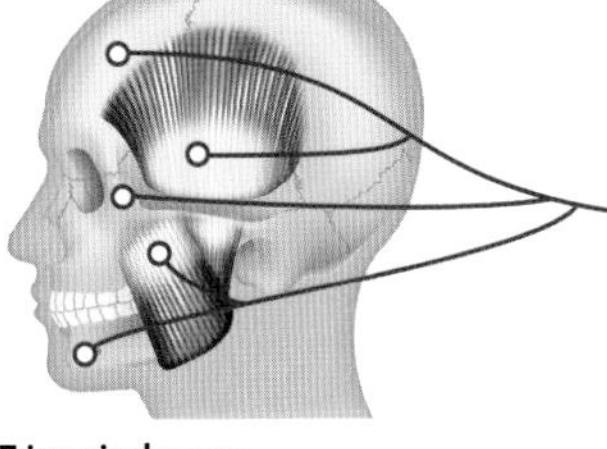

Trigeminal nerve (V, two sensory and one mixed branch)
Ophthalmic and maxillary branches of this nerve convey signals from eyes, teeth, and face, and other sensory fibres carry impulses from lower jaw; motor fibres control muscles involved with chewing

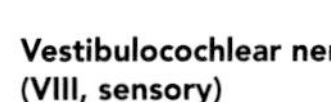

Vestibulocochlear nerve (VIII, sensory)
Vestibular branch of this nerve collects information from inner ear about head orientation and balance; cochlear branch is concerned with sound and hearing signals from ear

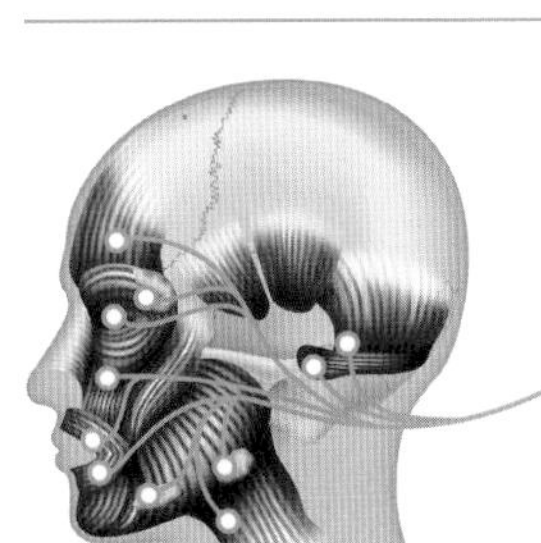

Facial nerve (VII, mixed)
Sensory fibres collect information from taste buds at front two-thirds of tongue; motor fibres are predominantly responsible for muscle movements controlling facial expression and also function of salivary gland and lacrimal gland, which secretes tears and lubricates the surface of the eye and conjunctiva of the eyelid

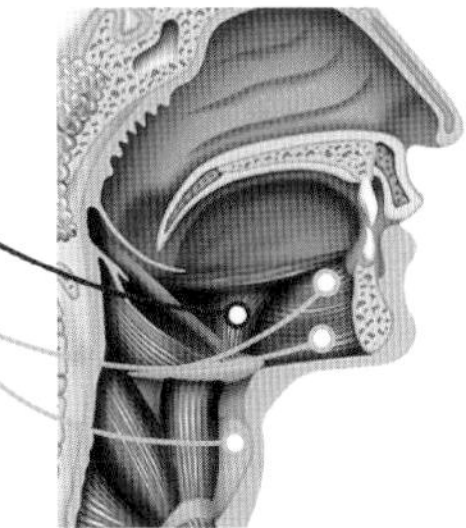

Glossopharyngeal and hypoglossal nerves (IX, XII, both mixed)
Motor fibres of these nerves control most of the muscles involved with tongue movement and swallowing; sensory fibres convey information on taste, touch, and temperature from tongue and pharynx and can trigger gag reflex if stimulated

CRANIAL NERVE CONNECTIONS

The cranial nerves I and II connect to the cerebrum, while cranial nerves III to XII connect to the brainstem. The fibres of sensory cranial nerves each project from a cell body that is located outside the brain itself, in sensory ganglia or elsewhere along the trunks of sensory nerves.

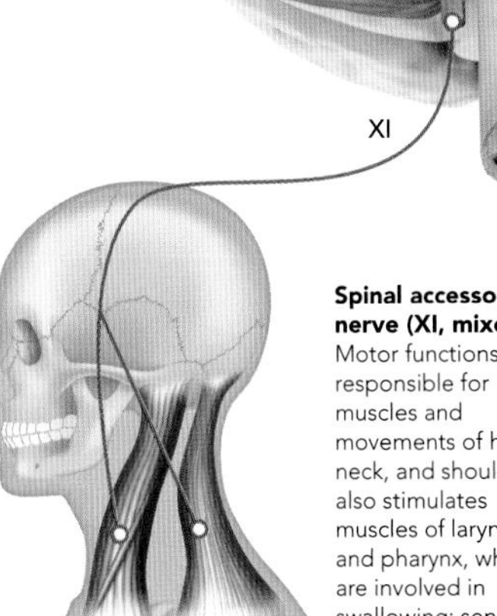

Spinal accessory nerve (XI, mixed)
Motor functions responsible for muscles and movements of head, neck, and shoulders; also stimulates muscles of larynx and pharynx, which are involved in swallowing; sensory functions unknown

Vagus nerve (X, mixed)
Longest and most branched of all cranial nerves, with autonomic, sensory, and motor fibres; serves lower part of head, throat, neck, chest, and abdomen, and plays role in many functions, including swallowing, breathing, heartbeat, and production of stomach acid

BRAIN SIZE, ENERGY USE, AND PROTECTION

THE BRAIN ACCOUNTS FOR AROUND 2 PER CENT OF TOTAL BODY WEIGHT, BUT CONSUMES A DISPROPORTIONATE AMOUNT OF FUEL TO SUPPORT ITS MANY ACTIVITIES. IT HAS SEVERAL FORMS OF PROTECTION – THE LAYERS OF MEMBRANE SURROUNDING IT, A BONY SKULL, AND FLUID PRODUCED IN ITS CHAMBERS (VENTRICLES) TO ABSORB THE IMPACT OF SHOCKS.

WEIGHT AND VOLUME

The average adult human brain weighs about 1.5kg (3 ¼lb). Its volume and shape are similar to those of an average-sized cauliflower, and the consistency of its tissues is similar to stiff jelly. The size of a person's brain bears little relation to their intelligence, and every brain, whatever its weight and volume, has roughly the same number of neurons and synapses. After the age of 20 or so, brain mass decreases by about 1g (1/32 oz) per year. New neurons are made throughout life, but not enough to replace those that die off with age. This is generally no cause for concern, as there are plenty of neurons left to carry out the brain's functions.

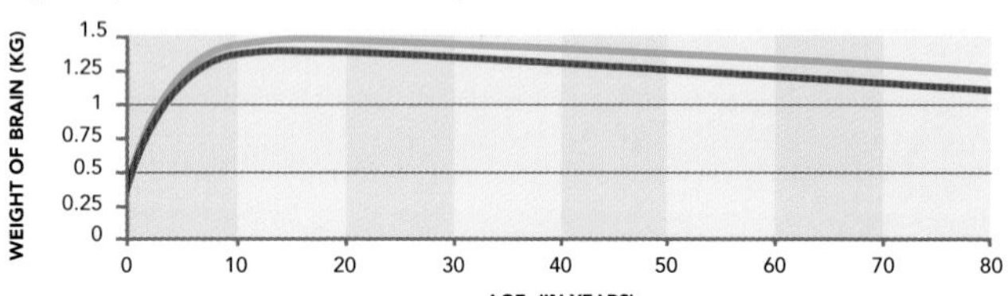

BRAIN WEIGHT
The brain's weight increases from birth and reaches its maximum during adolescence. As the body grows, neurons increase in size and form new connections. The male brain is consistently heavier than the female brain from birth.

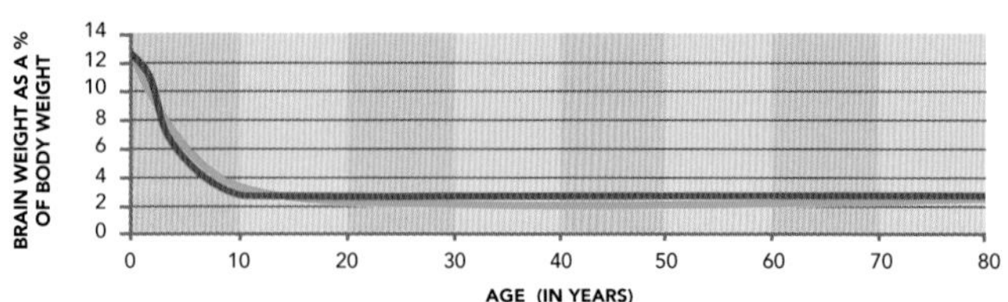

BRAIN WEIGHT AND BODY WEIGHT
This graph shows brain weight as a percentage of total body weight over the course of a lifetime. Proportionally, a baby's brain is around six times larger than an adult's. Despite being lighter than the male brain overall, the female brain after the age of 13 is actually heavier than the male brain as a proportion of the entire body's weight.

KEY
FEMALE
MALE

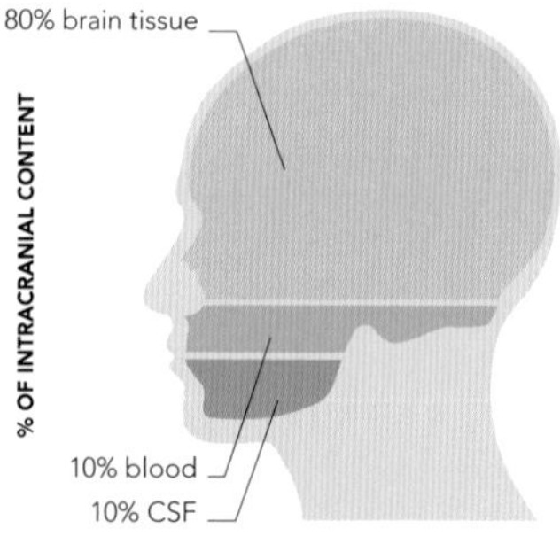

% OF INTRACRANIAL CONTENT
80% brain tissue
10% blood
10% CSF

INTRACRANIAL CONTENT
Brain tissue comprises grey and white matter, which consists of neurons and supporting glial cells respectively. A series of ventricles is filled with cerebrospinal fluid (CSF) and the brain is also richly supplied with blood vessels.

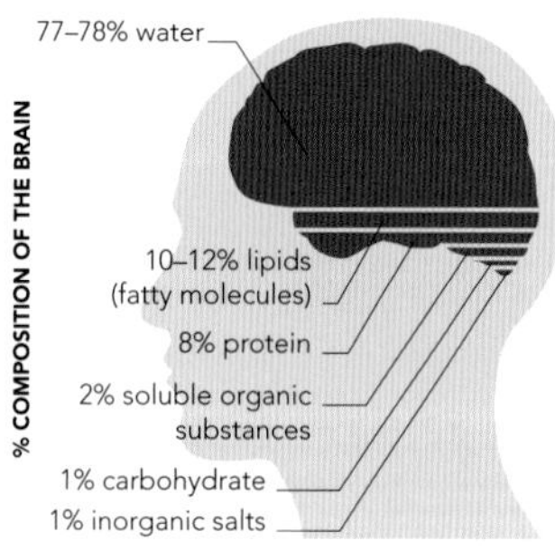

COMPOSITION OF THE BRAIN
The brain consists mainly of water, which occurs in the cytoplasm of neurons and glial cells, as well as being a major constituent of blood. The brain is also rich in lipids – fatty molecules that make up cell membranes.

LENGTH, WIDTH, AND HEIGHT

The brain is housed within the intracranial cavity, so measurements of the skull effectively relate to the size of the brain. The actual length, width, and height of an individual human brain can be measured using MRI scanning. There is considerable variation in the size of the adult human brain, but the average dimensions are given against the diagrams below. Bear in mind that, because of the numerous complex folds within the cerebrum, the brain has a much larger surface area than is apparent from its overall shape.

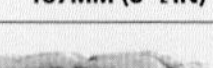

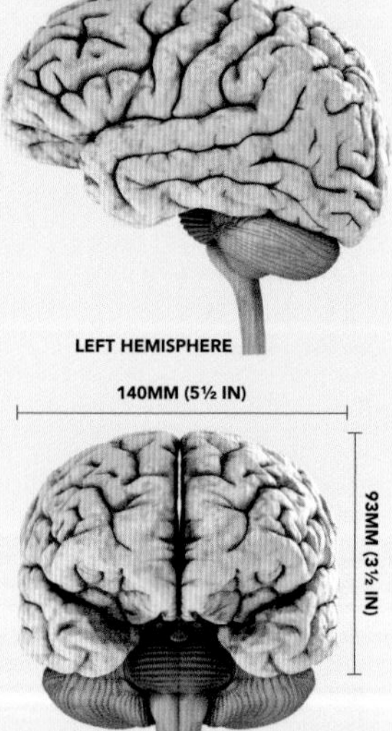

BRAIN VOLUME AND LIFESTYLE

A recent study linked alcohol consumption to brain shrinkage. Participants disclosed their drinking habits, and MRI scanning was used to measure each person's ratio of brain volume to skull size. It was found that abstainers had greater brain volumes than former drinkers, light drinkers, moderate drinkers, or heavy drinkers. On average, abstainers had 1.6 per cent greater brain volume than heavy drinkers. Interestingly, the effects were most marked among elderly women. In another study, participants between the ages of 60 and 79 took up either regular aerobic exercise or toning and stretching exercises for six months. MRI scans of each participant taken both before and after the six-month period showed an increase in the brain volumes of those practising aerobic exercise, suggesting that aerobic exercise can help to maintain the health of the brain in older adults.

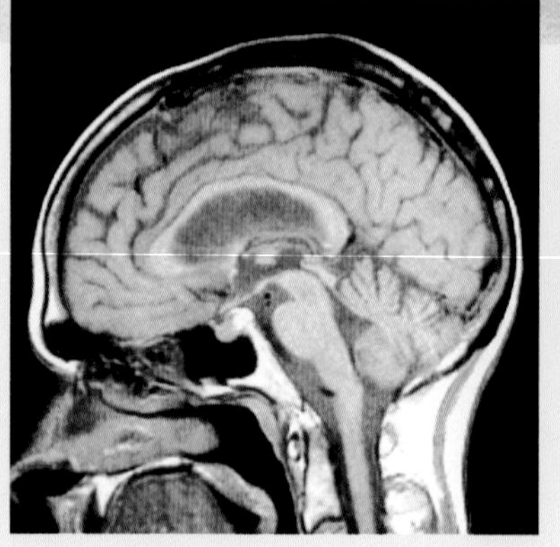

BRAIN OF A NORMAL MALE

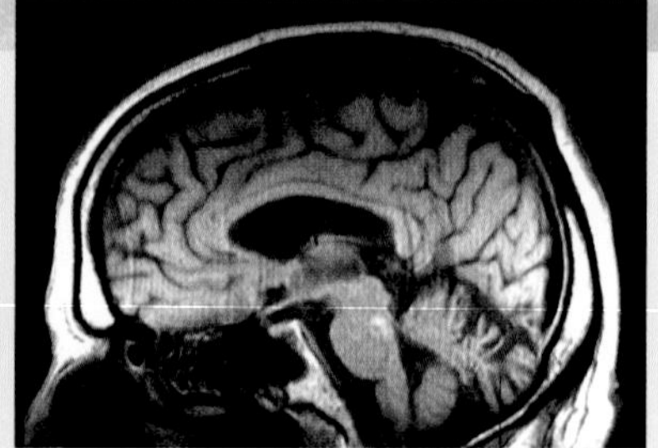

BRAIN OF AN ALCOHOLIC

cerebellar degeneration

ALCOHOLISM AND BRAIN ATROPHY
Alcoholism can lead to cerebellar degeneration as shown above. The low quality of the scan was due to the man's withdrawal symptoms, preventing him from sitting still.

OXYGEN AND GLUCOSE SUPPLY

Glucose is the brain's sole fuel, except under conditions of starvation, when it breaks down protein. The brain is by far the body's hungriest organ. Although it accounts for just 2 per cent of the body's weight, it requires a staggering 20 per cent of its total glucose supplies. This is obtained from dietary carbohydrate, which is transported to the brain via the bloodstream. It consumes roughly 120g (4oz) of glucose (about 420kcal) per day. Because the brain cannot store glucose, it must be readily available at all times via the blood supply. Without oxygen or glucose, the brain can last for only about 10 minutes before irreparable damage occurs. This is why prompt resuscitation is needed in cases of cardiac arrest.

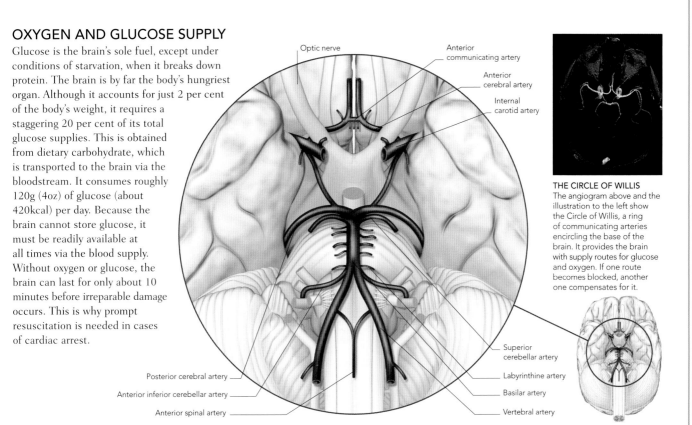

Optic nerve
Anterior communicating artery
Anterior cerebral artery
Internal carotid artery
Superior cerebellar artery
Labyrinthine artery
Basilar artery
Vertebral artery
Posterior cerebral artery
Anterior inferior cerebellar artery
Anterior spinal artery

THE CIRCLE OF WILLIS
The angiogram above and the illustration to the left show the Circle of Willis, a ring of communicating arteries encircling the base of the brain. It provides the brain with supply routes for glucose and oxygen. If one route becomes blocked, another one compensates for it.

PROTECTING THE BRAIN

The brain has several defence mechanisms to protect it from damage. The bony skull acts as a box, containing the brain and buffering it against blows. The meninges are three layers of membranes that line the skull, enclosing the brain and providing extra layers of protection between the skull and the brain. Cerebrospinal fluid circulates within the brain, nourishing brain tissue and working as a shock absorber to reduce the impact of knocks.

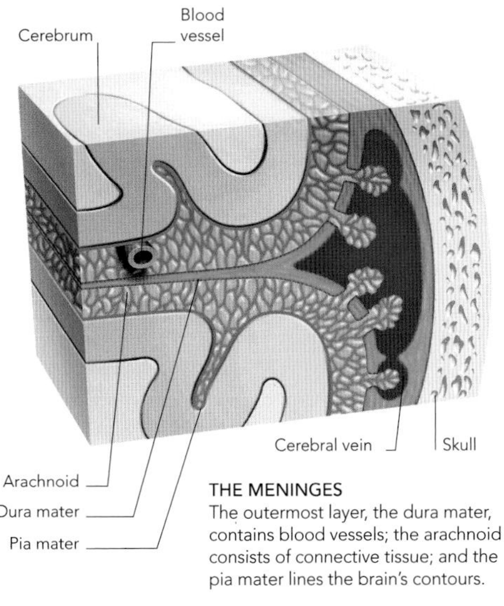

THE MENINGES
The outermost layer, the dura mater, contains blood vessels; the arachnoid consists of connective tissue; and the pia mater lines the brain's contours.

CEREBROSPINAL FLUID FLOW

Brain tissue floats in cerebrospinal fluid (CSF) within the skull. CSF absorbs shocks from blows to the brain. It is produced in a series of connected chambers within the brain known as the ventricles, and is renewed four to five times per day. It contains proteins and glucose to nourish brain cells, as well as white blood cells to protect against infection. It moves through the the ventricles, propelled by the pulsation of the cerebral arteries.

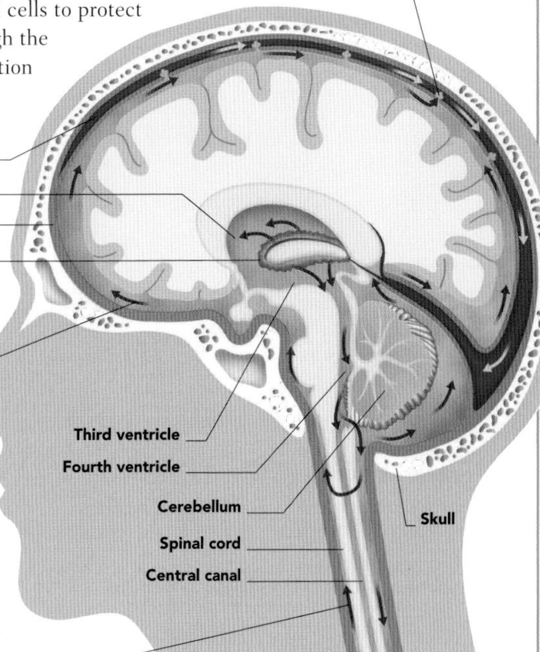

1 Site of fluid production (choroid plexus)
CSF is produced in the clusters of thin-walled capillaries (the choroid plexus) that line the walls of the ventricles.

2 Direction of flow
CSF flows from the lateral ventricles into the third and fourth ventricles. It then continues up the back of the brain, down around the spinal cord, and to the front of the brain, as indicated by the arrows.

3 Circulation around spinal cord
Helped by vertebral movement, fluid travels downwards along the back of the spinal cord, into the central canal, and upwards along the front of the cord.

4 Site of reabsorption (arachnoid granulations)
After travelling around the brain, the fluid is finally reabsorbed into the bloodstream through tiny arachnoid granulations (projections from the arachnoid layer of the meninges into the sagittal sinus).

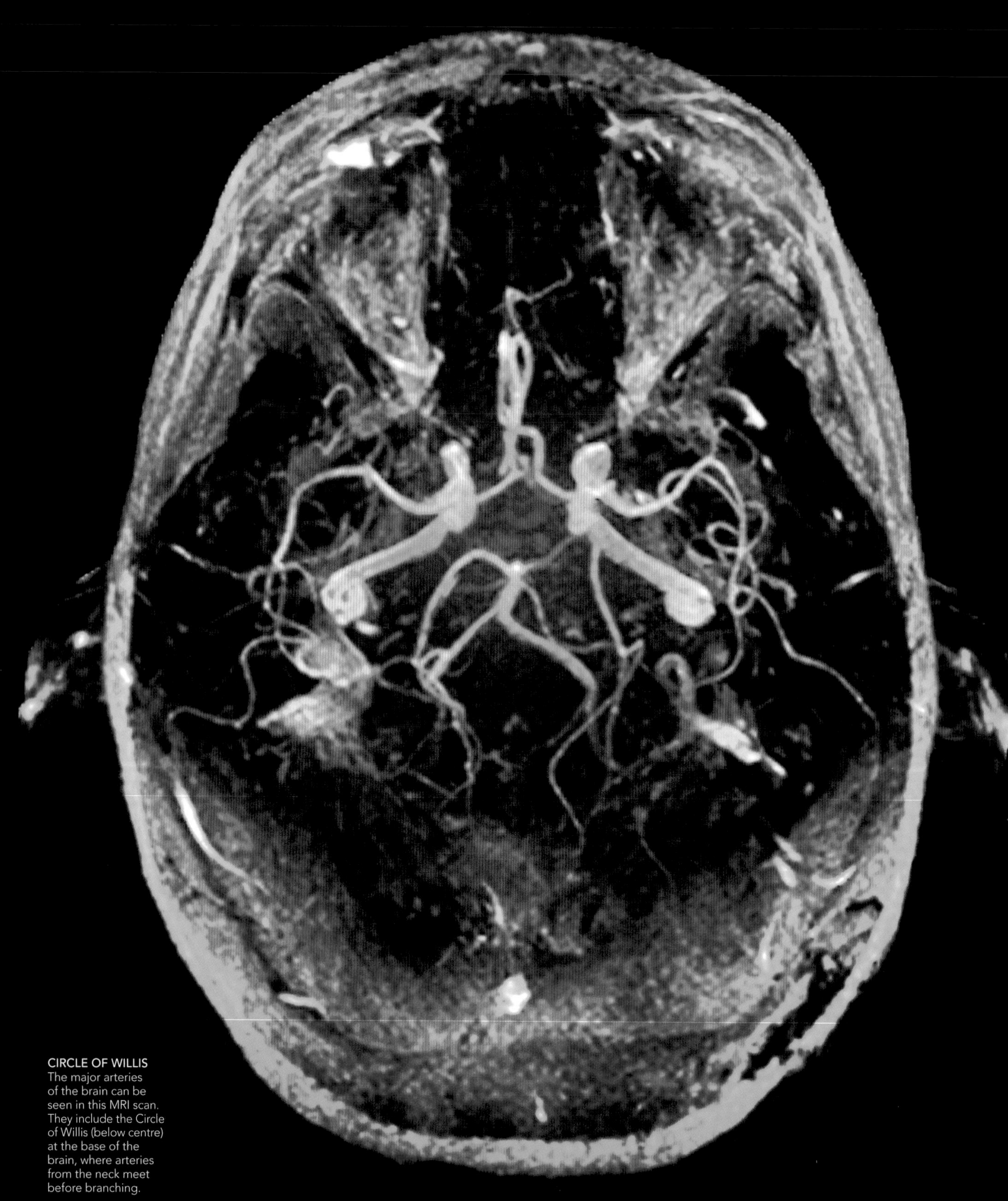

CIRCLE OF WILLIS
The major arteries of the brain can be seen in this MRI scan. They include the Circle of Willis (below centre) at the base of the brain, where arteries from the neck meet before branching.

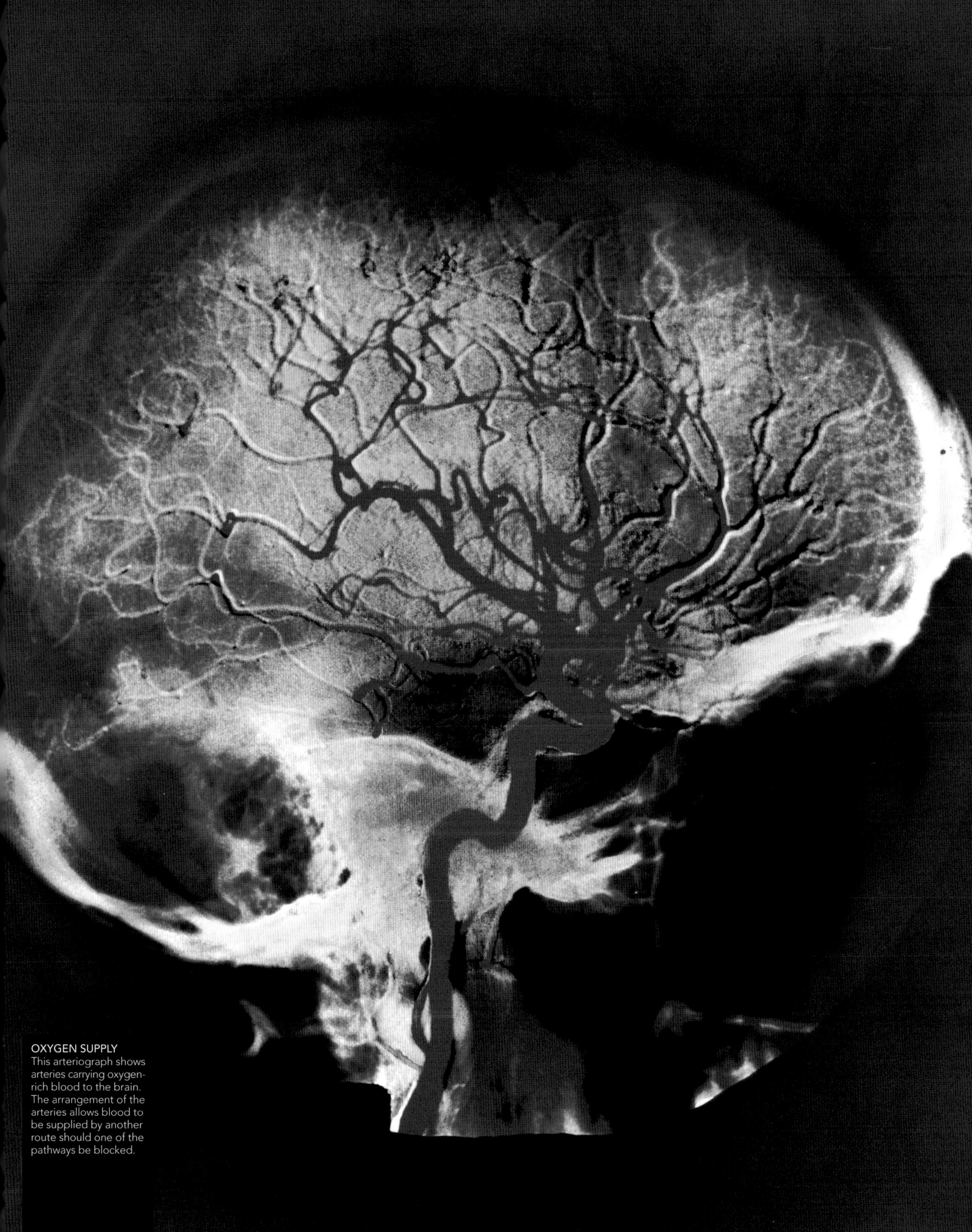

OXYGEN SUPPLY
This arteriograph shows arteries carrying oxygen-rich blood to the brain. The arrangement of the arteries allows blood to be supplied by another route should one of the pathways be blocked.

EVOLUTION

BRAINS EVOLVED TO ENABLE ANIMALS TO RESPOND TO ENVIRONMENTAL CHANGES. THE HUMAN BRAIN HAS EVOLVED TO ITS PRESENT COMPLEXITY THROUGH SEVERAL STAGES, MANY OF WHICH ARE COMMON TO ALL ANIMALS. ITS ORIGINS CAN BE SEEN IN THE BRAINS OF OTHER SPECIES, IN WHICH MORE PRIMITIVE STRUCTURES REMAIN.

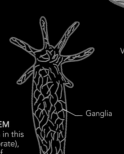

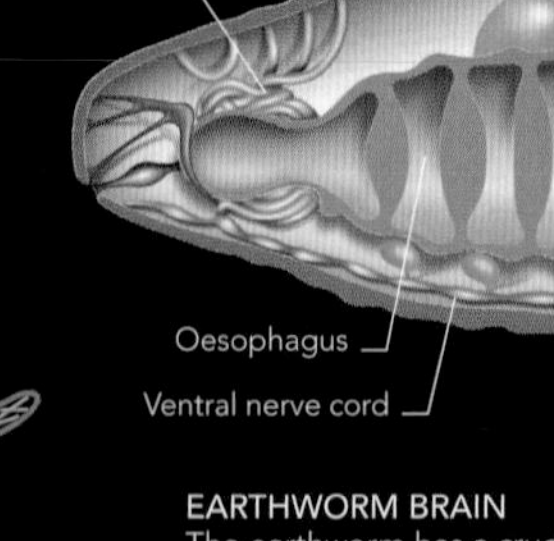

EVOLUTION OF THE INVERTEBRATE BRAIN

All animals have to respond to changes in their internal and external environment in order to survive. To do this, they have evolved cells that are sensitive to stimuli such as light and vibrations. The sensory cells are, in turn, connected to other cells that can move the organism or change its state in response to the stimulus. This system of interconnected nervous tissue is a crude form of brain. In invertebrates, such as worms, the nervous system is distributed throughout the creature's body, as a loose network of reactive fibres. Some of these networks contain small masses of nerves, known as ganglia. These are the forerunners of the structures that, in some species, have become the central nervous system or brain.

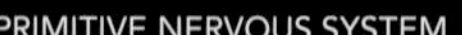

PRIMITIVE NERVOUS SYSTEM
The simplest system, as seen in this hydra (a tiny aquatic invertebrate), consists of a loose network of sensory cells with clumps of interconnected cells called ganglia.

EARTHWORM BRAIN
The earthworm has a crude brain, the cerebral ganglion, which is connected to a cord of nervous tissue (the ventral nerve cord) that runs the length of its body. Nerve fibres from the cord extend into each segment, so muscle contraction along the body can be co-ordinated to produce movement in response to stimuli.

EVOLUTION OF THE VERTEBRATE BRAIN

Through the course of evolution, the brain has undergone considerable changes. Compared to the primitive nervous systems of invertebrates, the brain of vertebrates is a well-developed, highly interconnected organ. The central nervous system is connected to the rest of the body via a peripheral nervous system that includes the fibres running to and from the sensory organs. The basic vertebrate brain – also sometimes referred to as the "reptilian brain" – corresponds to the cluster of nuclei that lies just above the brainstem in humans. They include the modules that produce arousal, sensation, and reaction to stimuli. It is unlikely, however, that these nuclei alone are sufficient to produce consciousness. This basic vertebrate brain does not include more advanced features, such as the limbic system or cerebral cortex, which exist only in the brains of mammals.

KEY TO VERTEBRATE BRAIN AREAS

- Cerebellum
- Optic lobe
- Cerebrum
- Pituitary gland
- Medulla
- Olfactory bulb

FISH
A fish's cerebrum receives sensory signals from the sense organs and combines them with information from the internal organs and nerves to guide action. Fish have a large cerebellum in order to co-ordinate movement and gauge pressure.

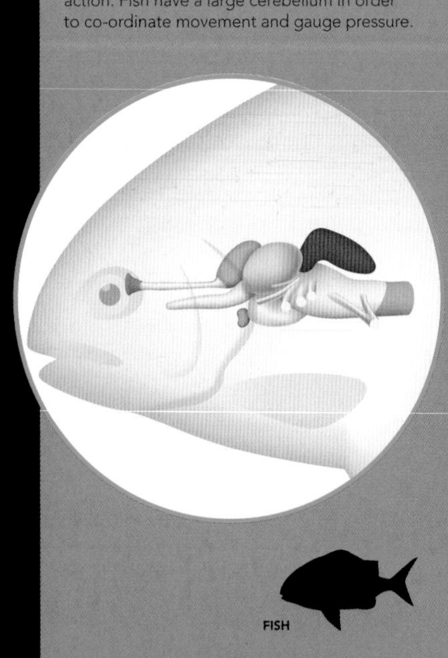

AMPHIBIANS
The amphibian brain resembles the fish brain except that the cerebrum is roofed over with nervous tissue. The main function of this region is to perceive smell, as reflected by the large olfactory bulb. The forebrain is much larger than the cerebellum.

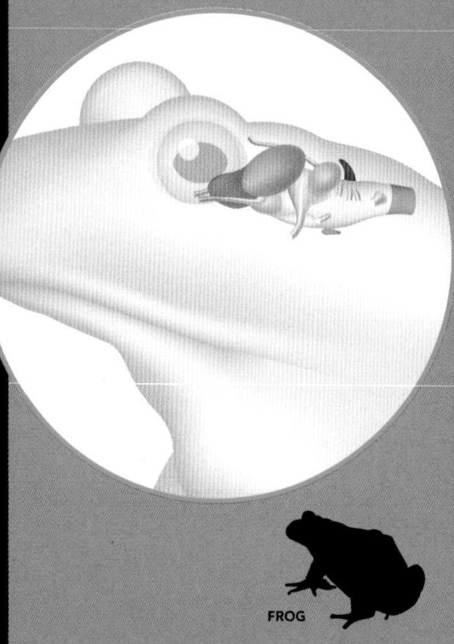

REPTILES
Modern reptiles show greater development in the basal parts of the forebrain, and the cerebrum is much larger than the optic lobe. The olfactory bulb is large in comparison with the other structures of the brain and is well developed.

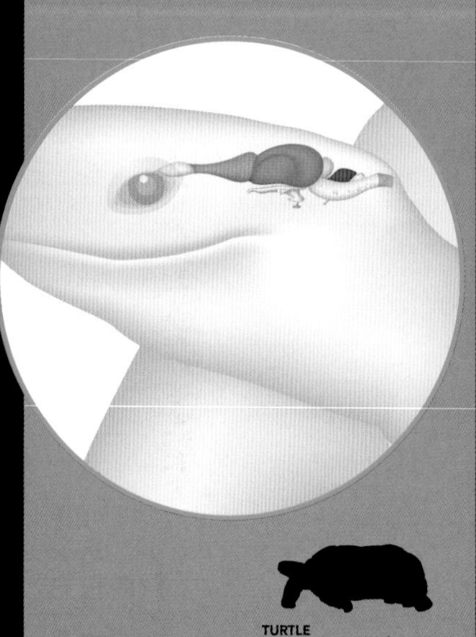

MAMMAL BRAINS

The mammalian brain comprises a cluster of structures that evolved on top of the basic vertebrate brain, known as the limbic system, and a wrinkled covering called the cortex, which interconnects with the limbic structures beneath. The limbic system is the part of the brain that produces emotions. These are responses to stimuli that go beyond the basic "grab" or "avoid" reactions in the vertebrate brain, and produce subtle and complex actions that are not always predictable. The limbic system also contains structures that encode experiences as memories, to be recalled for use in guiding future actions. The emotional and memory faculties greatly increase the range and complexity of behaviour that a mammal displays, because it is not governed purely by instinct.

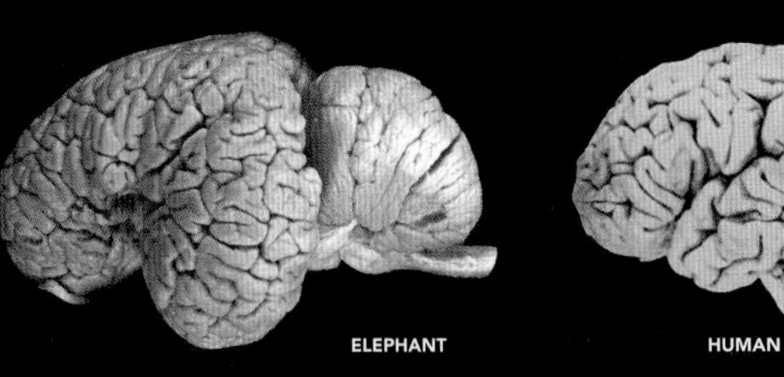

ELEPHANT

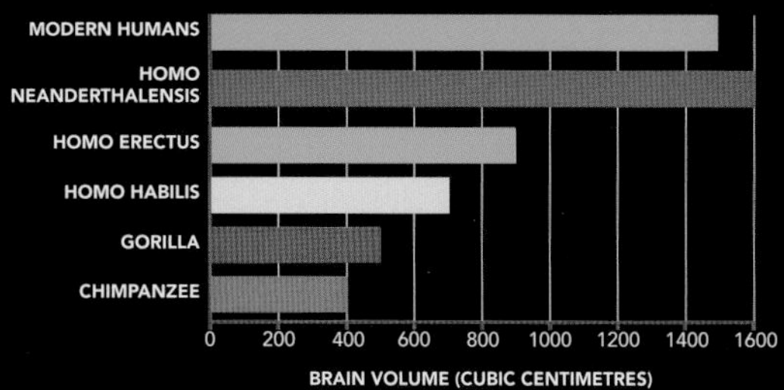

HUMAN

BRAIN SIZE AND SHAPE

One striking aspect of mammalian brain evolution is the development of the cortex. This outer layer has evolved to serve the particular needs of each species, and therefore varies dramatically between one animal and another. Compared to other mammals, animals such as humans, elephants, and dolphins have a disproportionately large cortex.

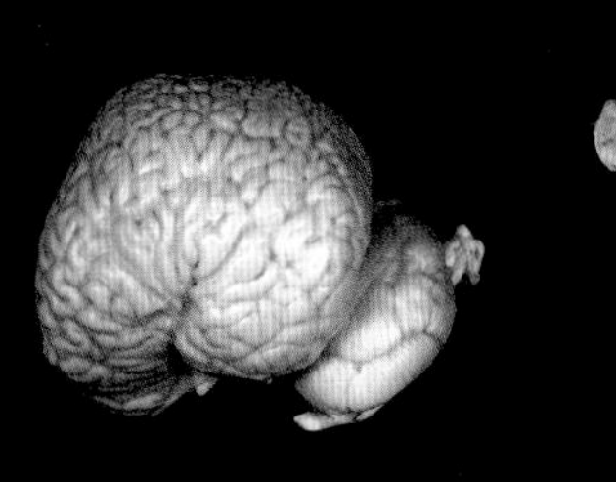

DOLPHIN

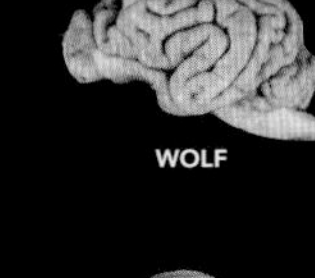

WOLF

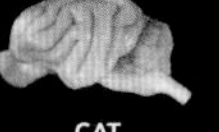

CAT

HOMINID BRAINS

The brains of hominids (modern humans and their ancestors) underwent a surge of evolutionary changes that left them, in some ways, distinctly different even from their near relatives, such as chimpanzees and gorillas. The main distinction between human and other mammalian brains is the size and density of the cortex, and particularly of the frontal lobe, which is responsible for complex thought, conscious judgement, and self-reflection. No one knows why the human brain evolved as it did – it may have been due to some change in diet forced by the environment, or the product of living in groups (see p.138) that depended on close interdependence for survival.

MODERN HUMANS
HOMO NEANDERTHALENSIS
HOMO ERECTUS
HOMO HABILIS
GORILLA
CHIMPANZEE
0 200 400 600 800 1000 1200 1400 1600
BRAIN VOLUME (CUBIC CENTIMETRES)

DOES SIZE MATTER?

The growth of the human brain over the course of evolution is thought to be the reason why we are so dominant. However, size alone is not the only factor that matters for intelligence or survival – the way brains are wired up may be more important. Neanderthals had bigger brains than humans, but were less innovative and were finally superseded by other hominids.

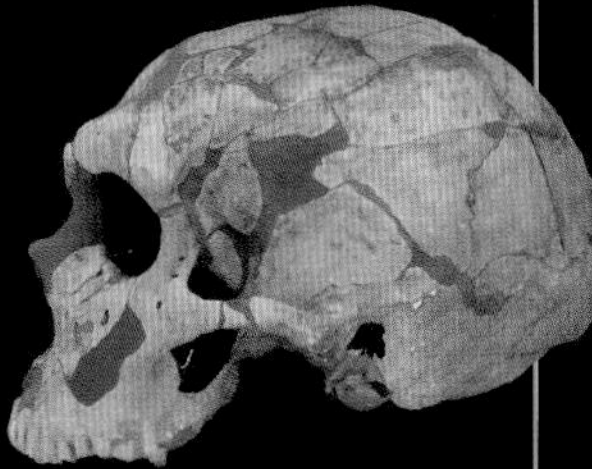

NEANDERTHAL SKULL

BIRDS

Birds' brains are similar to that of reptiles except that the cerebellum is highly developed to control balance and position in flight. Despite the size of the olfactory bulb, most birds have a poor sense of smell, with some exceptions, such as the kiwi.

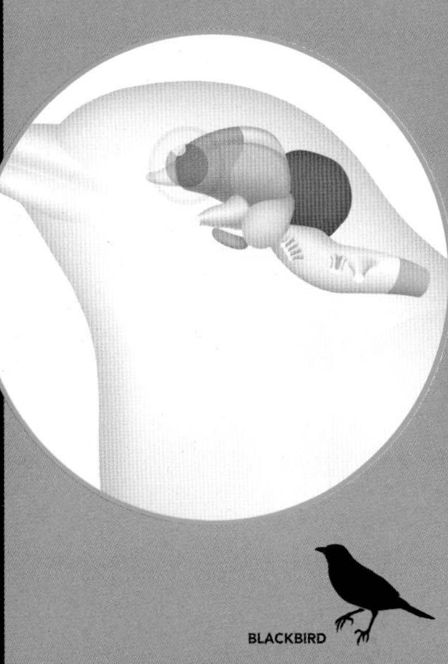

BLACKBIRD

MAMMALS

In mammals, the cerebellum is relatively small compared to the forebrain. The cerebrum is covered in wrinkled cortex; these wrinkles allow a greater volume of cortex to fit into the skull, compared to the smooth surface of the reptilian brain.

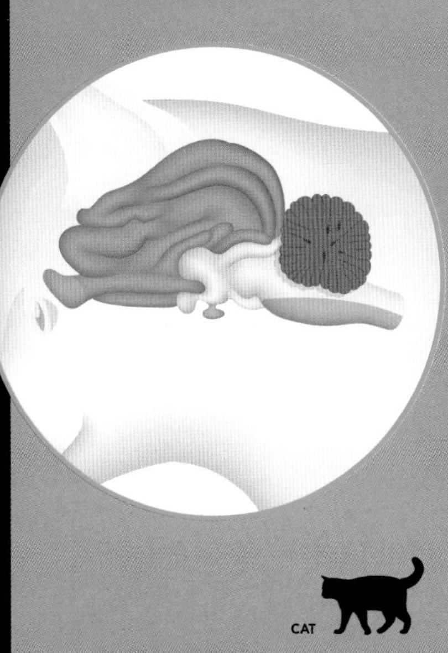

CAT

MAN

The human brain is completely dominated by the cerebrum, and the cortex is intricately folded to allow the maximum amount to be contained in the skull. The cerebellum remains large and active, however, to enable complex motor activity.

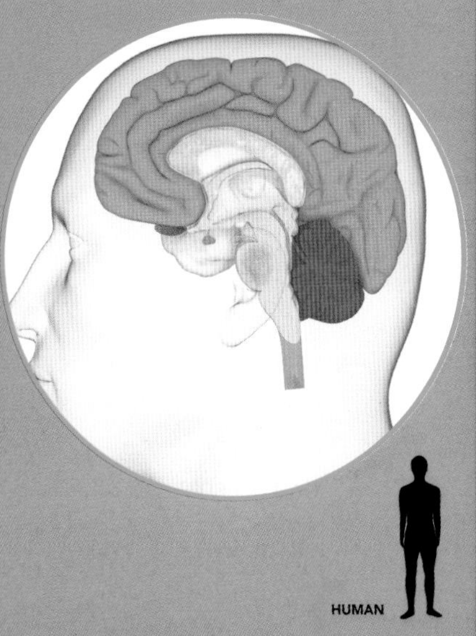

HUMAN

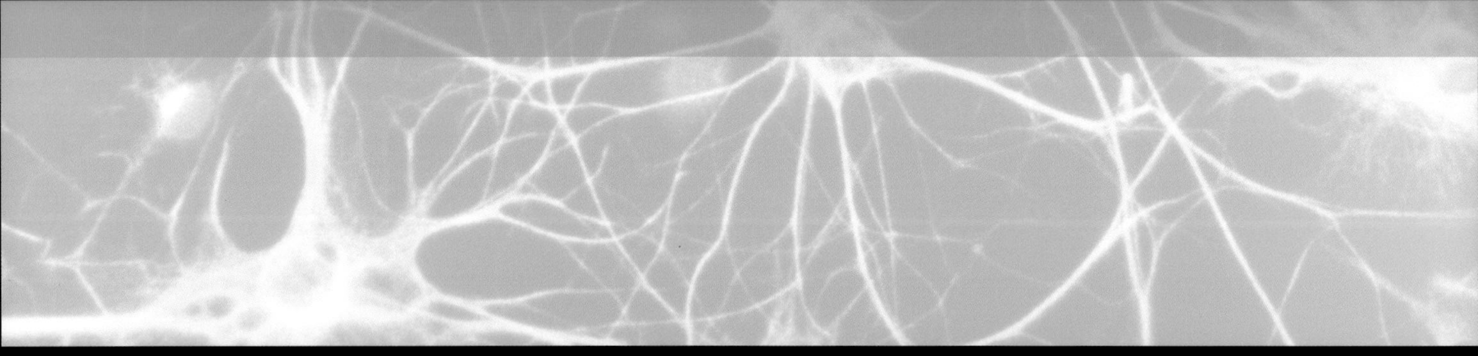

BRAIN ANATOMY IS HIDDEN, SECRET, AND MORE COMPLEX THAN ANY OTHER PART OF THE BODY. THE BASIC BUILDING BLOCK OF THE BRAIN IS THE CELL. SIGNALLING CELLS KNOWN AS NEURONS FORM LARGER STRUCTURES CALLED NUCLEI TO CARRY OUT PARTICULAR FUNCTIONS. THEY ALSO CLUSTER TOGETHER TO FORM THE THICK, LAMINATED SHEET OF GREY MATTER FORMING THE COVERING OF THE BRAIN CALLED THE CORTEX. A DEEP FISSURE IN ITS SURFACE DIVIDES THE BRAIN INTO TWO HALVES (THE HEMISPHERES), EACH WITH FIVE LOBES. THESE MAJOR DIVISIONS "SPECIALIZE" IN

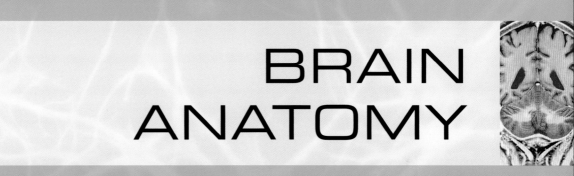

BRAIN ANATOMY

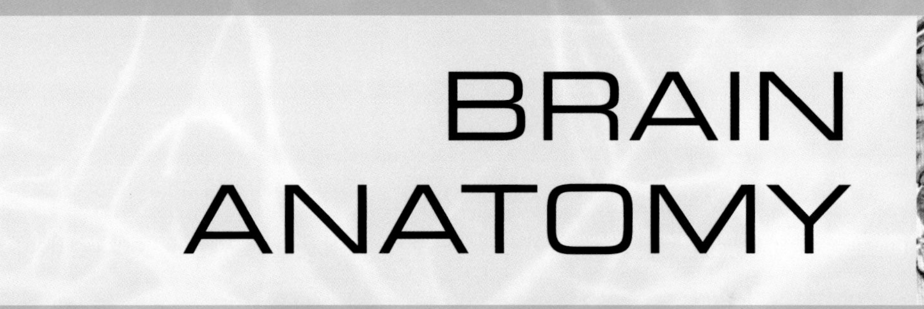

BRAIN STRUCTURES

THE BRAIN HAS A COMPLEX AND MANY-LAYERED ANATOMY. PEELING BACK THE DOMINANT CEREBRAL HEMISPHERES REVEALS A FURTHER SET OF STRUCTURES WITHIN. SOME ARE DISCRETE MASSES, SUCH AS THE CEREBELLUM AND THALAMUS, WHILE OTHERS ARE ZONES OF NERVE FIBRES OR NERVE CELLS WITHIN LARGER STRUCTURES, DISCERNIBLE ONLY BY MICROSCOPIC EXAMINATION.

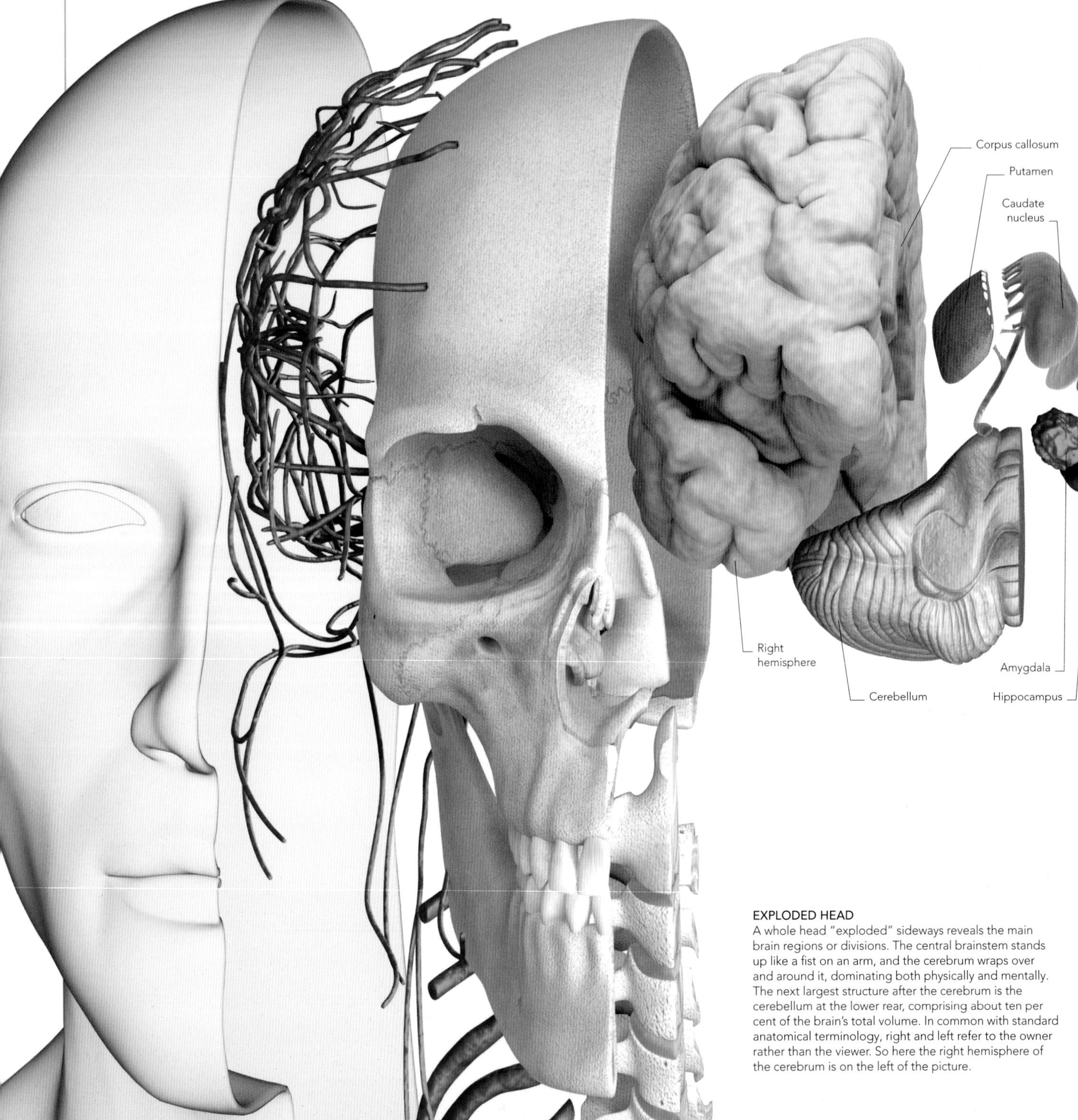

EXPLODED HEAD
A whole head "exploded" sideways reveals the main brain regions or divisions. The central brainstem stands up like a fist on an arm, and the cerebrum wraps over and around it, dominating both physically and mentally. The next largest structure after the cerebrum is the cerebellum at the lower rear, comprising about ten per cent of the brain's total volume. In common with standard anatomical terminology, right and left refer to the owner rather than the viewer. So here the right hemisphere of the cerebrum is on the left of the picture.

THE BRAIN HIERARCHY

The brain's major parts can be classified or categorized in several ways. In all of these systems, the dominant part is the cerebrum, the large pinky-grey wrinkled structure that forms more than three-quarters of the brain's total volume. The cerebrum is divided into left and right hemispheres, which are linked by a "bridge" of nerve fibres, the corpus callosum. The cerebrum, which includes the hippocampus and amygdala, is also known as the telencephalon. Together with the parts it wraps around – the thalamus, hypothalamus, and associated parts, collectively known as the diencephalon – it comprises the major brain "division" known as the forebrain (prosencephalon). Below the forebrain is the midbrain (mesencephalon), a small division that includes groups of nerve-cell bodies known as nuclei, such as the basal ganglia. Below the midbrain is the hindbrain (rhombencephalon), with the pons as its uppermost part, and beneath it the cerebellum and the medulla, which tapers to merge with the spinal cord.

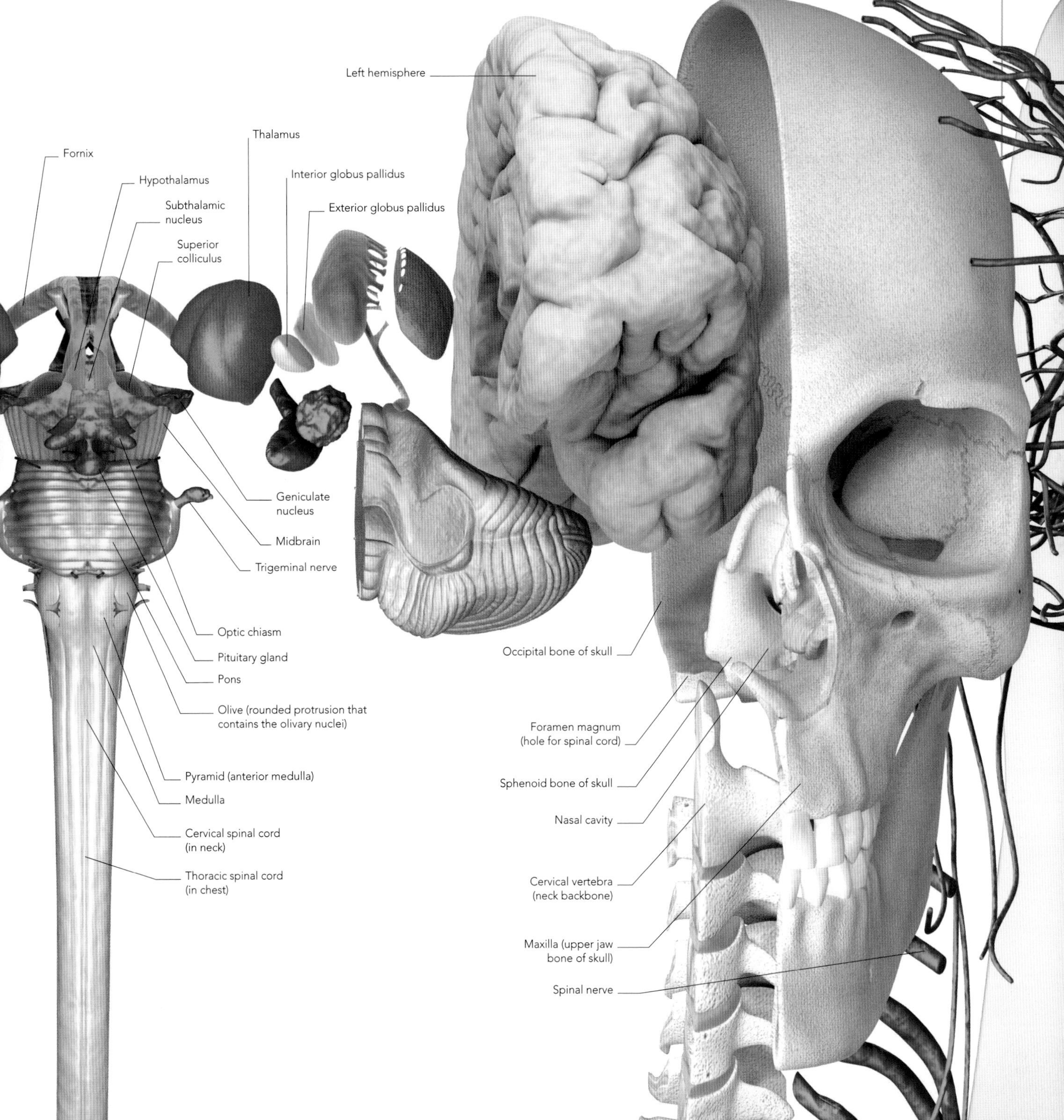

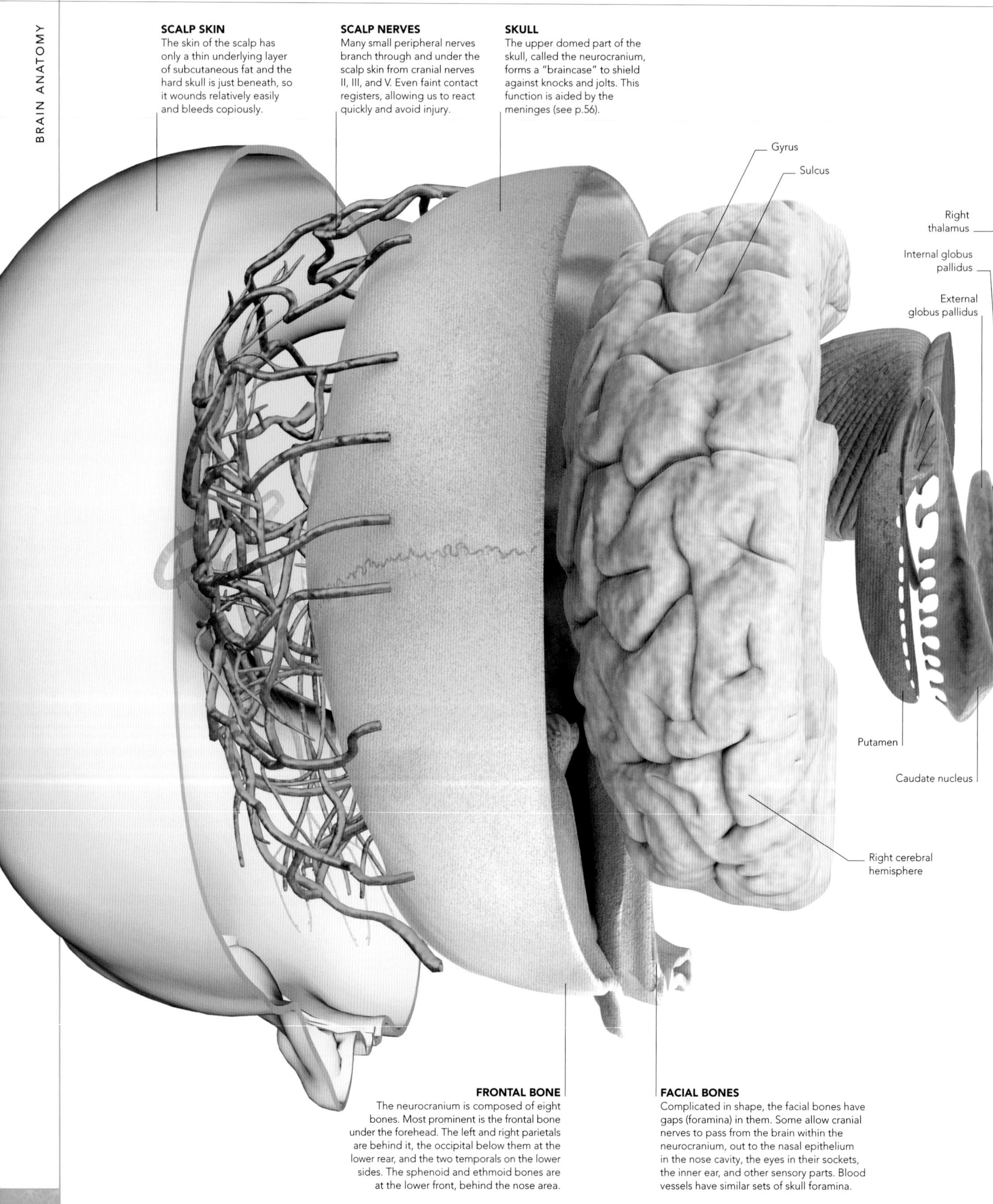

SCALP SKIN
The skin of the scalp has only a thin underlying layer of subcutaneous fat and the hard skull is just beneath, so it wounds relatively easily and bleeds copiously.

SCALP NERVES
Many small peripheral nerves branch through and under the scalp skin from cranial nerves II, III, and V. Even faint contact registers, allowing us to react quickly and avoid injury.

SKULL
The upper domed part of the skull, called the neurocranium, forms a "braincase" to shield against knocks and jolts. This function is aided by the meninges (see p.56).

FRONTAL BONE
The neurocranium is composed of eight bones. Most prominent is the frontal bone under the forehead. The left and right parietals are behind it, the occipital below them at the lower rear, and the two temporals on the lower sides. The sphenoid and ethmoid bones are at the lower front, behind the nose area.

FACIAL BONES
Complicated in shape, the facial bones have gaps (foramina) in them. Some allow cranial nerves to pass from the brain within the neurocranium, out to the nasal epithelium in the nose cavity, the eyes in their sockets, the inner ear, and other sensory parts. Blood vessels have similar sets of skull foramina.

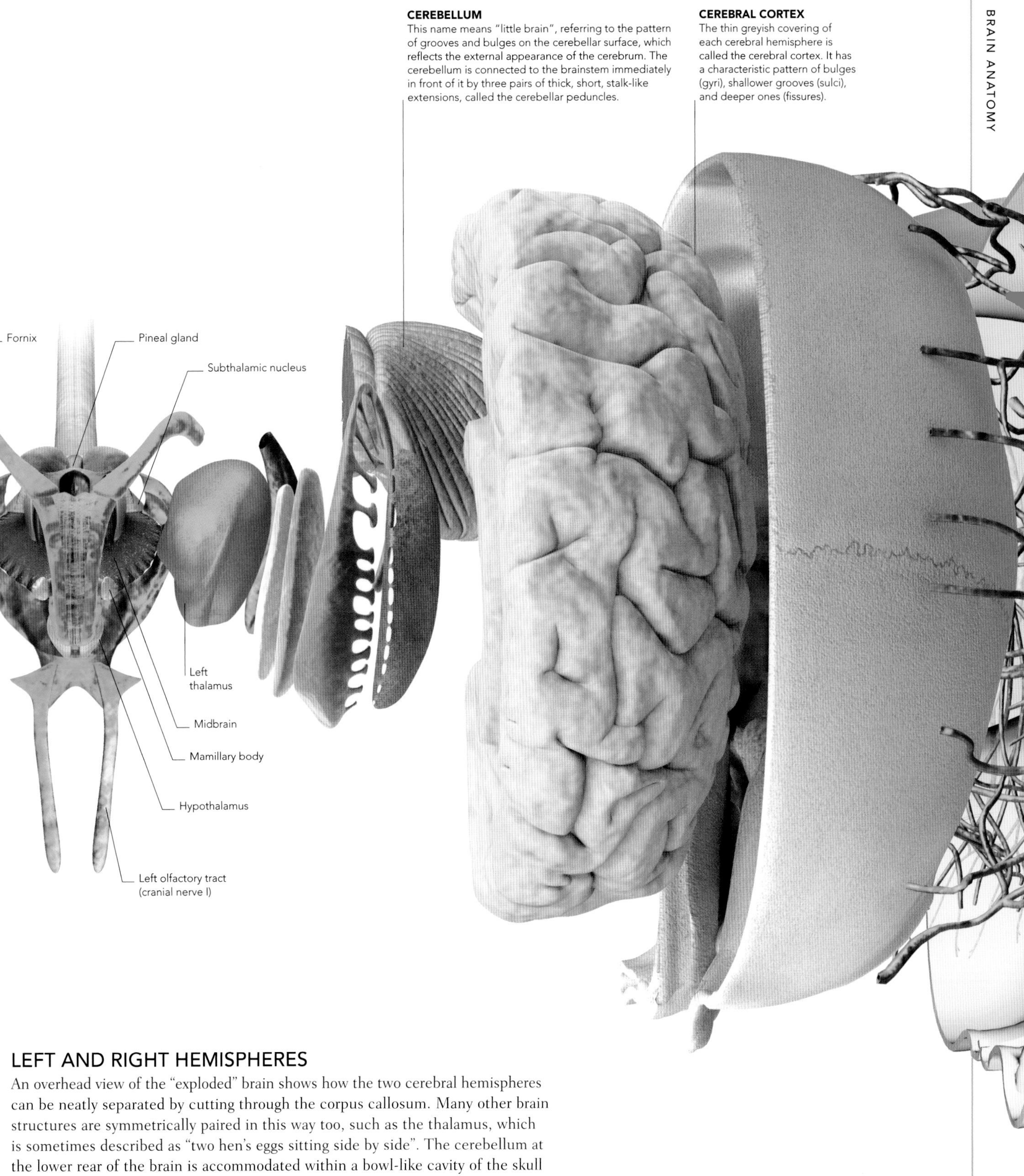
CEREBELLUM
This name means "little brain", referring to the pattern of grooves and bulges on the cerebellar surface, which reflects the external appearance of the cerebrum. The cerebellum is connected to the brainstem immediately in front of it by three pairs of thick, short, stalk-like extensions, called the cerebellar peduncles.
CEREBRAL CORTEX
The thin greyish covering of each cerebral hemisphere is called the cerebral cortex. It has a characteristic pattern of bulges (gyri), shallower grooves (sulci), and deeper ones (fissures).
Fornix
Pineal gland
Subthalamic nucleus
Left thalamus
Midbrain
Mamillary body
Hypothalamus
Left olfactory tract (cranial nerve I)

LEFT AND RIGHT HEMISPHERES

An overhead view of the "exploded" brain shows how the two cerebral hemispheres can be neatly separated by cutting through the corpus callosum. Many other brain structures are symmetrically paired in this way too, such as the thalamus, which is sometimes described as "two hen's eggs sitting side by side". The cerebellum at the lower rear of the brain is accommodated within a bowl-like cavity of the skull known as the posterior cranial fossa. The cranial nerves (numbered I to XII, see p.43) enter the brain directly rather than connecting to the spinal cord.

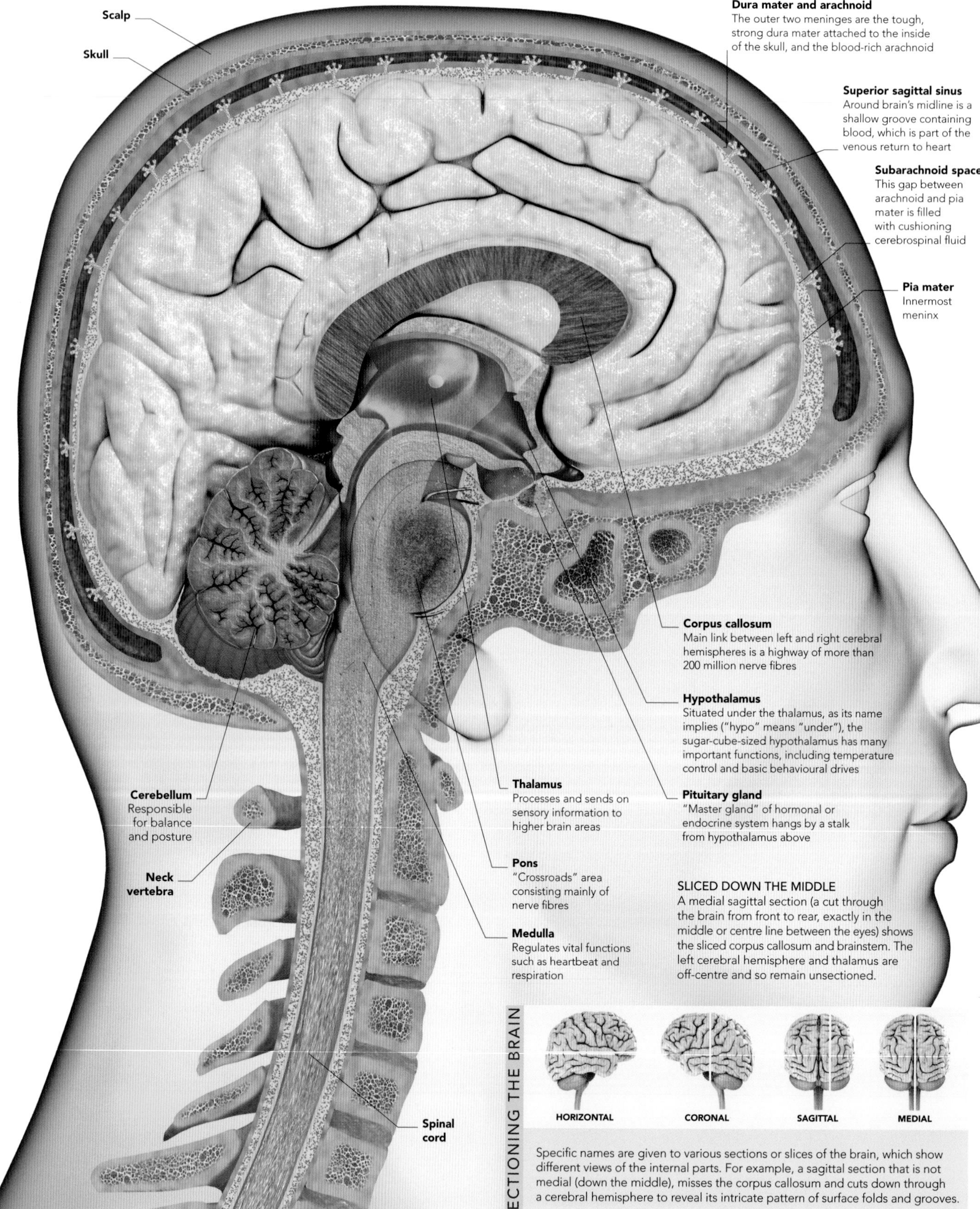

Scalp
Skull
Dura mater and arachnoid
The outer two meninges are the tough, strong dura mater attached to the inside of the skull, and the blood-rich arachnoid
Superior sagittal sinus
Around brain's midline is a shallow groove containing blood, which is part of the venous return to heart
Subarachnoid space
This gap between arachnoid and pia mater is filled with cushioning cerebrospinal fluid
Pia mater
Innermost meninx
Corpus callosum
Main link between left and right cerebral hemispheres is a highway of more than 200 million nerve fibres
Hypothalamus
Situated under the thalamus, as its name implies ("hypo" means "under"), the sugar-cube-sized hypothalamus has many important functions, including temperature control and basic behavioural drives
Cerebellum
Responsible for balance and posture
Thalamus
Processes and sends on sensory information to higher brain areas
Pituitary gland
"Master gland" of hormonal or endocrine system hangs by a stalk from hypothalamus above
Neck vertebra
Pons
"Crossroads" area consisting mainly of nerve fibres
Medulla
Regulates vital functions such as heartbeat and respiration
Spinal cord

SLICED DOWN THE MIDDLE

A medial sagittal section (a cut through the brain from front to rear, exactly in the middle or centre line between the eyes) shows the sliced corpus callosum and brainstem. The left cerebral hemisphere and thalamus are off-centre and so remain unsectioned.

SECTIONING THE BRAIN

HORIZONTAL | CORONAL | SAGITTAL | MEDIAL

Specific names are given to various sections or slices of the brain, which show different views of the internal parts. For example, a sagittal section that is not medial (down the middle), misses the corpus callosum and cuts down through a cerebral hemisphere to reveal its intricate pattern of surface folds and grooves.

BRAIN ZONES AND PARTITIONS

THE BRAIN'S PHYSICAL STRUCTURE BROADLY REFLECTS ITS MENTAL ORGANIZATION. IN GENERAL, HIGHER MENTAL PROCESSES OCCUR IN THE UPPER REGIONS, WHILE THE BRAIN'S LOWER REGIONS TAKE CARE OF BASIC LIFE SUPPORT.

VERTICAL ORGANIZATION

The uppermost brain region, the cerebral cortex, is mostly involved in conscious sensations, abstract thought processes, reasoning, planning, working memory, and similar higher mental processes. The limbic areas (see pp.64–65) on the brain's innermost sides, around the brainstem, deal largely with more emotional and instinctive behaviours and reactions, as well as long-term memory. The thalamus is a preprocessing and relay centre, primarily for sensory information coming from lower in the brainstem, bound for the cerebral hemispheres above. Moving down the brainstem into the medulla are the so-called "vegetative" centres of the brain, which sustain life even if the person has lost consciousness.

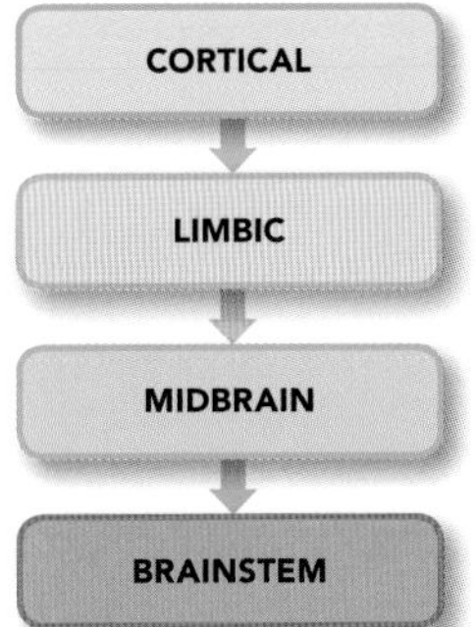

LESS CONSCIOUS, MORE AUTOMATIC
The brain's vertical zonation moves from high-level mental activity in the cerebral cortex gradually through to more basic or "primitive" lower functions, especially the autonomic centres of the medulla in the lower brainstem that deal with vital body functions, such as breathing and heartbeat.

LEFT AND RIGHT

Structurally, the left and right cerebral hemispheres look broadly similar. Functionally, however, speech and language, stepwise reasoning and analysis, and certain communicating actions are based mainly on the left side in most people. Since nerve fibres cross from left to right at the base of the brain, this dominant left side receives sensory information from, and sends messages to, muscles in the right side of the body – including the right hand. Meanwhile, the right hemisphere is more concerned with sensory inputs, auditory and visual awareness, creative abilities, and spatial–temporal awareness (what happens in our surroundings, second by second).

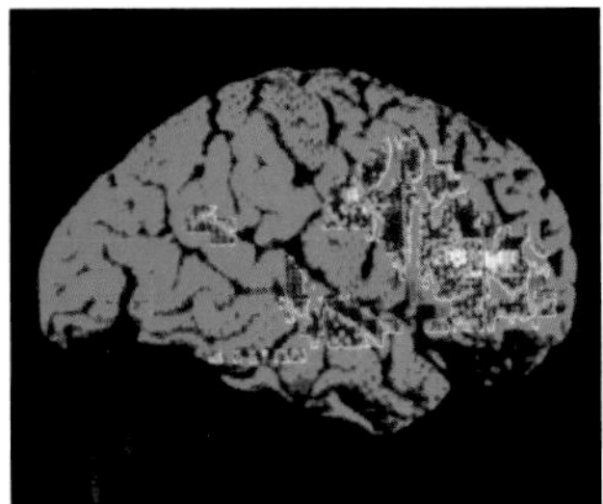

LEFT-HANDED PERSON
In a PET brain scan where yellow and red show increasing activity, a left-handed person involved in word recognition has busy areas at the right front cerebral cortex.

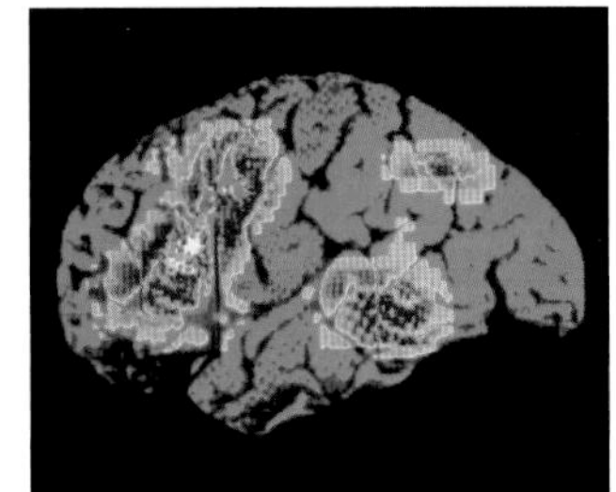

RIGHT-HANDED PERSON
On the same test in a right-handed subject, the left side of the cortex shows a similar pattern, with activity largely in the frontal region and the temporal and parietal areas.

ANARCHIC HAND SYNDROME

In anarchic hand syndrome (AHS), a person has one hand that is no longer under conscious control and seems to move on its own, almost as if possessed by another intelligence. The problem is usually due to an abnormality in the motor centre of the cortex on the opposite side of the brain to the hand. Nerve signals sent from here to control the hand do not register any conscious intention for the action.

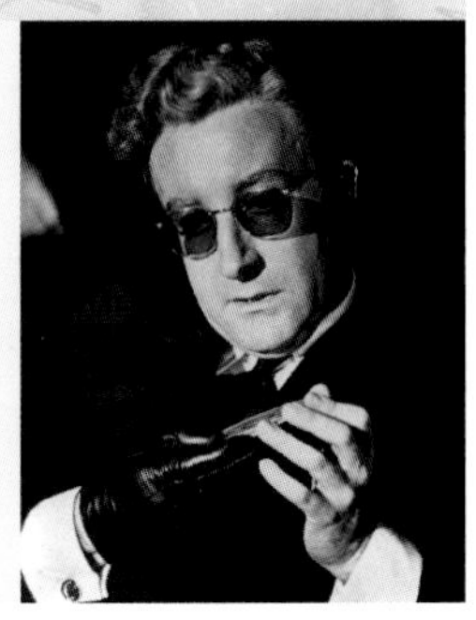

DR STRANGELOVE
In this 1964 film the "hero" struggled with AHS as his leather-gloved right hand even tried to kill him.

THE ASYMMETRICAL BRAIN

In recent years, new and more accurate scanning techniques, especially MRI (see p.13), have shown that on average, brains are not as symmetrical in their left–right structure as was once believed. The scanning computer can be programmed to exaggerate any subtle departures from an exact mirror image. For example, near the lateral sulcus (Sylvian fissure), the part of the temporal lobe for understanding speech is slightly larger on the left than on the right. The lateral sulcus itself is also usually different in shape, being longer and less curved on the left than the right. This is partly due to a twisting effect known as Yakovlevian torque, which warps the right side of the brain forwards.

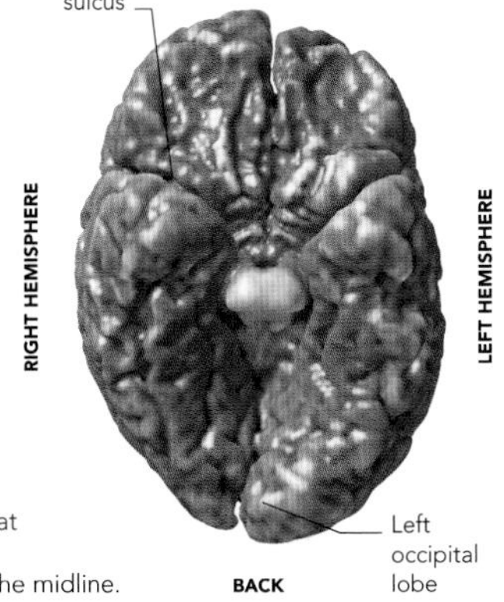

SEEN FROM BELOW
An asymmetry-enhanced MRI scan of the brain's underside reveals left–right differences, including a right frontal lobe that protrudes more than its counterpart, and a longer left occipital lobe that twists across the midline.

THE HOLLOW BRAIN

The brain has an internal system of chambers (ventricles), which are filled with a liquid – cerebrospinal fluid (CSF) – produced by the ventricle linings. The upper two chambers are the left and right lateral ventricles, one in each cerebral hemisphere, with horn-like forward- and side-facing projections. Small openings connect them to the third ventricle in the midbrain, which in turn links to the fourth ventricle in the pons and medulla. CSF flows slowly and continuously through the ventricles, then out via small openings into the subarachnoid space around the brain and the spinal cord.

VENTRICLES
Two large lateral ventricles communicate along ducts with the third ventricle (yellow, upper centre), which lies between and below them.

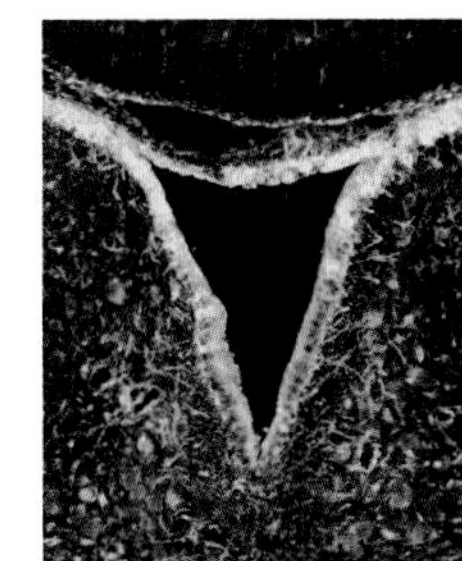

CEREBROSPINAL FLUID
CSF is made by the ventricle lining (green). It physically cushions the brain, distributes nutrients, and collects wastes.

THE NUCLEI OF THE BRAIN

IN THE BRAIN, NUCLEI ARE DISCRETE COLLECTIONS OF THE CELL BODIES OF NEURONS (NERVE CELLS). THEIR NERVE FIBRES OR AXONS SPREAD OUTWARDS TO PROJECT, OR LINK, TO VARIOUS OTHER BRAIN PARTS. THE BRAIN HAS MORE THAN 30 SETS OF NUCLEI, MOSTLY PAIRED LEFT AND RIGHT.

MAIN NUCLEI AND THEIR FUNCTIONS	
Basal	A system of nuclei (including some listed here) involved in motor control and learning.
Caudate	Involved in motor control and learning, especially processing feedback.
Subthalamic	Implicated in impulsive actions, including obsession–compulsion.
Thalamus	A major processing and relay area for inputs to the cerebral cortex (see pp.66–67).
Amygdala	Part of the limbic system, the amygdala is involved in learning, memory, and emotions.
Facial nucleus	One of several paired brainstem nuclei for cranial nerves, in this case nerve VII (facial).

GENERAL STRUCTURE

To the naked eye, most brain nuclei resemble "islands" of grey matter (nerve-cell bodies) within the white matter of nerve fibres. Many nuclei are unencapsulated, that is, not contained within a membrane or covering, so they may lack sharp delineation from surrounding tissues. An older term for some of these nuclei is "ganglia". However, this is now usually reserved for similar structures in the peripheral nervous system, where groups of nerve-cell bodies are generally encapsulated into a discrete structure.

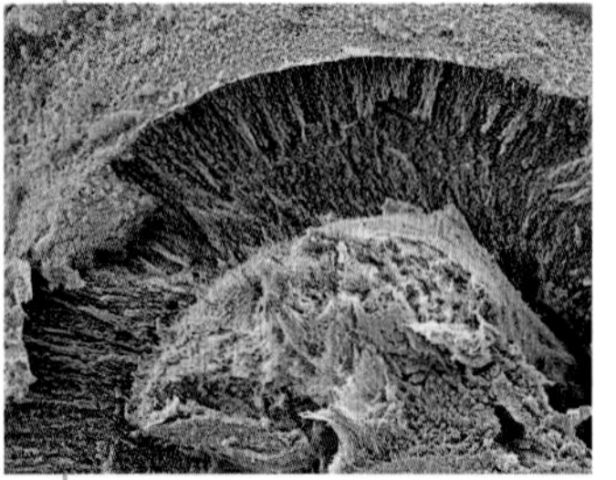

CORPUS STRIATUM
This micrograph shows the nerve cell bodies (dark) and nerve fibres (pale) that make this brain region look striped or striated.

THE BASAL NUCLEI

The basal nuclei (also known as the basal ganglia) is the collective name for several pairs of nuclei at the "base" of the cerebral hemispheres – adjacent to their inner surfaces, around and below the thalamus. They include the putamen, caudate nuclei, globus pallidus, subthalamic nuclei, and substantia nigra. The putamen and caudate nuclei are together called the dorsal striatum, due to the striped or striated appearance of their tissues. Together with the globus pallidus, or "pale sphere", the putamen and caudate nuclei are known as the corpus striatum.

THE SUBTHALAMIC NUCLEI AND GLOBUS PALLIDUS

As the name implies, each one of the paired subthalamic nuclei is situated beneath the thalamus. They are also immediately above the substantia nigra. Each nucleus is about the size and shape of a partly squashed pea and is almost surrounded by nerve fibres passing to, from, or around it. Most of the incoming (afferent) nerve fibres are from the globus pallidus, along with some from the cerebral cortex and the substantia nigra. The majority of the outgoing (efferent) nerve fibres carry signals to the globus pallidus and the substantia nigra. The globus pallidus and the putamen are sometimes termed the lentiform or lenticular nucleus.

SUBSTANTIA NIGRA

The substantia nigra or "black substance" paired nuclei are among the lowest, or most basal, of the basal nuclei. Each is situated just beneath a subthalamic nucleus. The dark colour that is characteristic of these nuclei is caused by the body pigment melanin (also found in the skin) that is part of the biochemical pathways involving the neurotransmitter dopamine. Degeneration of substantia nigra neurons is seen in Parkinson's disease (see p.234).

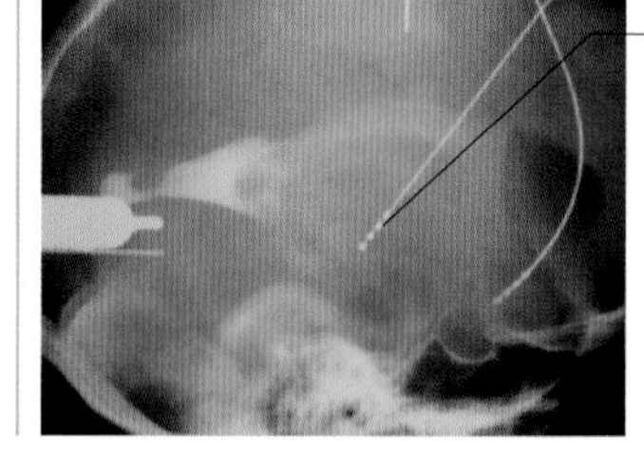

STIMULATION
Deep brain stimulation of basal nuclei, such as the substantia nigra, using electrodes is part of research into and treatment for Parkinson's.

CONNECTIONS AND FUNCTIONS

Most brain nuclei have multiple nerve connections, both inputs and outputs, and carry out wide-ranging functions. The C-shaped caudate nuclei above and to the side of the thalamus, and next to the lateral ventricle, have a head part, main body, and tapering tail. They are involved in motor (muscle) control and also in learning and memory. The rounded putamen, the outermost of the main basal ganglia, partly follows the shape of the caudate nucleus and is intricately linked anatomically to it. It, too, is heavily involved in motor control and movements, and in learning. The putamen has major nerve connections with the globus pallidus and substantia nigra. All of the basal ganglia work together as an integrated brain system to help ensure physical movements are smooth and co-ordinated. Problems with one or more of the nuclei can lead to movement disorders such as tremors, tics, Parkinson's disease (see p.234), Tourette's syndrome (see p.243), and Huntington's disease (see p.234). The subthalamic nuclei also have roles in impulsive actions and movement intentions.

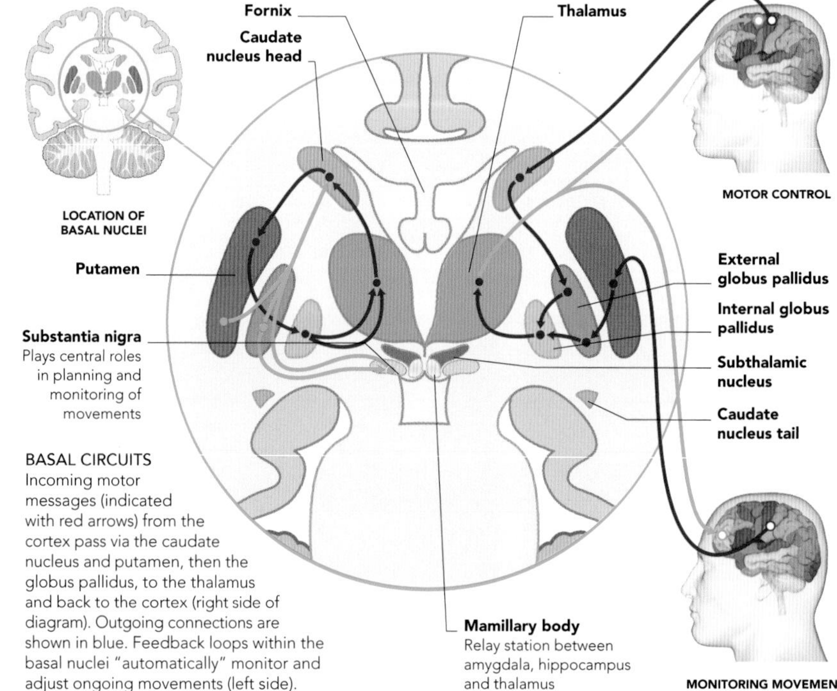

BASAL CIRCUITS
Incoming motor messages (indicated with red arrows) from the cortex pass via the caudate nucleus and putamen, then the globus pallidus, to the thalamus and back to the cortex (right side of diagram). Outgoing connections are shown in blue. Feedback loops within the basal nuclei "automatically" monitor and adjust ongoing movements (left side).

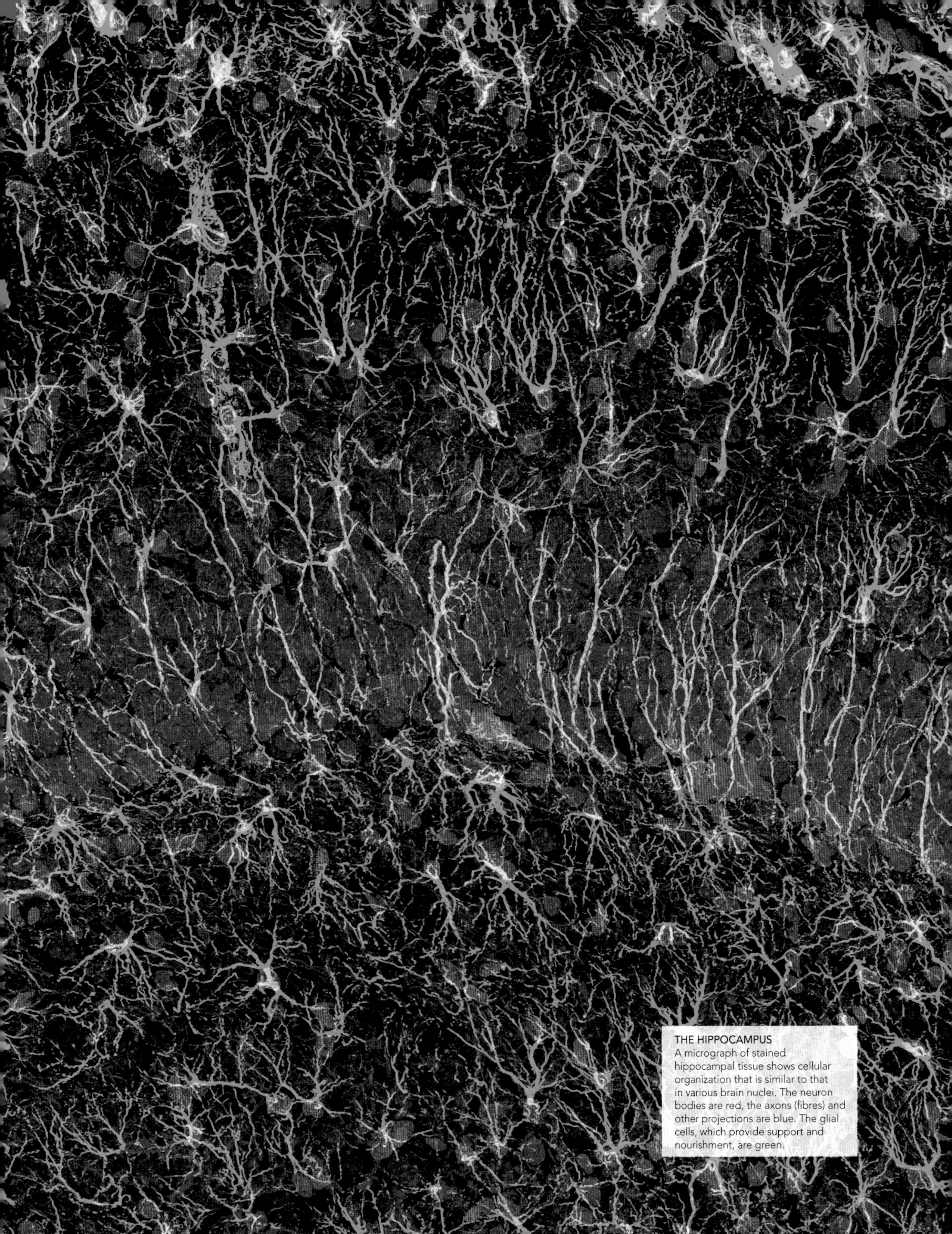

THE HIPPOCAMPUS
A micrograph of stained hippocampal tissue shows cellular organization that is similar to that in various brain nuclei. The neuron bodies are red, the axons (fibres) and other projections are blue. The glial cells, which provide support and nourishment, are green.

THE THALAMUS, HYPOTHALAMUS, AND PITUITARY GLAND

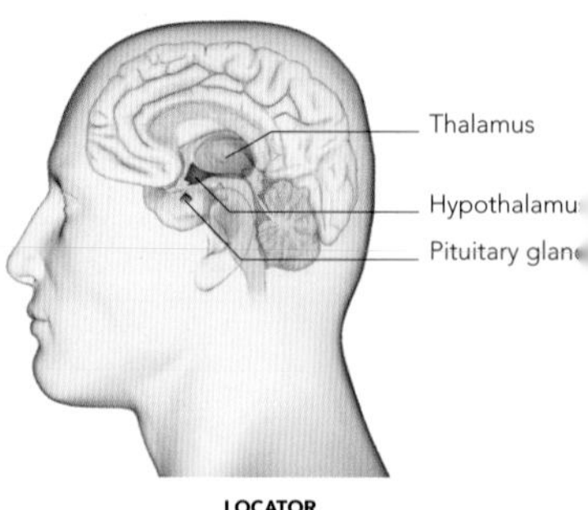

THE THALAMUS IS SITUATED AT THE ANATOMICAL CORE OF THE BRAIN. ITS POSITION MAKES IT PERFECTLY SITUATED TO ACT AS A RELAY STATION BETWEEN THE SENSE ORGANS AND THE BRAIN. SITTING BENEATH THE THALAMUS, THE HYPOTHALAMUS AND THE PITUITARY GLAND LINK THE CENTRAL NERVOUS SYSTEM AND THE ENDOCRINE SYSTEM.

THE THALAMUS

Paired, egg-shaped masses that sit side by side make up the thalamus. In a typical brain, each mass is about 3cm ($1\frac{1}{4}$ in) long and 1.5cm ($\frac{1}{2}$ in) across. There are no direct nerve connections from one mass to the other – in fact, the fluid-filled chamber of the third ventricle lies between them. The thalamus is the major relay station for nerve signals coming from all the senses except smell. It screens, sorts, and pre-processes this continuing torrent of sensory information and sends it onwards to the cerebral cortex.

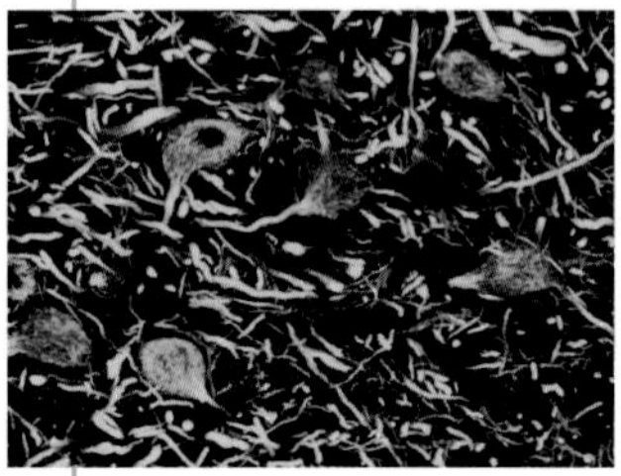

THALAMIC NEURONS
Densely interconnected neuron bodies and nerve fibres (green) receive physical and nutritional support from glial cells (red).

INSIDE THE THALAMUS
Each side (one of which is shown here) contains more than 20 nuclei consisting of "grey matter" – that is, collections of nerve-cell bodies. These nuclei, sometimes called thalamic bodies, are in groups separated by sheets of white matter (myelinated nerve fibres) known as laminae. The whole thalamus is enveloped in a similar white-matter wrapping.

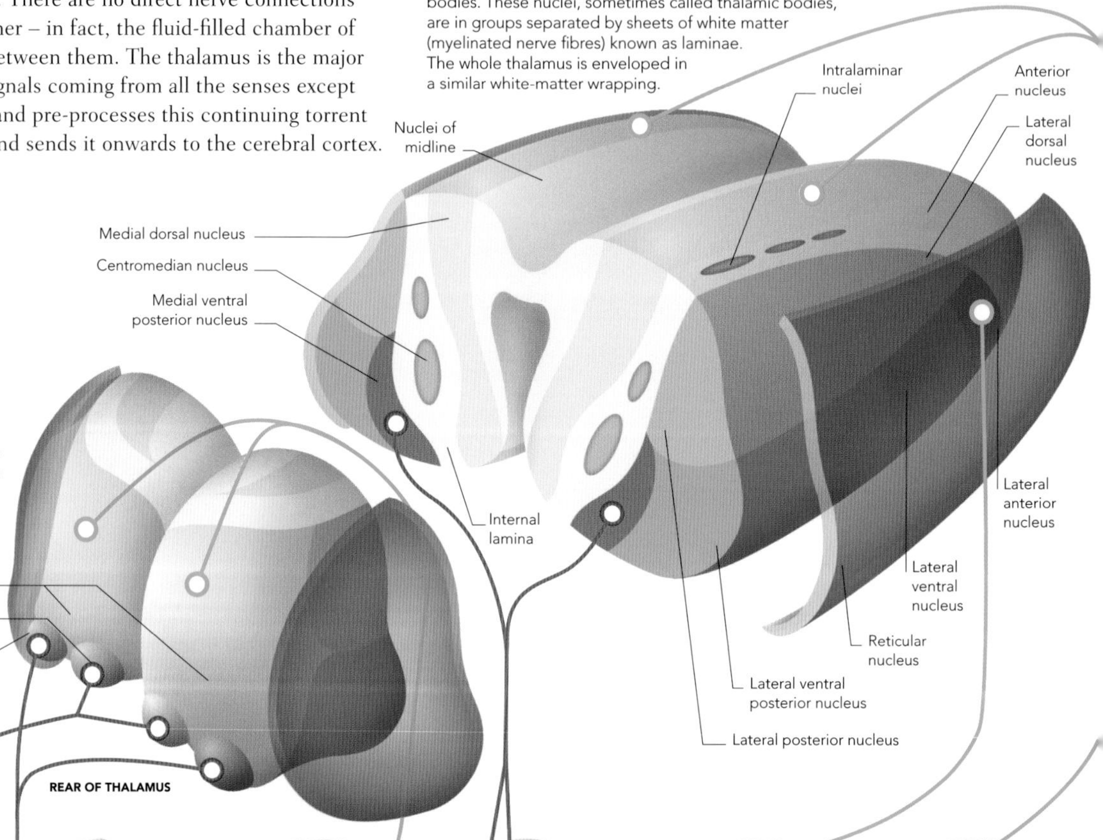

FRONT OF THALAMUS
Intralaminar nuclei
Anterior nucleus
Lateral dorsal nucleus
Nuclei of midline
Medial dorsal nucleus
Centromedian nucleus
Medial ventral posterior nucleus
Internal lamina
Lateral anterior nucleus
Lateral ventral nucleus
Reticular nucleus
Lateral ventral posterior nucleus
Lateral posterior nucleus
Lateral nuclei (pulvinars)
Medial geniculate nucleus
Lateral geniculate nucleus
REAR OF THALAMUS

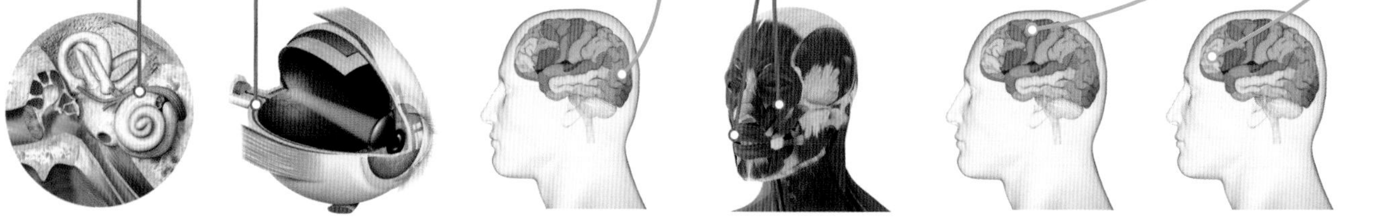

INNER EAR
Medial geniculate nuclei are the chief recipients of nerve impulses from the cochleas of the inner ears, which they forward to the auditory cerebral cortex (Brodmann areas 41 and 42, see p.67).

RETINA
Information from the retinas, about what the eyes see, arrives at the lateral geniculate nuclei. After processing, it passes to the primary visual cortex (area 17) and visual association cortex.

VISUAL CORTEX
Working with the lateral geniculate nuclei, each much larger lateral nucleus (or pulvinar) sends accessory sensory information to several parts of the visual cortex (see pp.82–83).

FACE AND MOUTH
Sensory information from the facial skin and interior of the mouth travels along the trigeminal nerve and the trigemino-thalamic tract to the medial ventral posterior nuclei.

PREMOTOR CORTEX
The thalamus has both incoming (afferent) and outgoing (efferent) nerve fibres. Many nerve fibres to the lateral anterior nuclei are afferent, from the premotor area of the cerebral cortex.

PREFRONTAL CORTEX
Most of the incoming signals for the medial dorsal nuclei are from the cerebral prefrontal cortex, and also from the hypothalamus when concerning emotions.

THE HYPOTHALAMUS

Not much larger than the end segment of the little finger, weighing just 4g ($^{5}/_{32}$ oz), and comprising only 0.4 per cent of total brain volume, the hypothalamus has many and varied vital roles – in conscious behaviour, emotions and instincts, and automatic control of body systems and processes. It consists of more than a dozen paired nuclei (regions of interlinked nerve-cell bodies) clustered into the floor of the diencephalon and separated by the lateral ventricle. Its secretory cells make hormones (called releasing factors) that enter the bloodstream, and its neurosecretory cells produce hormone-like substances that travel along nerve axons down to the pituitary gland (see below).

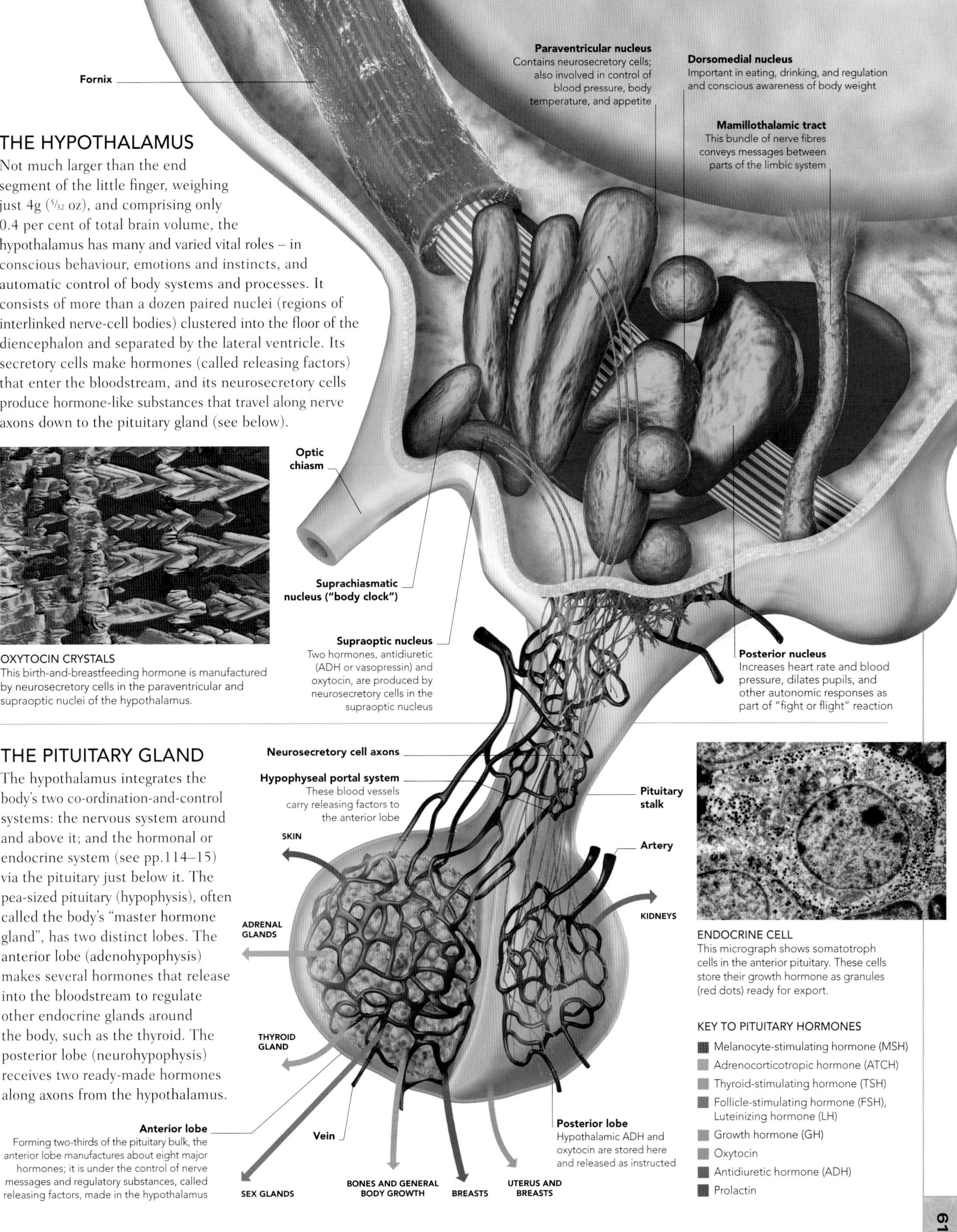

Fornix
Paraventricular nucleus
Contains neurosecretory cells; also involved in control of blood pressure, body temperature, and appetite
Dorsomedial nucleus
Important in eating, drinking, and regulation and conscious awareness of body weight
Mamillothalamic tract
This bundle of nerve fibres conveys messages between parts of the limbic system
Optic chiasm
Suprachiasmatic nucleus ("body clock")
Supraoptic nucleus
Two hormones, antidiuretic (ADH or vasopressin) and oxytocin, are produced by neurosecretory cells in the supraoptic nucleus
Posterior nucleus
Increases heart rate and blood pressure, dilates pupils, and other autonomic responses as part of "fight or flight" reaction
Neurosecretory cell axons
Hypophyseal portal system
These blood vessels carry releasing factors to the anterior lobe
Pituitary stalk
Artery
SKIN
KIDNEYS
ADRENAL GLANDS
THYROID GLAND
Anterior lobe
Forming two-thirds of the pituitary bulk, the anterior lobe manufactures about eight major hormones; it is under the control of nerve messages and regulatory substances, called releasing factors, made in the hypothalamus
Vein
Posterior lobe
Hypothalamic ADH and oxytocin are stored here and released as instructed
SEX GLANDS
BONES AND GENERAL BODY GROWTH
BREASTS
UTERUS AND BREASTS

OXYTOCIN CRYSTALS
This birth-and-breastfeeding hormone is manufactured by neurosecretory cells in the paraventricular and supraoptic nuclei of the hypothalamus.

THE PITUITARY GLAND

The hypothalamus integrates the body's two co-ordination-and-control systems: the nervous system around and above it; and the hormonal or endocrine system (see pp.114–15) via the pituitary just below it. The pea-sized pituitary (hypophysis), often called the body's "master hormone gland", has two distinct lobes. The anterior lobe (adenohypophysis) makes several hormones that release into the bloodstream to regulate other endocrine glands around the body, such as the thyroid. The posterior lobe (neurohypophysis) receives two ready-made hormones along axons from the hypothalamus.

ENDOCRINE CELL
This micrograph shows somatotroph cells in the anterior pituitary. These cells store their growth hormone as granules (red dots) ready for export.

KEY TO PITUITARY HORMONES

- Melanocyte-stimulating hormone (MSH)
- Adrenocorticotropic hormone (ATCH)
- Thyroid-stimulating hormone (TSH)
- Follicle-stimulating hormone (FSH), Luteinizing hormone (LH)
- Growth hormone (GH)
- Oxytocin
- Antidiuretic hormone (ADH)
- Prolactin

THE BRAINSTEM AND CEREBELLUM

THE BRAINSTEM IS PERHAPS MISNAMED. IT IS NOT A STEM LEADING TO THE SEPARATE BRAIN ABOVE, BUT AN INTEGRAL PART OF THE BRAIN ITSELF. IT IS SHAPED RATHER LIKE A WIDENING UPRIGHT STALK, ON TOP OF WHICH ARE THE THALAMUS AND THE DOME OF THE CEREBRAL HEMISPHERES. CURLED AROUND THE LOWER BRAINSTEM, AT THE REAR OF THE BRAIN, SITS THE CEREBELLUM.

BRAINSTEM ANATOMY

The brainstem includes almost all of the brain except for the highest parts, which make up the forebrain (cerebrum and diencephalon, see p.52). Its uppermost region is the midbrain comprising an upper "roof" or tectum incorporating the superior and inferior colliculi or bulges at the rear, and the tegmentum to the front. Below the midbrain is the hindbrain. At its front is the large bulge of the pons. Behind and below this is the medulla, which narrows to merge with the uppermost end of the body's main nerve, the spinal cord. The cerebellum joins to the rear of the medulla by three pairs of stalks, known as the cerebellar peduncles.

INTERNAL STRUCTURE

Within the brainstem are groupings of nerve-cell bodies known as nuclei (see pp.58–59) and numerous bundles of nerve fibres or axons, called nerve tracts. For example, the pontine nuclei of the front or ventral pons are involved in learning and remembering motor skills – they act as relay stations for nerve signals from the motor cortex, which are travelling to the cerebellum behind the pons (see panel, opposite).

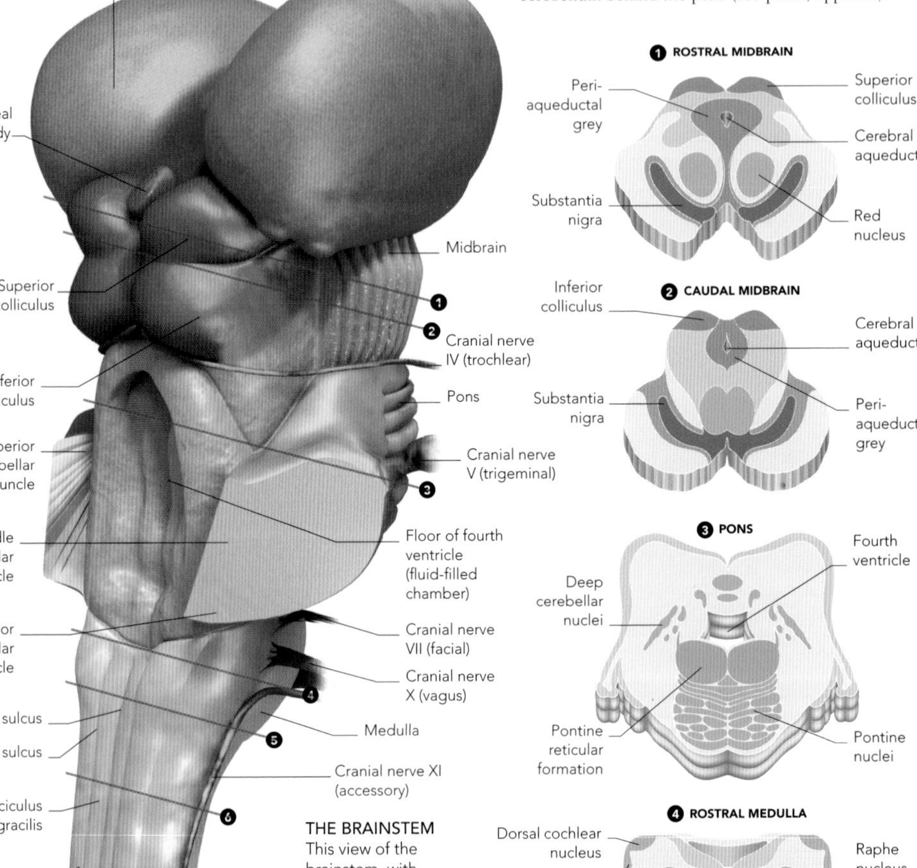

THE BRAINSTEM
This view of the brainstem, with the cerebellum removed, reveals the medulla and bundles of axons called fascicles. The cranial nerves join various parts of the brainstem.

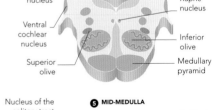

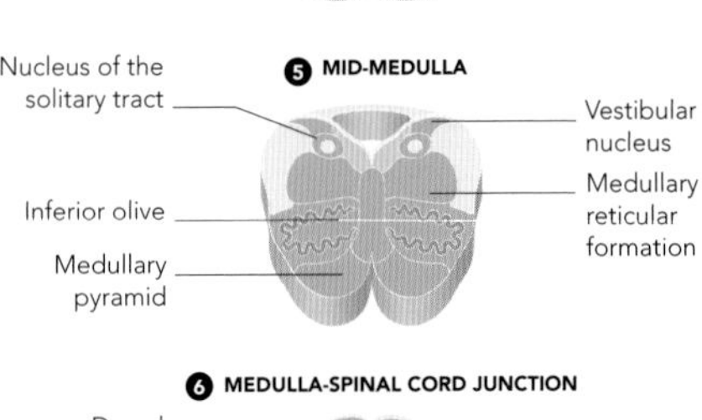

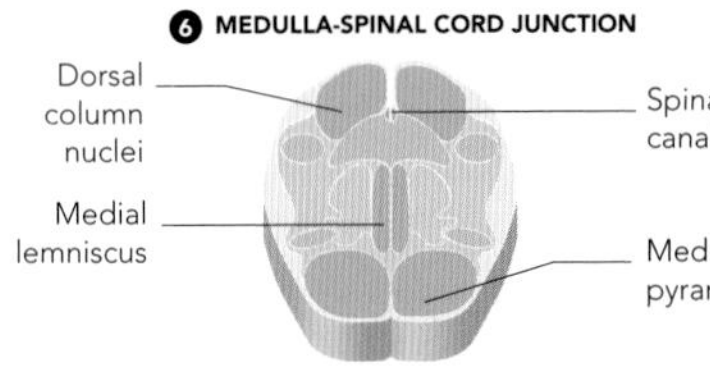

BRAINSTEM SECTIONS
The horizontal cross-sections of the brainstem shown here match the numbers in the illustration above left. Nuclei are shown in green; the white matter of nerve fibre tracts is pale. In each section, the rear of the body is uppermost.

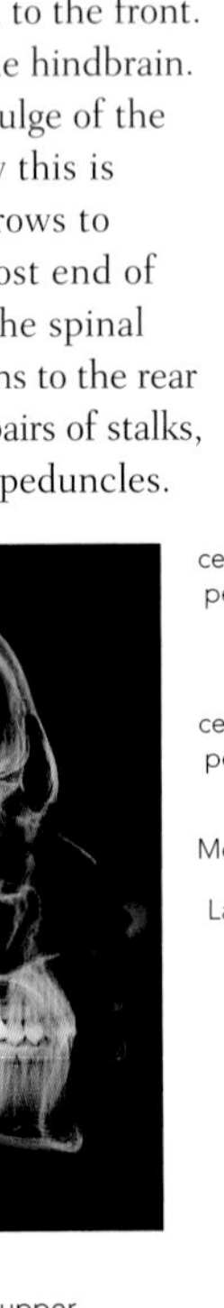

CONNECTING THE BRAIN
This MRI scan shows how the upper brainstem is at about level with the eyes, and its lower region joins the spinal cord at a gap through the base of the skull, the foramen magnum.

360-DEGREE VIEW

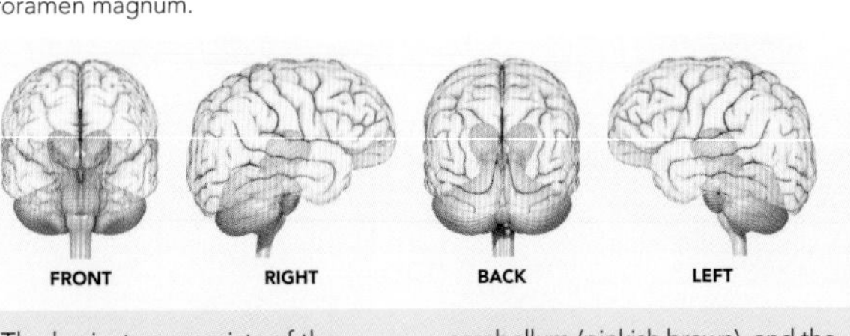

The brainstem consists of the structures shown here inferior to, or below, the thalamus (green). Major landmarks are the pons (blue), the cerebellum (pinkish brown), and the medulla (creamy beige). In some categorizations, the thalamus is included as part of the brainstem.

BRAINSTEM FUNCTIONS

The brainstem is highly involved in mid- to low-order mental activities, for example, the almost "automatic" scanning movements of the eyes as we watch something pass by, rather than higher activities such as abstract thought. It is also the site of subconscious or autonomic control mechanisms, of which we are usually unaware. The medulla, in particular, houses groups of nuclei that are centres for respiratory (breathing), cardiac (heartbeat), and vasomotor (blood pressure) monitoring and control, as well as for vomiting, sneezing, swallowing, and coughing.

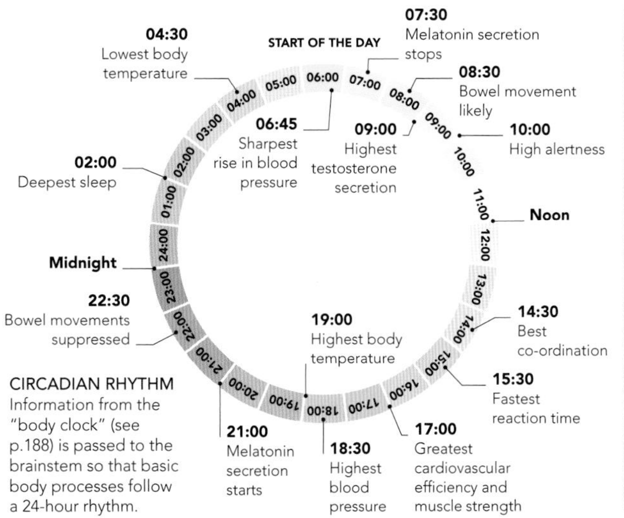

CIRCADIAN RHYTHM
Information from the "body clock" (see p.188) is passed to the brainstem so that basic body processes follow a 24-hour rhythm.

LOCKED-IN SYNDROME

Damage to certain parts of the brainstem, especially the forward-facing area of the pons, can produce a condition known as "locked-in" or ventral pontine syndrome. The sufferer is aware of their surroundings and able to see and hear, but cannot activate any voluntary muscles – those that are under conscious control – and so is unable to move or react. Damage may be due to injury or the lack of blood supply during a stroke. In some cases, the eye muscles continue to function, allowing communication by eye movements.

THE CEREBELLUM

The "little brain" is the lower, rearmost part of the entire brain. It resembles the wrinkled appearance of the cerebrum above, but its grooves and bulges are finer and organized into more regular patterns. Major anatomical parts of the cerebellum include: the long, slim vermis ("worm") in the centre; two flocculonodular lobes beneath, one on each side; and outside these, two much larger lateral lobes, each of which is divided into several lobules. The two lateral lobes are reminiscent of the two hemispheres of the cerebrum and are sometimes termed cerebellar hemispheres. The cerebellum's main functions are to co-ordinate bodily movements through integrated control of muscles, including balance and posture, and equilibrium.

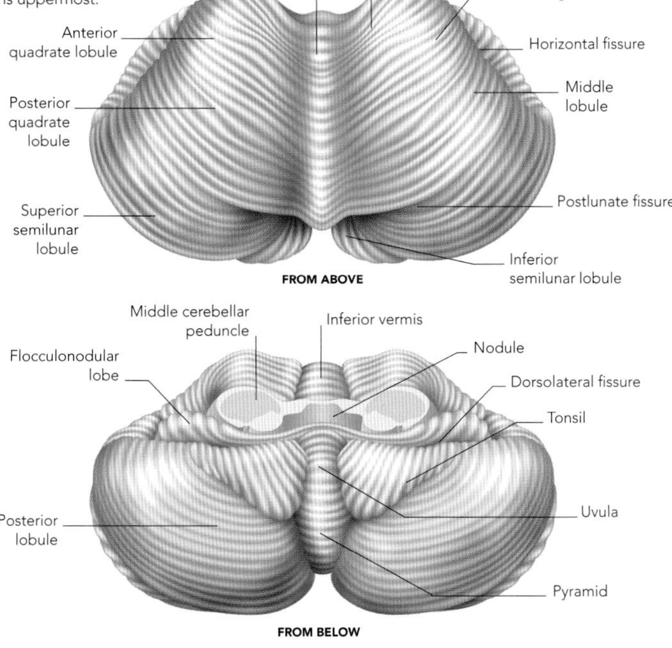

THE CEREBELLUM
The grooves in the cerebellar surface are termed fissures, and the bulges are known as folia. In each image, the front is uppermost.

INTERNAL STRUCTURE

The cerebellum has a similar layered microstructure to the cerebrum. The outer layer, or cerebellar cortex, is grey matter composed of nerve-cell bodies and their dendrite projections. Beneath this is a medullary area of white matter consisting largely of nerve fibres. Towards the centre are collections of more nerve-cell bodies known as deep cerebellar nuclei. Nerve fibres run from these nuclei to the cerebral cortex high above. In a cross-section at almost any angle through the cerebellum, the white matter between the cortex and deep nuclei forms a complex branching pattern known as the arbor vitae.

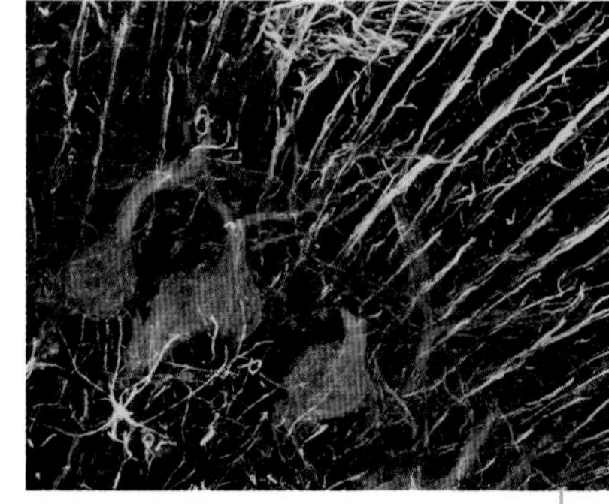

CEREBELLUM CELLS
The main types of nerve cells in the cerebellar cortex are known as Purkinje cells (red), supported by glial cells (green).

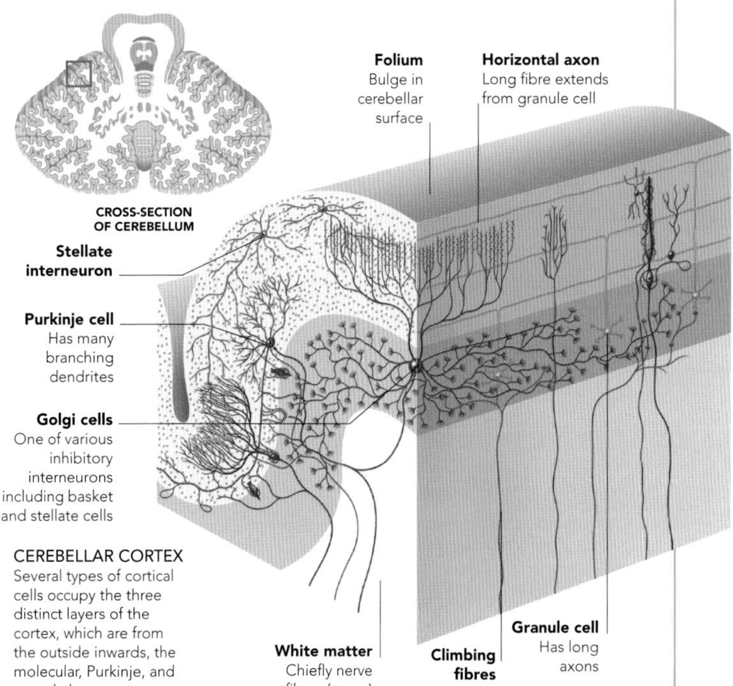

CEREBELLAR CORTEX
Several types of cortical cells occupy the three distinct layers of the cortex, which are from the outside inwards, the molecular, Purkinje, and granule layers.

THE LIMBIC SYSTEM

THE LIMBIC SYSTEM IS INVOLVED IN INSTINCTIVE BEHAVIOURS, DEEP-SEATED EMOTIONS, AND BASIC IMPULSES SUCH AS SEX, ANGER, PLEASURE, AND GENERAL SURVIVAL. IT ALSO FORMS A LINK BETWEEN CENTRES OF HIGHER CONSCIOUSNESS, IN THE CEREBRAL CORTEX, AND THE BRAINSTEM, WHICH REGULATES THE BODY'S SYSTEMS.

Fornix

Corpus callosum

Mamillary bodies

AT THE BRAIN'S CORE
Situated approximately in the anatomical centre or core of the brain, the limbic system is a varied collection of structures extending from the cerebrum inwards and down to the brainstem.

COMPONENTS OF THE LIMBIC SYSTEM

The limbic system includes the areas of the cortex and adjacent parts known as the limbic lobe (see opposite page), along with the amygdala, hypothalamus, thalamus, mamillary bodies, and other deeper, more central brain structures. The system is also "hard-wired" into parts of the sensory system, especially the sense of smell. Nerve fibres link all of these parts intimately and also connect them to other areas of the brain, particularly the lower frontal cortex, with its roles in expectation, reward, and decision-making.

Fornix
This tract of nerve fibres connects the mamillary bodies and hippocampus

Cingulate gyrus
Part of limbic cortex just above corpus callosum

Column of fornix

Mamillary bodies
Small lumps of nerve cells, these relay signals to thalamus, contributing to alertness and memory formation

Olfactory bulbs
Tracts of sensory nerve cells extend from nasal cavity into the brain; they part-process smell information before it enters conscious awareness

Hypothalamus
Chief link and mediator between nervous system and hormonal or endocrine system (see p.61)

Pons

Hippocampus
Named after its vague S-shaped resemblance to a seahorse, this part is involved in memory and spatial awareness

Midbrain
The limbic system extends nerve fibres from thalamus and other higher parts into this uppermost part of the brainstem and also to the basal nuclei

Parahippocampal gyrus
This area of cortex flanking the hippocampus is active when viewing scenes and places

Amygdala
Almond-shaped neuron clusters that are heavily involved in memory and emotional responses

LIMBIC STRUCTURES
The name of this system is derived from the Latin *limbus*, meaning "border" or "edge". Its major structures form a circular, belt-like transition zone between the relatively plain-looking main cerebral cortex and the more distinctive bodies, tracts, and nuclei of the inner, lower brain.

360-DEGREE VIEW

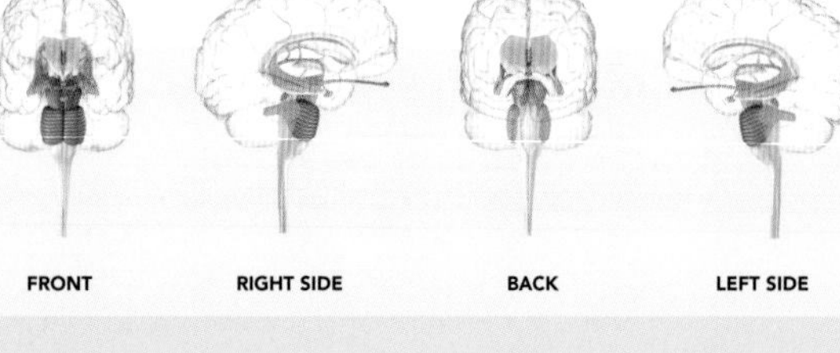

These views of the limbic system show how it is situated in the centre of the brain, and occupies parts of the inner or medial surfaces of the cerebral cortex. The cingulate gyrus, the hippocampus, and the parahippocampal gyrus – all part of the cerebral cortex – arch around and down below the corpus callosum.

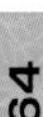

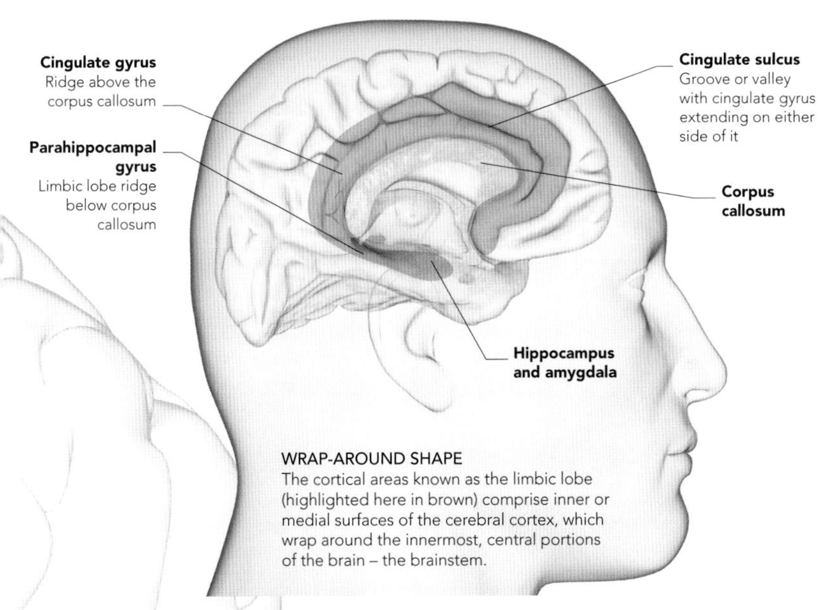

WRAP-AROUND SHAPE
The cortical areas known as the limbic lobe (highlighted here in brown) comprise inner or medial surfaces of the cerebral cortex, which wrap around the innermost, central portions of the brain – the brainstem.

THE LIMBIC LOBE

The structures of the limbic system are surrounded by an area of the cortex referred to as the limbic lobe. The lobe forms a collar- or ring-like shape on the inner surfaces of the cerebral hemispheres, both above and below the corpus callosum. The upper part is the cingulate gyrus, on either side of the cingulate sulcus. The lower part is the parahippocampal gyrus, delineated below by the collateral fissure and rhinal sulcus. The cingulate and parahippocampal gyri are together known as the fornicate gyrus. As such, the limbic lobe comprises the inward-facing parts of other cortical lobes, including the temporal, parietal, and frontal, where the left and right lobes curve around to face each other. The hippocampus and amygdala are not integral to this split-ring shape, but are considered as anatomically part of the limbic lobe as well as components of the limbic system.

THE HIPPOCAMPUS

The hippocampus is strung along the upper edge of the parahippocampal gyrus. The hippocampus interlocks with another ridge, known as the dentate gyrus – together the two form the hippocampal–dentate complex. It is part of the cerebral cortex, but it has only between one and three layers of cells, rather than the usual six layers found in most of the more “advanced” regions of the cortex.

The main functions of the hippocampus include spatial awareness, and memory formation and recall. In particular, the hippocampus helps to select transient information for memorizing and then pass it through to longer-term memory areas. Damage to it can prevent a person forming new memories, even though memories from before the damage are intact.

NEURONS
A light micrograph of a section through the hippocampus reveals neurons that have been labelled with green fluorescent protein. Also seen are ion channels (coloured gold) that allow the exchange of sodium and calcium ions across the cell membrane. This exchange propagates nerve impulses.

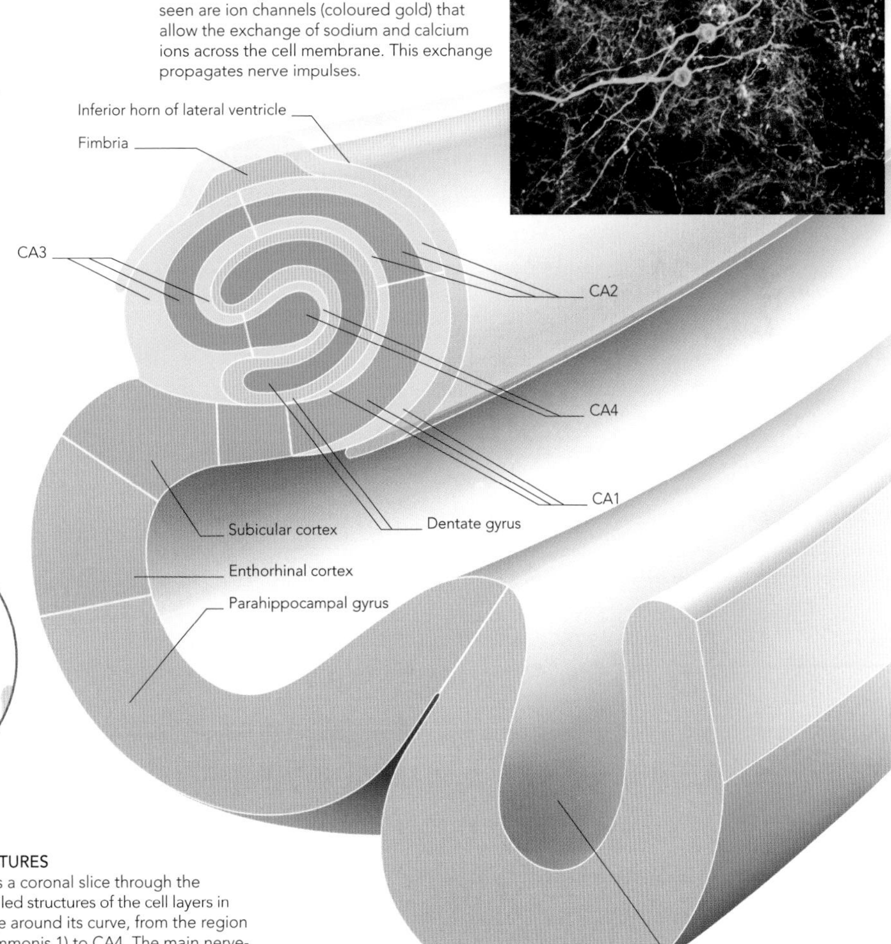

HIPPOCAMPAL STRUCTURES
This cross-section shows a coronal slice through the hippocampus. The detailed structures of the cell layers in the hippocampus change around its curve, from the region known as CA1 (cornis ammonis 1) to CA4. The main nerve-signal inputs are from the parahippocampal gyrus, the fornix, and the hippocampus in the opposite hemisphere.

THE CEREBRAL CORTEX

THE CEREBRAL CORTEX IS THE OUTER LAYER OF THE BRAIN'S MOST DOMINANT PART, THE CEREBRUM. IT IS THE BULGING WRINKLED SURFACE WE SEE WHEN LOOKING AT THE BRAIN FROM ANY ANGLE. IT IS COMMONLY KNOWN AS GREY MATTER FROM ITS COLOUR, WHICH CONTRASTS WITH THE WHITE MATTER IN THE LAYER BELOW.

THE CEREBRAL LOBES

Bulges and grooves help to divide the cortex into between four and six paired lobes, according to the anatomical system used. The main and deepest groove is the longitudinal fissure that separates the cerebral hemispheres. Both the extent and the names of the lobes are also partly related to the overlying bones of the skull, known as the neurocranium. For example, the two frontal lobes are approximately beneath the frontal bone, and likewise for the occipital lobes under the occipital bone. In some naming systems, the limbic lobe (see p.65) and the insula, or central lobe, are distinguished as separate from other lobes.

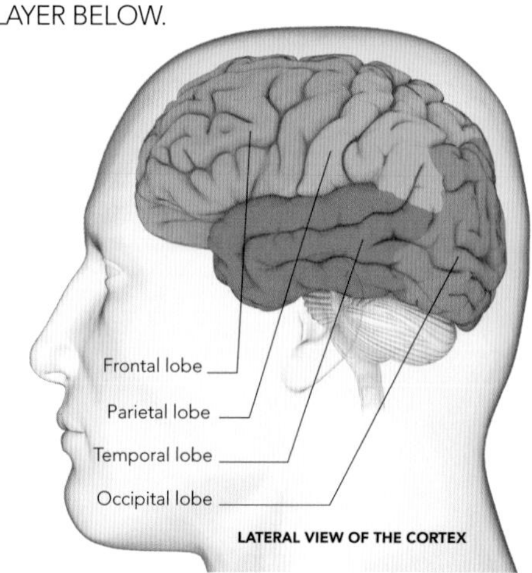

LATERAL VIEW OF THE CORTEX

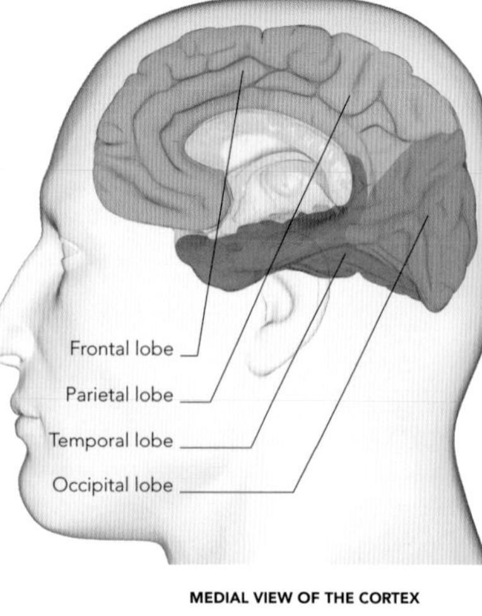

MEDIAL VIEW OF THE CORTEX

LOBE DIVISIONS
The cortex can be divided into four areas called lobes (shown here). In some classifications, the forward part of the frontal lobe is separated as the prefrontal lobe, but the term prefrontal cortex is more generally accepted.

CORTICAL LANDMARKS

Rounded bulges of the cortex are known as gyri; grooves are termed sulci when relatively shallow and fissures when deeper. The overall patterns of gyri and sulci are similar but rarely identical among normal brains – individual variations occur. They are also similar for the left and right of an individual's brain, although there are minor asymmetries (see p.57).

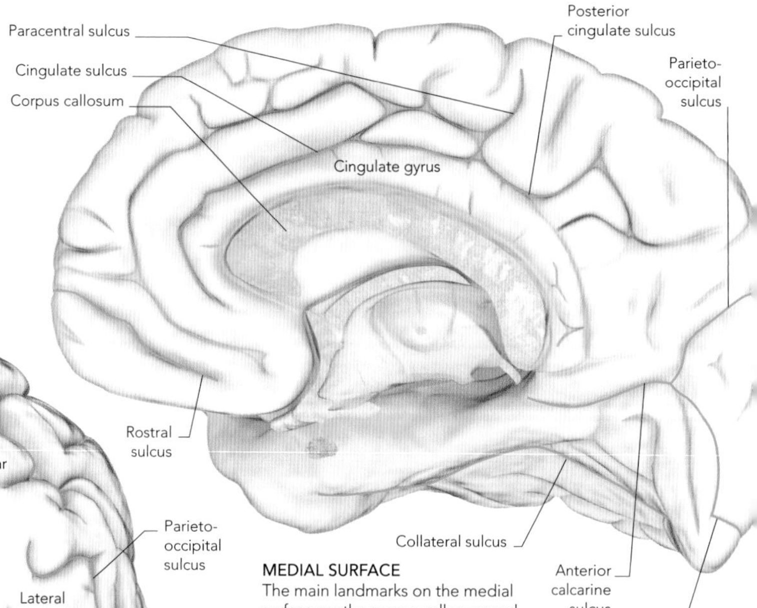

Central sulcus
Precentral sulcus
Intraparietal sulcus
Postcentral sulcus
Superior frontal sulcus
Superior frontal gyrus
Precentral gyrus
Postcentral gyrus
Supramarginal gyrus
Angular gyrus
Middle frontal gyrus
Inferior frontal gyrus
Parieto-occipital sulcus
Lateral occipital gyrus
Superior temporal gyrus
Middle temporal gyrus
Inferior temporal gyrus
Orbital gyri
Lateral sulcus (Sylvian fissure)
Superior temporal sulcus
Inferior temporal sulcus
Preoccipital notch

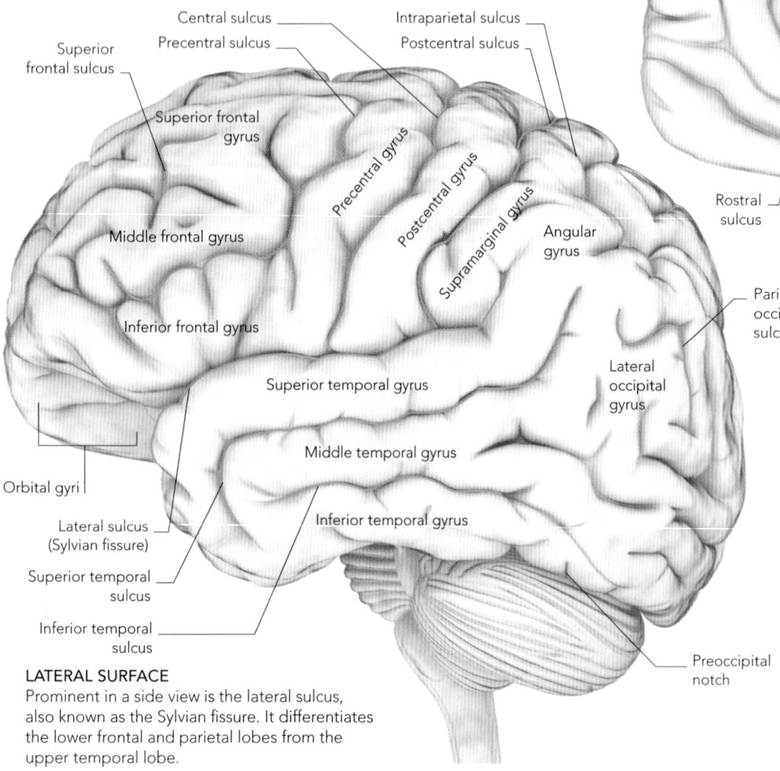

LATERAL SURFACE
Prominent in a side view is the lateral sulcus, also known as the Sylvian fissure. It differentiates the lower frontal and parietal lobes from the upper temporal lobe.

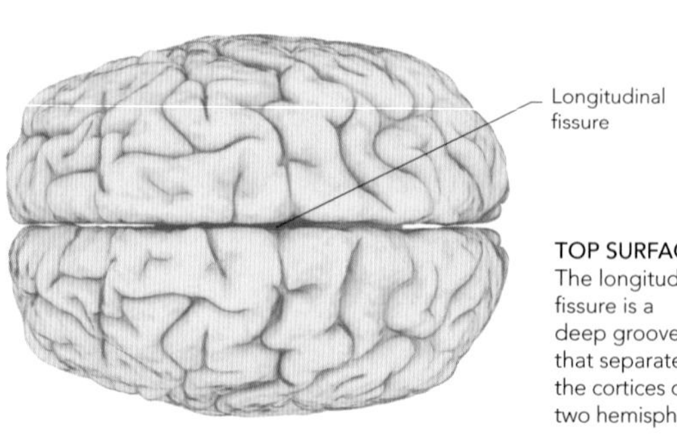

Paracentral sulcus
Cingulate sulcus
Corpus callosum
Posterior cingulate sulcus
Parieto-occipital sulcus
Cingulate gyrus
Rostral sulcus
Collateral sulcus
Anterior calcarine sulcus
Posterior calcarine sulcus

MEDIAL SURFACE
The main landmarks on the medial surface are the corpus callosum and the cingulate gyrus, which forms part of the limbic lobe (see p.65).

Longitudinal fissure

TOP SURFACE
The longitudinal fissure is a deep groove that separates the cortices of the two hemispheres.

FUNCTIONAL AREAS

The cortex can be "mapped" in three ways. One is by gross anatomy, as defined by sulci and gyri (see opposite page). A second is by microscopic anatomy – the shapes and types of cells and their connections, as pioneered by Korbinian Brodmann (see panel, below). The map of areas shown here is named after him. The third method is by neurological function, in which small areas are correlated with what they do. For example, the lobe at the back of the brain is mainly devoted to vision, and within it smaller areas are responsible for various aspects of visual processing determining colour, shape, or motion, among others. The earliest parts of this functional "map" were created by matching damage in a person's brain (usually after their death) with cognitive deficits they displayed when alive. Now it is mainly done by stimulating small areas and noting the effect, or by functional brain imaging. The three "maps" only partially coincide.

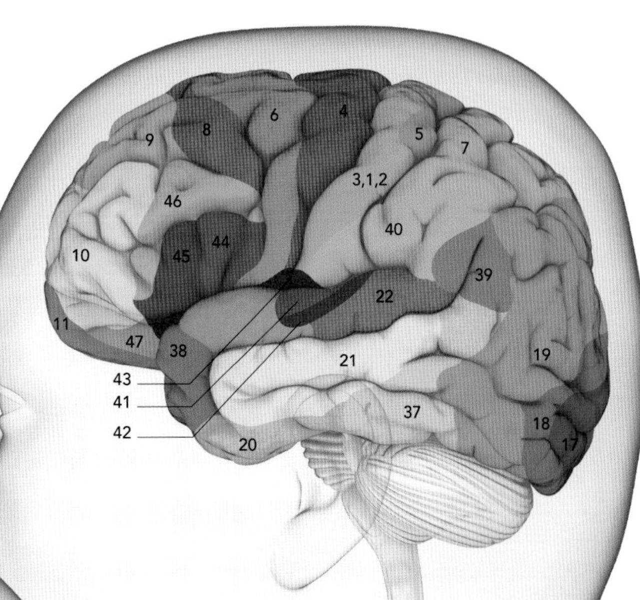

LATERAL BRODMANN AREAS
Korbinian Brodmann (see panel, below) created a map of the cortex based on the arrangement of nerve-cell bodies (soma). Several Brodmann areas extend from the lateral surface to the medial surface. Some areas are also commonly known by other names, such as areas 44 and 45, which is known as Broca's area.

MEDIAL BRODMANN AREAS
On the medial surface of the right cortex, these areas directly face their counterparts on the left medial cortex. Area 38 extends underneath the brain, from the medial surface to the lateral surface. It is an important junctional zone that links areas associated with hearing, vision, memory, and emotional awareness and reactions.

APPROXIMATE FUNCTIONS

AUDITION
Temporal lobe
22, 41, 38, 42

BODY SENSATION
Parietal lobe
1, 2, 3; 5, 39, 7, 40, 31

EMOTION
Anterior cingulate and orbital cortex
11, 32, 12, 33, 24, 38, 25

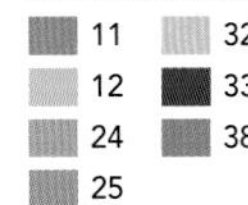

GUSTATION
Insula
43

OLFACTION
Medial temporal cortex
28, 34

MEMORY
Medial temporal lobe, posterior cingulate cortex
23, 30, 26, 35, 27, 36, 29

MOTOR
Frontal lobe
4, 44, 6, 45, 8, 46, 9, 47, 10

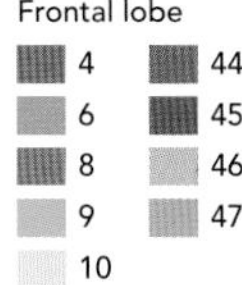

VISION
Occipital cortex and temporal cortex
17, 21, 18, 37, 19, 38, 20

KORBINIAN BRODMANN

A German neurologist, Brodmann (1868–1918) made a detailed study of the cortex, looking at the way its layers, tissues, and individual neurons and other cells vary in their structure and size. He identified and numbered different areas in the brains of humans, monkeys, and other mammals, ending the considerable confusion in naming parts of the cortex that existed at the time.

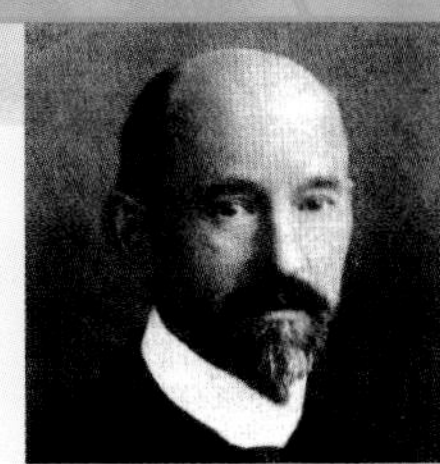

ASSOCIATION AREAS

Some parts of the cortex, called association areas, are composed of neurons that are connected to two or more functional areas. This means that they receive different types of information: for example, visual and auditory. Their role is to combine this information. It is part of the construction process that allows us to see the world as an integrated whole rather than discrete bits. The adjoining edges of the visual and parietal areas, for example, combine visual information with body awareness to work out the position of a visually perceived object in relation to the body. The frontal cortex may be considered an association area as it receives information from all other areas of the brain and combines it. The product of this mix is thoughts, judgements, and conscious feelings.

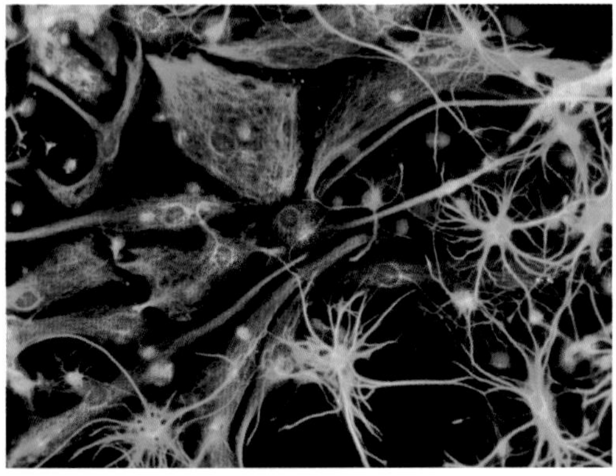

GLIAL CELLS
In this light micrograph, star-shaped astrocytes (lighter green) can be seen along with other support cells, or neuroglia. They make up the brain's connective tissue and provide protection to neurons. Connective tissue supports the neurons transmitting information between cortical areas.

Frontal lobes
The front of the brain gathers input from all other areas to produce complex cognition including thoughts, judgements, and long-term plans

Orbito-frontal cortex
Input from the limbic system is combined with other information here to create values used in decision-making

INCOMING INFORMATION
Association areas receive input from various parts of the brain and combine it to form – or start to form – complex, multifaceted perceptions.

STRUCTURE OF THE CORTEX

The highly convoluted sheet of grey matter that constitutes the cerebral cortex varies in thickness from about 2 to 5mm (1/16 to 3/16 in). Estimates of its cell numbers vary from 10 billion to more than 50 billion neurons and about five to ten times this number of glial (supporting) and other cells. The neurons are organized into six layers, known generally from the outside inwards as the molecular, external granular, external pyramidal, internal granular, internal pyramidal, and multiform layers (see opposite). Each Brodmann area (see p.67) also has distinct types and shapes of neurons. For example, primary motor area 4 is rich in pyramidal cells. The neurons in the cortex are arranged with the body of the cell on top and axons below. The body is greyish, while axons are coated with fat (myelin) and look whitish. This accounts for the grey colour that distinguishes the cortex from internal brain areas.

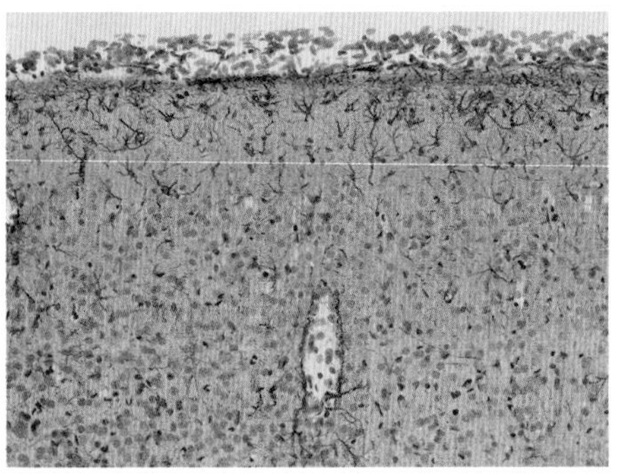

CORTEX TISSUE

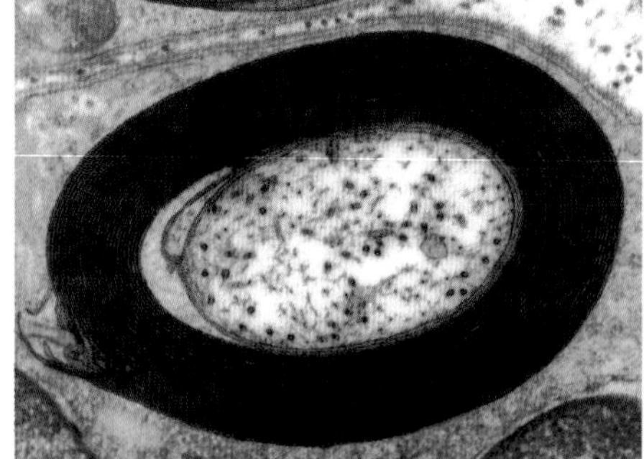

NERVE FIBRE

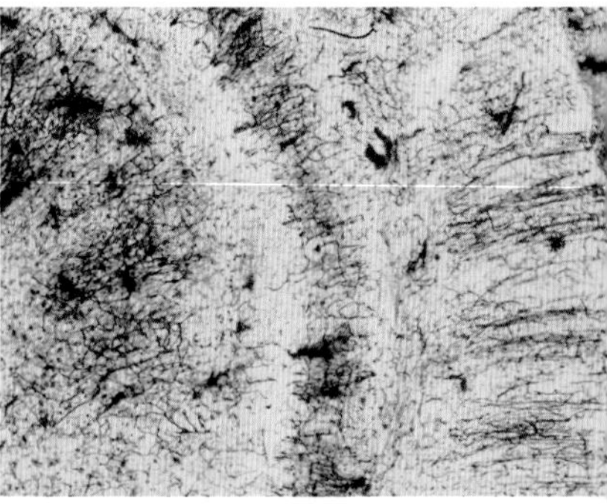

CEREBRAL LAYERS

Parietal lobes
Inputs arrive here from visual, auditory, and emotional areas to produce body-centred understanding of the current environment

Temporo-parietal junction
This area puts together perceptual information to give a "whole" knowledge of what is happening at any moment

Cerebellum
The back of the brain combines input from perceptual areas to guide fine motor actions

CORTICAL FUNCTIONING

Most of the human cortex comprises six layers, each of which contains a distinct pattern of neuron types. Cortical neurons receive and send signals to other brain areas, including other parts of the cortex. This to and fro of messages keeps all parts of the brain aware of what is going on elsewhere. Neurons in the cortex are "head down" – their receiving parts (dendrites) point up to the surface, while threads that carry messages to other cells (axons) are oriented down. Some axons extend below the cortex and form part of the "white matter" – connective tissue that carries information to distant brain areas. Other axons travel through the lower layers of cortex to connect with other cortical cells.

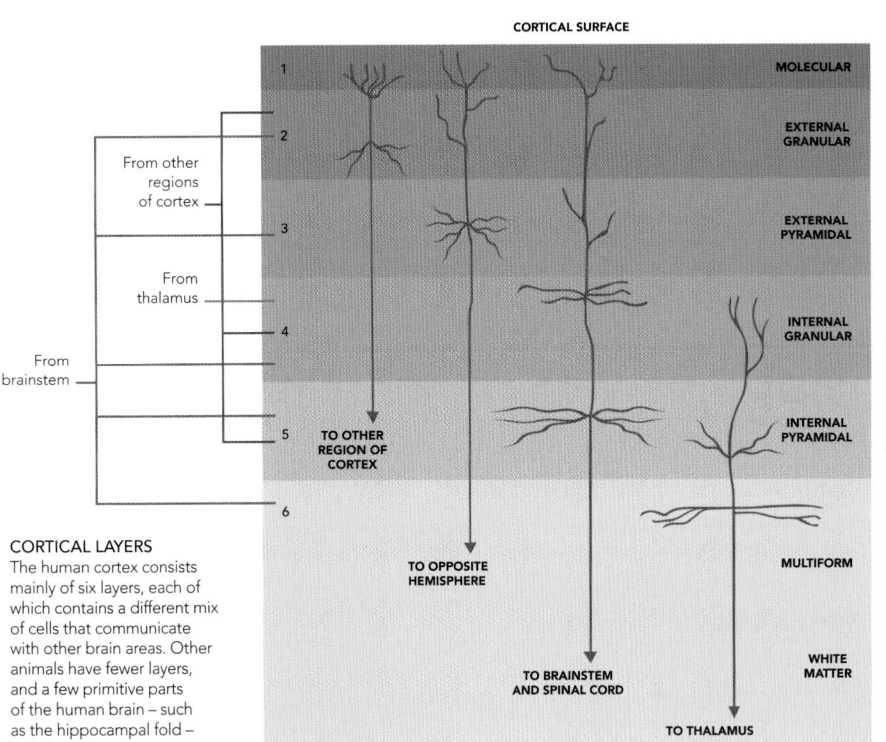

CORTICAL LAYERS
The human cortex consists mainly of six layers, each of which contains a different mix of cells that communicate with other brain areas. Other animals have fewer layers, and a few primitive parts of the human brain – such as the hippocampal fold – have just three.

THE FOLDED BRAIN

The scrunched-up structure of the cortex is one of the features that distinguishes the human brain most clearly from that of other species. Most of the cortical surface is tucked into grooves, and if it could be flattened out, it would cover the size of a small tablecloth. The dense cortical folding seen in humans may have evolved along with the shift from walking on all fours to bipedalism. To allow an upright stance, our ancestors evolved a narrow pelvis, which hampered childbirth. It might be that babies with small heads were more likely to survive, and that their head size was due to a genetic mutation that caused the brain to fold up, allowing the skull to stay relatively small. Apart from packing in more neurons, cortical folding creates shorter nerve pathways, which in turn create faster data processing.

FLAT CORTEX
Computer software can "flatten" the surface of a brain to show the tissue that is normally hidden in the sulci. Here the green areas are the surface (gyri) and the red areas are those normally tucked inside.

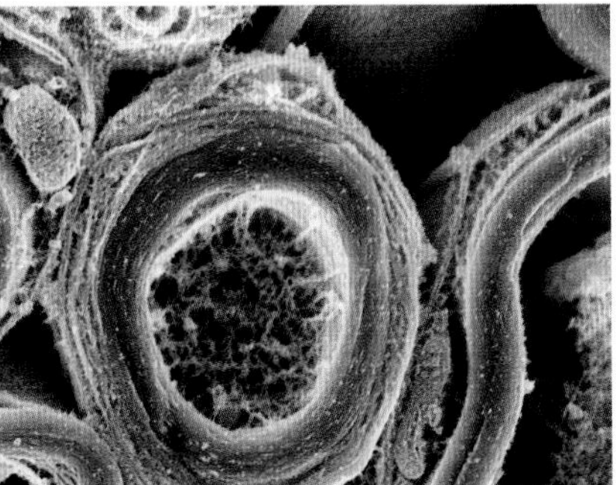

OLIGODENDROCYTE CELL

CORTEX COMPONENTS
Relatively low magnification of cortical tissue shows neurons (far left, blue-grey) packed among supporting glial cells (red). Higher magnification reveals an individual axon at the cortex base (second from left). Different laboratory stains show four of the six cortical layers (third from left) and fatty myelin wrapped around an axon.

BRAIN CELLS

THERE ARE OVER A THOUSAND TYPES OF BRAIN CELL, WHICH FALL INTO TWO BROAD GROUPS: NEURONS AND GLIAL CELLS. NEURONS SEND ELECTRICAL SIGNALS, OR "FIRE", IN RESPONSE TO STIMULI. THERE ARE ABOUT 86 BILLION NEURONS IN AN AVERAGE HUMAN BRAIN AND TEN TIMES AS MANY GLIAL CELLS.

NEURONS

Like hepatocyte cells in the liver, osteocytes in bone, or erythrocytes (red cells) in blood, each neuron is a self-contained functioning unit. Its internal components, the organelles, include a nucleus harbouring the genetic material (DNA), energy-providing mitochondria, and protein-making ribosomes. As in most other types of cells, the organelles are concentrated in the main cell body. In addition, characteristic features of neurons are neurites – long, thin, finger- or thread-like extensions from the cell body (soma). There are two main types: dendrites and axons. Usually dendrites receive nerve signals, while axons send them onwards.

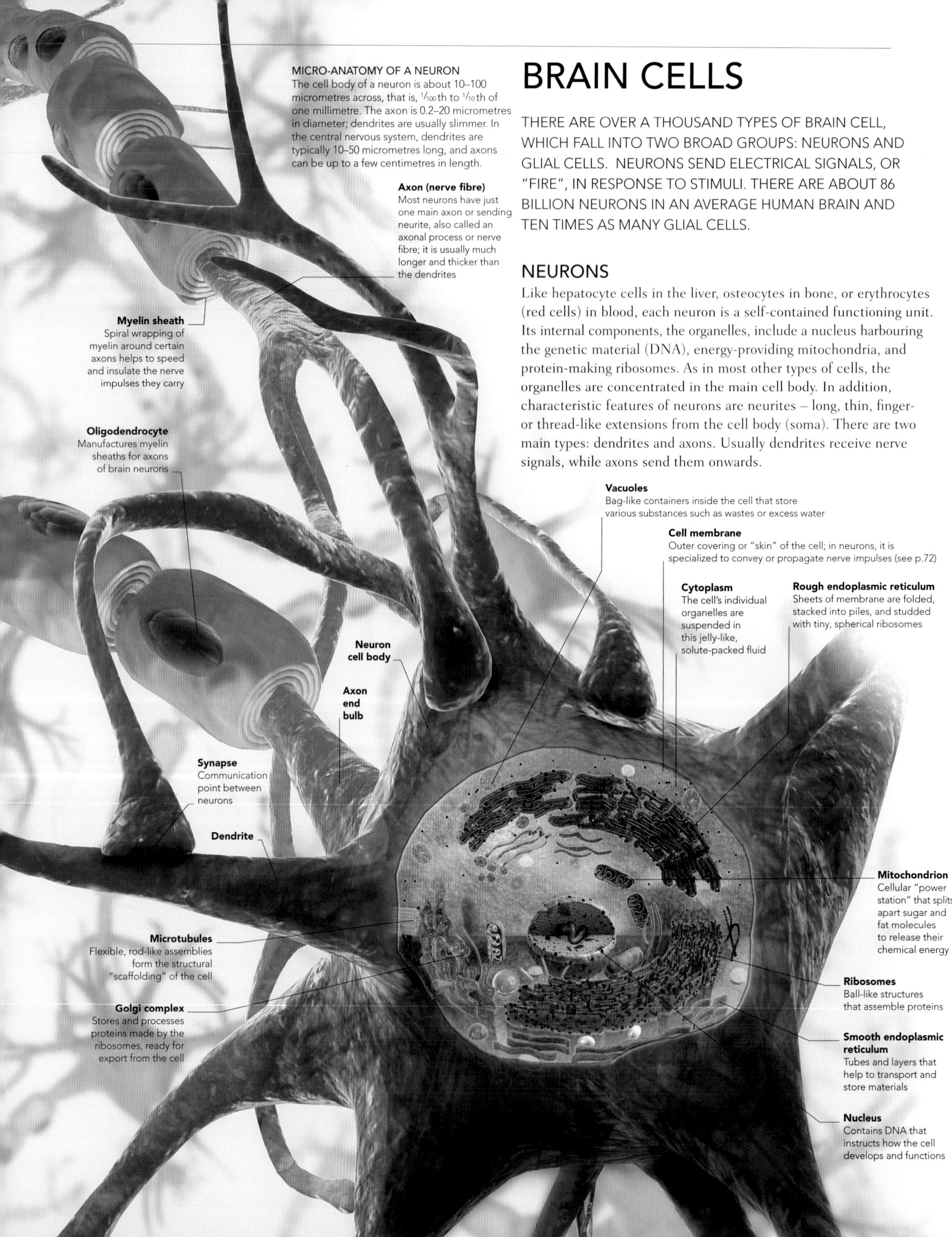

Axon (nerve fibre)
Most neurons have just one main axon or sending neurite, also called an axonal process or nerve fibre; it is usually much longer and thicker than the dendrites
Myelin sheath
Spiral wrapping of myelin around certain axons helps to speed and insulate the nerve impulses they carry
Oligodendrocyte
Manufactures myelin sheaths for axons of brain neurons
Neuron cell body
Axon end bulb
Synapse
Communication point between neurons
Dendrite
Microtubules
Flexible, rod-like assemblies form the structural "scaffolding" of the cell
Golgi complex
Stores and processes proteins made by the ribosomes, ready for export from the cell
Vacuoles
Bag-like containers inside the cell that store various substances such as wastes or excess water
Cell membrane
Outer covering or "skin" of the cell; in neurons, it is specialized to convey or propagate nerve impulses (see p.72)
Cytoplasm
The cell's individual organelles are suspended in this jelly-like, solute-packed fluid
Rough endoplasmic reticulum
Sheets of membrane are folded, stacked into piles, and studded with tiny, spherical ribosomes
Mitochondrion
Cellular "power station" that splits apart sugar and fat molecules to release their chemical energy
Ribosomes
Ball-like structures that assemble proteins
Smooth endoplasmic reticulum
Tubes and layers that help to transport and store materials
Nucleus
Contains DNA that instructs how the cell develops and functions

MICRO-ANATOMY OF A NEURON
The cell body of a neuron is about 10–100 micrometres across, that is, $\frac{1}{100}$th to $\frac{1}{10}$th of one millimetre. The axon is 0.2–20 micrometres in diameter; dendrites are usually slimmer. In the central nervous system, dendrites are typically 10–50 micrometres long, and axons can be up to a few centimetres in length.

TYPES OF NEURON

Neurons can be categorized structurally according to the location of the cell body in relation to the axon and dendrites, and also the number of dendrites and axon branches (see illustration, below). In some regions of the brain, peripheral nervous system, and sense organs, neuron types are organized and easily recognized. For example, the retina of the eye contains ranks of bipolar neurons (see p.80). However, in many other regions, the neurons are mixed in shape and form a complex, interconnected web. In the cortex, one neuron may receive signals from many thousands of other neurons via its multitudinous branching dendrites. Signals are conducted to the soma, around this, and then away along the axon – always by the cell membrane, not through the cytoplasm.

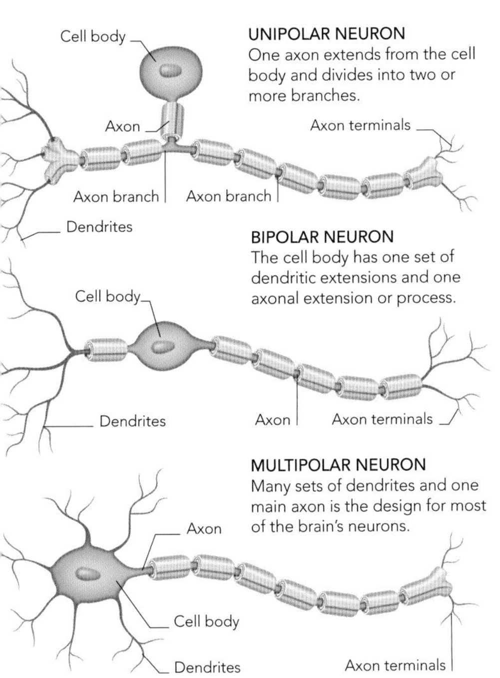

UNIPOLAR NEURON
One axon extends from the cell body and divides into two or more branches.

BIPOLAR NEURON
The cell body has one set of dendritic extensions and one axonal extension or process.

MULTIPOLAR NEURON
Many sets of dendrites and one main axon is the design for most of the brain's neurons.

NEURON REGENERATION

Each neuron has its own immensely complex, highly individual shape and sets of connections, via synapses, to other neurons. Its links are shaped by its history and how it is used over time, as some of its connections weaken and fade while others strengthen. This uniqueness makes any disease or damage very serious. The neuron is unlikely to reform all of its extensions and their links. Even if regrowth occurs, it is slow and at first random, as the dendrites and axon "feel" their way according to the nerve signals being received and sent.

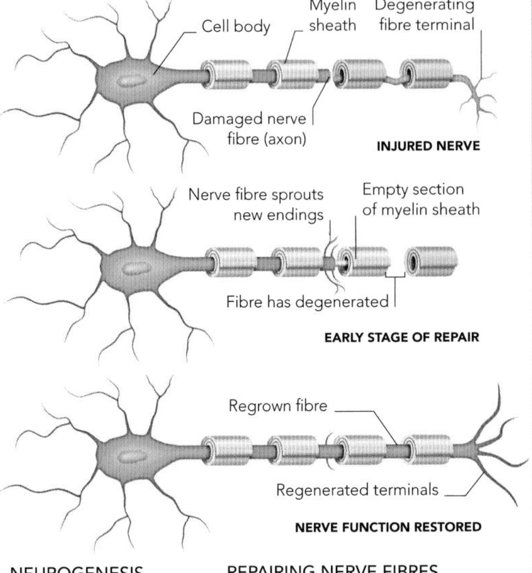

NEUROGENESIS
The brain can form new nerve cells. Neural progenitor cells (shown in this micrograph) are a stage in specialization between stem cells and fully formed nerve cells. At this stage they can specialize into neurons or support cells.

REPAIRING NERVE FIBRES
Nerve cell repair is a very slow process, if it occurs at all. The damaged or severed end of the axon (fibre) can be encouraged to send out new sprout growths by treating it with substances called nerve growth factors. A sprout that finds an empty myelin sheath may then grow through it.

GLIAL CELLS

Glial cells give physical support to neurons (glia means "glue" in Greek) but they are also thought to influence neurons' electrical activity. They provide physical support for the thin dendrites and axons that wind their way around the neural network, and supply nutrition for neurons in the form of sugars and raw materials for growth and repair. There are several types of glial cells. Oligodendrocytes make myelin sheathing, a task performed in peripheral nerves by Schwann cells. Microglia destroy invading microbes and clear up debris from degenerating neurons. Astrocytes are thought to affect neuronal behaviour and play a role in memory and sleep.

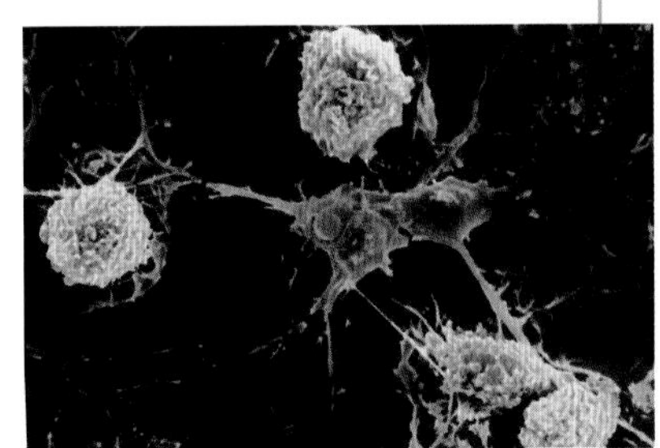

OLIGODENDROCYTES UNDER ATTACK
In multiple sclerosis (MS) oligodendrocytes (purple), which normally make insulating myelin sheaths around nerve axons in the brain and spinal cord, are attacked and destroyed by microglia (yellow).

SYNAPSES

Synapses are communication sites where neurons pass nerve impulses among themselves. Many neurons do not actually touch one another, but pass their signals via chemicals (neurotransmitters) across an incredibly thin gap, called the synaptic cleft (see p.72–73). Micro-anatomically, synapses are divided into types according to the sites where the neurons almost touch. These sites include the soma, dendrites, axons, and tiny narrow projections called dendritic spines found on certain kinds of dendrites (see illustration, right). Axospinodendritic synapses form more than 50 per cent of all synapses in the brain; axodendritic synapses constitute about 30 per cent.

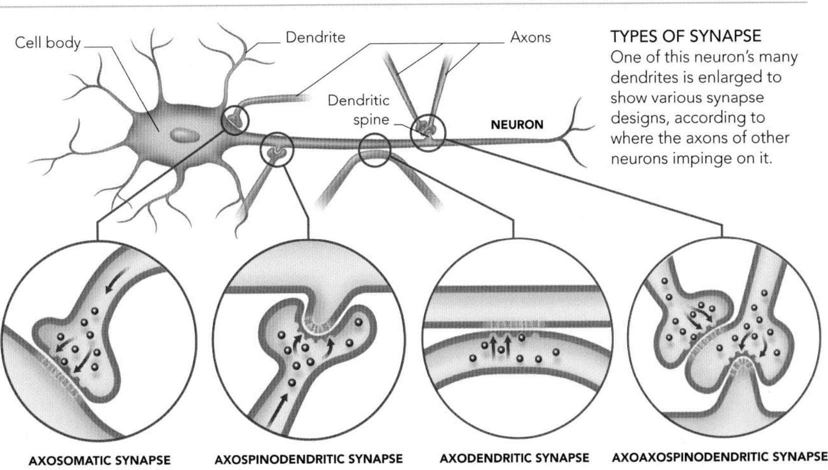

TYPES OF SYNAPSE
One of this neuron's many dendrites is enlarged to show various synapse designs, according to where the axons of other neurons impinge on it.

NERVE IMPULSES

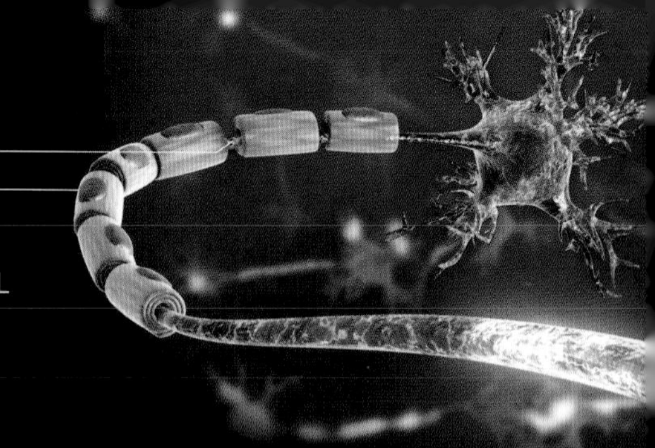

Neurofibral node

Myelin-coated internode

A NERVE IMPULSE OR SIGNAL CAN BE THOUGHT OF AS A TINY, BRIEF "SPIKE" OF ELECTRICITY TRAVELLING THROUGH A NEURON. AT A MORE FUNDAMENTAL LEVEL, IT CONSISTS OF CHEMICAL PARTICLES MOVING ACROSS THE CELL'S OUTER MEMBRANE, FROM ONE SIDE TO THE OTHER.

ANATOMY OF AN IMPULSE

Nerve signals are composed of series of discrete impulses, also known as action potentials. A single impulse is caused by a travelling "wave" of chemical particles called ions, which have electrical charges and are mainly the minerals sodium, potassium, and chloride. In the brain, and throughout the body, most impulses in most neurons are of the same strength – about 100 millivolts (0.1 volt). They are also of the same duration – around one millisecond ($^{1}/_{1,000}$ of a second) – but travel at varying speeds. The information they convey depends on how frequently they pass in terms of impulses per second, where they came from, and where they are heading.

SPEED OF CONDUCTION

Impulses travel at widely differing speeds, from 1 to more than 100m/s (3–330ft/s), depending on the type of nerve carrying them. They are fastest in myelinated axons. Here the impulse "jumps" rapidly between the myelin-coated sections from one gap (neurofibral node), to the next node.

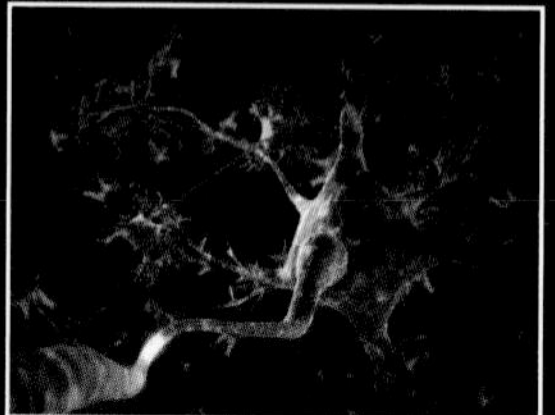

IMPULSE HEADS TOWARDS SYNAPSE

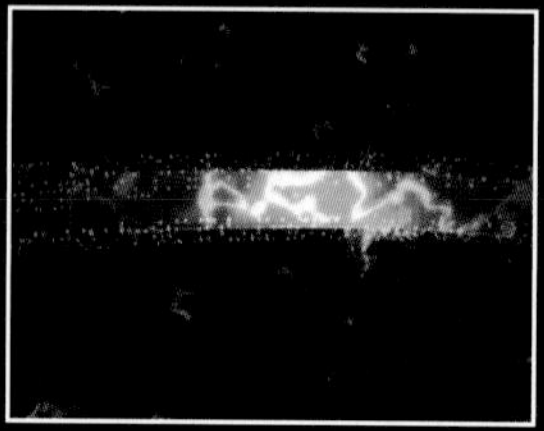

AXON IS POLARIZED AT REST

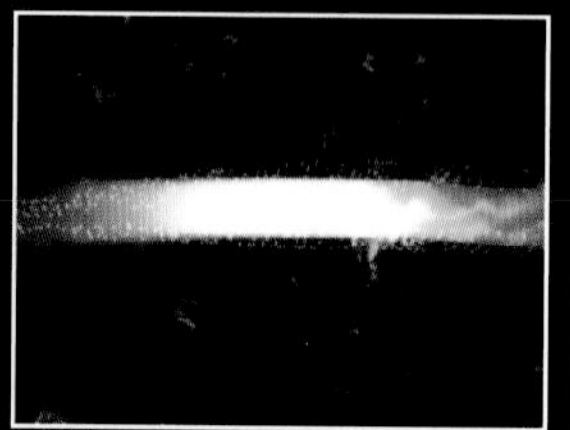

AXON DEPOLARIZES AS IMPULSE PASSES

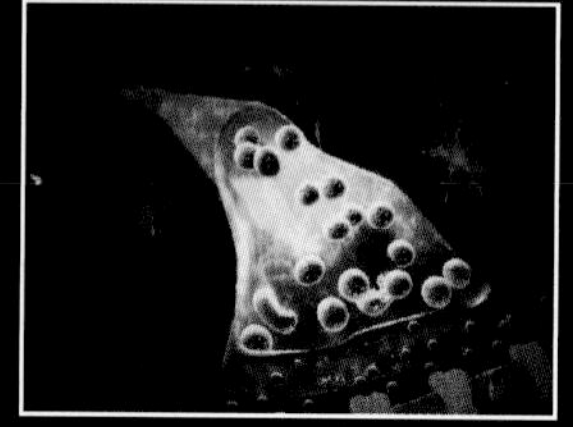

IMPULSE ARRIVES AT SYNAPSE

CHANGING FORM

A nerve impulse is always based on chemical particles. As it passes along a dendrite or axon, it consists of moving electrically charged ions, but at a synapse, it relies more on the structural shape of the chemical neurotransmitter.

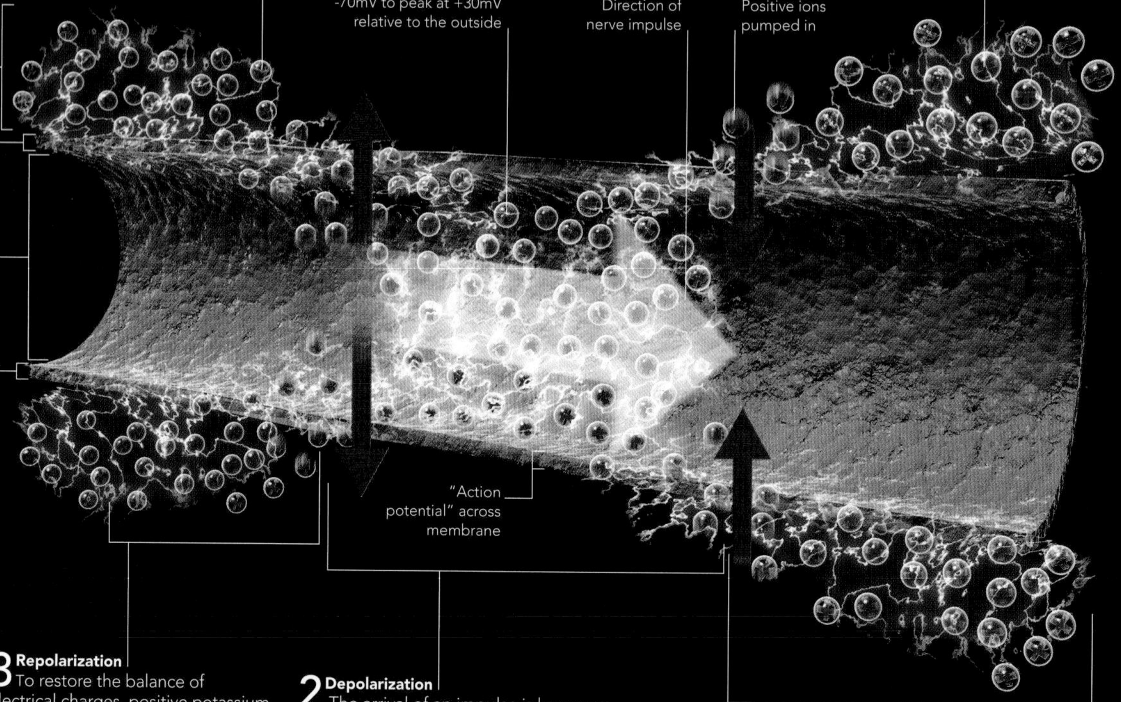

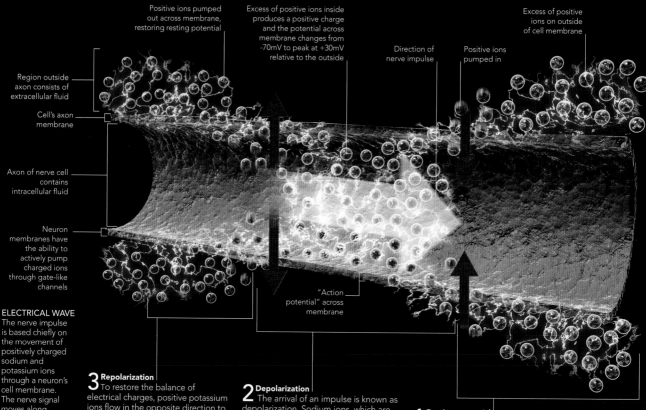

Positive ions pumped out across membrane, restoring resting potential

Excess of positive ions inside produces a positive charge and the potential across membrane changes from -70mV to peak at +30mV relative to the outside

Direction of nerve impulse

Positive ions pumped in

Excess of positive ions on outside of cell membrane

Region outside axon consists of extracellular fluid

Cell's axon membrane

Axon of nerve cell contains intracellular fluid

Neuron membranes have the ability to actively pump charged ions through gate-like channels

"Action potential" across membrane

ELECTRICAL WAVE

The nerve impulse is based chiefly on the movement of positively charged sodium and potassium ions through a neuron's cell membrane. The nerve signal moves along the membrane as a wave of depolarization and repolarization.

3 Repolarization To restore the balance of electrical charges, positive potassium ions flow in the opposite direction to the sodium ions. This stimulates adjacent areas of the membrane behind the depolarized area, disrupting their resting potentials.

2 Depolarization The arrival of an impulse is known as depolarization. Sodium ions, which are positive, flow quickly through sodium-ion channels in the neuron's axon membrane, from outside to inside. The inside is now positive compared to the outside.

1 Resting potential When no impulse is passing, there are more potassium and negative ions inside the neuron's axon membrane, and more sodium and other positive ions outside. This causes a polarization or difference in electrical potential across the membrane, with the outside positive.

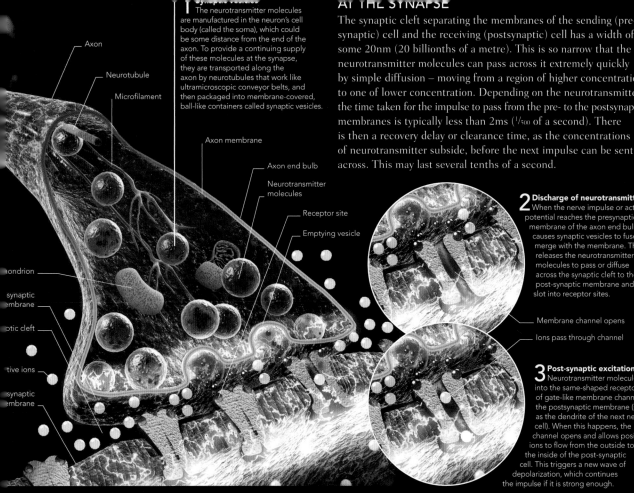

1 The neurotransmitter molecules are manufactured in the neuron's cell body (called the soma), which could be some distance from the end of the axon. To provide a continuing supply of these molecules at the synapse, they are transported along the axon by neurotubules that work like ultramicroscopic conveyor belts, and then packaged into membrane-covered, ball-like containers called synaptic vesicles.

AT THE SYNAPSE

The synaptic cleft separating the membranes of the sending (presynaptic) cell and the receiving (postsynaptic) cell has a width of some 20nm (20 billionths of a metre). This is so narrow that the neurotransmitter molecules can pass across it extremely quickly by simple diffusion – moving from a region of higher concentration to one of lower concentration. Depending on the neurotransmitter, the time taken for the impulse to pass from the pre- to the postsynaptic membranes is typically less than 2ms ($^1/_{500}$ of a second). There is then a recovery delay or clearance time, as the concentrations of neurotransmitter subside, before the next impulse can be sent across. This may last several tenths of a second.

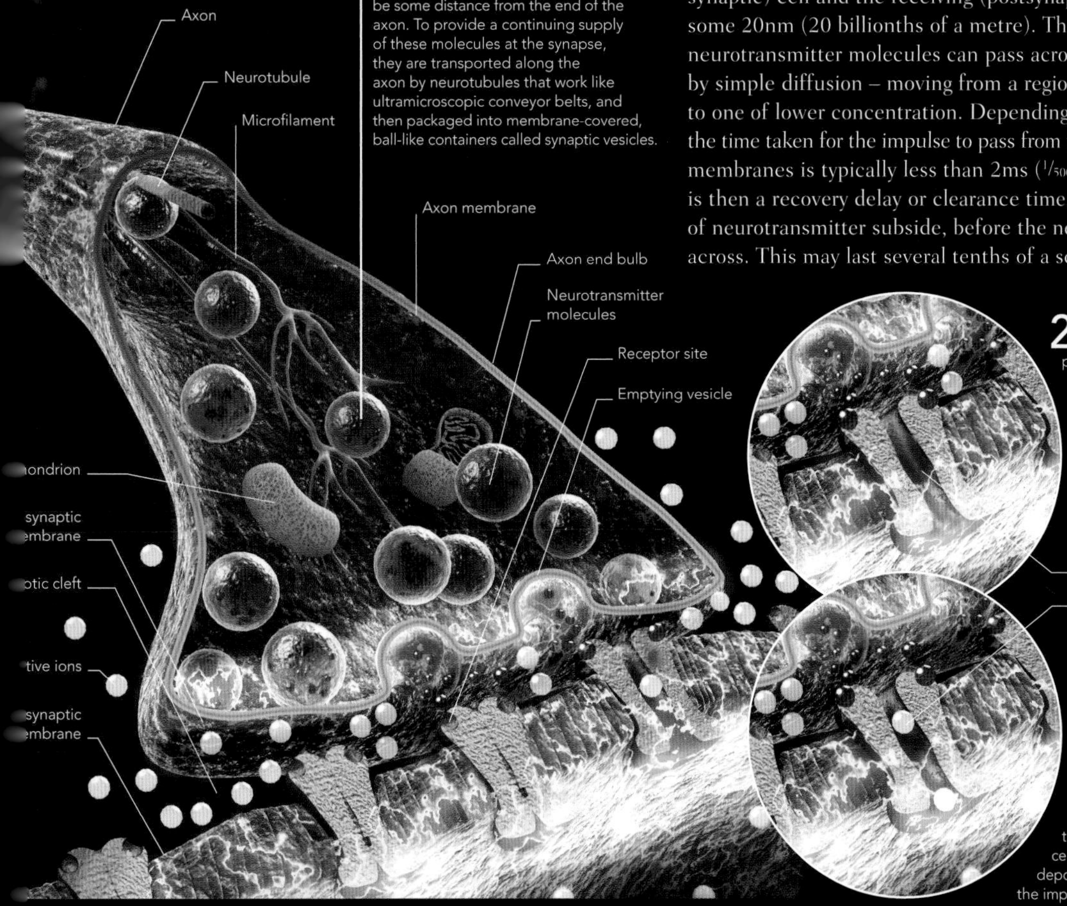

Axon

Neurotubule

Microfilament

Axon membrane

Axon end bulb

Neurotransmitter molecules

Receptor site

Emptying vesicle

ondrion

synaptic embrane

otic cleft

tive ions

synaptic embrane

2 Discharge of neurotransmitter When the nerve impulse or action potential reaches the presynaptic membrane of the axon end bulb, it causes synaptic vesicles to fuse or merge with the membrane. This releases the neurotransmitter molecules to pass or diffuse across the synaptic cleft to the post-synaptic membrane and slot into receptor sites.

Membrane channel opens

Ions pass through channel

3 Post-synaptic excitation Neurotransmitter molecules slot into the same-shaped receptor sites of gate-like membrane channels in the postsynaptic membrane (such as the dendrite of the next nerve cell). When this happens, the channel opens and allows positive ions to flow from the outside to the inside of the post-synaptic cell. This triggers a new wave of depolarization, which continues the impulse if it is strong enough.

NEUROTRANSMITTERS

Neurotransmitters are chemicals that allow signals to pass between a neuron and another cell. There are several groups of neurotransmitter molecules. One contains only acetylcholine. A second is known as biogenic amines, or monoamines, and includes dopamine, histamine, noradrenaline, and serotonin. The third group is composed of amino acids, such as GABA, glutamic acid, aspartic acid, and glycine. Many of these substances have other roles in the body. For example, histamine is involved in the inflammatory response. Amino acids (apart from GABA) are also very common, being the building blocks for hundreds of kinds of protein molecules.

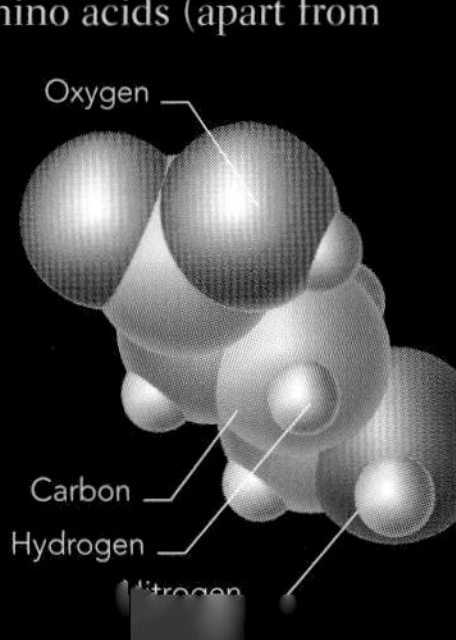

GABA MOLECULE
GABA is the chief inhibitory neurotransmitter throughout much of the human brain and nervous system.

SMALL MOLECULE NEUROTRANSMITTERS

Several common examples of neurotransmitters are listed together with their typical effects at synapses.

NEUROTRANSMITTER CHEMICAL NAME	USUAL POST-SYNAPTIC EFFECT
Acetylcholine	Mostly excitatory
Gamma-aminobutyric acid (GABA)	Inhibitory
Glycine	Inhibitory
Glutamate	Excitatory
Aspartate	Excitatory
Dopamine	Excitatory and inhibitory
Noradrenaline	Mostly excitatory
Serotonin	Inhibitory
Histamine	Excitatory

EXCITATION AND INHIBITION

A particular neurotransmitter can either excite a receiving nerve cell, helping to depolarize the axon hillock (where the soma and axon meet) and continue a nerve impulse, or inhibit it by preventing depolarization from taking place. Which of

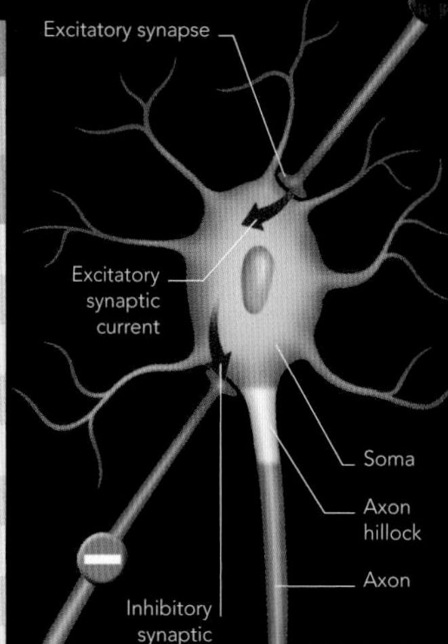

FIRE OR NOT?
Whether a receiving nerve cell "fires" a new impulse depends on the balance of the excitatory and inhibitory currents.

BRAIN MAPPING AND SIMULATION

CREATING AN ARTIFICIAL BRAIN IS A LONG-HELD DREAM, AND STEPS ARE BEING MADE TO MAKE IT POSSIBLE THANKS TO ADVANCES IN COMPUTER POWER. TWO GLOBAL PROJECTS ARE NOW UNDERWAY TO REPRODUCE A DIGITAL SIMULATION OF THE HUMAN ORGAN. IF THIS IS ACHIEVED IT WILL EFFECTIVELY BE A BRAIN, ALTHOUGH WHETHER IT WILL BE CONSCIOUS AND WHAT SORT OF EXPERIENCE IT MIGHT HAVE ARE UNKNOWN.

THE CONNECTOME

The connections between neurons form the "wiring" of the brain, and in order to recreate a working simulation it is essential to know in detail the route taken by information passing from one neuron to another. A global initiative called the Connectome project charts these pathways using a form of MRI scanning called diffusion tensor imaging. The connecting fibres of the brain are skeins of myelin-coated axons, which snake out from one cell to contact another. The overall pattern of neural pathways is similar in all of us, but differs in detail from person to person. It is these differences that make each of us unique. For instance, someone with relatively few pathways from their amygdala – the area deep in the brain that generates fear – to their prefrontal cortex is likely to be less nervous than someone whose neural wiring allows their forebrain to be deluged by doom alerts from the amygdala.

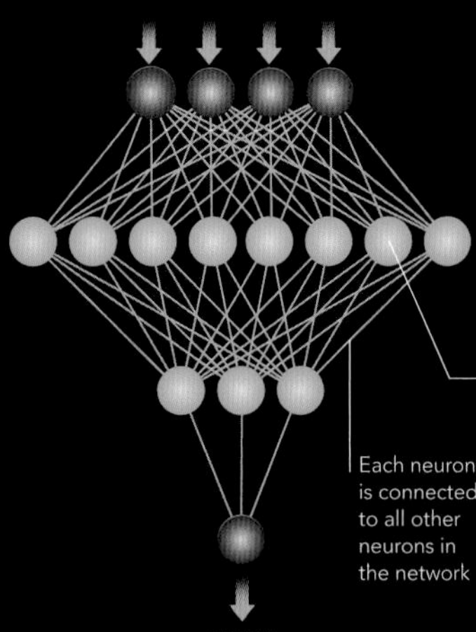

NEAT THEORY
Neural networks are a neat theoretical model of how the brain works. The virtual neurons form a mini-brain. When data is fed into the system, it changes in a way thought to be similar to the physical brain. Connections of different strengths are formed between all the neurons in the network.

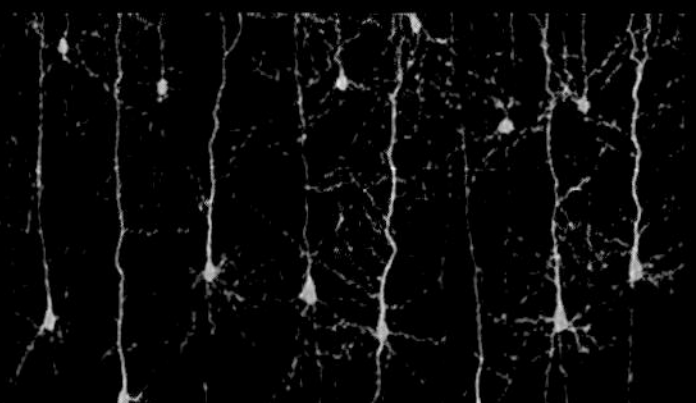

COMPLEX WEB
This image of cells in a minute section of neocortex reveals that the network of fibres in the brain is incredibly complex. To produce a model of a brain that really behaves like a human one involves tracing each and every fibre.

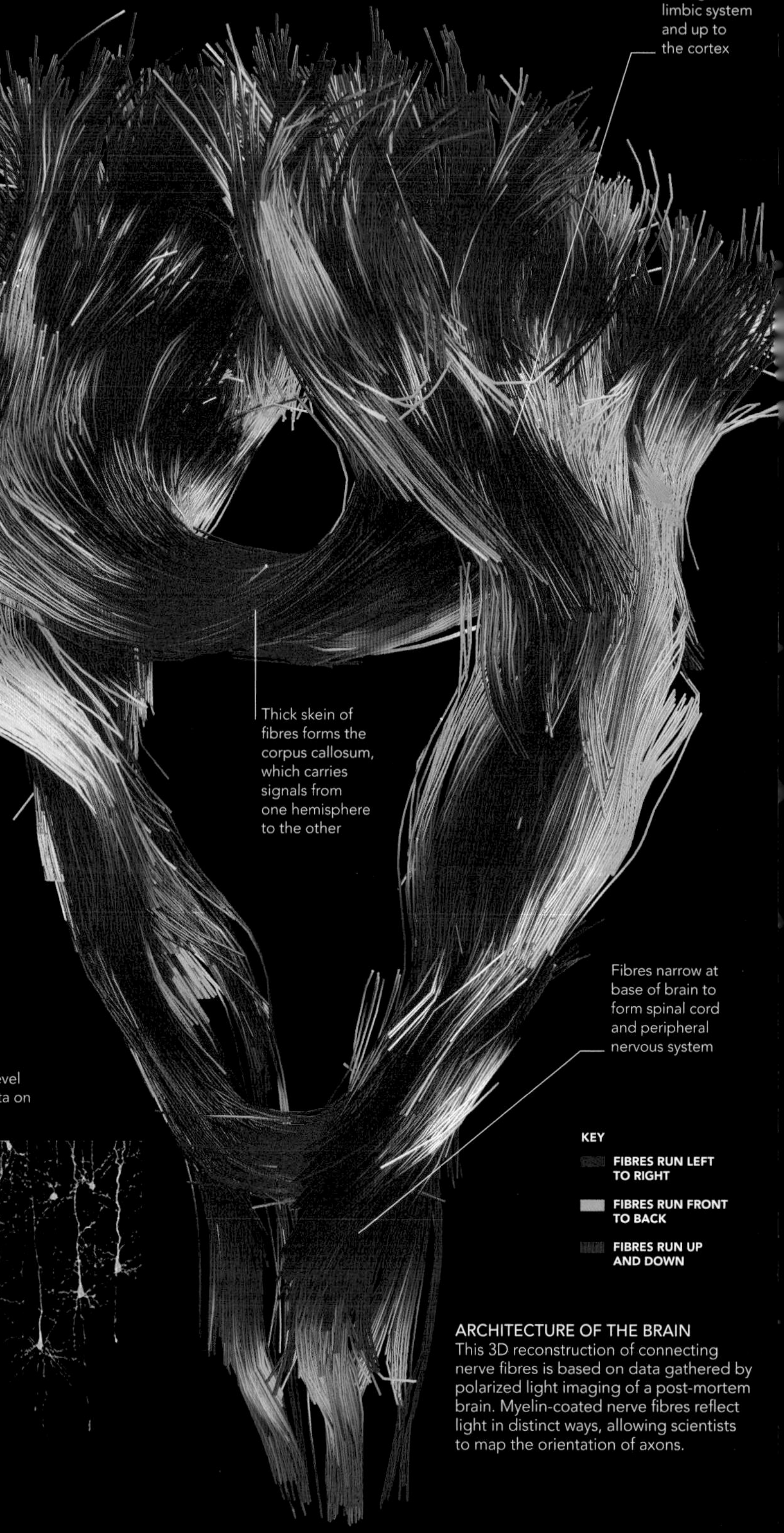

ARCHITECTURE OF THE BRAIN
This 3D reconstruction of connecting nerve fibres is based on data gathered by polarized light imaging of a post-mortem brain. Myelin-coated nerve fibres reflect light in distinct ways, allowing scientists to map the orientation of axons.

MAKING A BRAIN

Researchers are working on digital simulations of the brain by mapping its electrical circuitry, then modelling it by substituting electrical devices for biological mechanisms (see below). An electrical brain is unlikely to be conscious or to fulfil all the functions of a real brain because it would need to be embedded in a body and exist in an environment in which to learn. Nor does it include non-electrical elements, such as hormones.

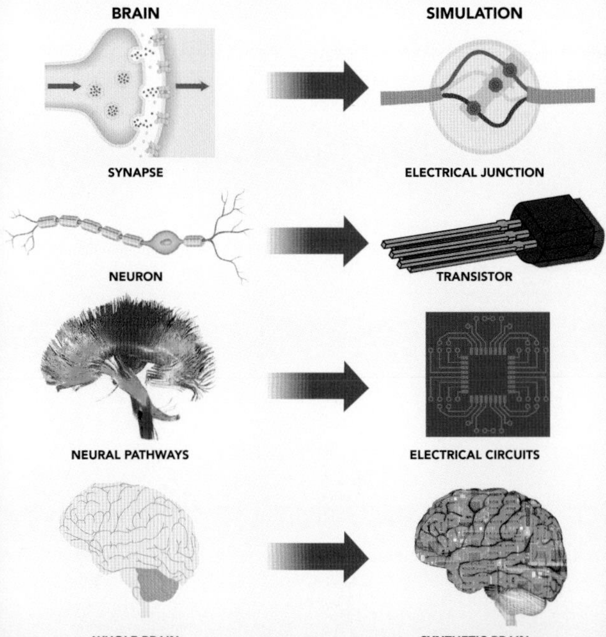

DIGITAL MODELLING

The biggest challenge facing neuroscientists is to simulate an entire human brain. The current approach is to identify every neuron in a normal brain and trace the connections between them. Bit by bit, the entire organ and its wiring will be determined and the information converted to a digital model, which will be stored on supercomputers. The system could then be run on demand, fed by digital input that mimics sensations triggered by the environment. This should, in theory, function like a real brain. In Europe, this mammoth task is being undertaken by the European Union flagship Human Brain Project (HBP), and a similar endeavour, Brain Research through Advancing Innovative Neurotechnologies (BRAIN), is underway in the USA.

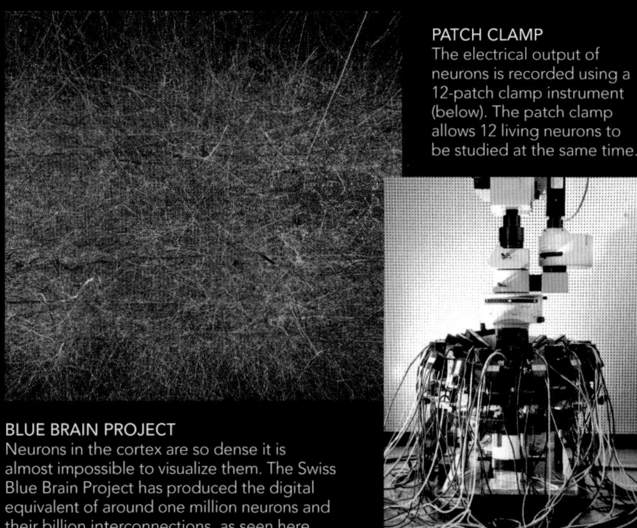

PATCH CLAMP
The electrical output of neurons is recorded using a 12-patch clamp instrument (below). The patch clamp allows 12 living neurons to be studied at the same time.

BLUE BRAIN PROJECT
Neurons in the cortex are so dense it is almost impossible to visualize them. The Swiss Blue Brain Project has produced the digital equivalent of around one million neurons and their billion interconnections, as seen here.

THE SELF-BUILD BRAIN

Another approach to brain simulation is to let a virtual brain grow digitally. The idea is to create a neural network – a system of computer-based information nodes organized to communicate with one another – that will restructure itself as it receives new data. NeuraBASE, for example, is a computer-based artificial-intelligence system that starts with virtual motor and sensory neurons, each of which responds to an element of information. Real-life stimuli are fed into the system, much as the brain is fed with experiences through the senses. The neurons in NeuraBASE form associations like neurons in the brain do. The virtual links form networks that become denser as more stimuli is fed in, just as biological brains learn through experience. Given enough computer resources NeuraBASE could in theory grow itself to function like a brain.

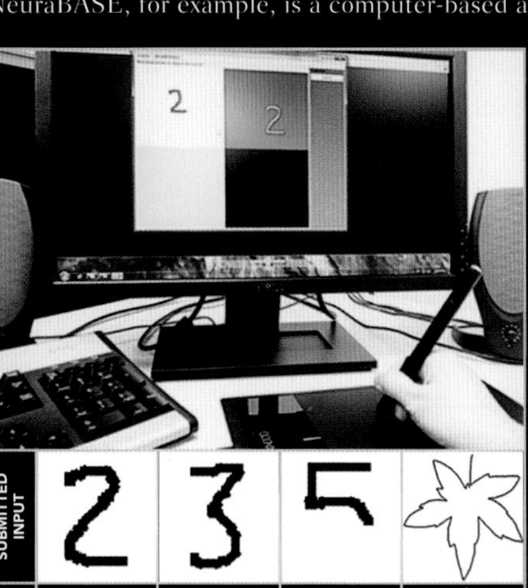

LEARNING PROGRAMME
NeuraBASE learns to recognize hand-drawn figures and reproduce them. It does not just copy the input but, like a human brain, it recognizes the idea encapsulated in the input even when – like the 5 here – it is incomplete.

AUTOMATA

Attempts to replicate brain-like systems go back a long way. Automata – apparently driven by internal intelligence – were popular entertainments in the 18th century and are the forerunners of today's robots. Lifelike figures had hidden clockwork mechanisms. These moved their limbs and allowed them to carry out seemingly intelligent actions like writing. Although the workings of such mechanical "brains" seem crude today, the idea – to make an artificial system that functions like a human being – is the same as that driving today's huge projects.

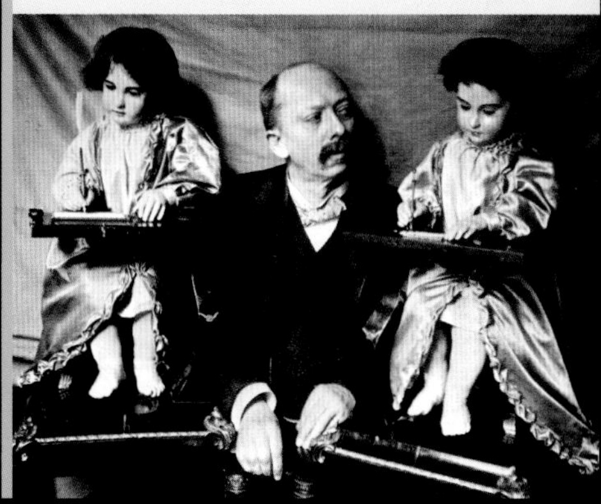

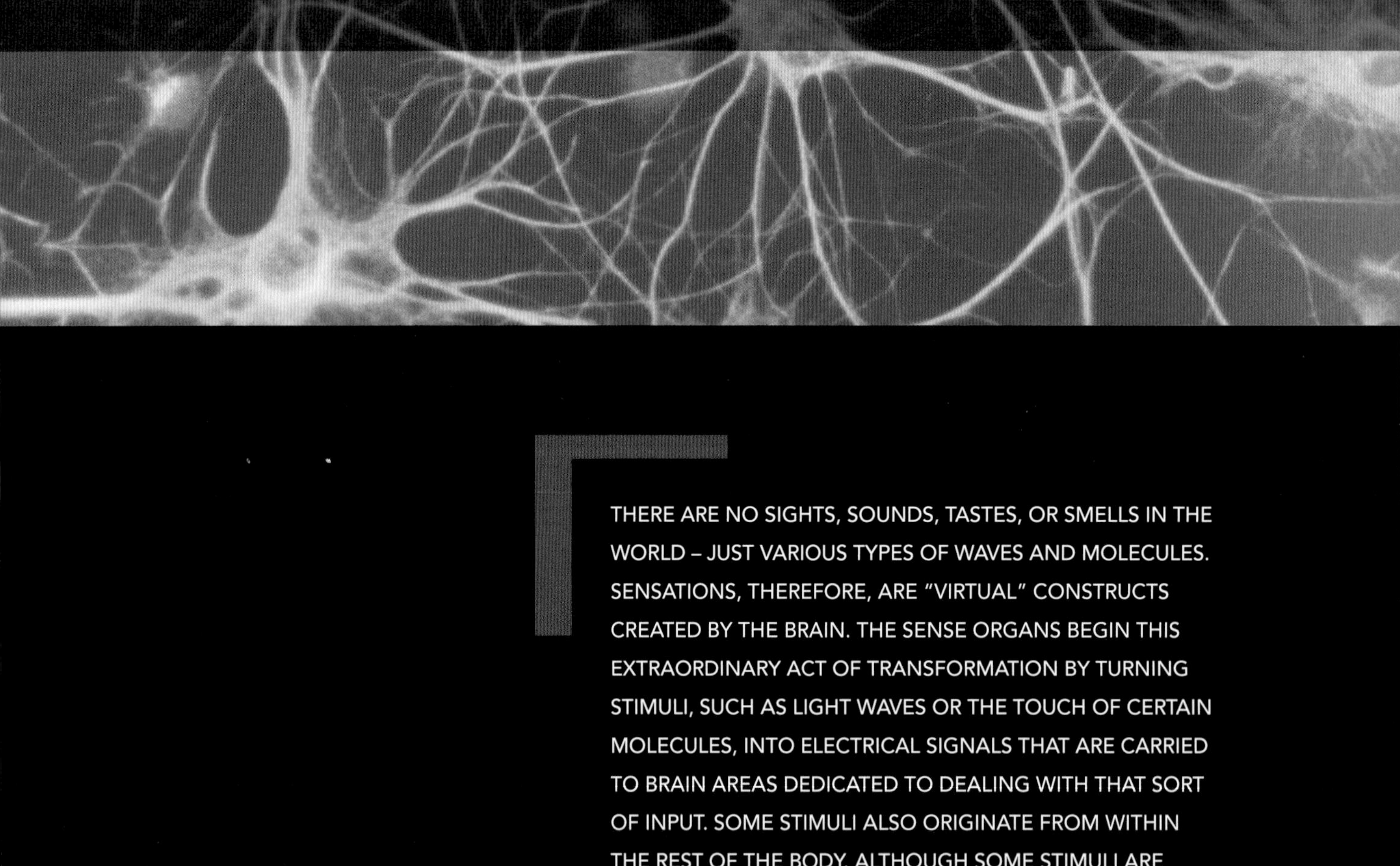

THERE ARE NO SIGHTS, SOUNDS, TASTES, OR SMELLS IN THE WORLD – JUST VARIOUS TYPES OF WAVES AND MOLECULES. SENSATIONS, THEREFORE, ARE "VIRTUAL" CONSTRUCTS CREATED BY THE BRAIN. THE SENSE ORGANS BEGIN THIS EXTRAORDINARY ACT OF TRANSFORMATION BY TURNING STIMULI, SUCH AS LIGHT WAVES OR THE TOUCH OF CERTAIN MOLECULES, INTO ELECTRICAL SIGNALS THAT ARE CARRIED TO BRAIN AREAS DEDICATED TO DEALING WITH THAT SORT OF INPUT. SOME STIMULI ALSO ORIGINATE FROM WITHIN THE REST OF THE BODY. ALTHOUGH SOME STIMULI ARE

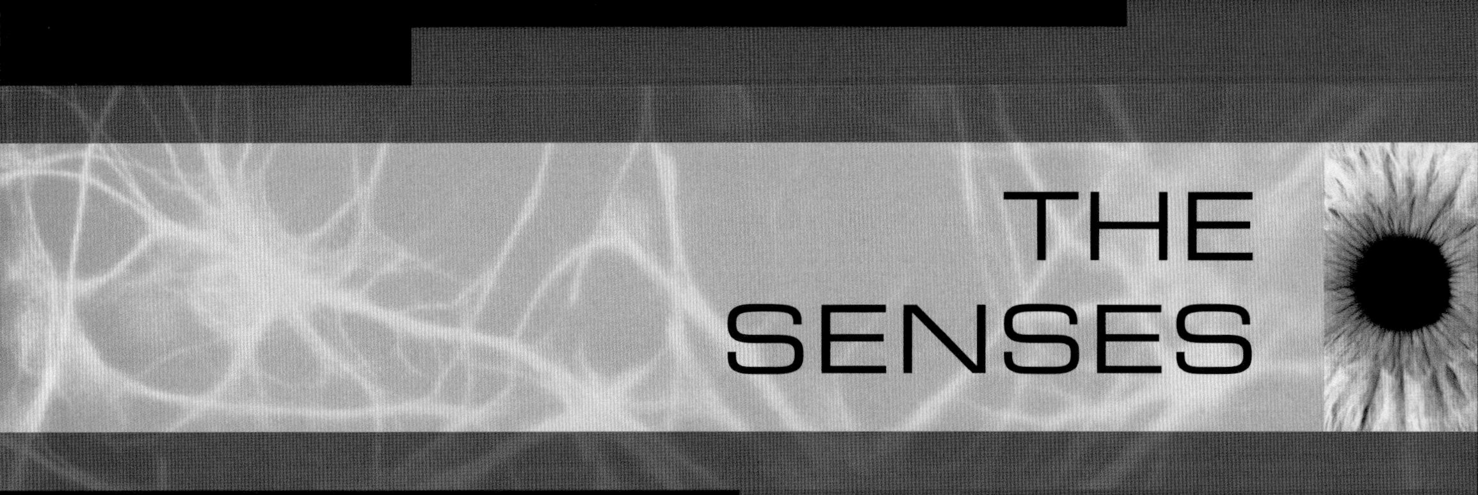

THE SENSES

HOW WE SENSE THE WORLD

THE BRAIN REACHES OUT TO THE ENVIRONMENT VIA OUR SENSE ORGANS, WHICH RESPOND TO VARIOUS STIMULI SUCH AS LIGHT, SOUND WAVES, AND PRESSURE. THE INFORMATION IS TRANSMITTED AS ELECTRICAL SIGNALS TO SPECIALIZED AREAS OF THE CEREBRAL CORTEX (THE OUTER LAYER OF THE CEREBRUM) TO BE PROCESSED INTO SENSATIONS SUCH AS VISION, HEARING, AND TOUCH.

MIXED SENSES

Sensory neurons respond to data from specific sense organs. Visual cortical neurons, for example, are most sensitive to signals from the eyes. But this specialization is not rigid. Visual neurons have been found to respond more strongly to weak light signals if accompanied by sound, suggesting they are activated by data from the ears as well as the eyes. What you see also influences what you hear. In a phenomenon known as the McGurk effect, if someone says "ba", while you watch someone mouthing "ga", you hear a third sound, "da". This is the brain's attempt to make sense of conflicting inputs. Other studies show that in people who are blind or deaf, some neurons that would normally process visual or auditory stimuli are "hijacked" by the other senses. For example, the visual cortex is used for touch in blind people.

HEARING PERSON PROCESSES SPEECH	DEAF PERSON PROCESSES SIGNING
LEFT SIDE OF BRAIN	LEFT SIDE OF BRAIN
RIGHT SIDE OF BRAIN	RIGHT SIDE OF BRAIN

"HEARING" WITHOUT SOUND
These fMRI scans of human brains show some sensory neurons that are activated by speech in hearing people being used in deaf people to process sign language.

SYNAESTHESIA

Most people are aware of only a single sensation in response to one type of stimulus. For example, sound waves make noise. But some people experience more than one sensation in response to a single stimulus. They may "see" sounds as well as hear them, or "taste" images. Called synaesthesia, this sensory duplication occurs when the neural pathway from a sense organ diverges and carries data on a type of stimulus to a part of the brain that normally processes another type.

NUMBER TEST
Some synaesthetes see numbers as having different colours. This enables them to see variations in shape (bottom) that are normally difficult to detect.

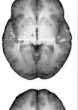

CONTROL GROUP | SYNAESTHETES

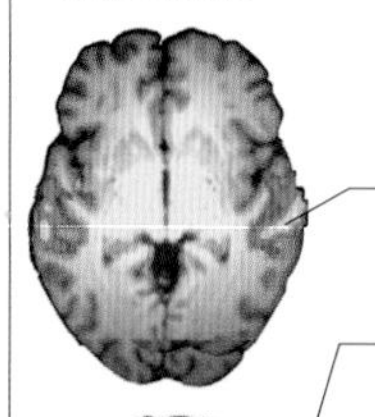

Larger area responds to sounds

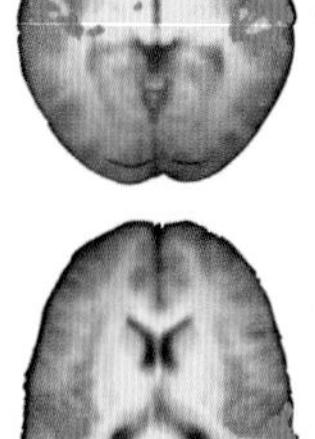

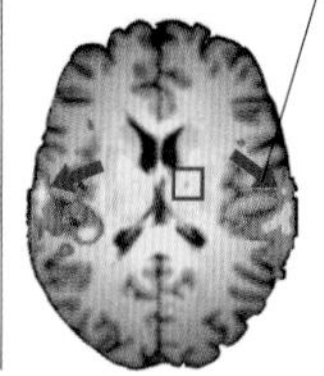

Increased activity

RICHER EXPERIENCE
These fMRI scans show brain activity in people listening to sounds. In response, those with synaesthesia generate more sensations than others, suggesting that the condition enriches everyday experiences by increasing sensation.

Touch area

Auditory area

Visual area

ROUTES TO SENSATION
Sense organs detect stimuli, turn the information into electrical signals, and transmit these to areas of the brain that are specialized to process specific types of sensory information into sensations such as sound, vision, taste, smell, touch, and pain. Some of this data is then "forwarded" to areas of the brain that make it conscious.

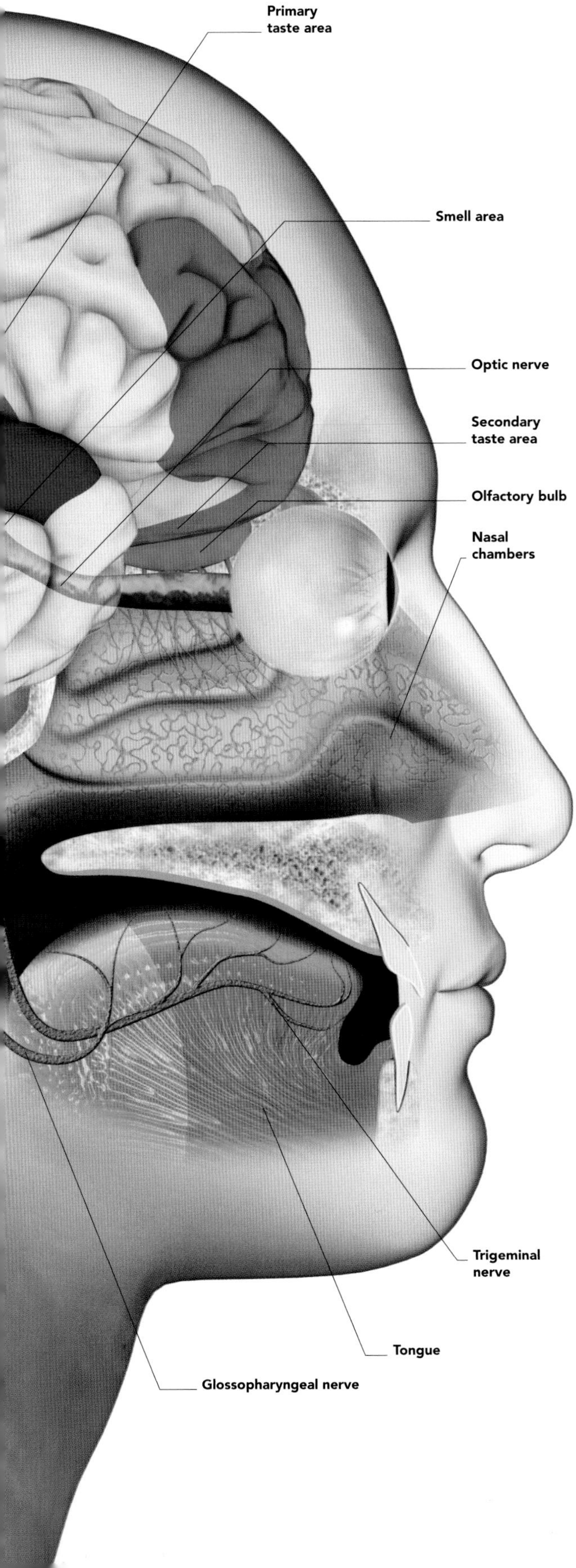

Primary taste area
Smell area
Optic nerve
Secondary taste area
Olfactory bulb
Nasal chambers
Trigeminal nerve
Tongue
Glossopharyngeal nerve

CONSCIOUS AND UNCONSCIOUS SENSATION

Our brains are bombarded with sensory information, but only a fraction of it reaches consciousness. Most sensory signals fizzle out unnoticed. Especially "loud" or important data grabs our attention (see pp.182–83), and we become conscious of it. Sensations we are not conscious of may still guide our actions. For example, unconscious sensations relating to our body position allow us to move without thinking about it. Also, sights and sounds we fail to notice (such as advertising material) may influence our behaviour.

BLINDSIGHT

Blindsight gives visual knowledge without conscious vision. It is likely that we all have it, but it is most easily measured in people who are blind due to cortical damage. Such people cannot knowingly see, but if something is put in front of them they can correctly "guess" what it looks like, without knowing how. Most blindsight studies use moving objects. The subjects say they can't see the objects, but they can usually "guess" the direction of movement correctly.

Moving object
Visual input
Optic nerve
Optic chiasm
Thalamus
Visual movement area
Visual cortex

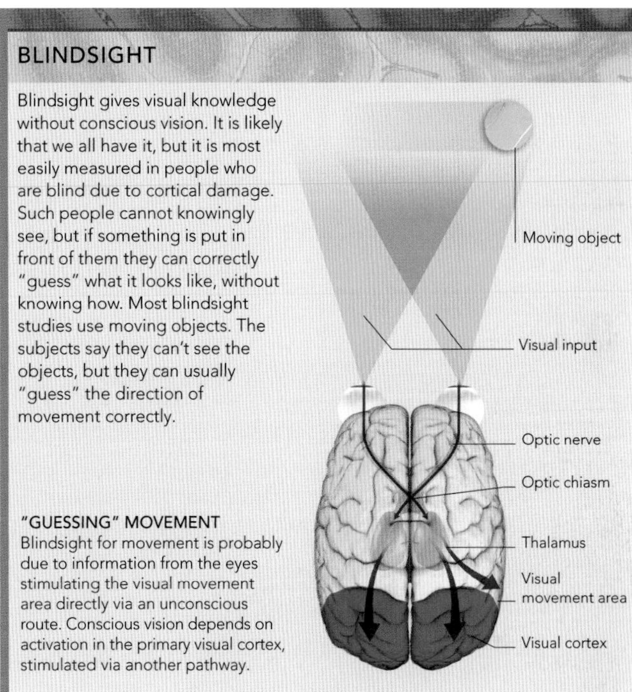

"GUESSING" MOVEMENT
Blindsight for movement is probably due to information from the eyes stimulating the visual movement area directly via an unconscious route. Conscious vision depends on activation in the primary visual cortex, stimulated via another pathway.

BOTTOM-UP AND TOP-DOWN PROCESSING

Sensations are triggered externally, by an occurrence that impacts on a sense organ, and internally, by memory or imagination. The former is known as "bottom-up", and the latter as "top-down" processing (see p.87). The two combine to create our experience of reality. Each person's experience of a given event is different. Physiological differences affect bottom-up processing. One person's colour-processing area in the brain may be highly sensitive, for example, so colours for them are more vibrant than average. Also, an individual's own memories, knowledge, and expectations affect their top-down processing.

A C 12 14

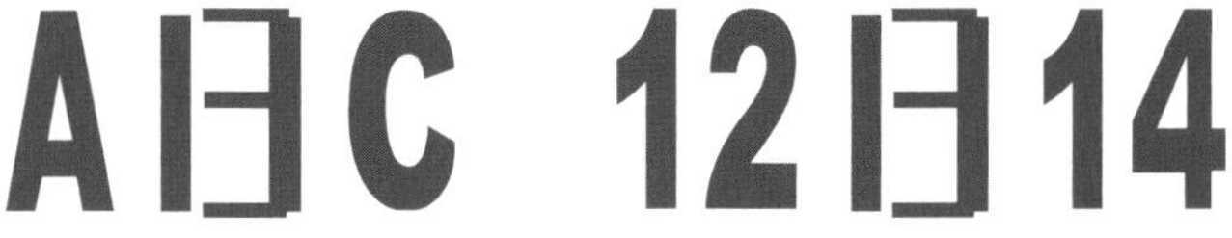

LETTER OR NUMBER?
The symbol in the centre is identical in these two images, and our "bottom-up" visual process sees it as such. However, expectation, or "top-down" visual processing, leads to us seeing it as different. The context in which it appears on the left causes us to see it as the letter "B", while we see it as "13" in the right-hand image.

THE EYE

THE EYE IS AN EXTENSION OF THE BRAIN. IT CONTAINS ABOUT 125 MILLION LIGHT-SENSITIVE NERVE CELLS, KNOWN AS PHOTORECEPTORS, WHICH GENERATE ELECTRICAL SIGNALS THAT ALLOW THE BRAIN TO FORM VISUAL IMAGES.

THE STRUCTURE OF THE EYE

The eyeball is a fluid-filled orb with a hole in the front (the pupil), a sheet of nerve cells (the retina), some of which are light-sensitive, at the back, and a lens in between. The pupil is surrounded by pigmented fibres (the iris) and covered by a sheet of clear tissue (the cornea) that merges with the tough outer surface or the "white" of the eye (the sclera). The optic nerve passes through a hole in the back of the eye (the optic disc) to enter the brain.

Optic nerve

OPTIC NERVE
This coloured MRI scan shows the thick bundle of fibres, the optic nerve, connecting each eye to the brain.

SEQUENCE OF VISION

Light passes through the cornea and enters the eye through the pupil. The iris controls how much enters by changing shape, so the pupil appears smaller in bright light and expands in shade. Light rays then pass through the lens, which bends (refracts) the light so it converges on the retina. If focusing on a near object, the lens thickens to increase refraction, but if the object is distant, the lens needs to flatten. The light then hits the photoreceptors in the retina, some of which fire, sending electrical signals to the brain via the optic nerve.

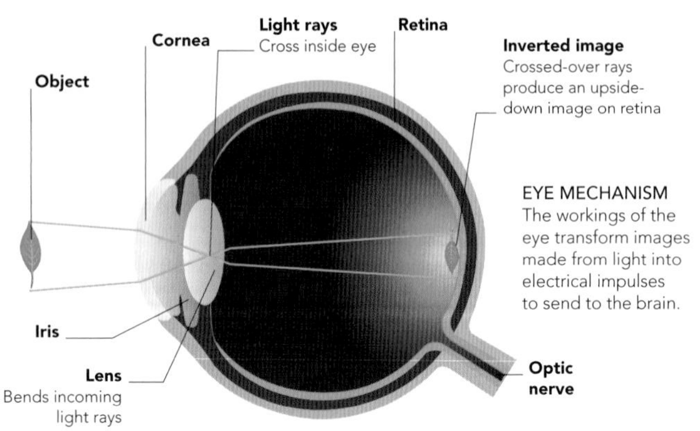

EYE MECHANISM
The workings of the eye transform images made from light into electrical impulses to send to the brain.

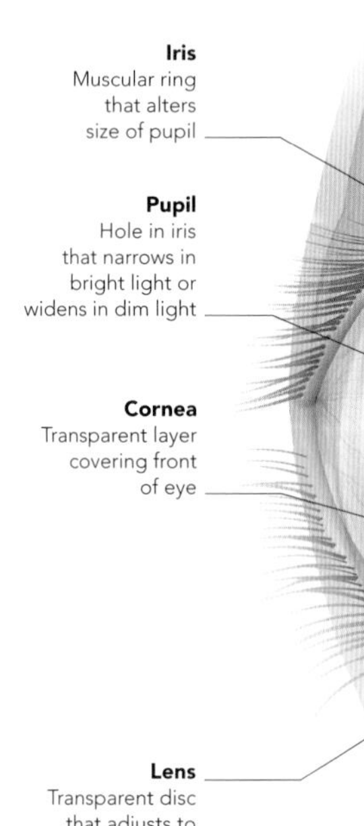

VISUAL PATHWAYS

Information from the eyes has to travel right to the back of the brain before it starts to be turned into conscious vision. En route, it passes through two major junctions, and half of it crosses from one side of the brain to the other. Signals from the two optic nerves first converge at a crossover junction called the optic chiasm. Fibres carrying information from the left side of each retina join up and proceed as the left optic tract, while fibres carrying information from the right side form the right optic tract. Each tract ends at the lateral geniculate nucleus, which is part of the thalamus, but their signals continue to the visual cortex via bands of nerve fibres, called the optic radiation.

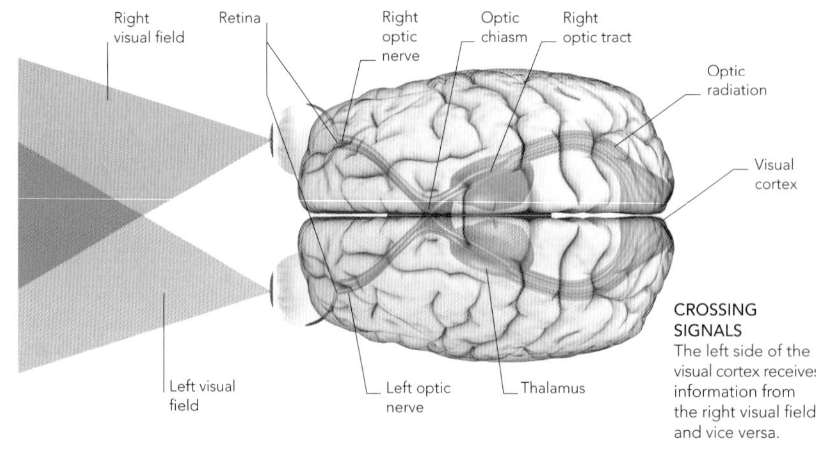

CROSSING SIGNALS
The left side of the visual cortex receives information from the right visual field and vice versa.

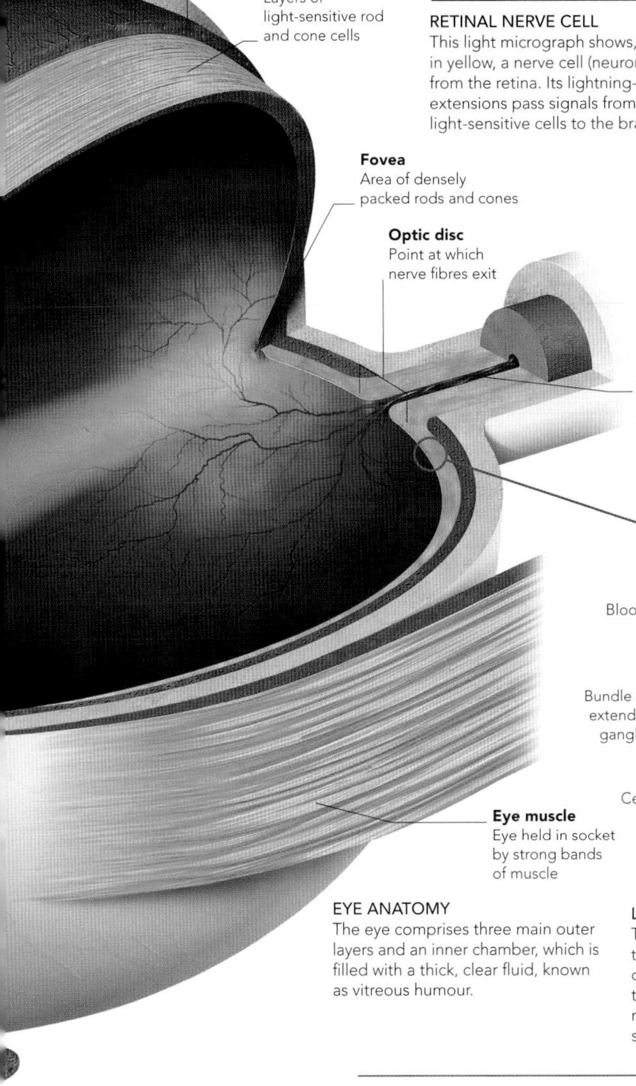

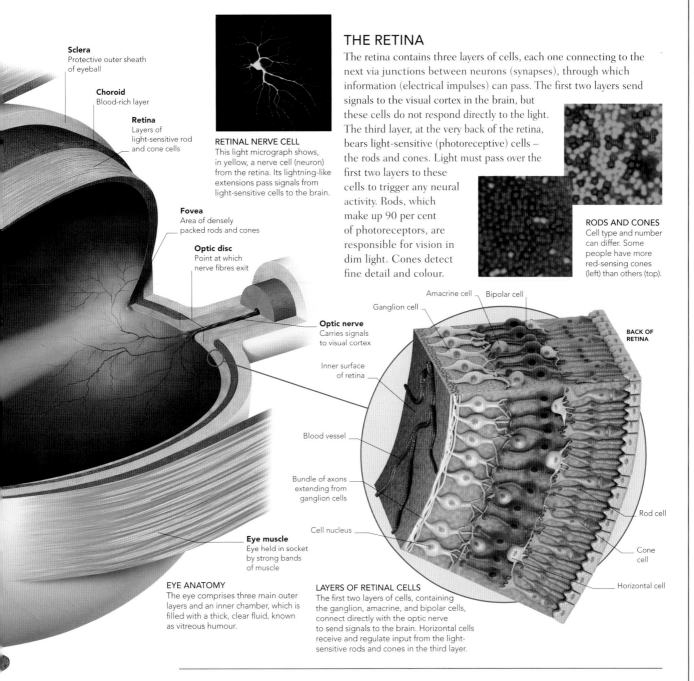

Sclera
Protective outer sheath of eyeball

Choroid
Blood-rich layer

Retina
Layers of light-sensitive rod and cone cells

Fovea
Area of densely packed rods and cones

Optic disc
Point at which nerve fibres exit

Optic nerve
Carries signals to visual cortex

Eye muscle
Eye held in socket by strong bands of muscle

EYE ANATOMY
The eye comprises three main outer layers and an inner chamber, which is filled with a thick, clear fluid, known as vitreous humour.

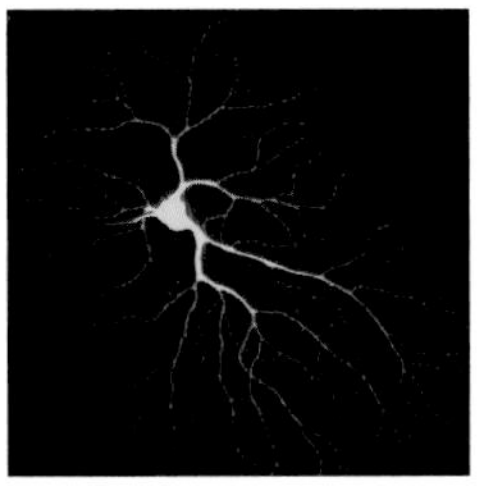

RETINAL NERVE CELL
This light micrograph shows, in yellow, a nerve cell (neuron) from the retina. Its lightning-like extensions pass signals from light-sensitive cells to the brain.

THE RETINA

The retina contains three layers of cells, each one connecting to the next via junctions between neurons (synapses), through which information (electrical impulses) can pass. The first two layers send signals to the visual cortex in the brain, but these cells do not respond directly to the light. The third layer, at the very back of the retina, bears light-sensitive (photoreceptive) cells – the rods and cones. Light must pass over the first two layers to these cells to trigger any neural activity. Rods, which make up 90 per cent of photoreceptors, are responsible for vision in dim light. Cones detect fine detail and colour.

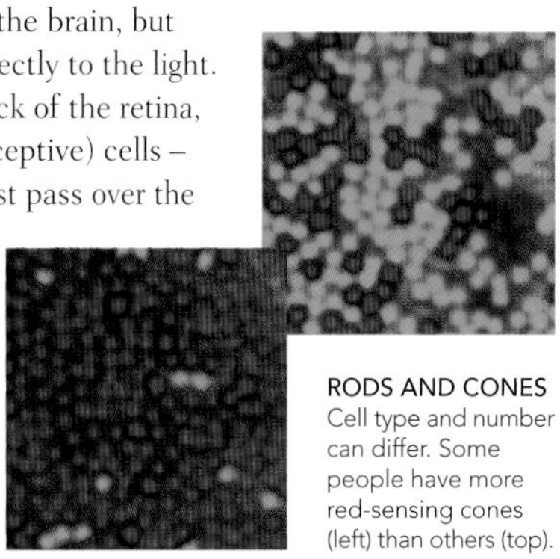

RODS AND CONES
Cell type and number can differ. Some people have more red-sensing cones (left) than others (top).

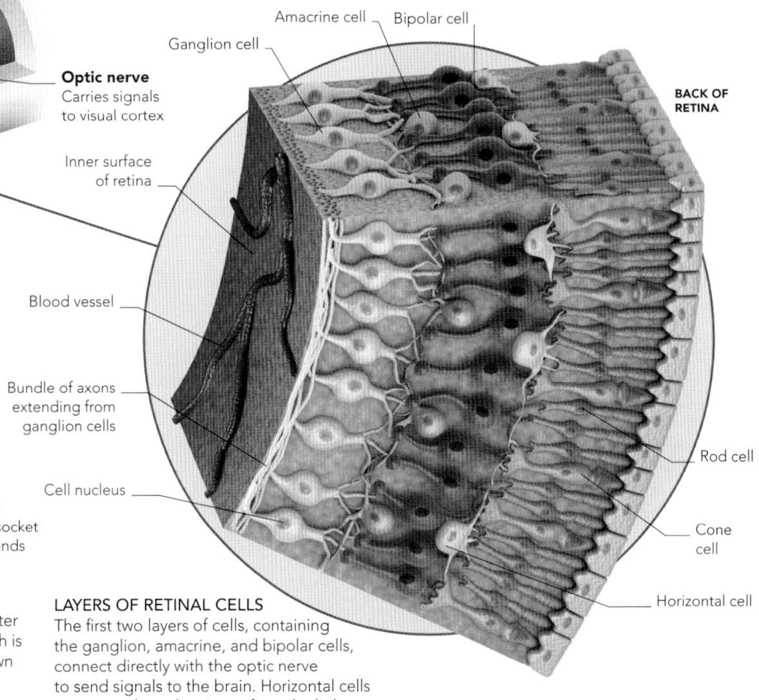

Amacrine cell
Bipolar cell
Ganglion cell
BACK OF RETINA
Inner surface of retina
Blood vessel
Bundle of axons extending from ganglion cells
Cell nucleus
Rod cell
Cone cell
Horizontal cell

LAYERS OF RETINAL CELLS
The first two layers of cells, containing the ganglion, amacrine, and bipolar cells, connect directly with the optic nerve to send signals to the brain. Horizontal cells receive and regulate input from the light-sensitive rods and cones in the third layer.

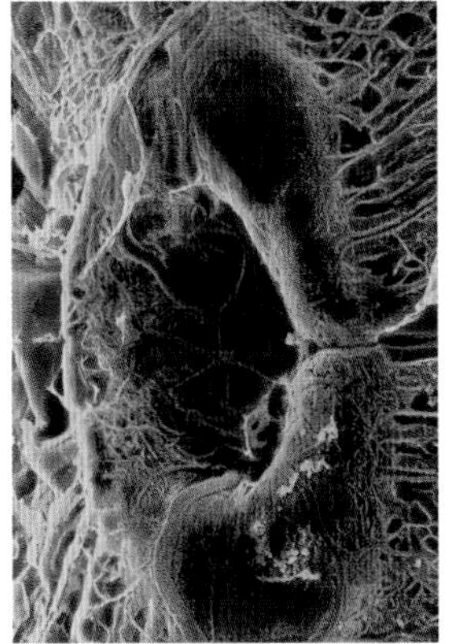

THE FOVEA

The central part of the retina allows for far sharper vision than the periphery because it contains more cones (which pick up detail and colour) than rods. Right in the centre of the retina is the fovea, a tiny pitted area where cones are most densely packed. In addition to being more numerous, foveal cones can also pass on more detail, as almost every one has a dedicated signal-sending pathway to the brain. Light-sensitive cells elsewhere on the retina must share these means of output.

FOVEAL MAGNIFICATION
This electron micrograph shows the part of the retina that gives sharpest vision, the foveal pit.

BLIND SPOT

Signal-carrying nerve fibres bundle together at the optic disc in the back of the eye to form the optic nerve. Consequently, this area has no light-sensitive cells, so it forms a "blind spot". We are unaware of this gap in our vision because the brain "fills in" the area we can't see.

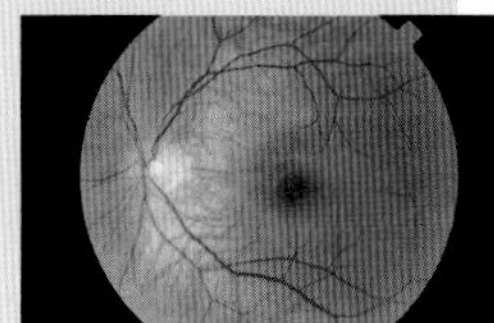

OPTIC DISC
This opthalmoscope image of a retina shows the optic disc, the site of the blind spot.

THE VISUAL CORTEX

THE VISUAL AREAS OF THE BRAIN ARE RIGHT AT THE BACK, SO INFORMATION FROM THE EYES HAS TO TRAVEL THE FULL DEPTH OF THE SKULL BEFORE IT BEGINS TO BE PROCESSED INTO SIGHT. VISUAL INFORMATION CAN GUIDE ACTIONS WITHIN ONE-FIFTH OF A SECOND, BUT IT TAKES ABOUT HALF A SECOND FOR US TO SEE AN OBJECT CONSCIOUSLY.

VISUAL AREAS

The visual cortex is divided into several functional areas, each of which specializes in a particular aspect of vision (see table, right). The process is similar to assembly-line production: raw material is checked in by V1, then sent on to other vision areas, which contribute shape, colour, depth, and motion. These components are then combined to form a whole image. The modular nature of vision means that if one of the sight areas is damaged, a particular visual component may be lost while the others remain intact. Cell death in the motion-detecting area, for example, may cause the world to be seen as a series of still snapshots.

AREAS OF THE VISUAL CORTEX

AREA	FUNCTION
V1	Responds to visual stimuli
V2	Passes on information and responds to complex shapes
V3A, V3D, VP	Registers angles and symmetry, and combines motion and direction
V4D, V4V	Responds to colour, orientation, form, and movement
V5	Responds to movement
V6	Detects motion in periphery of visual field
V7	Involved in perception of symmetry
V8	Probably involved in processing of colour

V6
V3A
V3D
V2
V1
V2
V4V
V8
VP

INTERIOR CORTEX
Some, but not all, of the visual processing areas curve around the back of the brain and into the groove between the hemispheres.

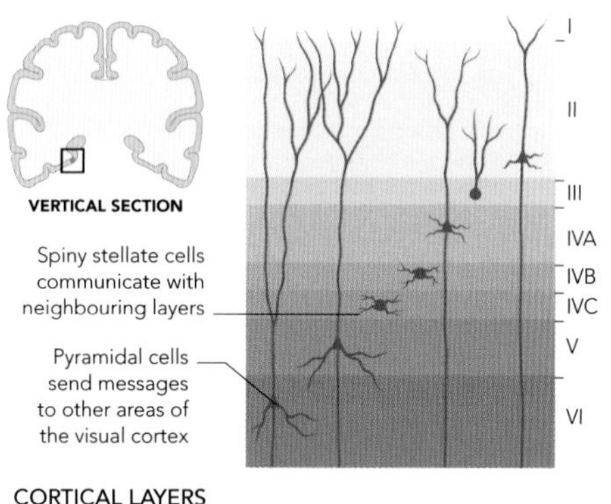

CORTICAL LAYERS
The primary visual cortex consists of several cell layers, numbered I to VI, each of which contains a special mix of cells. Each layer sends and receives signals to and from different parts of the brain.

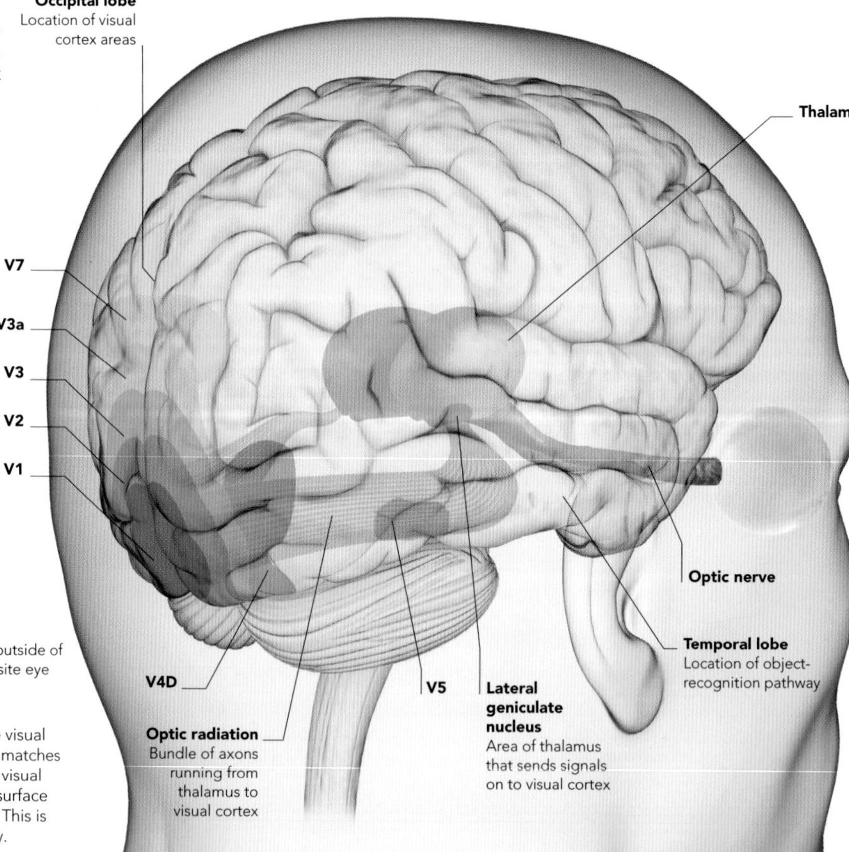

THE SEEING BRAIN
Signals from the eyes arrive at V1, which passes them to other visual areas for further processing (see also pp.84–85). Activation in V1 is not sufficient for conscious sight, but it is necessary for it. So long as we are consciously seeing something, V1 is kept activated.

THE MIND'S MIRROR

The criss-cross layout of the visual pathways (see p.80) causes the view seen by the eyes to be reversed, so it registers on the primary visual cortex (V1) as a mirror image. Signals from the left field of vision end up in the right hemisphere and vice versa. The information is passed between the two sides to give a shared view. In certain rare conditions, each side of the brain sees something different – the person appears to be in "two minds" (see p.11, p.205).

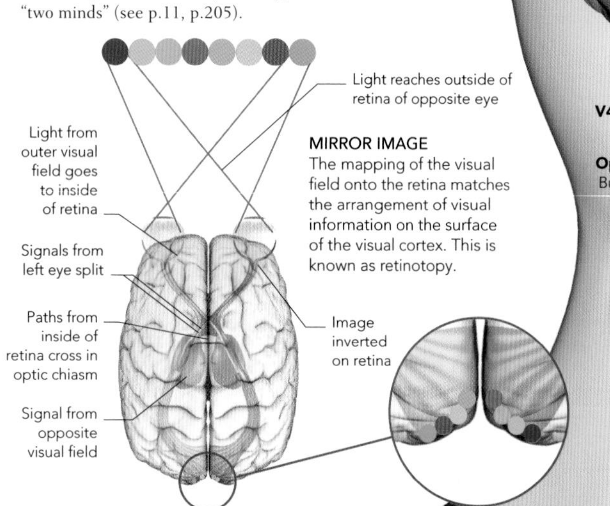

MIRROR IMAGE
The mapping of the visual field onto the retina matches the arrangement of visual information on the surface of the visual cortex. This is known as retinotopy.

DISTINGUISHING COLOURS

In theory, the human visual system can distinguish millions of colours but in practice the number of colours we see depends on whether we have learned to see them. Presented with a globe showing all possible colours, people can easily distinguish those for which they have distinct names. But if a range of hues is lumped together under a single name, they often find it hard to see the differences.

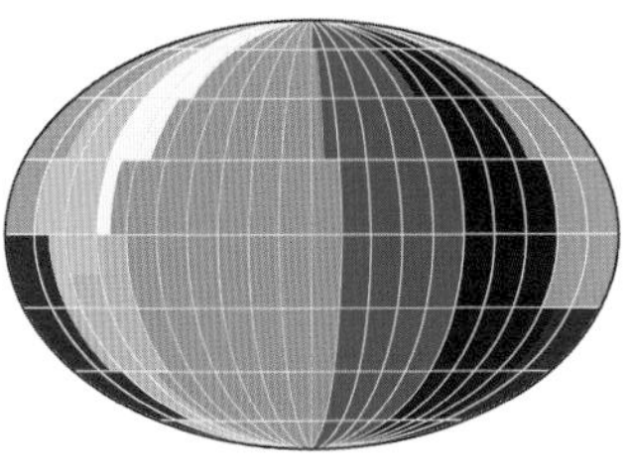

ENGLISH HUES
This globe shows the spectrum of colour, which is divided into eight basic categories (red, orange, green, blue, purple, yellow, and brown) in the English language.

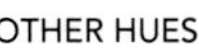

OTHER HUES
Studies suggest that language affects how people see the globe. For example, the Berinmo tribe of Papua New Guinea split colours into five categories, each of which relates to a different hue from those above.

RECOGNIZING OBJECTS

Conscious sight requires the brain to recognize what it is seeing. To achieve this, the image is forwarded from the occipital lobe to other brain areas concerned with emotion and memory. Here it gains information relating to its function, its identity, and its emotional significance. One of the first stops is in the object-recognition area, which runs along the bottom rim of the temporal lobe. Human faces are dealt with in a particular sub-region that has evolved to make fine distinctions. Its ability to distinguish tiny differences between individual faces makes nearly all of us "experts" at recognizing one another.

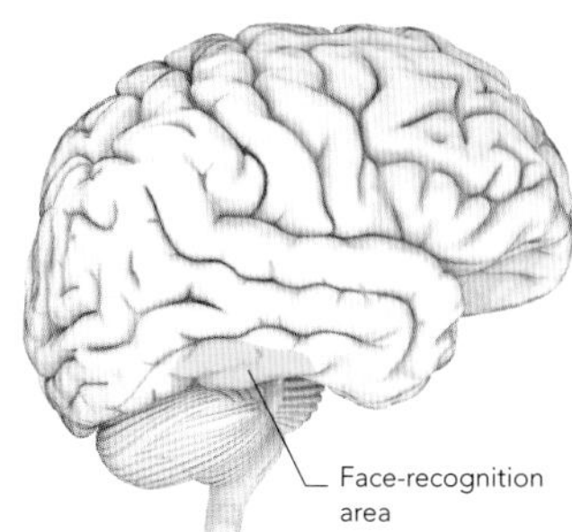

FACE-RECOGNITION AREA
Part of the brain's object-recognition path scrutinizes things of importance. This area processes objects that call for fine discrimination, such as faces.

GREEBLES

Greebles are organic-looking objects used in studies that, like faces, are each slightly different from one another. At first sight the differences are easily overlooked, but as people become familiar with Greebles their brains start processing the sight of them in the face-recognition area. This allows them to see the tiny differences very clearly and they become Greeble "experts".

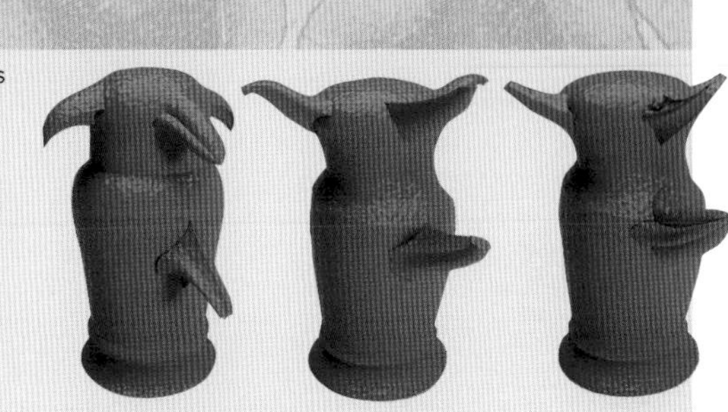

DEPTH AND DIMENSION

The brain uses two types of cues to produce our three-dimensional view of the world. One is the slightly different image recorded by each eye (spatial binocular disparity), and the other is the way the perceived shape of an object shifts as it moves. Both cues come together in an area of the brain called the anterior intraparietal area (AIP), which lies between the visual processing areas and the part of the brain devoted to monitoring our position in space.

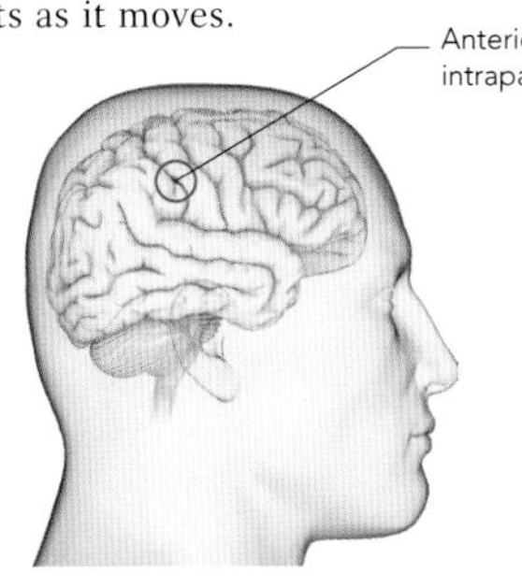

DEPTH AREA
The AIP combines two types of visual cue to calculate distance and depth. This information guides the movements involved in reaching out and grasping objects.

STEREOGRAM

Stereoscopic images make use of the way the brain processes visual information to trick it into seeing a three-dimensional image when in fact there is only a flat plane. One way to do this is to present, side by side, two minutely differing images of the same scene. The difference between them is that which would normally be perceived by each eye – a tiny shift of perspective equal to the distance between the eyes. These illusions were popular in Victorian times.

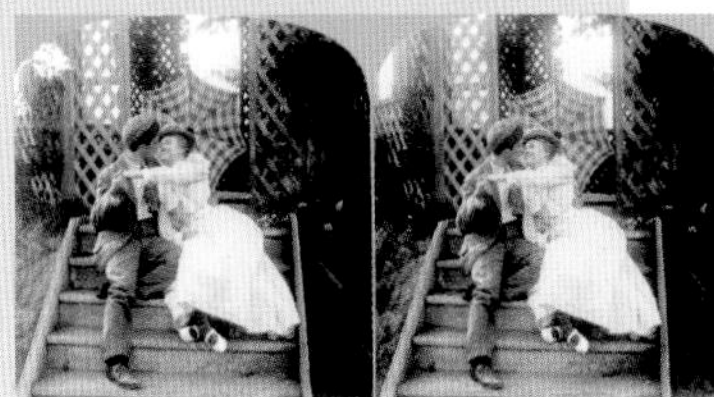

PHANTOM IMAGE
If you can force your eyes to cross or to diverge, so that each eye sees just one of the pictures, a ghostly third image appears in the centre in three dimensions.

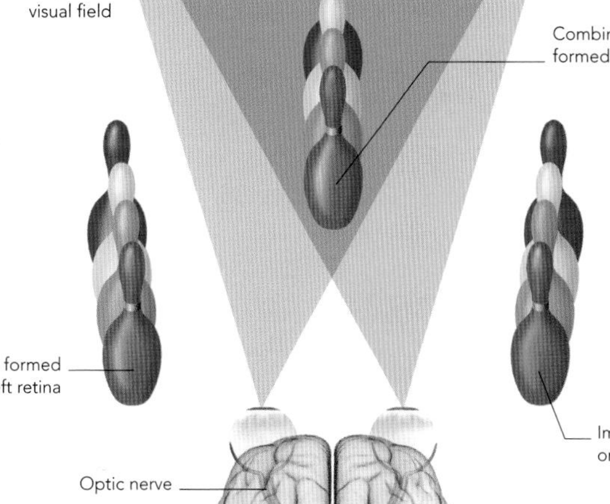

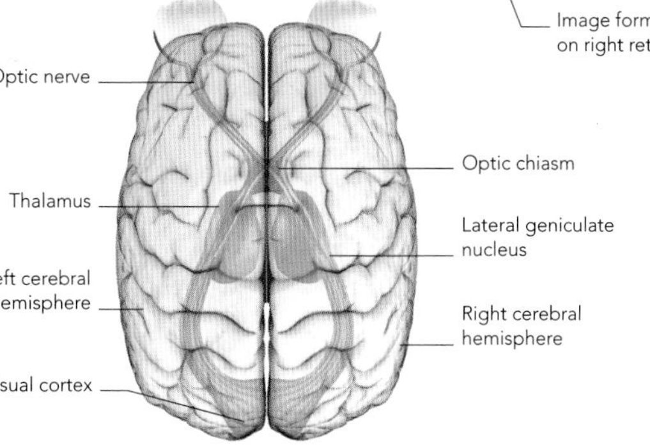

3-D VISION
The slightly differing views provided by each eye, combined with information about how shapes change as they move across the visual field, produce a three-dimensional view of the world.

VISUAL PATHWAYS

CONSCIOUS VISION IS THE FAMILIAR PROCESS OF SEEING SOMETHING, WHILE UNCONSCIOUS VISION USES INFORMATION FROM THE EYES TO GUIDE BEHAVIOUR WITHOUT OUR KNOWING IT IS HAPPENING. THE TWO TYPES OF VISION ARE PROCESSED ALONG SEPARATE PATHWAYS IN THE BRAIN. THE UPPER (DORSAL) ROUTE, IS UNCONSCIOUS AND GUIDES ACTION, WHILE THE LOWER (VENTRAL) PATH IS CONSCIOUS AND RECOGNIZES OBJECTS.

DORSAL AND VENTRAL ROUTES
Electrical signals from the eyes travel to the primary visual cortex, where the brain begins to process them into vision. The signals are then sent on to other brain regions via the two separate dorsal and ventral pathways.

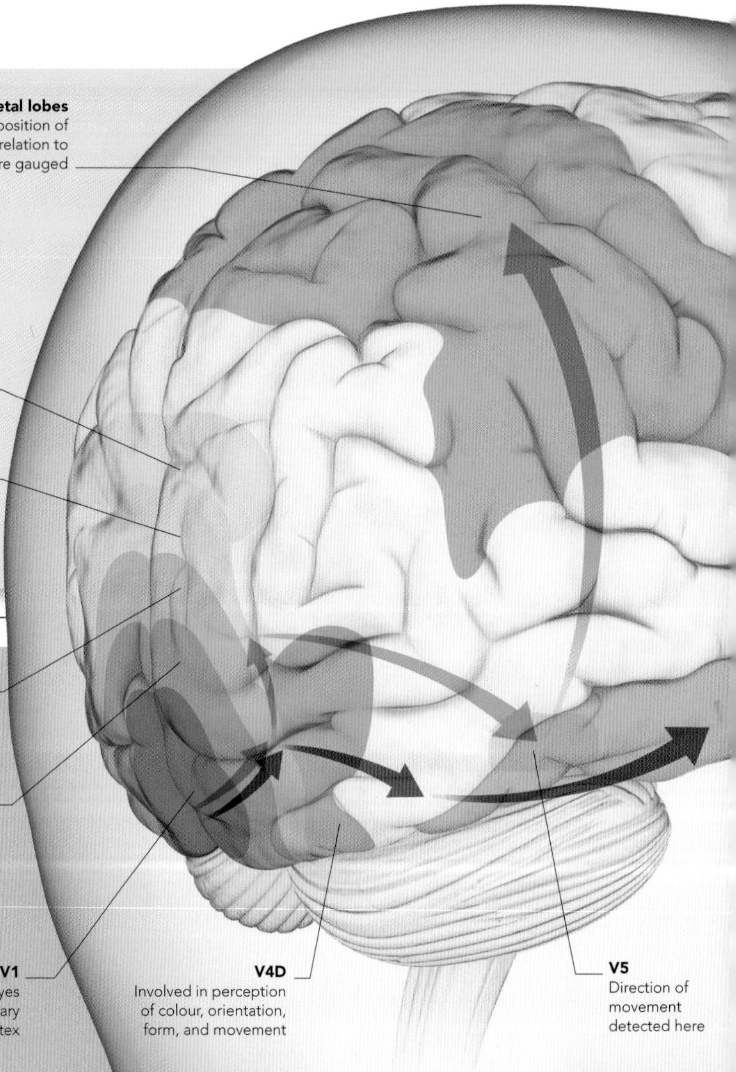

DORSAL

THE "WHERE" PATHWAY

The dorsal, or "where", pathway carries signals triggered by a visual stimulus – for example, the light bouncing off a nearby object – from the visual cortex to the parietal cortex. Along the way, it passes through areas that calculate the object's location in relation to the viewer and creates an action plan in relation to it. The dorsal path gathers information about motion and timing that is integrated into the action plan. All the information needed to, say, duck a flying object, is gathered along this path with no need for conscious thought.

VENTRAL

THE "WHAT" PATHWAY

The ventral, or "what", pathway follows a route that takes it first through a series of visual processing areas, each of which adds a specific aspect of perception, such as shape, colour, depth, and so on (see pp.88–89). The loosely formed representation then passes into the bottom edge of the temporal lobe, where it is matched or compared to visual memories in order to achieve recognition. Some information continues along this pathway to the frontal lobes, where it is assessed for meaning and significance. At this stage, it becomes a conscious perception.

Parietal lobes
Depth and position of object in relation to observer are gauged

V7
Contributes to perception of symmetry

V3a
Information on motion and direction is collated here

V3
Angles and orientation analysed – paths split

V2
Information passed on through secondary visual cortex – complex shapes are registered here

V1
Signals from eyes received in primary visual cortex

V4D
Involved in perception of colour, orientation, form, and movement

V5
Direction of movement detected here

RECOGNIZING FACES

Different types of visual stimuli are processed in different parts of the brain. Faces, which are recognized by the pattern of human facial features, activate the face-recognition area. This extracts information about facial expression and forwards it to relevant brain areas. When a face matches a memory, the information is sent to the frontal lobes for further processing.

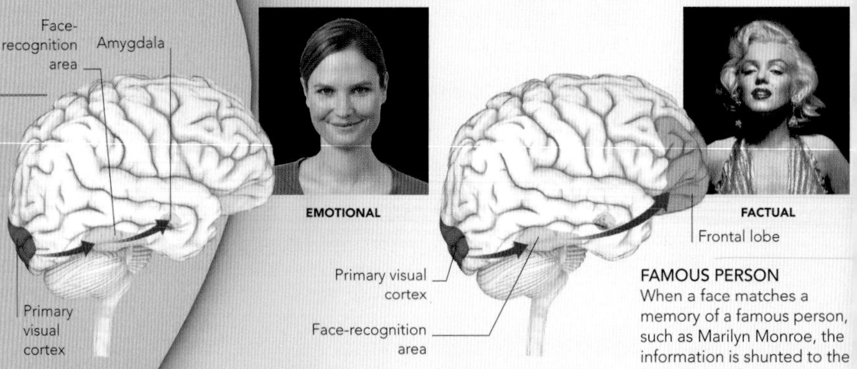

FAMILIAR PERSON
Emotional recognition is near-instant. The pathway runs from the visual cortex via the face area to the amygdala.

Face-recognition area
Amygdala
Primary visual cortex
EMOTIONAL
SEEING SOMEONE FAMILIAR

FACTUAL
Frontal lobe
Primary visual cortex
Face-recognition area
SEEING SOMEONE FAMOUS

FAMOUS PERSON
When a face matches a memory of a famous person, such as Marilyn Monroe, the information is shunted to the frontal lobes for processing.

Frontal lobe
Some information from dorsal route arrives in frontal lobes, where it is consciously perceived

Inferior temporal lobe
Fusiform gyrus involved in recognizing objects, especially faces

DAMAGE TO THE DORSAL PATHWAY

Damage to the dorsal visual pathway causes a number of disorders, all of which affect the ability to deal with objects in space. A person may, for example, be unable to see that two objects are in different places or to correctly see their spatial relationship, one to the other. They may find it impossible to reach out and grasp an object accurately or to know where it lies in relation to themselves. For example, a person may say something like, "I know there is a banana there but I don't know where it is". Patients may also suffer visual attention defects (see pp.182–83).

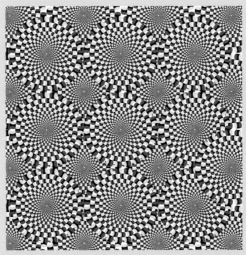

ILLUSORY MOTION
The brain frequently detects motion where there is actually none. Many different types of illusions can do this. Most of them depend on exciting motion-detecting neurons, causing them to fire and thus create the effect of movement.

STILL LIFE

The ability to see movement is vital for survival. Many animals, such as frogs, can only see things in motion. The motion area of the human brain is tiny and more than 90 per cent of neurons here are specialized to detect direction of movement. It is generally well-protected from injury but, very rarely, a person may lose motion vision due to a stroke. The effect is profoundly disturbing, reducing the world to a series of snapshots. Day-to-day life becomes difficult – crossing the road, for example, is perilous as approaching traffic appears first to be distant and then suddenly close. Pouring a cup of tea is difficult because the column of liquid seems to be frozen and then overflowing.

PROSOPAGNOSIA

If the face-recognition area is damaged, or fails for some reason to develop normally, people may be unable to recognize people they know – even their closest friends and members of their own family. Prosopagnosia is severely socially disabling. Affected people may get quite good at identifying people by features other than their face (by voice or clothing) but these techniques are slower and less reliable than normal face recognition. Face recognition relies on detailed information about distances between features. In the faces above, the shape of the features or the distance between them have been manipulated.People with prosopagnosia are unable to spot the differences.

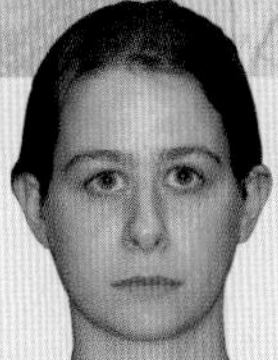

EYES CLOSE

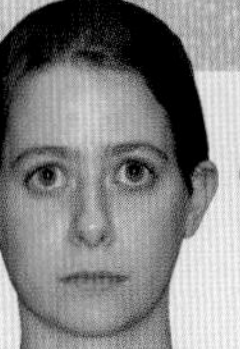

EYES ENLARGED

EYES APART

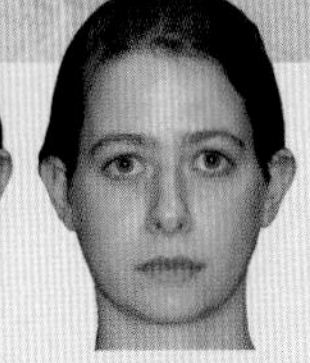

MOUTH ENLARGED

ALTERED IMAGES
These photographs have had features, such as mouth or eye size, altered or have been changed configurally – the eyes moved together or further apart.

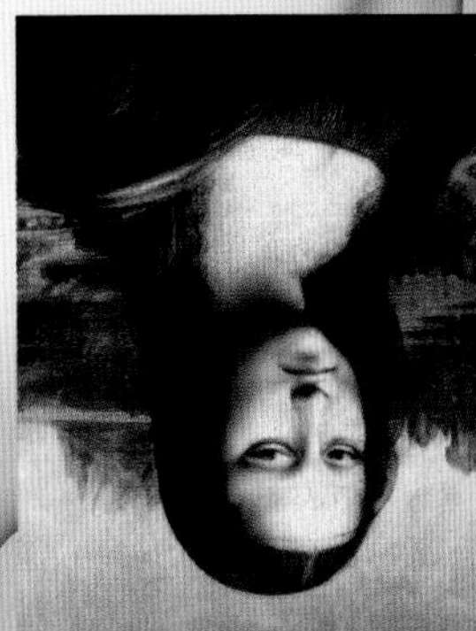

MONA LISA ILLUSION
The face-recognition area only processes stimuli that have the pattern of facial features. So a picture of an upturned face is not processed here but is dealt with by an area that is not sensitive to facial expression. The upturned image of Mona Lisa seems at first to be normal. Turn it the right way up, though, and the face area alerts you to something very wrong!

DAMAGE TO THE VENTRAL PATHWAY

Damage to the ventral pathway results in one or another form of visual agnosia – the inability to recognize what one is seeing. Prosopagnosia, the inability to recognize faces (see panel, above), is one type of agnosia, but there are many others. Visual agnosia is generally divided into two categories: apperceptive and associative. The first type results from damage to the parts of the pathway in the occipital lobe and manifests itself as an inability to form a properly constructed perception. Hence a person with apperceptive agnosia cannot copy or draw an object, even though they may be able to see the parts of it quite clearly. Associative agnosia is an inability to identify objects. The person sees the object and may be able to mime an appropriate action in relation to it – for example, using a fork to raise food to the mouth – yet be unable to say what it is.

LETTER

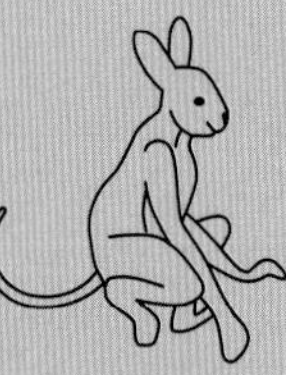

FANTASY OBJECT

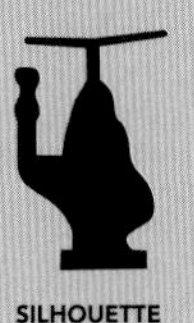

SILHOUETTE

AGNOSIA TESTS
Tests for agnosia include recognizing objects from their silhouettes, telling fantasy objects from real ones, or identifying an incomplete letter.

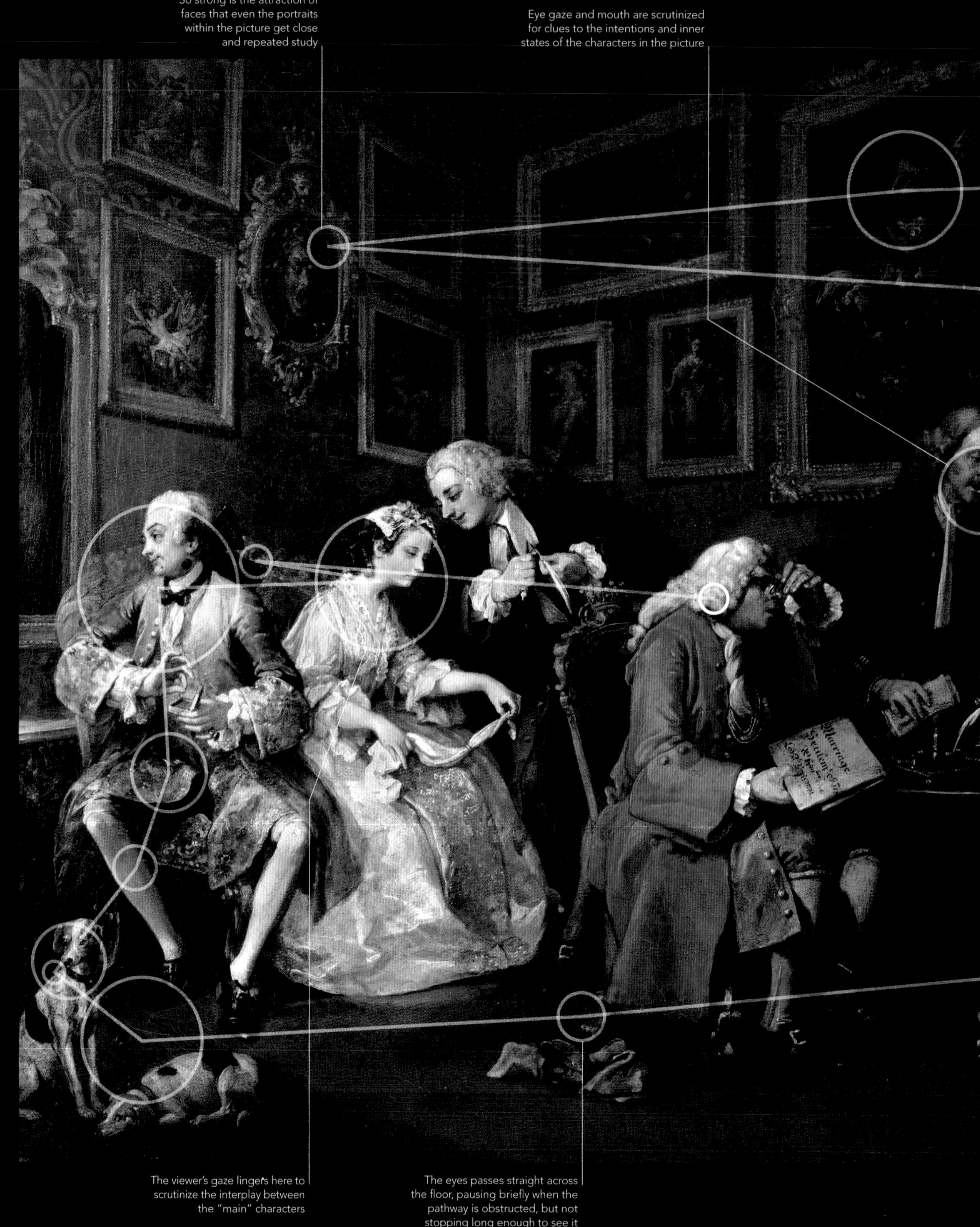

So strong is the attraction of faces that even the portraits within the picture get close and repeated study

Eye gaze and mouth are scrutinized for clues to the intentions and inner states of the characters in the picture

The viewer's gaze lingers here to scrutinize the interplay between the "main" characters

The eyes passes straight across the floor, pausing briefly when the pathway is obstructed, but not stopping long enough to see it

the possibility of others intruding on the scene and altering the human dynamics within it

VISUAL PERCEPTION

WE DO NOT SEE WHAT WE THINK WE SEE. WHEN WE LOOK AT A SCENE WE HAVE THE IMPRESSION OF SEEING ALL OF IT IN ONE GLANCE, BUT IN PRACTICE WE TYPICALLY PICK OUT JUST A FEW TINY DETAILS.

TOP-DOWN AND BOTTOM-UP PROCESSING

Visual perception is momentary, partial, and fragmentary. "Bottom-up" visual processing presets the brain with information about the whole field of vision, but "top-down" processes select which parts of a scene to make conscious. When we look at a picture, our eyes typically alight on a few thumbnail size areas that we scan in sequence repeatedly. The rest of the image remains a blur unless we deliberately turn our attention to it. Eye-tracking studies (see left) show that the parts of a scene that we look at most closely are those that relate to other people. Although this visual selection is determined by "higher" brain functions – those involved in social concerns rather than, say, ducking a low branch – people are often unaware of what they are looking at. When asked, they may say they are looking at one thing when in fact their eyes have been resting on another.

MAKING SENSE OF PICTURES

The brain works hard to make sense of visual information. Looking at a complex scene (see left) activates processes that distinguish target objects, such as people, from the background and then selects which bits of the target to focus on. These details are then scrutinized while the conscious brain pieces together the story. This interpretation begins unconsciously. Colours and shades are not recognized just by the type and amount of light reflected from them. The unconscious brain works out an object's most likely colour or shade from its context.

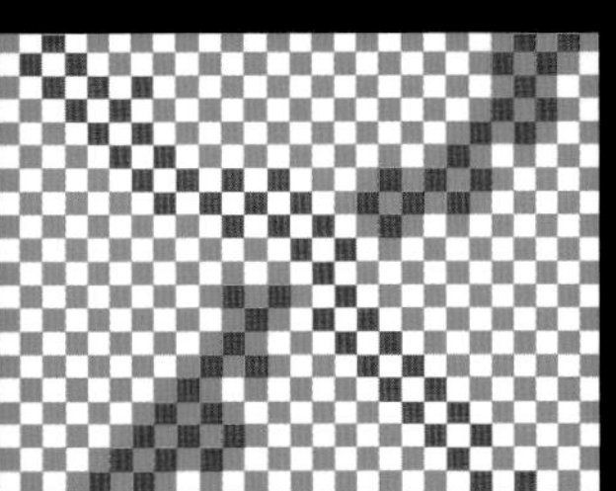

CYLINDER ILLUSION
The two squares A and B are identical shades but B looks lighter as we assume that the cylinder is casting a shadow over it.

COLOUR ILLUSION
The colour you see depends on those around it. Pink next to white looks paler than pink next to green. This is due to "lateral inhibition", which defines objects from their surroundings.

LAUGHTER PLAYS TRICKS ON THE EYES

Laughing literally changes the way you see the world. Normally when you look at a Necker cube, the image switches between two competing 3-D images, a situation known as binocular rivalry. This rivalry occurs because each eye sends a slightly different image to each side of the brain (see p.83), and the brain switches conscious awareness of one to the other. One theory on why switching stops during laughter is that amusement is a state in which information from both halves of the brain merges more than usual.

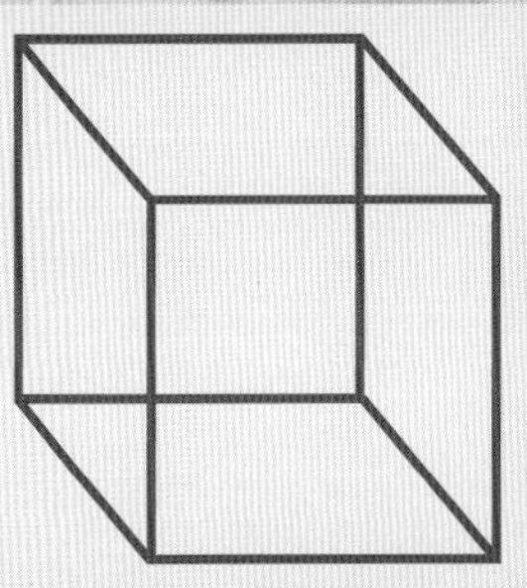

NECKER CUBE

TUNING IN TO DETAIL
The white lines on this image track the viewer's eyes as they navigate around the scene. The circles represent where the gaze rests – the larger the circle, the longer the eye lingers.

SEEING

SEEING SEEMS TO BE INSTANTANEOUS AND EFFORTLESS, AND VISUAL IMAGES ALWAYS APPEAR FULLY FORMED. UNCONSCIOUSLY, HOWEVER, THE BRAIN IS CONSTANTLY UNDERTAKING A MAJOR FEAT OF CONSTRUCTION TO PRESENT US WITH OUR VIEW OF THE WORLD.

VISUAL PERCEPTION

One way of thinking about visual perception is to see it as the end product that emerges from a long and complicated assembly line. The construction process begins in earnest when information from the eyes – the raw material – reaches the primary visual cortex at the back of the brain. This is then sent along two main pathways (see pp.84–85), through a number of cortical and subcortical areas. Each of these responds by creating neural activity that generates various aspects of vision such as colour, form, location, and movement. Eventually, the various elements are bound together and we become conscious of a meaningful sight.

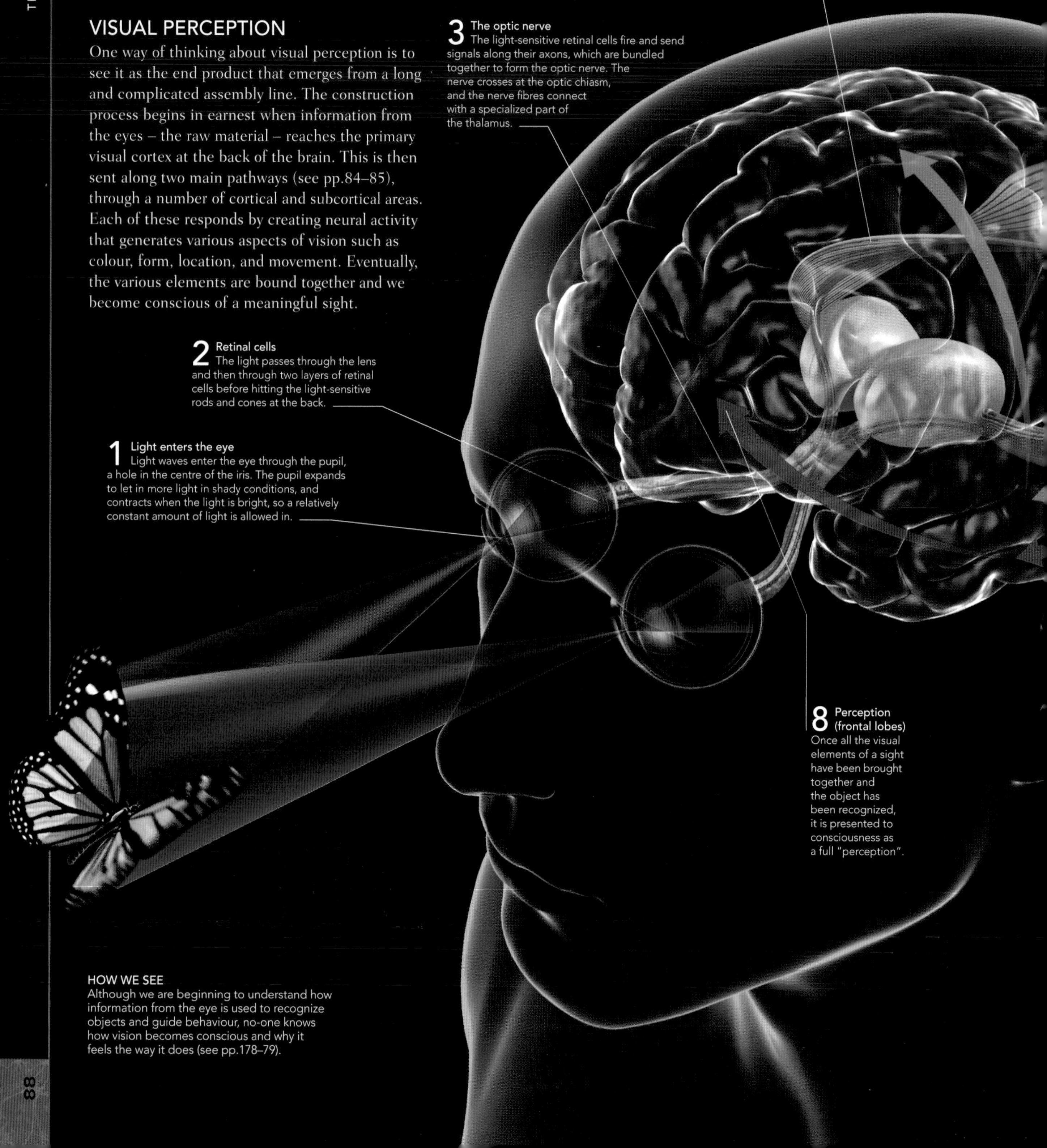

4 The optic radiation
The signals are then sent from the thalamus on to the visual cortex via a thick band of tissue known as the optic radiation.

3 The optic nerve
The light-sensitive retinal cells fire and send signals along their axons, which are bundled together to form the optic nerve. The nerve crosses at the optic chiasm, and the nerve fibres connect with a specialized part of the thalamus.

2 Retinal cells
The light passes through the lens and then through two layers of retinal cells before hitting the light-sensitive rods and cones at the back.

1 Light enters the eye
Light waves enter the eye through the pupil, a hole in the centre of the iris. The pupil expands to let in more light in shady conditions, and contracts when the light is bright, so a relatively constant amount of light is allowed in.

8 Perception (frontal lobes)
Once all the visual elements of a sight have been brought together and the object has been recognized, it is presented to consciousness as a full "perception".

HOW WE SEE
Although we are beginning to understand how information from the eye is used to recognize objects and guide behaviour, no-one knows how vision becomes conscious and why it feels the way it does (see pp.178–79).

registered by the primary visual cortex and then sent forwards along two pathways for further processing. The dorsal route takes it up through areas that are concerned with charting the location of the target object in relation to the viewer. Along this route, neuronal activity encodes the object's position, movement, and some aspects of its size and shape. The dorsal route ends in the parietal areas, which construct action plans relative to the viewed object. This process occurs unconsciously.

is an essential component of any "action plan" (see p.121), and the brain not only notes current motion, but also predicts where an object will be in a split second. This ensures any action plan in regard to it is well timed.

brain combines visual signals from both eyes – each of which has a slightly different view (see p.83) – along with information about how the shape of the image alters as the eyes move.

DORSAL

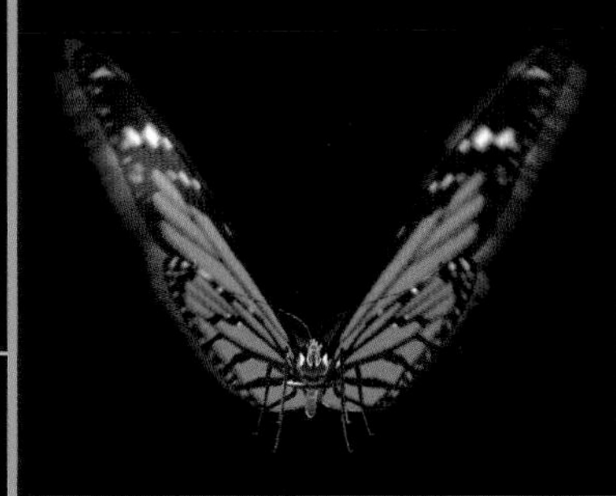

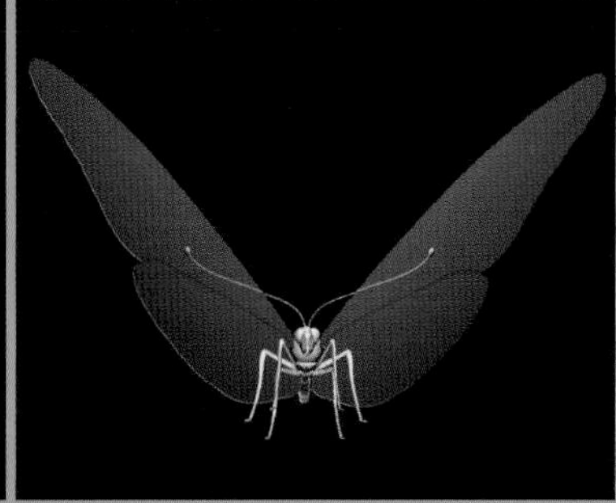

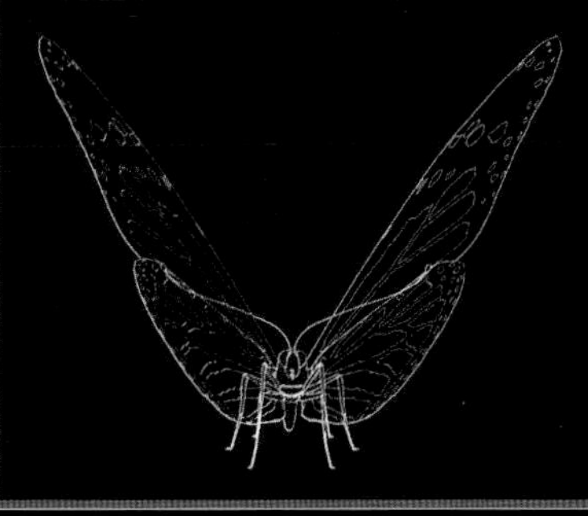

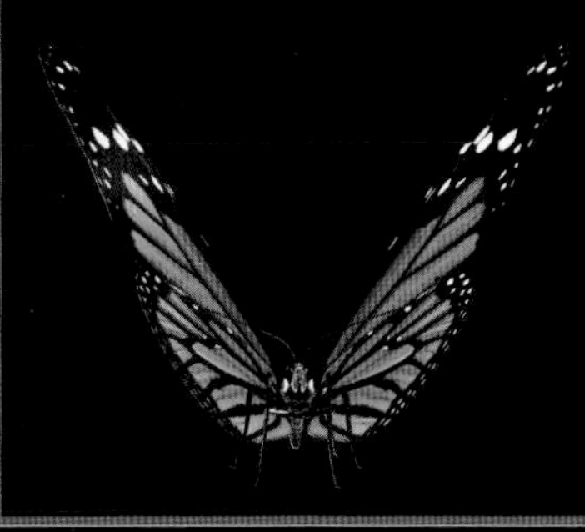

VENTRAL

6 THE VENTRAL ROUTE
The ventral route carries information from the primary visual cortex down through the temporal lobes, where the neural activity identifies the sights and "clothes" them with meaning. A face, for example, is distinguished and recognized here (see p.84), and information about it such as the name of the person is recalled from memory (see p.163). Information travelling along the ventral path is brought together with that from the dorsal path in the frontal lobes – resulting in conscious perception rather than action.

Form
The brain has many different ways of "seeing" form. These include registering the orientation of light waves hitting an object and processing information about the way the waves reflect from its surfaces or outlines.

Colour
Colour discrimination begins in the retinal cells, some of which are tuned to fire in response to specific light wavelengths. Colour processing continues in the brain, especially in an area known as V4 (see pp.82–83), which contains the majority of colour-sensing neurons.

7 Recognition path
In order to see something properly, a person needs to have some idea of what they are seeing. If an image is not recognized, it is less likely to be consciously registered and may be overlooked altogether. Recognition is not purely visual, but involves clothing the perception with knowledge – such as who or what it is, what their intention is (if it is sentient), why it is there, and what it is called. Some of these elements may be missing – you may see someone you know but fail to recall their name, for example. By contrast, the purely visual elements of a perception are nearly always intact.

SEEING WITH SOUND?

A device that turns visual information into sound has been reported to create visual experience in at least one user, who is otherwise blind. The device involves mounting a small camera on a person's head, which captures a moment-by-moment view of what would normally be the person's visual field. This information is then turned into a "soundscape" that is played into the user's ears. As the person learns to recognize the physical qualities matching the sounds – for example, that a single high-pitched tone signifies a vertical surface – they seem to cease to hear it as a noise and instead experience it much like normal vision. One woman claims that her experience of "hearing" the environment is sometimes indistinguishable from seeing it.

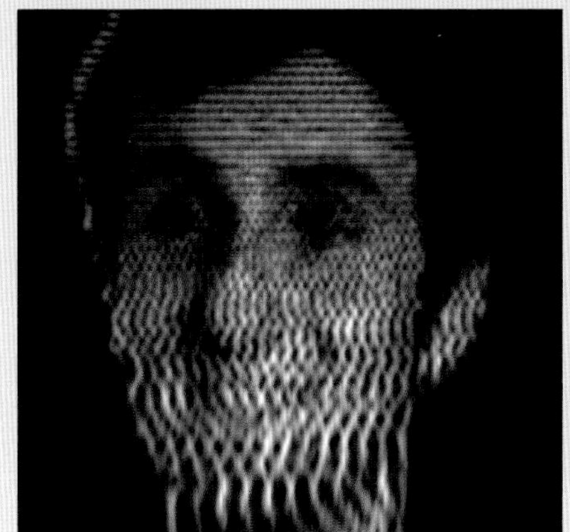

SOUNDSCAPE
This image is a computer reconstruction of one second of sound, as "seen" by the system that builds soundscapes from camera images.

THE EAR

THE EAR PICKS UP SOUND WAVES IN THE ENVIRONMENT AND TRANSLATES THIS INFORMATION INTO NERVE IMPULSES, WHICH ARE SENT TO THE BRAIN FOR PROCESSING. THE EAR ALSO SENSES THE MOTION AND POSITION OF THE BODY, WHICH ALLOWS THE BRAIN TO REGULATE BALANCE.

THE ANATOMY OF HEARING

The ear is divided into three sections: the outer ear, middle ear, and inner ear. The outer ear funnels sound waves along the ear canal to the eardrum (tympanic membrane) – the start of the middle ear. The sound waves cause the eardrum to vibrate, which in turn causes a chain of bones, known as the ear ossicles, to vibrate. One of these, the stapes, is attached to a membrane known as the oval window – the start of the inner ear. Beyond this is the maze of fluid-filled chambers of the spiral-shaped cochlea. The vibrations of the stapes on the oval window are converted into pressure waves, which travel in the fluid within the cochlea to the organ of Corti. Sensory hair cells on this organ transform the pressure waves into electrical impulses, which travel through the auditory nerve (specifically, the cochlear branch of the vestibulocochlear nerve) to the brain.

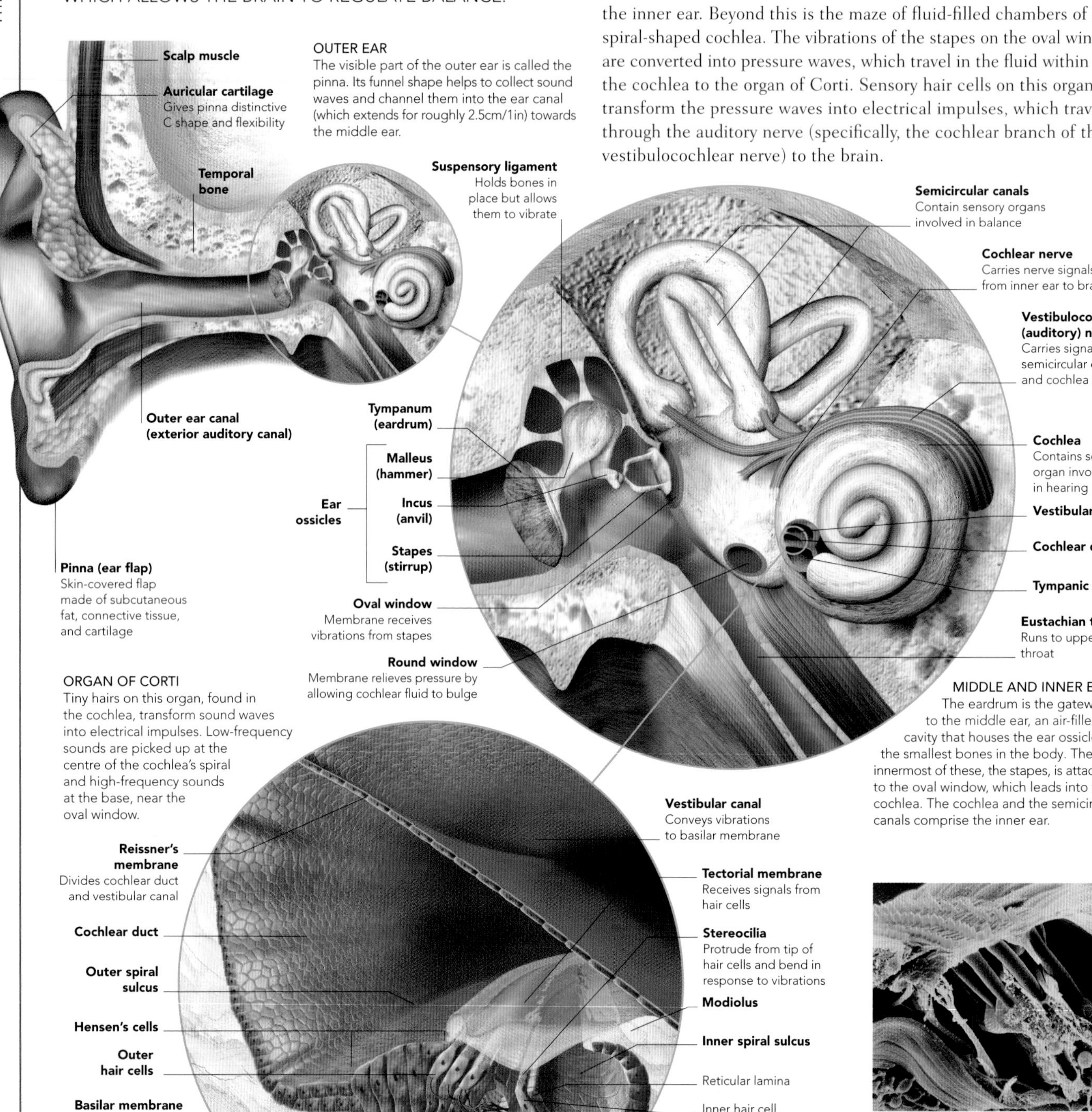

OUTER EAR
The visible part of the outer ear is called the pinna. Its funnel shape helps to collect sound waves and channel them into the ear canal (which extends for roughly 2.5cm/1in) towards the middle ear.

MIDDLE AND INNER EAR
The eardrum is the gateway to the middle ear, an air-filled cavity that houses the ear ossicles – the smallest bones in the body. The innermost of these, the stapes, is attached to the oval window, which leads into the cochlea. The cochlea and the semicircular canals comprise the inner ear.

ORGAN OF CORTI
Tiny hairs on this organ, found in the cochlea, transform sound waves into electrical impulses. Low-frequency sounds are picked up at the centre of the cochlea's spiral and high-frequency sounds at the base, near the oval window.

HAIRS ON THE ORGAN OF CORTI
This coloured electron micrograph shows sound-sensing hairs. There are 20,000 or so outer hairs (yellow). Around 3,500 inner hairs (red) lead to the auditory nerve.

THE AUDITORY CORTEX

Sound information, in the form of electrical impulses, travels from the ear along the auditory nerve to the auditory cortex (situated in the temporal lobe, beneath the temples) for processing. In one of its three areas, the primary auditory cortex, different auditory neurons respond to specific sound frequencies. Also, some respond to the intensity of a sound rather than its frequency, and others respond to more complex sounds, such as clicks, animal noises, and bursts of noise. It is thought that the secondary auditory cortex plays a part in processing harmony, rhythm, and melody, while the tertiary auditory cortex is involved in integrating the variety of sounds into a whole impression.

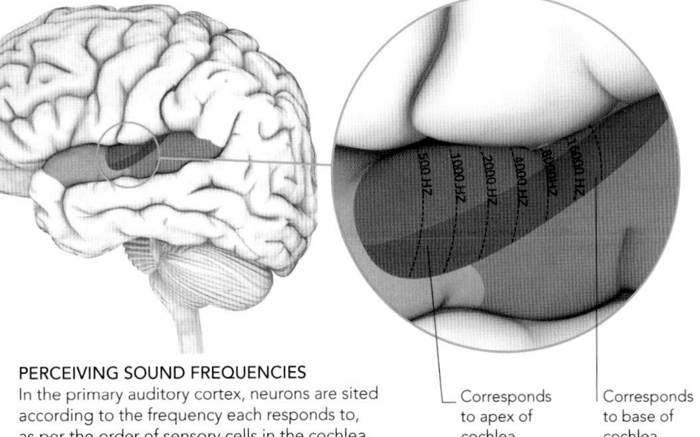

PERCEIVING SOUND FREQUENCIES
In the primary auditory cortex, neurons are sited according to the frequency each responds to, as per the order of sensory cells in the cochlea.

AUDITORY RANGES	
SPECIES	**FREQUENCY (HERTZ)**
Elephant	16–12,000
Goldfish	20–3,000
Human	64–23,000
Dog	67–45,000
Porpoise	75–150,000
Bullfrog	100–3,000
Owl	200–12,000
Bat	2,000–110,000

AUDITORY RANGES

Many animals can hear sounds that humans cannot, both at higher and lower frequencies. Some animals pick up frequencies significantly higher than those humans can detect. For example, bats using echolocation can detect reflected sounds in the 14,000–100,000 Hertz range. The lower limit of the human auditory frequency range is fixed throughout life, but the upper limit begins to fall from adolescence. The maximum frequency heard by a normal middle-aged adult is between 14,000 and 16,000 Hertz.

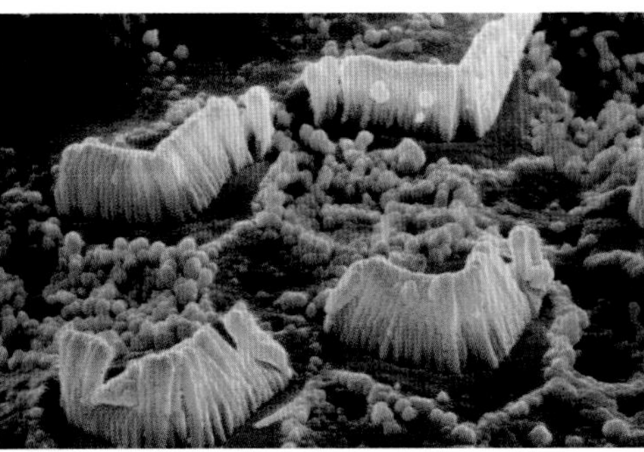

HAIR CELLS AND FREQUENCY
This coloured electron micrograph shows V-shaped sensory hair cells on the organ of Corti (see opposite page), each with multiple strands (yellow) or stereocilia. Cells are arranged within the cochlea according to the frequency of the sound each is able to detect.

THE COCHLEAR IMPLANT

Rather than restore hearing, this device helps the wearer to have a perception of sound with no time-lag, which can help with lip-reading. A microphone picks up sounds and passes them to a sound processor, which turns them into digital electrical signals. The transmitter conveys the signals, in the form of radio waves, to the implanted receiver, located beneath the skin. This receiver communicates via electrodes with the sensory hair cells in the cochlea, which pass the information on to the brain.

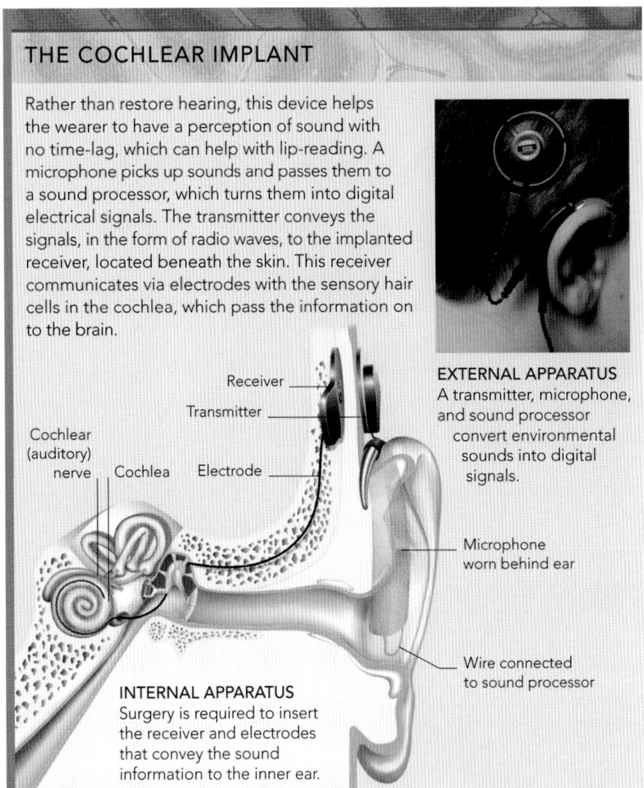

EXTERNAL APPARATUS
A transmitter, microphone, and sound processor convert environmental sounds into digital signals.

INTERNAL APPARATUS
Surgery is required to insert the receiver and electrodes that convey the sound information to the inner ear.

AUDITORY DISORDERS

Hearing loss is common but total deafness is rare and usually results from a congenital problem. Mild or severe hearing loss can result from ear disease, injury, or degeneration of the hearing system with age. Hearing loss is either conductive (a fault in the transferral of sound from the outer to inner ear) or sensorineural (sometimes known as nerve deafness, involving damage to the auditory nerves, or to the sensory parts of the inner ear). Common hearing disorders include otitis media and otosclerosis. Otitis media mainly affects young children and is an inflammation of the middle ear caused by a bacterial infection. Otosclerosis occurs when there is abnormal bone growth on the stapes bone of the middle ear, which stops it from vibrating and conducting sound waves on to the inner ear.

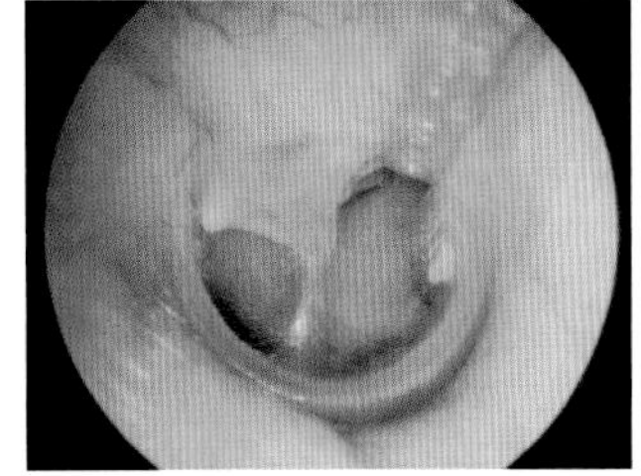

PERFORATED EARDRUM
The eardrum may become perforated due to infection, injury, or sudden exposure to an explosive noise that causes excessive vibration. Perforations can heal naturally.

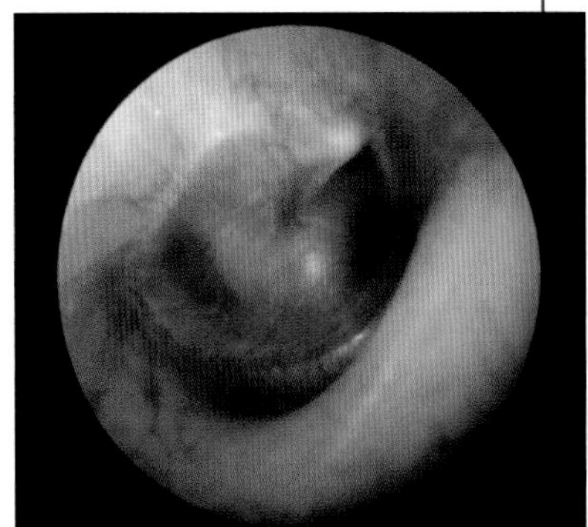

NORMAL EARDRUM
The eardrum consists of a thin layer of fibrous tissue continuous with the skin of the outer ear and the mucous membrane of the middle ear.

MAKING SENSE OF SOUND

SOUND VIBRATIONS ARE TURNED INTO ELECTRICAL IMPULSES IN THE COCHLEA. FROM THERE, THEY TRAVEL TO THE AUDITORY CORTEX AND ITS ASSOCIATION AREAS VIA THE MEDULLA AND THE THALAMUS.

PERCEPTION OF SOUND

Sounds start as vibrations entering the ears. In the inner ear, receptor cells in the cochlea transform these vibrations into electrical signals, which pass along the cochlear nerve to the medulla in the brainstem, and then to the inferior colliculus. The cochlear nerve fibres divide so that most of the input from each ear can go to both hemispheres. At this stage, the source of the sound is determined by areas of the brainstem that compare input from both ears and analyse the delay (of about 1/1,500 of a second) between the receipt of the signal by the ear nearest to the source and the ear furthest away. The signals reach the auditory cortex via the thalamus, where frequency, quality, intensity, and meaning are perceived. The left auditory cortex is more concerned with the meaning and identification of sound; the right, with quality.

THE COCKTAIL-PARTY EFFECT

The brain not only receives signals from the ears, it also sends signals to them, creating a circuit that modulates input. Background noise is dimmed, and the longer a person concentrates on a single strand of conversation, the greater the effect of filtering. This makes it easy to hear words you are interested in but may reduce the background so much that important messages fail to get through. If your brain registers an important sound, such as your name, it will instantly identify the source of that sound and upgrade it from heard to listened to. This is known as the cocktail-party effect.

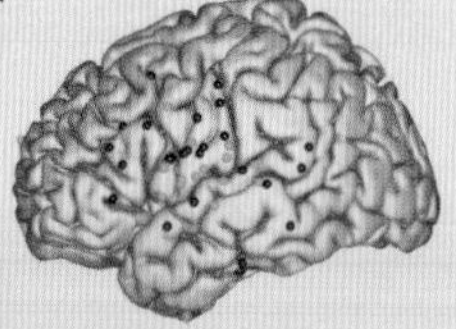

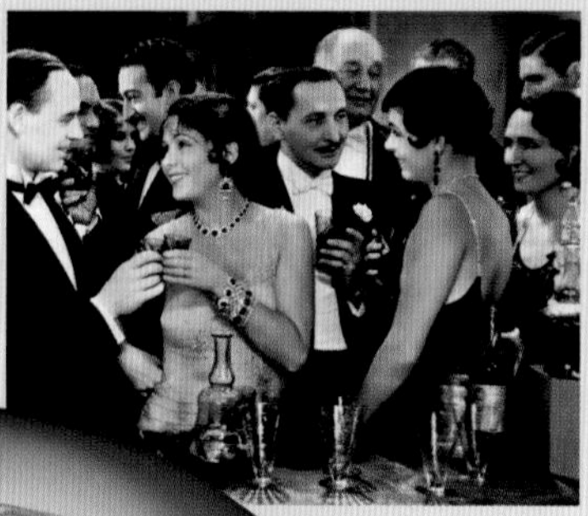

HEAR OR LISTEN
When in a noisy environment, such as at a party, the brain can tune in to listen to a particular conversation while still hearing the noise of background speech. Green areas in the scan above register the sound of speech while red areas process speech to the level of understanding – it is "listened to" as well as heard.

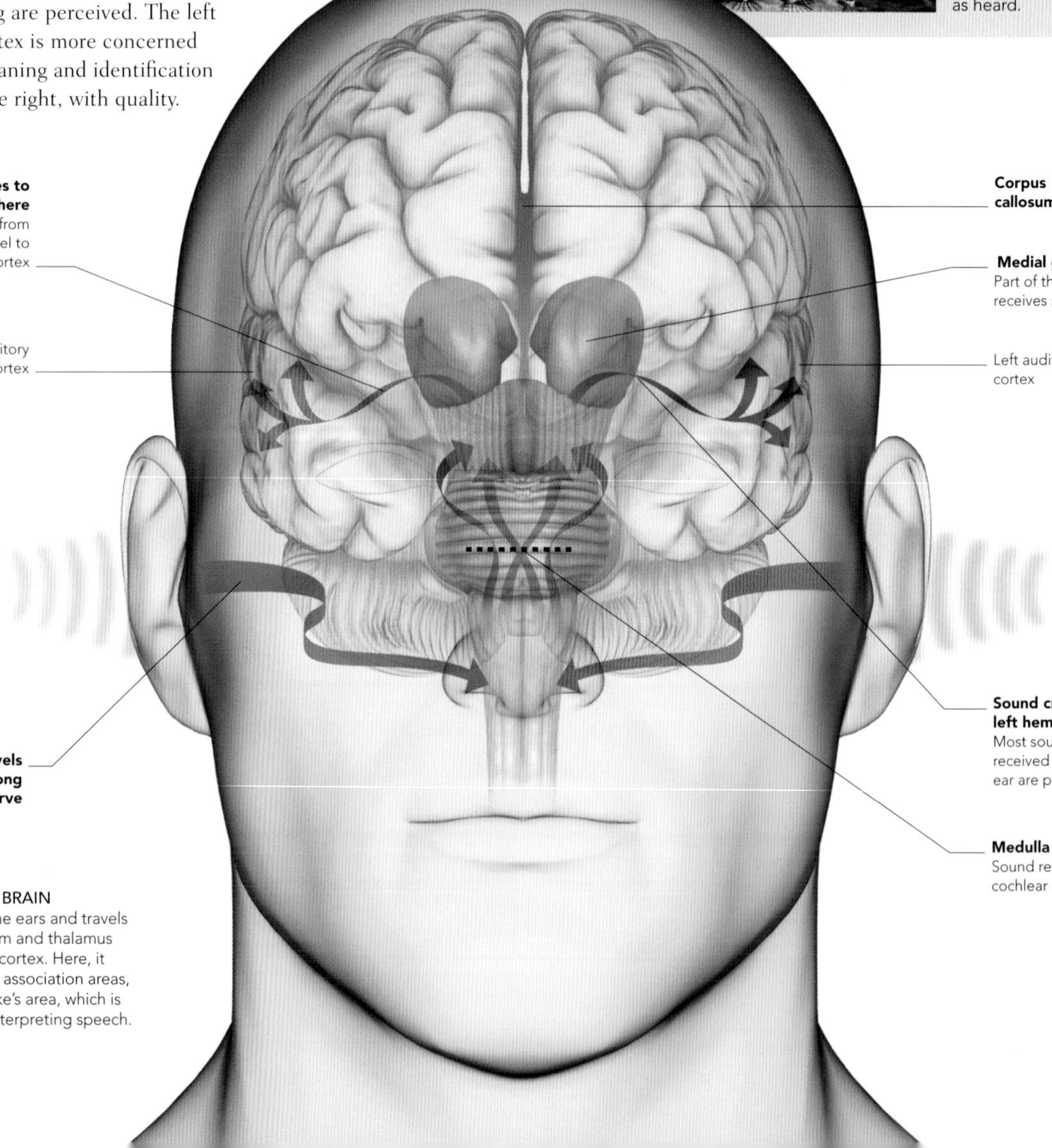

Sound crosses to right hemisphere Most signals from left cochlea travel to right side of cortex

Right auditory cortex

Corpus callosum

Medial geniculate body Part of thalamus that receives signal

Left auditory cortex

Sound travels through ear along cochlear nerve

Sound crosses to left hemisphere Most sound signals received from right ear are processed here

Medulla in brainstem Sound received in cochlear nucleus

THE HEARING BRAIN
Sound enters the ears and travels via the brainstem and thalamus to the auditory cortex. Here, it is processed by association areas, such as Wernicke's area, which is involved with interpreting speech.

NOISE OR MUSIC?

Sound consists of waves, or vibrations, whose characteristics are determined by the source of the sound. The main characteristics influencing our perception of sound are frequency (number of vibrations per second) and amplitude (the size of the waves' "peaks" and "troughs"). Frequency influences pitch, and amplitude governs loudness. Irregular sound-wave patterns tend to be experienced as noise; in contrast, music produces regular patterns.

Music is hard to define precisely, but the quality of musical notes depends upon their sound source – a musical instrument – and how it is being played. Another important factor in music is timbre, or the "quality" of a sound. Timbre depends upon how many different frequencies of the note are heard at once; multiple frequencies or overtones (harmony) make a richer timbre. The auditory cortex responds to different qualities in music. The primary region responds to frequencies and the secondary area to harmony and rhythm, while the tertiary area adds higher levels of appreciation and integration.

FREQUENCY (HERTZ)

TONE

NOISE

TIME (SECONDS)

NOISE OR NOTE
Analysis of the wave forms of sounds reveals pure tones to be regular in frequency and amplitude, while noise is irregular.

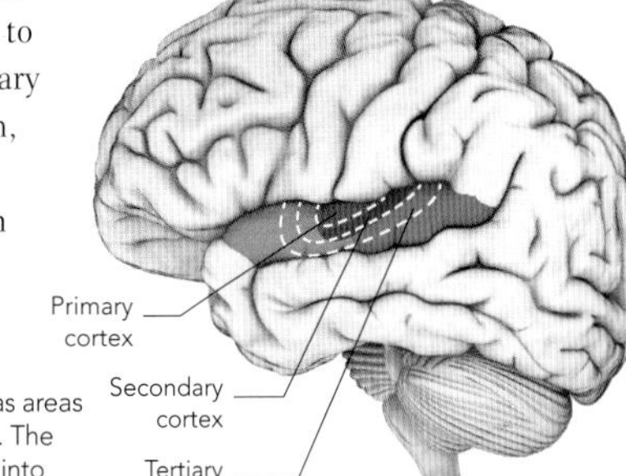

AUDITORY CORTEX
The inner primary auditory cortex has areas associated with specific frequencies. The secondary and tertiary regions tune into more complex aspects of sound perception.

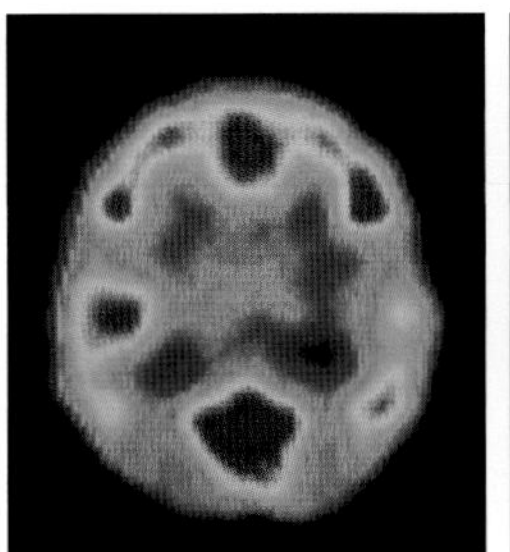

ACTIVITY DURING SPEECH
Speech tends to produce more intense activity in the left-hand side of the auditory cortex.

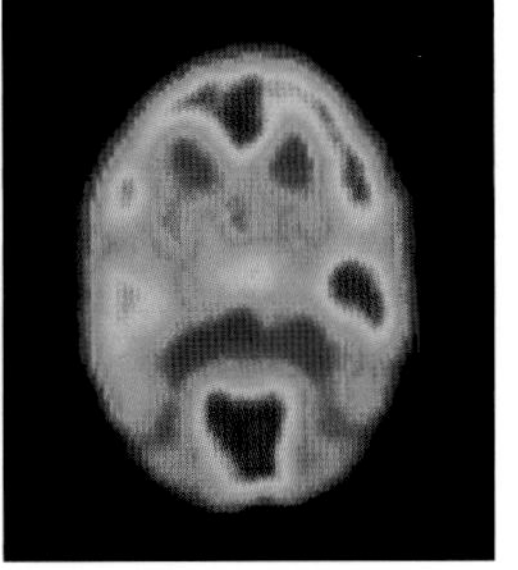

ACTIVITY DURING MUSIC
Music produces more pronounced activity on the right-hand side of the auditory cortex.

THE MOZART EFFECT

The French child-development expert Alfred Tomatis first described the "Mozart effect" in 1991. He claimed that listening to the music of the 18th-century classical composer Mozart could help the mental development of children under three. Researchers have also demonstrated that students listening to Mozart could improve their performance on tasks involving spatial reasoning and show a temporary increase in IQ. Recent research has given mixed results, but the idea has gained in popularity. The Mozart effect may, however, have more to do with changes in mood and arousal affecting mental performance than any direct impact on intelligence.

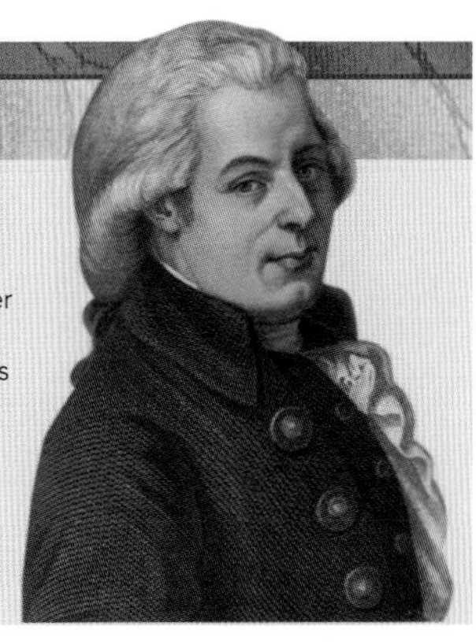

DEVELOPMENT OF HEARING

The development of hearing is a gradual process that begins in the womb and is complete by about the end of the first year of a baby's life. Research shows that the unborn child is capable of hearing by about the fourth month of gestation, but the auditory apparatus is not fully formed until about the sixth month. At birth, hearing is the most developed of the senses, so it is of prime importance to the baby in exploring its world. Studies have shown how the baby learns to recognize sounds in its first few months, gradually becomes able to distinguish between speech and non-speech sounds, and then begins to understand words. Children also lose the ability to hear differences between sounds that are not important in their native language. Many Japanese children, for example, can no longer hear the difference between "l" and "r", which they could distinguish at an earlier age.

DEVELOPMENT BEFORE AND AFTER BIRTH

The human fetus has some basic hearing capacity from the age of about 18 weeks. This ability matures and develops over the next few weeks, with low-frequency sounds outside the mother's body being heard better than those of high frequency. From birth up to four months, the baby starts to respond to loud or sudden sounds, beginning to localize them by turning the head. From three to six months, the baby begins to recognize and also make sounds. Between six and 12 months, he or she begins to babble, recognizes basic words like "mummy", and starts to recognize voices. The baby begins to form words from the age of about one year. Each child reaches these milestones in hearing and speech development at different times, but very slow development may indicate some problem with the hearing apparatus.

Ears start to form

Can hear sounds

Auditory apparatus completely formed

Can hear voices

Can recognize voices

Can recognize familiar and unfamiliar sounds

Can distinguish between speech and other sounds

Learns to segment speech

0 1 2 3 4 5 6 7 8 9 | 1 2 3 4 5 6 7 8 9 10 11 12 13 14 15 16

IN THE WOMB (AGE IN MONTHS) | AFTER BIRTH (AGE IN MONTHS)

HEARING

HEARING INVOLVES MECHANICAL VIBRATIONS FROM THE ENVIRONMENT – SPEECH, MUSIC, AND EVERYDAY NOISE – JOURNEYING THROUGH THE OUTER, MIDDLE, AND INNER EAR. THE VIBRATIONS ARE TRANSFORMED TO ELECTRICAL SIGNALS, WHICH TRAVEL TO THE BRAIN TO BE INTERPRETED AS SOUND.

PATHWAY OF SOUND

The ear is a complex, exquisitely designed instrument for the capture of sound and its transport to the brain. Once mechanical vibrations from sound sources reach the inner ear, they are transformed into electrical impulses that shoot along the cochlear nerve to the brainstem. Here they follow complex pathways up to the thalamus before arriving at the auditory cortex. Processing in the brain allows perception of the meaning, direction, and volume of a sound.

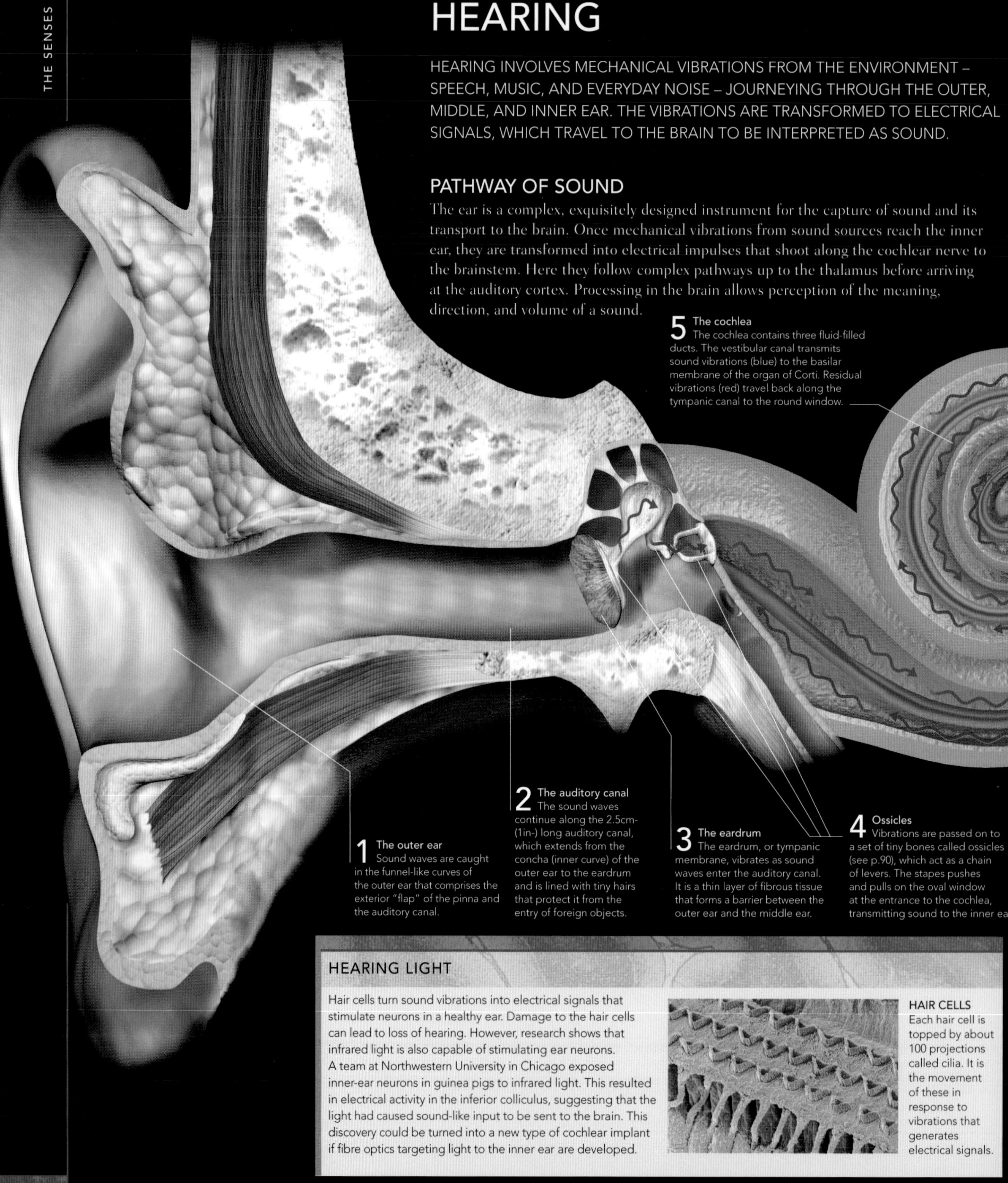

5 The cochlea The cochlea contains three fluid-filled ducts. The vestibular canal transmits sound vibrations (blue) to the basilar membrane of the organ of Corti. Residual vibrations (red) travel back along the tympanic canal to the round window.

1 The outer ear Sound waves are caught in the funnel-like curves of the outer ear that comprises the exterior "flap" of the pinna and the auditory canal.

2 The auditory canal The sound waves continue along the 2.5cm- (1in-) long auditory canal, which extends from the concha (inner curve) of the outer ear to the eardrum and is lined with tiny hairs that protect it from the entry of foreign objects.

3 The eardrum The eardrum, or tympanic membrane, vibrates as sound waves enter the auditory canal. It is a thin layer of fibrous tissue that forms a barrier between the outer ear and the middle ear.

4 Ossicles Vibrations are passed on to a set of tiny bones called ossicles (see p.90), which act as a chain of levers. The stapes pushes and pulls on the oval window at the entrance to the cochlea, transmitting sound to the inner ear.

HEARING LIGHT

Hair cells turn sound vibrations into electrical signals that stimulate neurons in a healthy ear. Damage to the hair cells can lead to loss of hearing. However, research shows that infrared light is also capable of stimulating ear neurons. A team at Northwestern University in Chicago exposed inner-ear neurons in guinea pigs to infrared light. This resulted in electrical activity in the inferior colliculus, suggesting that the light had caused sound-like input to be sent to the brain. This discovery could be turned into a new type of cochlear implant if fibre optics targeting light to the inner ear are developed.

HAIR CELLS Each hair cell is topped by about 100 projections called cilia. It is the movement of these in response to vibrations that generates electrical signals.

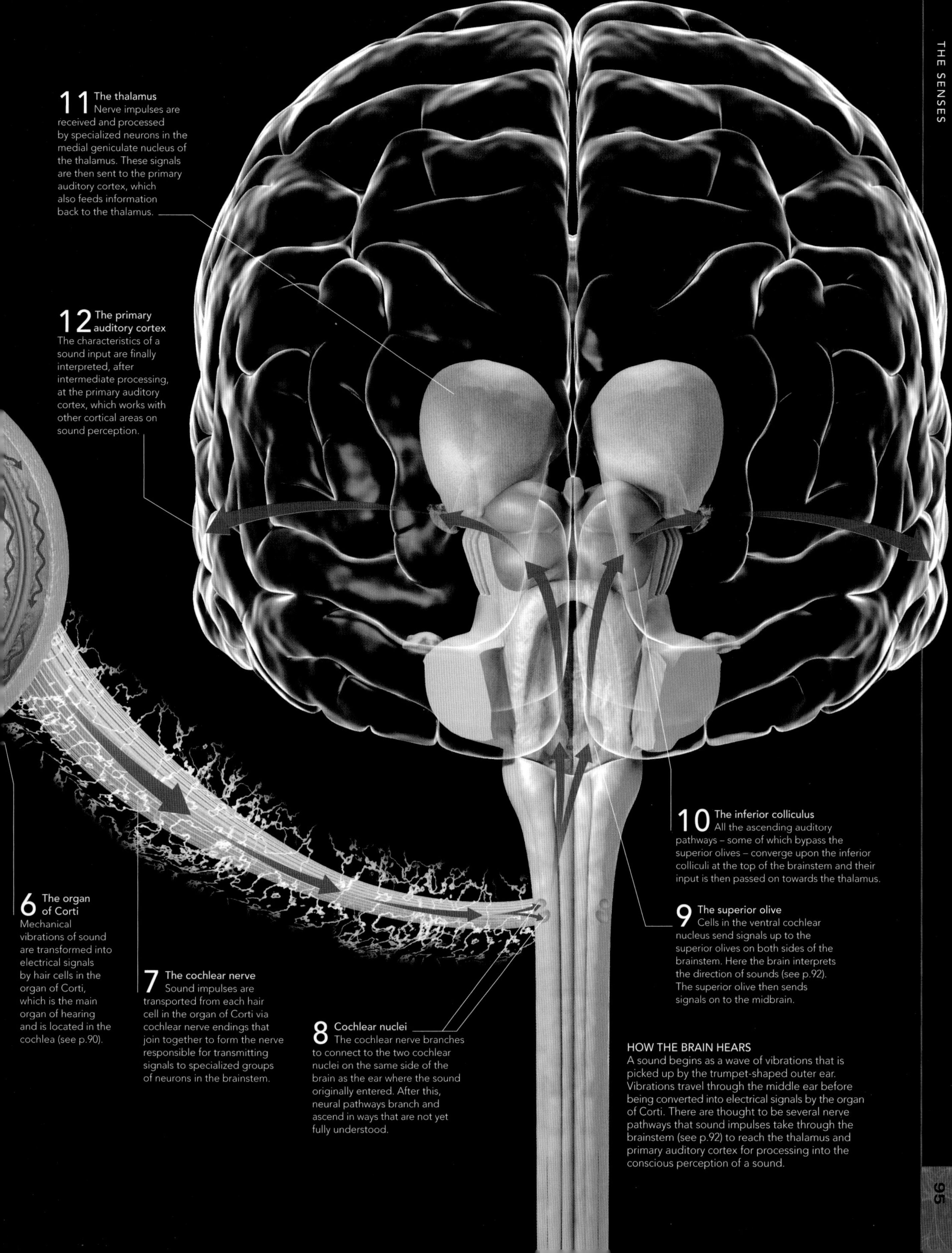

11 The thalamus Nerve impulses are received and processed by specialized neurons in the medial geniculate nucleus of the thalamus. These signals are then sent to the primary auditory cortex, which also feeds information back to the thalamus.

12 The primary auditory cortex The characteristics of a sound input are finally interpreted, after intermediate processing, at the primary auditory cortex, which works with other cortical areas on sound perception.

10 The inferior colliculus All the ascending auditory pathways – some of which bypass the superior olives – converge upon the inferior colliculi at the top of the brainstem and their input is then passed on towards the thalamus.

6 The organ of Corti Mechanical vibrations of sound are transformed into electrical signals by hair cells in the organ of Corti, which is the main organ of hearing and is located in the cochlea (see p.90).

9 The superior olive Cells in the ventral cochlear nucleus send signals up to the superior olives on both sides of the brainstem. Here the brain interprets the direction of sounds (see p.92). The superior olive then sends signals on to the midbrain.

7 The cochlear nerve Sound impulses are transported from each hair cell in the organ of Corti via cochlear nerve endings that join together to form the nerve responsible for transmitting signals to specialized groups of neurons in the brainstem.

8 Cochlear nuclei The cochlear nerve branches to connect to the two cochlear nuclei on the same side of the brain as the ear where the sound originally entered. After this, neural pathways branch and ascend in ways that are not yet fully understood.

HOW THE BRAIN HEARS

A sound begins as a wave of vibrations that is picked up by the trumpet-shaped outer ear. Vibrations travel through the middle ear before being converted into electrical signals by the organ of Corti. There are thought to be several nerve pathways that sound impulses take through the brainstem (see p.92) to reach the thalamus and primary auditory cortex for processing into the conscious perception of a sound.

SMELL

ALTHOUGH VISION HAS BECOME THE DOMINANT SENSE IN HUMANS, THE SENSE OF SMELL (OLFACTION) REMAINS IMPORTANT TO SURVIVAL BECAUSE IT CAN WARN US OF HAZARDOUS SUBSTANCES IN OUR ENVIRONMENT. THE SENSES OF SMELL AND TASTE ARE CLOSELY LINKED.

DETECTING SMELL

Like the sense of taste, smell is a chemical sense. Specialized receptors in the nasal cavity detect incoming molecules, which enter the nose on air currents and bind to receptor cells. Sniffing sucks up more odour molecules into the nose, allowing you to "sample" a smell. It is a reflex action that occurs when a smell attracts your attention, and can help to warn of danger, such as smoke from a fire or rotting food. Olfactory receptors located high up in the nasal cavity send electrical impulses to the olfactory bulb, in the limbic area of the brain, for processing.

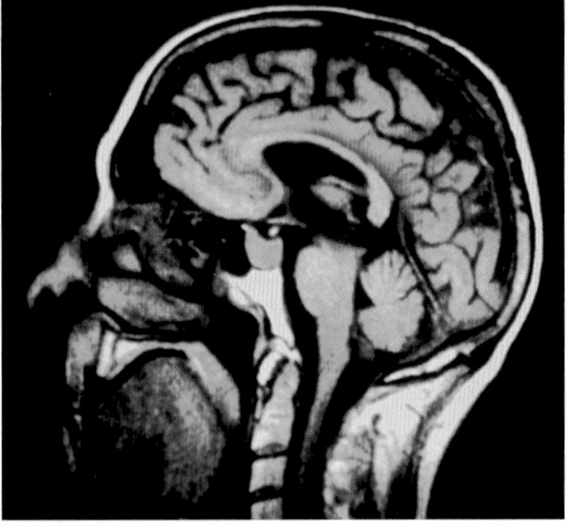

SMELL CENTRES IN THE BRAIN
The olfactory bulb is the smell gateway to the brain. Here, data about smells is processed in the forebrain (yellow), then sent to various areas of the brain, including the olfactory cortex adjacent to the hippocampus (red).

SMELL PATHWAYS

Odours are initially registered by receptor cells in the nasal cavity. These send electrical impulses along dedicated pathways to the olfactory bulb (each nostril connects to one olfactory bulb). The olfactory bulb is part of the brain's limbic system, the seat of our emotions, desires, and instincts, which is why smells can trigger strong emotional reactions. Once processed by the olfactory bulb, data is transmitted via three olfactory pathways to higher centres in the brain that process it in different ways. This process is called "orthonasal" smelling, in which smell data travels along pathways directly from the nose (see opposite). In "retronasal" smelling (see p.101), odours also have a flavour component that enters the olfactory pathways via the mouth.

SAME-SIDE PROCESSING
Unlike data gathered by the other sense organs, odours are processed on the same, not opposite, side of the brain as the nostril the sensory data was sent from.

RECEPTOR ARRAYS

There are around 1,000 types of receptor cell in the nasal cavity, but we can distinguish around 20,000 different smells so, clearly, there is more to smell reception than "one receptor, one smell". Research shows that each receptor has zones on it, each of which responds to a number of smell molecules. Also, multiple receptors respond to the same smell molecule – it may be that each receptor binds to a different part of it. A specific smell will activate a specific pattern or "array" across the receptors, so that each smell has its own "signature". When the receptors forming a specific pattern are activated, this signature is sent to the brain for processing.

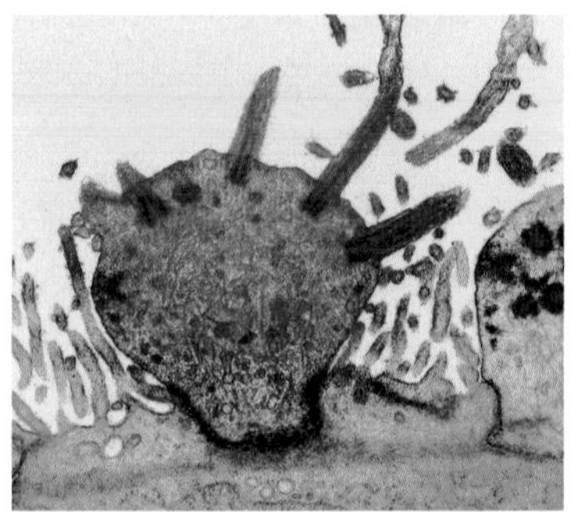

OLFACTORY RECEPTOR CELL
This coloured electron micrograph shows tiny cilia projecting from a receptor cell. Odour molecules bind to the cilia and activate the receptor.

THE CHEMISTRY OF SMELL

There is still much to be learned about the relationship between chemical structure and smell. Scientists have identified eight primary odours (rather like the three primary colours): camphorous, fishy, malty, minty, musky, spermatic, sweaty, and urinous. Smells are often produced by a combination of many different smell molecules, often from different categories. Comparisons of the structures of smell molecules within each category have shown some similarities – for example, minty smelling compounds often share a similar molecular structure. However, tiny differences in molecular structure can produce very different smells. Octanol, a fatty alcohol, smells like oranges, while octanoic acid, a saturated fatty acid that differs from octanol by only one oxygen atom, smells like sweat.

SMELL AND MOLECULAR STRUCTURE
These two molecules differ significantly in their chemical structure, yet both of them conjure the same characteristic "mothball" smell of camphor. One theory is that it is not the shape of molecules that causes them to smell, but the frequency at which their atoms vibrate.

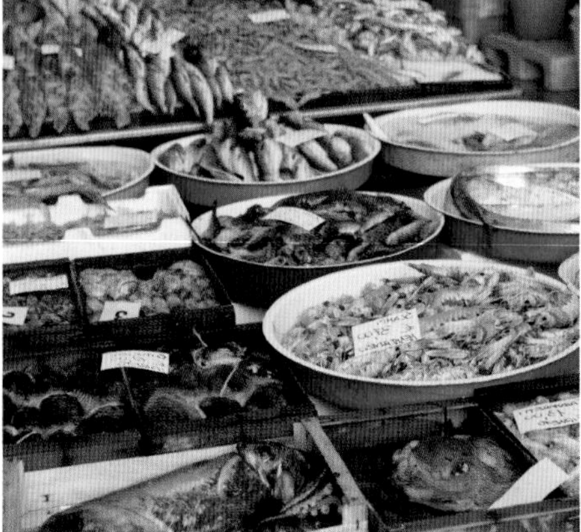

PRIMARY SMELLS
Scientists investigating the perception of smell have attempted to identify primary odours, which can be combined with one another to produce the much larger range of smells that we experience. To date, eight primary odours have been identified, including the distinctive smell of fish.

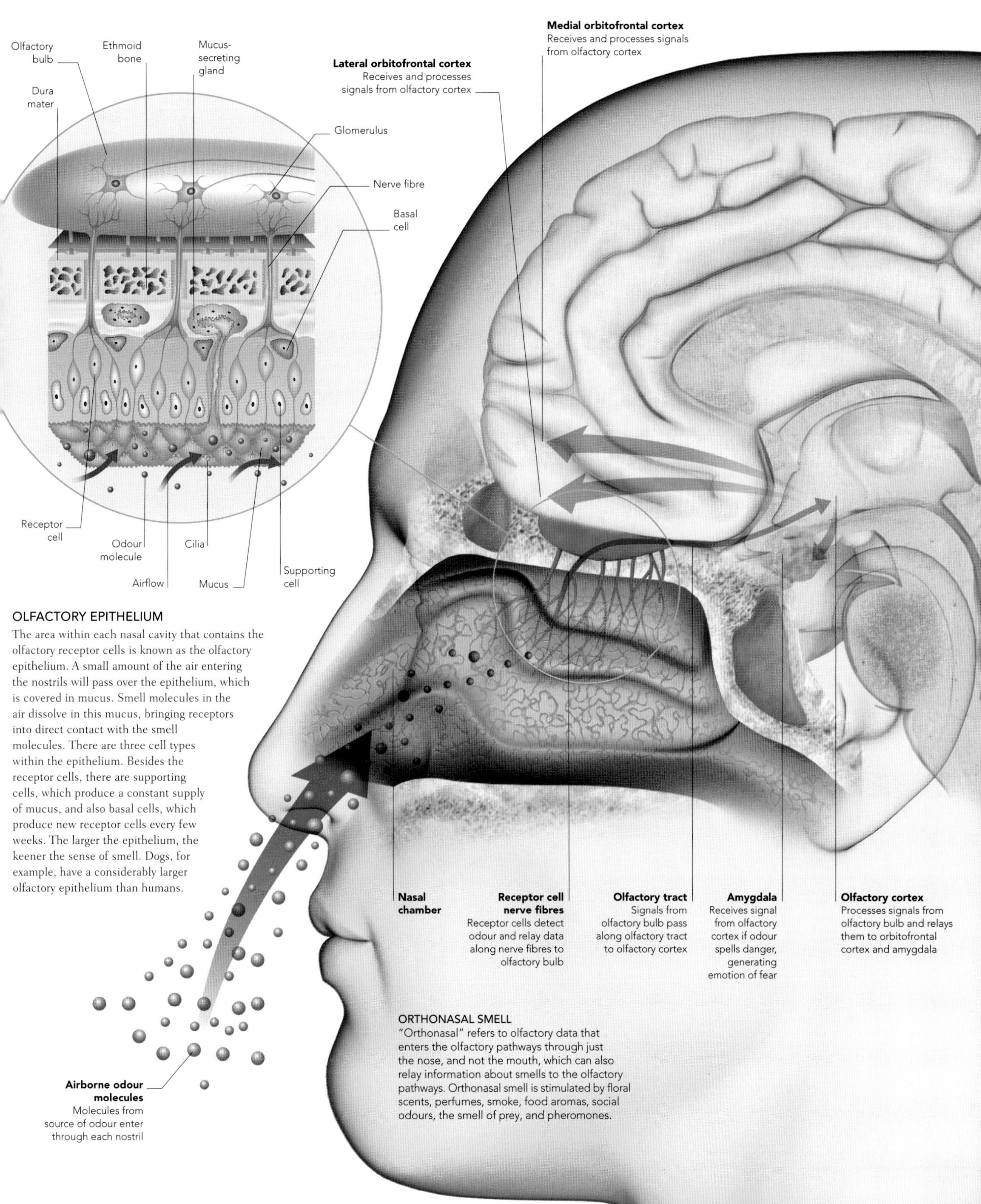

Olfactory
bulb

Dura
mater

Ethmoid
bone

Mucus-
secreting
gland

Glomerulus

Nerve fibre

Basal
cell

Receptor
cell

Odour
molecule

Cilia

Airflow

Mucus

OLFACTORY EPITHELIUM

The area within each nasal cavity that contains the olfactory receptor cells is known as the olfactory epithelium. A small amount of the air entering the nostrils will pass over the epithelium, which is covered in mucus. Smell molecules in the air dissolve in this mucus, bringing receptors into direct contact with the smell molecules. There are three cell types within the epithelium. Besides the receptor cells, there are supporting cells, which produce a constant supply of mucus, and also basal cells, which produce new receptor cells every few weeks. The larger the epithelium, the keener the sense of smell. Dogs, for example, have a considerably larger olfactory epithelium than humans.

**Nasal
chamber**

**Receptor cell
nerve fibres**
Receptor cells detect
odour and relay data
along nerve fibres to
olfactory bulb

Olfactory tract
Signals from
olfactory bulb pass
along olfactory tract
to olfactory cortex

Amygdala
Receives signal
from olfactory
cortex if odour
spells danger,
generating
emotion of fear

Olfactory cortex
Processes signals from
olfactory bulb and relays
them to orbitofrontal
cortex and amygdala

ORTHONASAL SMELL

"Orthonasal" refers to olfactory data that enters the olfactory pathways through just the nose, and not the mouth, which can also relay information about smells to the olfactory pathways. Orthonasal smell is stimulated by floral scents, perfumes, smoke, food aromas, social odours, the smell of prey, and pheromones.
Molecules from
source of odour enter
through each nostril

PERCEIVING SMELL

SMELL IS MORE LIKELY TO EVOKE EMOTION AND MEMORY THAN THE OTHER SENSES. THE FACT THAT OLFACTORY AREAS OF THE BRAIN EVOLVED EARLY ON AND ARE WIRED INTO THE PRIMITIVE BRAIN SUGGESTS THAT SMELL IS VITAL FOR OUR SURVIVAL, AS WELL AS THE SURVIVAL OF OTHER ANIMALS.

THE EVOLUTION OF SMELL

The smell brain, centred around the olfactory bulb in the limbic system, is of ancient origin, having evolved about 50 million years ago in fish. The sense of smell was overtaken in importance by the sense of vision when humans began to walk on two legs, although it is still dominant for many animals. But smell is an important aspect of survival for humans, shown in the fact that we take prompt action if we smell gas or smoke, for example. It also plays an important role in sexual selection, emotional responses, and forming preferences for food and drink. All of these factors were probably of key importance in the lives of our ancestors.

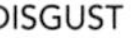

DISGUST
When a bad odour is detected, such as that of rotting meat, it is natural to both feel and express disgust. Avoidance of the source of the odour follows, and it is almost impossible to eat food that smells bad.

OLFACTION IN ANIMALS

Although humans can smell some odours at a concentration as low as one part per trillion, our sense of smell is weak compared to that of other animals. The size of the surface area of the olfactory epithelium (see p.97) and the density of smell receptor cells indicate how sensitive an animal's sense of smell is. Dogs, for example, can identify a particular human from just a few odour molecules. Northern dogs, such as huskies and jackals, are renowned for their sense of smell. Hunting dogs and greyhounds have a weaker sense of smell – in the chase, they don't have time to distinguish prey from background smells.

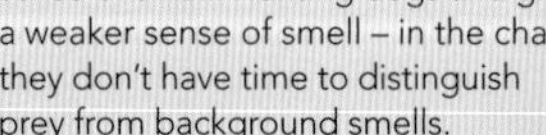

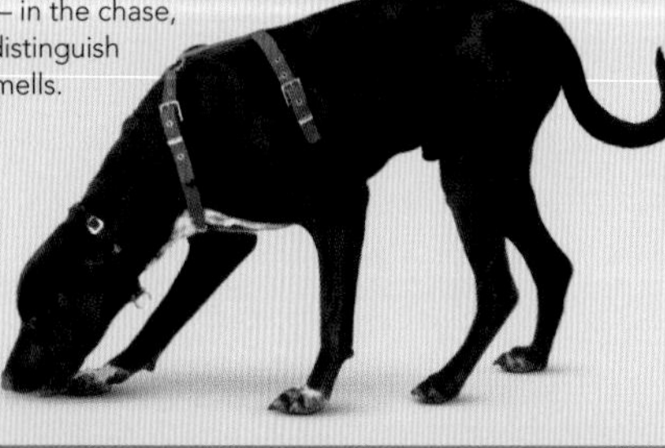

SNIFFER DOG
A breed combining the behavioural characteristics of a domestic dog and a jackal's sense of smell makes an ideal sniffer dog for security work.

SMELL ACROSS SPECIES

SPECIES	NUMBER OF OLFACTORY RECEPTOR CELLS	AREA OF OLFACTORY EPITHELIUM
Human	12 million	10 square cm (1½ square in)
Cat	70 million	21 square cm (3¼ square in)
Rabbit	100 million	Data not available
Dog	1 billion	170 square cm (26½ square in)
Bloodhound	4 billion	381 square cm (59 square in)

SMELL PREFERENCES

Whether we find a smell nice, nasty, or neutral is very subjective and depends upon familiarity, intensity, and perception as pleasant or unpleasant. It is not clear if preferences are innate or learned, but much experimental evidence supports the latter possibility. Associative learning links pleasant smells to pleasant experiences, and vice versa. For example, people who fear the dentist do not like the clove-like smell of eugenol, which is used in dental cement; those without a fear of the dentist react positively or neutrally to this odour.

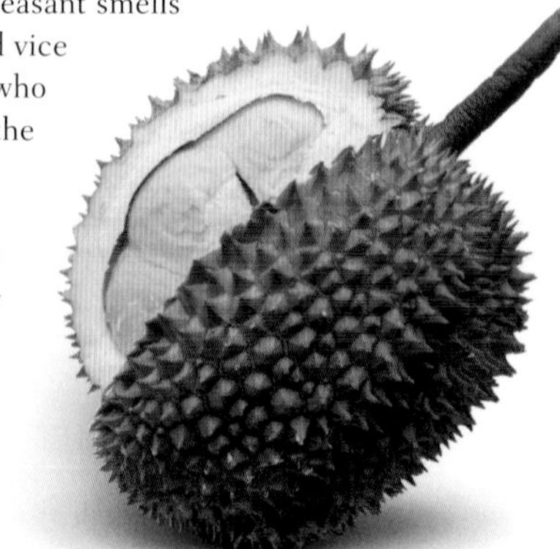

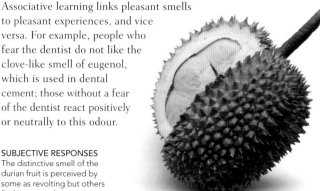

SUBJECTIVE RESPONSES
The distinctive smell of the durian fruit is perceived by some as revolting but others find it extremely tempting.

THE SIX WORST SMELLS IN THE WORLD

SMELL	DESCRIPTION
Decaying flesh	Repulsive to most people, perhaps as it evokes thoughts of death
Skunk odour	Horrible to most, but a few people find it "interesting"
Vomit	Often associated with illness, which may heighten disgust
Faeces or urine	Caused by gas released as bacteria break down food residue
Decaying food	Triggers an "adaptive" response to food that could cause illness
Isonitriles	Chemicals in non-lethal weapons described as "world's worst smell"

STEREOSCOPIC AND BLIND SMELL

It is generally believed that the human sense of smell has atrophied in relation to our other senses, but recent research shows that humans can still effectively track a scent. Using both nostrils to sample a smell, the human brain uses both sets of data to accurately pinpoint the location of the source of the odour. Therefore, as with vision and hearing, smell can be "stereoscopic", relying on both nostrils for a full understanding of a scent. "Blind" smell refers to the ability of the brain to detect a smell without being consciously aware of it, which has been demonstrated in experiments using fMRI scans showing how olfactory areas are activated without the participant's knowledge.

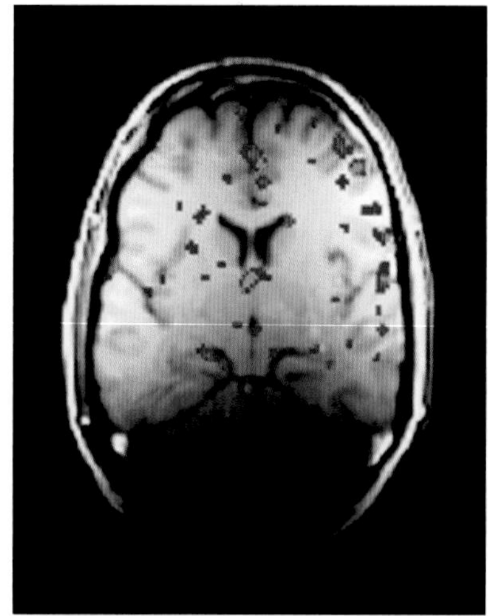

BLIND SMELL ACTIVATION
This fMRI scan shows widespread activity throughout the brain in areas including the thalamus (just above centre), on exposure to an odour at concentrations that cannot be detected consciously.

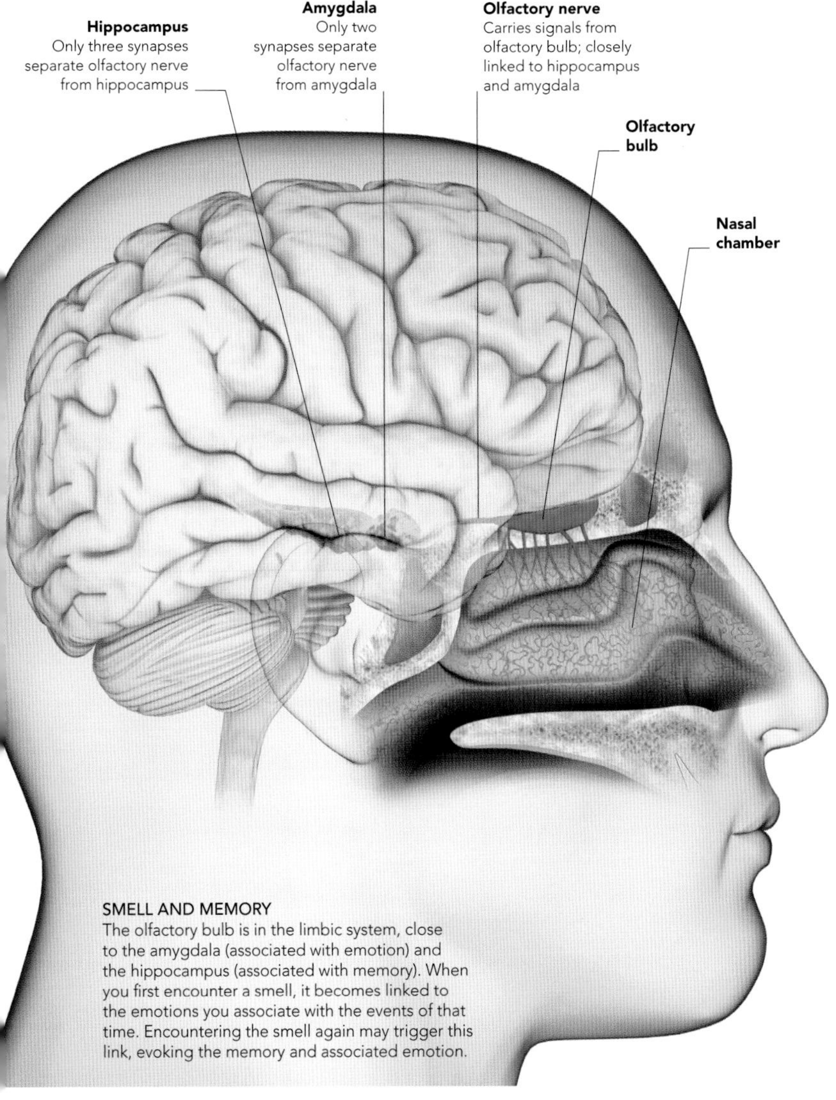
Hippocampus
Only three synapses separate olfactory nerve from hippocampus
Amygdala
Only two synapses separate olfactory nerve from amygdala
Olfactory nerve
Carries signals from olfactory bulb; closely linked to hippocampus and amygdala
Olfactory bulb
Nasal chamber

SMELL AND MEMORY
The olfactory bulb is in the limbic system, close to the amygdala (associated with emotion) and the hippocampus (associated with memory). When you first encounter a smell, it becomes linked to the emotions you associate with the events of that time. Encountering the smell again may trigger this link, evoking the memory and associated emotion.

SMELL AND MEMORY

An event is associated with input from all the senses, co-ordinated by the hippocampus. Re-experiencing any of the sight, smell, or sound inputs may trigger a memory of the event, but smell seems most strongly associated with memory. This may be because olfactory regions are linked to all emotional areas in the limbic system. Research shows that a memory of a visual image is likely to fade within days, but the memory of a smell may persist for up to a year or even decades. The hippocampus may not even be crucial for the link, because people who sustain damage to this region can still recall scents from their childhood, even though suffering from general memory loss.

THE MADELEINE EFFECT

The madeleine effect is named after an episode in Marcel Proust's epic *Remembrance of Things Past*. As a mature adult, the novel's hero eats a madeleine soaked in lime-blossom tea and is mentally transported to his childhood and the house of his aunt, who used to serve madeleines before Sunday mass. Long before the effect was investigated scientifically, Proust recognized that taste and olfactory memories can take us further back than visual or auditory cues.

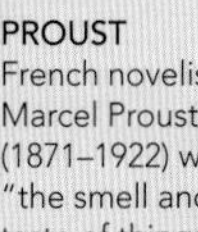

PROUST
French novelist Marcel Proust (1871–1922) wrote "the smell and taste of things remain poised a long time, ready to remind us…".

SMELL AND COMMUNICATION

Animals emit compounds called pheromones that are used as communication signals and detected by an accessory olfactory system in the brain. Humans recognize each other in a similar way – for example, infants prefer the smell of their mother's breast to that of other women. Research into the existence of pheromones in humans has found that women's menstrual cycles can synchronize when one woman is exposed to odourless compounds (supposing that these are pheromones) emitted from the underarms of another woman. In animals, the accessory olfactory system is linked to the vomeronasal region (VMO), an area in the nasal cavity that responds to pheromones. The VMO's existence in humans remains debatable.

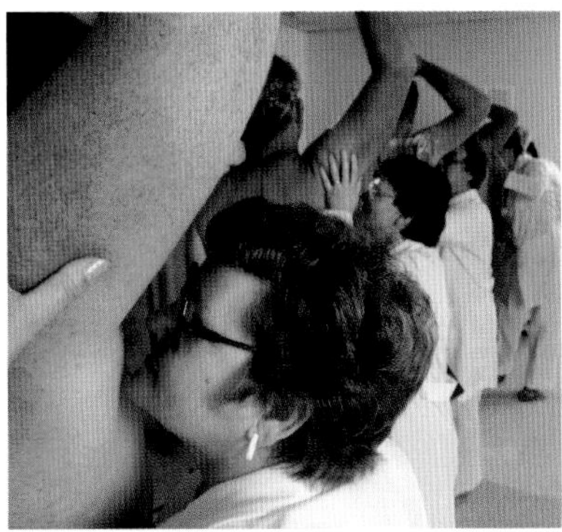

MALE BODY SMELL
Male sweat contains androstenone, a musky compound. When sprayed on a waiting-room chair, most women choose that one. Androstadienone, another compound, affects men, making them more helpful. It is likely to stem from the need for men to hunt co-operatively.

USING SMELL COMMERCIALLY
Some estate agents claim that the smells of baking bread, cinnamon, and coffee can help to sell a house by evoking a good feeling in potential purchasers. Equally, they advise banishing pets, so that animal smells do not put off buyers.

TASTE

LIKE SMELL, TASTE HAS A SURVIVAL VALUE – POISONOUS SUBSTANCES TEND TO TASTE BAD (USUALLY BITTER) WHILE THOSE THAT ARE NOURISHING TASTE PLEASURABLE (USUALLY SWEET OR SAVOURY). TOGETHER, TASTE AND SMELL ALLOW ANIMALS TO EVALUATE AND RECOGNIZE WHAT THEY EAT AND DRINK.

THE EVOLUTION OF TASTE

The sense of taste enables animals, including humans, to make the most of the variety of foods available to them. Many plants that look tempting are toxic, so genes that enable us to detect (and therefore avoid) these toxins have an obvious survival value. One such gene that has been identified affords taste sensitivity to phenylthiocarbamide (PTC), an organic compound that resembles many toxic compounds found in plants.

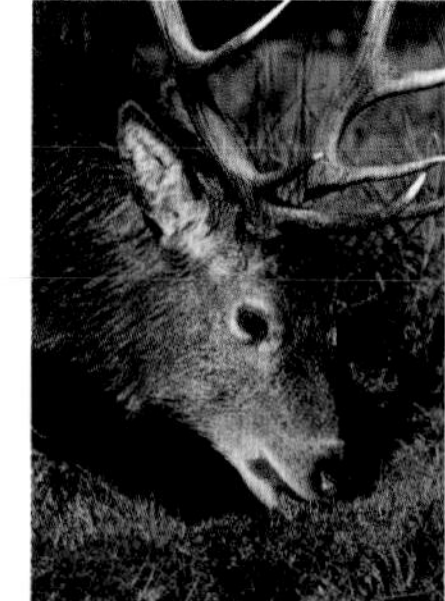
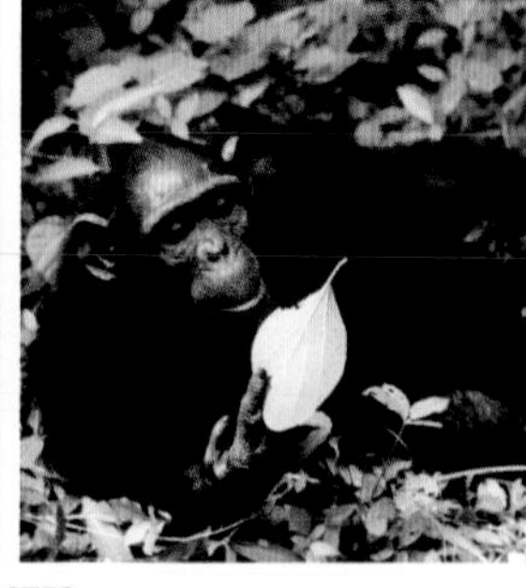

EVOLVED TO REACT TO TASTES
Herbivores, such as deer, have fewer bitter-taste genes than omnivores, so are less selective and therefore benefit from an increased food supply. They can tolerate more toxins because they have larger livers than omnivores, such as chimpanzees.

THE TONGUE

The tongue is the main sensory organ for taste detection. It is the body's most flexible muscular organ, as revealed by its work in both nutrition and communication. It has three interior muscles and three pairs of muscles connecting it to the mouth and throat. Its surface is dotted with tiny, pimple-like structures called papillae. Other parts of the mouth, such as the palate, pharynx, and epiglottis can also detect taste stimuli.

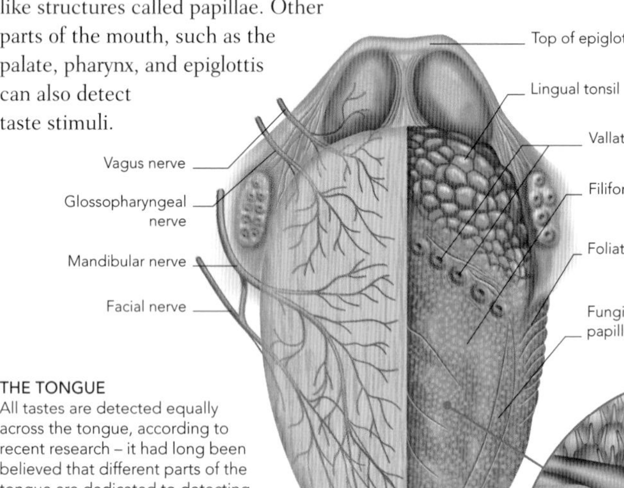

THE TONGUE
All tastes are detected equally across the tongue, according to recent research – it had long been believed that different parts of the tongue are dedicated to detecting specific tastes. The tongue is well supplied with nerves that carry taste-related data to the brain.

SUPERTASTERS

Around a quarter of the population are "supertasters", which means they have an overall higher level of tasting ability. They are very sensitive to a chemical called propylthiouracil (PROP), finding it incredibly bitter. Half the remaining population find PROP moderately bitter, and the final quarter cannot taste it at all. Supertasters find bitter compounds such as coffee too strong. They seem to have more fungiform papillae on the tongue, which may explain the increased sensitivity.

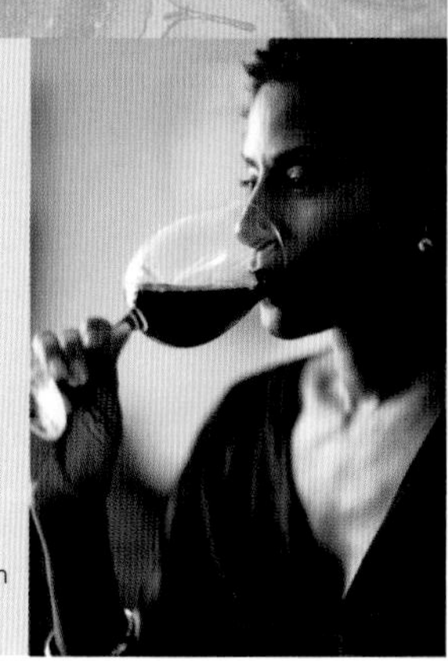

THE FIVE BASIC FLAVOURS	
Along with the basic tastes, people can detect other substances, such as fatty acids, through receptors in the upper airways. This suggests that taste is a part of smell, just as smell is a part of taste.	
NAME	**DESCRIPTION**
Sweet	Often linked to energy-rich, high-calorie foods.
Sour	May be a danger sign, signalling unripe or "off" foods.
Salty	Most chemical salts, including sodium chloride, taste salty.
Bitter	May be linked to natural toxins, so is best avoided.
Umami	Savoury ("umami" means "delicious" in Japanese).

Tongue epithelium
Filiform papilla
Fungiform pailla
Vallate papilla
Mucus-secreting gland
Connective tissue

PAPILLAE
Papillae contain taste buds and are distributed across the tongue. Four types of papillae have been distinguished – vallate, filiform, foliate, and fungiform. Each type bears a different amount of taste buds. Fungiform and filiform are the smallest papillae, and vallate are the largest, and together form a V-shape across the rear of the tongue.

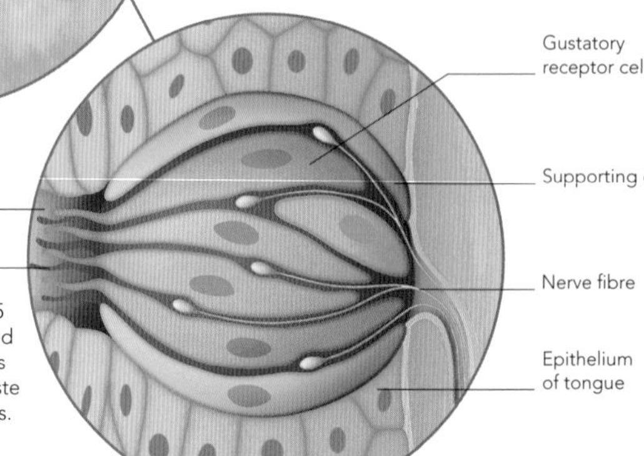

TASTE BUDS
A taste bud is composed of a group of about 25 receptor cells alongside supporting cells, layered together much like a bunch of bananas. The tips of the cells form a small pore, through which taste molecules enter and contact receptor molecules. These are borne on taste hairs (tiny projections called microvilli) that extend into the pore.

TASTE AND SMELL BRAIN AREAS

Taste and smell are both chemical senses – receptors in the nose and mouth bind to incoming molecules, generating electrical signals to send to the brain. Both sets of signals pass along the cranial nerves. Smell-related (olfactory) signals travel from the nose to the olfactory bulb, then along the olfactory nerve to the olfactory cortex in the temporal lobe for processing (see also pp.96–97). The pathway of taste-related (gustatory) data travels from the mouth along branches of the trigeminal and glossopharyngeal nerves to the medulla, continues to the thalamus, then to primary gustatory areas of the cerebral cortex.

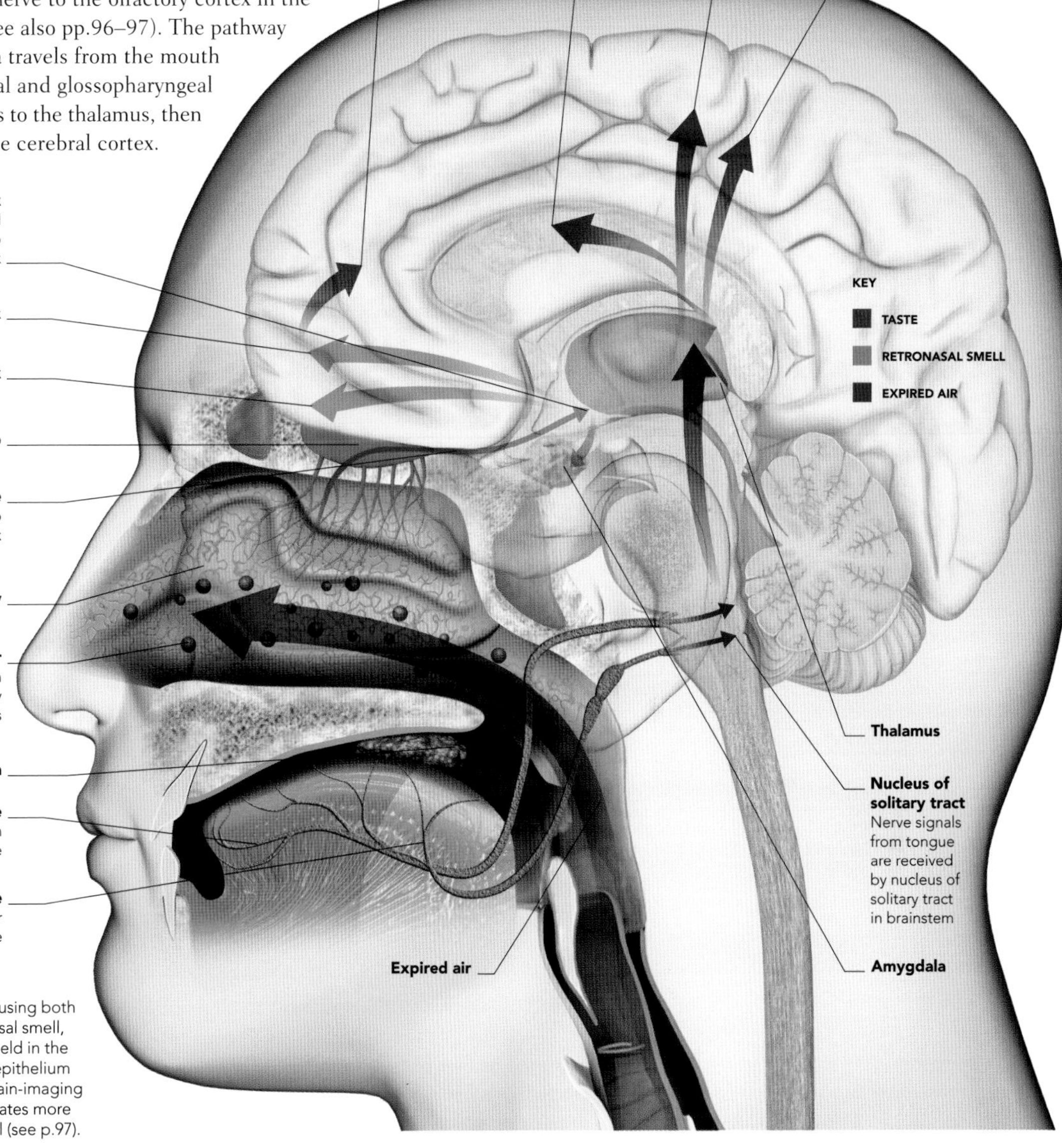

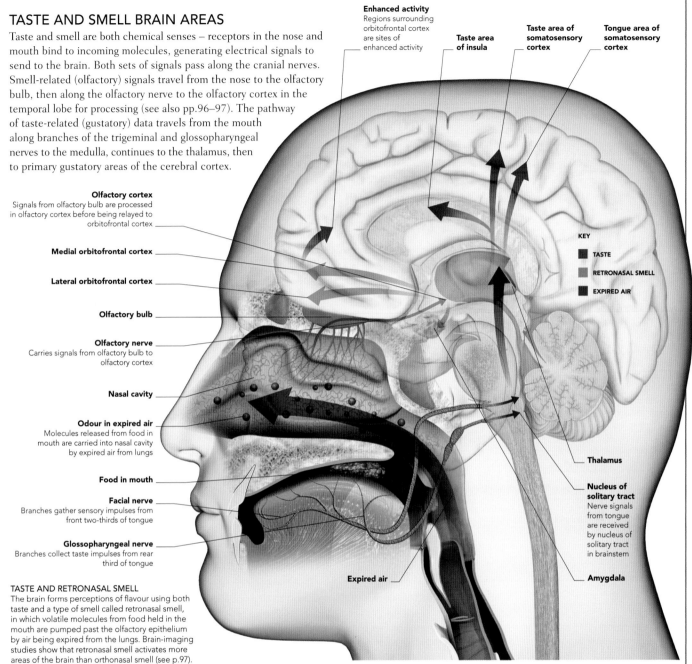

Enhanced activity
Regions surrounding orbitofrontal cortex are sites of enhanced activity

Taste area of insula

Taste area of somatosensory cortex

Tongue area of somatosensory cortex

Olfactory cortex
Signals from olfactory bulb are processed in olfactory cortex before being relayed to orbitofrontal cortex

Medial orbitofrontal cortex

Lateral orbitofrontal cortex

Olfactory bulb

Olfactory nerve
Carries signals from olfactory bulb to olfactory cortex

Nasal cavity

Odour in expired air
Molecules released from food in mouth are carried into nasal cavity by expired air from lungs

Food in mouth

Facial nerve
Branches gather sensory impulses from front two-thirds of tongue

Glossopharyngeal nerve
Branches collect taste impulses from rear third of tongue

Expired air

KEY
TASTE
RETRONASAL SMELL
EXPIRED AIR

Thalamus

Nucleus of solitary tract
Nerve signals from tongue are received by nucleus of solitary tract in brainstem

Amygdala

TASTE AND RETRONASAL SMELL
The brain forms perceptions of flavour using both taste and a type of smell called retronasal smell, in which volatile molecules from food held in the mouth are pumped past the olfactory epithelium by air being expired from the lungs. Brain-imaging studies show that retronasal smell activates more areas of the brain than orthonasal smell (see p.97).

TASTE ASSOCIATIONS

When a food makes you ill (spoiled seafood, for example), the association can linger for a long time, making even the thought of that food repulsive. The phenomenon, known as flavour-aversion learning, has been demonstrated by researchers at Harvard Medical School who fed rats a sweet liquid with a substance that made them briefly ill. Thereafter, the rats avoided the liquid despite its tempting sweetness. When a food is paired with nausea, flavour-aversion learning has a survival value in teaching animals to avoid attractive-looking foods that may be toxic. It is a robust form of learning – occurring after one episode only, but lasting for many years.

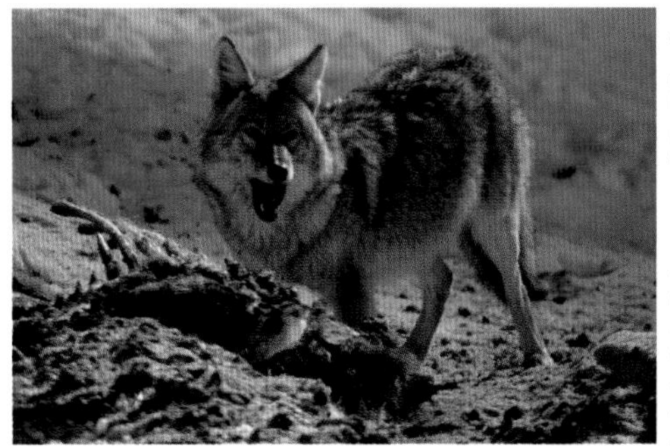

TASTE AVERSION
As an alternative to killing coyotes that prey on domestic sheep, some farmers in the western United States place lamb bait laced with an illness-inducing drug around their ranches. The coyotes learn to avoid lamb meat and therefore stop approaching sheep.

TOUCH

THERE ARE MANY KINDS OF TOUCH SENSATION. THESE INCLUDE LIGHT TOUCH, PRESSURE, VIBRATION, AND TEMPERATURE AS WELL AS PAIN (SEE PP.106–107), AND AWARENESS OF THE BODY'S POSITION IN SPACE (PROPRIOCEPTIONS, SEE PP.104–105). THE SKIN IS THE BODY'S MAIN SENSE ORGAN FOR TOUCH.

TOUCH RECEPTORS

There are around 20 types of touch receptor that respond to various types of stimuli. For instance, light touch, a general category that covers sensations ranging from a tap on the arm to stroking a cat's fur, is detected by four different types of receptor cells: free nerve endings, found in the epidermis; Merkel's discs, found in deeper layers of the skin; Meissner's corpuscles, which are common in the palms, soles of the feet, eyelids, genitals, and nipples; and, finally, the root hair plexus, which responds when the hair moves. Pacinian and Ruffini corpuscles respond to more intense pressure. The sensation of itching is produced by repetitive, low-level stimulation of nerve fibres in the skin, while feeling ticklish involves more intense stimulation of the same nerve endings when the stimulus moves over the skin.

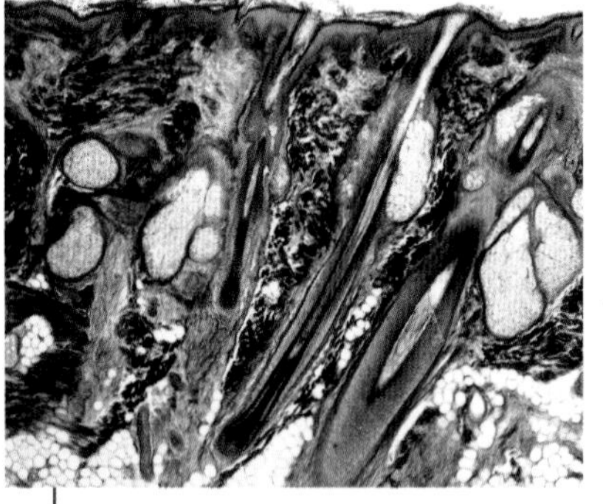

SKIN STRUCTURE
Skin is the largest sense organ and allows us to interact fully with our surroundings. This light micrograph reveals how it is embedded with nerves, receptors, glands, hair follicles, and a rich blood supply.

Hair When body is cold, hair is pulled up by dedicated erector pili muscle, which is located in dermis

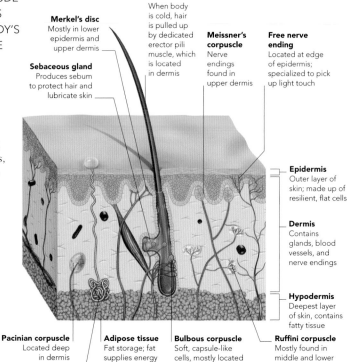

Merkel's disc Mostly in lower epidermis and upper dermis

Meissner's corpuscle Nerve endings found in upper dermis

Free nerve ending Located at edge of epidermis; specialized to pick up light touch

Sebaceous gland Produces sebum to protect hair and lubricate skin

Epidermis Outer layer of skin; made up of resilient, flat cells

Dermis Contains glands, blood vessels, and nerve endings

Hypodermis Deepest layer of skin, contains fatty tissue

Pacinian corpuscle Located deep in dermis

Adipose tissue Fat storage; fat supplies energy and absorbs shocks

Bulbous corpuscle Soft, capsule-like cells, mostly located in mucous membranes

Ruffini corpuscle Mostly found in middle and lower layers of dermis

Sweat gland Produces sweat that passes to skin's surface via sweat duct

TYPES OF RECEPTORS
The variety of touch receptors gives rise to a wide range of sensations. They are distributed throughout the body in the skin, conjunctiva, the bladder, and in muscles and joints.

TYPES OF TOUCH

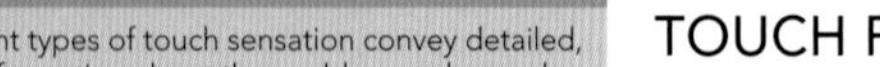

The different types of touch sensation convey detailed, complex information about the world around us and can act as a warning signal. Touch is essential for experiencing the texture and "feel" of objects. It also plays a vital role in communicating with others.

SENSATION	RECEPTORS
Light touch	The skin is not deformed by light touch, for example a handshake or a kiss. Free nerve endings in the skin respond to light-touch stimuli.
Touch pressure	Pressure entailing short-lived skin deformation stimulates Pacinian corpuscles and Ruffini corpuscles, located deep in the skin.
Vibration	Pacinian corpuscles and Meissner's corpuscles (mechanoreceptors, detecting mechanical movements) respond to vibrations.
Heat and cold	Receptors are sensitive to either hot or cold, not temperature itself. Heat and cold receptors occur in specific spots on the skin.
Pain	Pain signals come from damaged tissue and stimulate nociceptors (see pp.106–107), which consist of free nerve endings.
Proprioception	Receptor cells located in muscles and joints send information to the brain about the position and movement of the body.

TOUCH PATHWAY

When a sense receptor is activated, it sends information about touch stimuli as electrical impulses along a nerve fibre of the sensory nerve network to the nerve root on the spinal cord. The data enters the spinal cord and continues upwards to the brain. The processing of sensory data is begun by nuclei in the upper (dorsal) column of the spinal cord. From the brainstem, sensory data enters the thalamus, where processing continues. The data then travels to the postcentral gyrus of the cerebral cortex, the location of the somatosensory cortex. Here, it is finally translated into a touch perception.

1 FIRST ORDER TO SECOND ORDER
First-order neurons carry data from the upper thigh to the spinal cord from touch receptors. Their cell bodies are found in the dorsal root ganglia of the spinal cord. On entering the spinal cord, they connect with second-order neurons, most of which are located in the grey matter of the spinal cord, before travelling up the spinal cord along the pathway known as the ascending anterior spinothalamic tract.

FRONT OF SPINAL CORD
White matter
Grey matter
Ventral horn
Signal passes into spinal cord
Sensory information from upper thigh
Dorsal root ganglion cell
Dorsal root axon
Dorsal horn
BACK OF SPINAL CORD

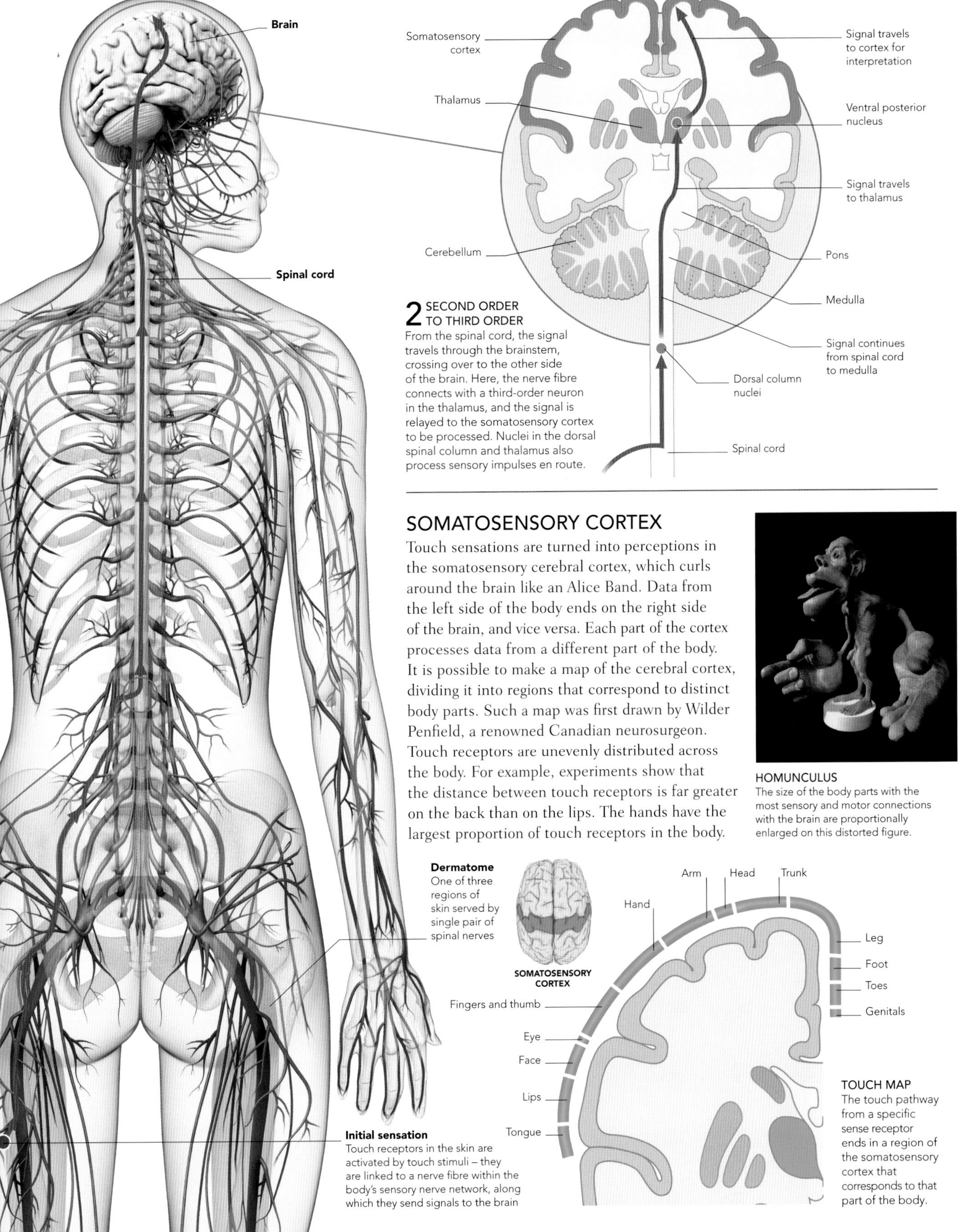

2 SECOND ORDER TO THIRD ORDER
From the spinal cord, the signal travels through the brainstem, crossing over to the other side of the brain. Here, the nerve fibre connects with a third-order neuron in the thalamus, and the signal is relayed to the somatosensory cortex to be processed. Nuclei in the dorsal spinal column and thalamus also process sensory impulses en route.

SOMATOSENSORY CORTEX

Touch sensations are turned into perceptions in the somatosensory cerebral cortex, which curls around the brain like an Alice Band. Data from the left side of the body ends on the right side of the brain, and vice versa. Each part of the cortex processes data from a different part of the body. It is possible to make a map of the cerebral cortex, dividing it into regions that correspond to distinct body parts. Such a map was first drawn by Wilder Penfield, a renowned Canadian neurosurgeon. Touch receptors are unevenly distributed across the body. For example, experiments show that the distance between touch receptors is far greater on the back than on the lips. The hands have the largest proportion of touch receptors in the body.

HOMUNCULUS
The size of the body parts with the most sensory and motor connections with the brain are proportionally enlarged on this distorted figure.

Dermatome
One of three regions of skin served by single pair of spinal nerves

Initial sensation
Touch receptors in the skin are activated by touch stimuli – they are linked to a nerve fibre within the body's sensory nerve network, along which they send signals to the brain

TOUCH MAP
The touch pathway from a specific sense receptor ends in a region of the somatosensory cortex that corresponds to that part of the body.

THE SIXTH SENSE

PROPRIOCEPTION – FROM *PROPRIO*, THE LATIN FOR "SELF" – IS SOMETIMES REFERRED TO AS THE SIXTH SENSE. IT IS THE SENSING OF BODY POSITION, MOVEMENT, AND POSTURE, INVOLVING FEEDBACK TO THE BRAIN FROM THE BODY. HOWEVER, THIS INFORMATION IS NOT ALWAYS MADE CONSCIOUS.

WHAT IS PROPRIOCEPTION?

Proprioception is our sense of how our bodies are positioned and moving in space. This "awareness" is produced by part of the somatic sensory system, and involves structures called proprioceptors in the muscles, tendons, joints, and ligaments that monitor changes in their length, tension, and pressure linked to changes in position. Proprioceptors send impulses to the brain. Upon processing this information, a decision can be made – to change position or to stop moving. The brain then sends signals back to the muscles based on the input from the proprioceptors – completing the feedback cycle.

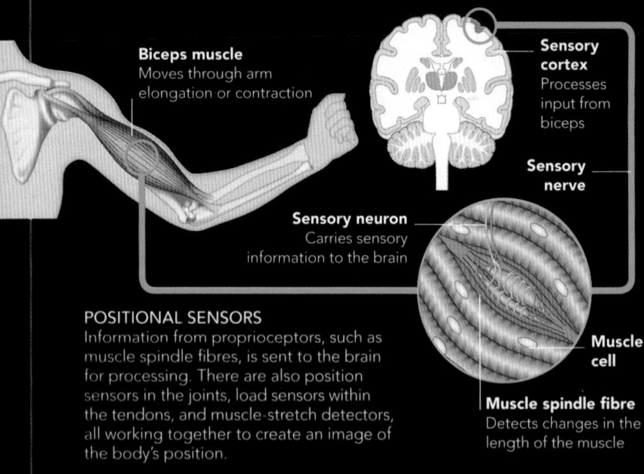

POSITIONAL SENSORS
Information from proprioceptors, such as muscle spindle fibres, is sent to the brain for processing. There are also position sensors in the joints, load sensors within the tendons, and muscle-stretch detectors, all working together to create an image of the body's position.

FIELD SOBRIETY TESTS

Proprioception is impaired when people are under the influence of alcohol or certain other drugs. The degree of impairment can be tested by field sobriety tests, which have long been used by the police in cases of suspected drink-driving. Typical tests include asking someone to touch their index finger to their nose with their eyes closed, to stand on one leg for 30 seconds, or to walk heel-to-toe in a straight line for nine steps.

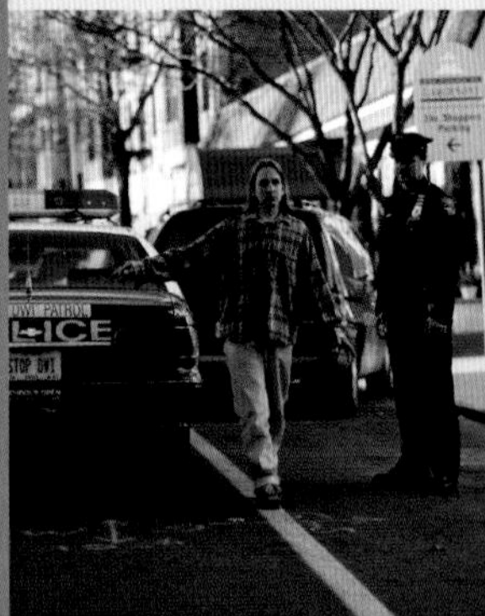

TYPES OF PROPRIOCEPTION

Proprioceptive information is either made conscious or processed unconsciously. For example, keeping and adjusting balance is generally an unconscious process. Conscious proprioception usually involves some kind of cortical processing, resulting in decision-making. This normally ends in a command to the muscles to perform a movement. The sheer amount of proprioceptive input means that much is processed unconsciously.

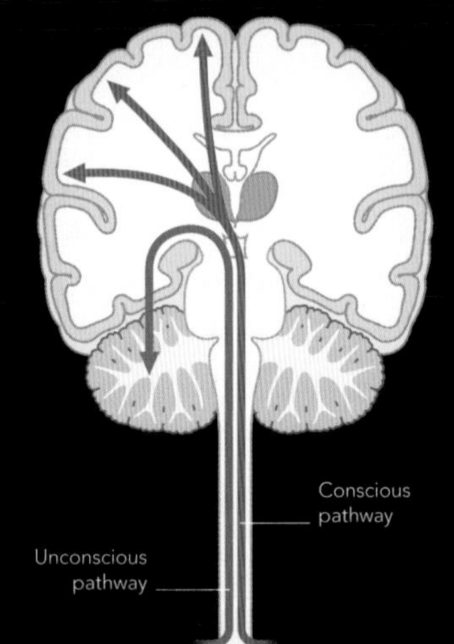

PROPRIOCEPTION PATHWAYS
Conscious proprioception uses the dorsal column–medial lemniscus pathway, which passes through the thalamus, and ends in the parietal lobe of the cortex. Unconscious proprioception involves spinocerebellar tracts, and ends in the cerebellum, the part of the brain at the back of the skull involved with the control of movement.

PHANTOM LIMBS

When someone has a part of the body amputated or removed – be it a limb, an extremity, or an organ, such as the appendix – they sometimes continue to have sensations, often including pain, in that area. Research has linked this to changes in the sensory cortex. Specifically, the somatosensory cortex undergoes a remapping process in which the areas near the "dead" area "take over", so that stimuli in these areas are felt as sensations in the area that has been lost. This reorganization of the cortex has been confirmed through imaging studies.

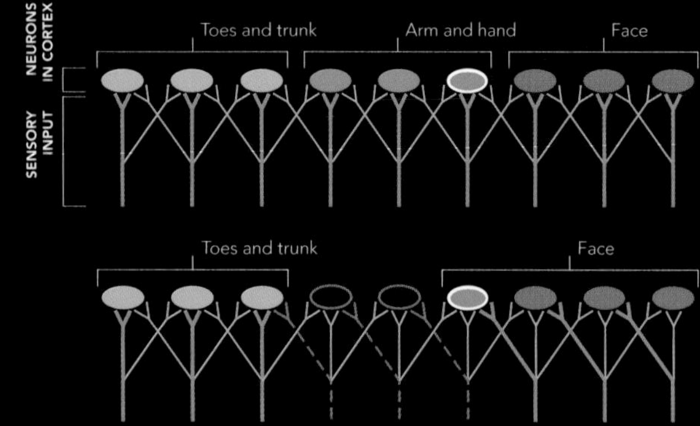

BEFORE AMPUTATION
Sensory inputs from the arm and hand are connected to the appropriate region of the sensory cortex. Other parts of the body are also connected to specific, neighbouring cortical regions.

AFTER AMPUTATION
There is no sensory input from the amputated arm and hand, but the pathway to the cortex remains. Input from another part of the body takes over, reshaping the sensory map, which may produce sensations.

PHANTOM-LIMB-PAIN TREATMENT

Research has shown that the development of phantom-limb pain is linked to the plasticity of the sensory cortex. Trying to reverse the changes in the cortex can actually reduce the pain sensation for the patient. For instance, use of an electric prosthetic limb that is moved by signals from the patient's muscles was helpful. Brain scans revealed that this was linked with reversion of the cortex to its original state, maybe by replacing some of the original input.

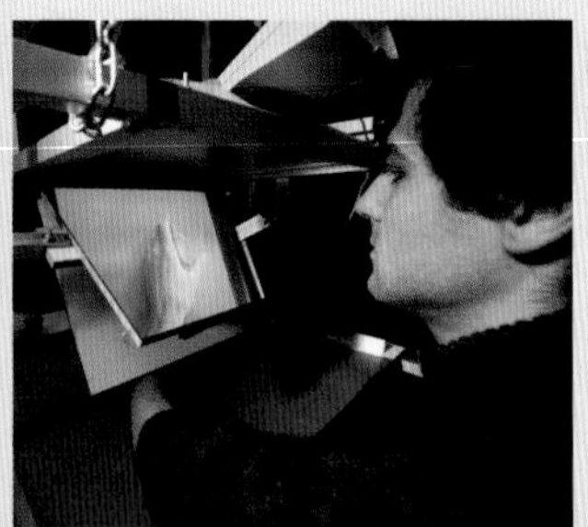

MIRROR TREATMENT
When a patient's remaining arm is shown as a mirror image and moved, it looks as though the missing arm is moving. Somehow, this illusion can relieve phantom-limb pain.

FINE BALANCE
Proprioceptors in the muscles, tendons, and skin work together with hair cells in the vestibule and semicircular canals of the inner ear to maintain balance. A gymnast will work on all aspects of strength, movement, and body co-ordination to achieve feats involving fine balance.

PAIN SIGNALS

PAIN IS PRIMARILY A WARNING SIGNAL. IT TELLS YOU THERE IS SOMETHING WRONG AND FORCES YOU TO TAKE ACTION. PAIN USUALLY OCCURS AS A RESULT OF STIMULATION OF SPECIALIZED NERVE FIBRES THAT EXTEND THROUGHOUT THE BODY.

PAIN PATHWAYS

Pain-transmitting nerve fibres permeate almost every part of the body. When stimulated by an injury, they send electrical signals from the site of the stimulus to the spinal cord. The signals then cross over the cord and continue up to the brain. This crossover means that pain from one side of the body activates the opposite side of the brain. As they pass through the medulla in the brainstem, pain signals trigger automatic bodily responses. The signals then arrive at the thalamus and are distributed to various regions of the brain to be processed.

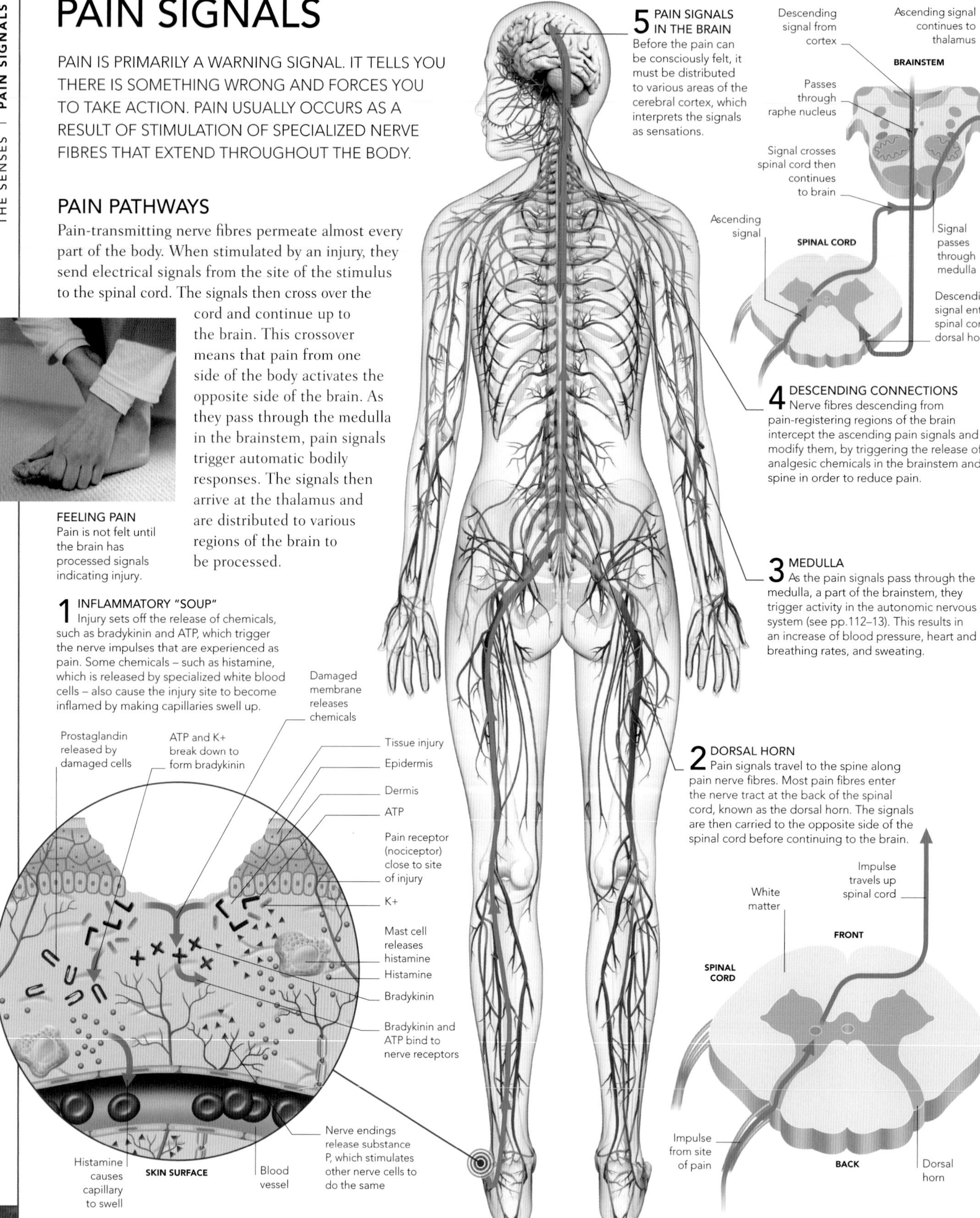

FEELING PAIN
Pain is not felt until the brain has processed signals indicating injury.

1 INFLAMMATORY "SOUP"
Injury sets off the release of chemicals, such as bradykinin and ATP, which trigger the nerve impulses that are experienced as pain. Some chemicals – such as histamine, which is released by specialized white blood cells – also cause the injury site to become inflamed by making capillaries swell up.

2 DORSAL HORN
Pain signals travel to the spine along pain nerve fibres. Most pain fibres enter the nerve tract at the back of the spinal cord, known as the dorsal horn. The signals are then carried to the opposite side of the spinal cord before continuing to the brain.

3 MEDULLA
As the pain signals pass through the medulla, a part of the brainstem, they trigger activity in the autonomic nervous system (see pp.112–13). This results in an increase of blood pressure, heart and breathing rates, and sweating.

4 DESCENDING CONNECTIONS
Nerve fibres descending from pain-registering regions of the brain intercept the ascending pain signals and modify them, by triggering the release of analgesic chemicals in the brainstem and spine in order to reduce pain.

5 PAIN SIGNALS IN THE BRAIN
Before the pain can be consciously felt, it must be distributed to various areas of the cerebral cortex, which interprets the signals as sensations.

THE CHEMISTRY OF PAIN RELIEF

The body has a natural opioid (pain relief) system that acts in much the same way as opiate drugs, such as heroin and morphine. Natural opioids, which include endorphins and encephalins, are produced by the thalamus and pituitary gland during stress and pain. These substances are also produced in situations associated with feeling a natural "high", such as strenuous exercise and sexual activity. Nerve endings in the brain and throughout the body have special receptors on them that bind to opiate substances. The opiates then dampen the pain signals carried in those nerve endings, thus reducing pain.

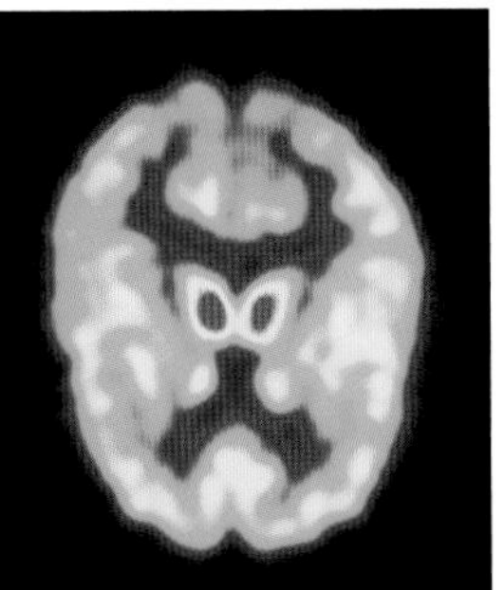

OPIOID RECEPTORS
This PET scan shows the concentration of opioid receptors in a normal brain. Red areas show where they are highest, through yellow and green, to blue, which indicates the lowest concentration.

PAIN FIBRES

There are two main types of nerve fibre that detect pain: A-delta and C. A-delta fibres are thin and carry sharp, localized pain signals to the brain. The site of the injury will be within a millimetre of these nerve fibres, so the site is easily identified. These nerve fibres are covered in a fatty, myelin sheath that aids the transmission of signals. C-fibres are not insulated by a myelin sheath. The source of pain transmitted by a C-fibre is difficult to pinpoint as its nerve endings spread out over a relatively large area.

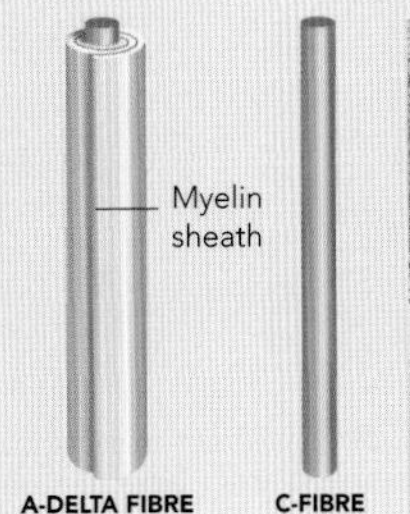

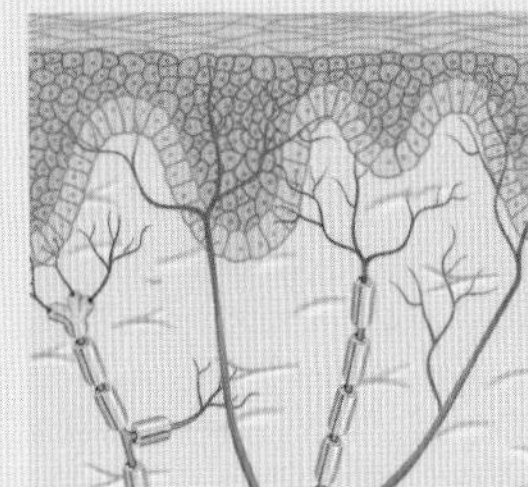

C-FIBRES AND A-DELTA FIBRES
A-delta fibres are found mostly in subcutaneous tissue. C-fibres accompany all the blood vessels, lymphatic, sensory, and motor nerves, and the peripheral autonomic nerves.

TYPES OF PAIN

Pain usually arises when pain receptors are stimulated by heat, cold, vibration, overstretching, or by chemicals released from damaged cells. Specialized nerve fibres (see panel, above) transmit this information to the brain. However, certain types of pain are processed and experienced in different ways, for example the facial nerves connect directly to the cranial nerves (see below), whereas visceral pain, from internal organs such as the heart (see right), can be difficult to locate. Damage to the nervous system itself, such as a trapped nerve, is known as neuropathic pain (see bottom).

FACIAL PAIN

Stimulation of trigeminal nerves usually causes facial pain. It often affects only one side of the face and can be felt on the skin or in the mouth and teeth. It comes and goes unpredictably and its nature is variously described as stabbing, lacerating, electric shock-like, and shooting. It can range in severity from mild to excruciating. There are frequently "trigger points" on the skin, which, if touched, will bring on a violent pain spasm. People may experience pain daily for weeks and months, then it may disappear for months or even years.

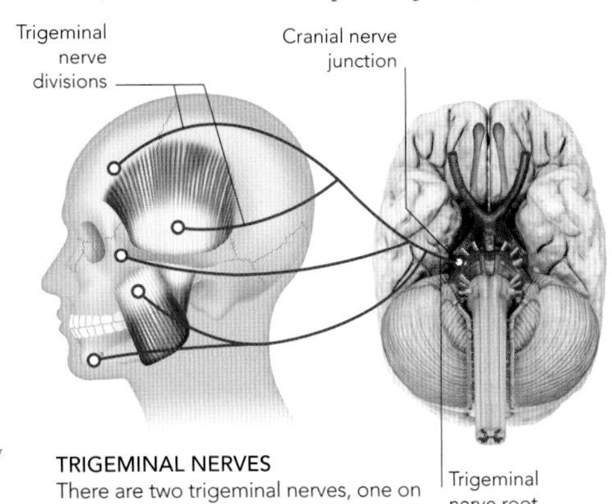

TRIGEMINAL NERVES
There are two trigeminal nerves, one on each side of the face, each has branches to the forehead, cheek, and jaw.

REFERRED PAIN

Referred pain occurs when nerve fibres from areas of high sensory input (such as the skin) and nerve fibres from areas of low sensory input (such as internal organs) enter the spinal cord at the same location. As the brain expects to be receiving the data from high-sensory areas, it misinterprets the location of the pain.

Spinal cord
Ganglion
Sensory nerve fibres Converge upon entry into spine
Area of pain
Heart attack
Skin
Pain receptors

HEART ATTACK
Pain-signalling nerves from the heart converge with those from the arm as they enter the spinal cord. The brain interprets the signals as coming from the arm rather than the heart.

NEUROPATHIC PAIN

Pain that is caused by damage or malfunction in the nervous system itself rather than injury is known as neuropathic pain. A pain-transmitting nerve may be severed, or be stimulated so often that it gets into the "habit" of sending pain signals to the brain. Pain-registering neurons in the cortex can become sensitized so that they produce the experience of pain even when there is no external cause.

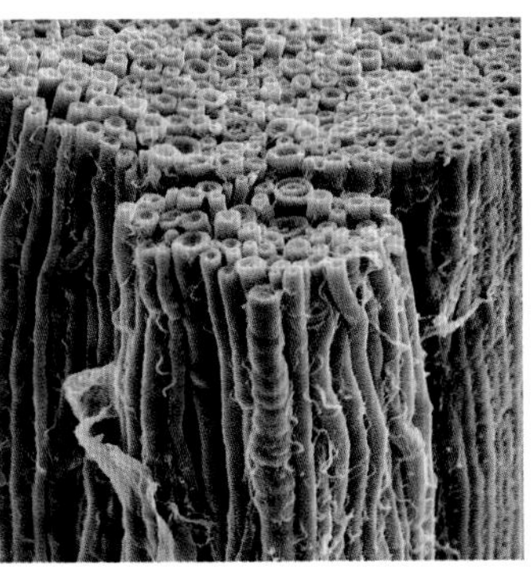

SEVERED NERVE BUNDLE
This coloured electron micrograph shows a severed bundle of nerves. These may continue to send pain signals to the brain even when the cause of the damage itself is long gone.

EXPERIENCING PAIN

THE FEELING OF PAIN IS NOT ACTUALLY CAUSED BY AN INJURY IN ITSELF. IN ORDER TO EXPERIENCE PAIN, IT MUST BE MADE CONSCIOUS. THIS REQUIRES ACTIVITY IN BRAIN AREAS INVOLVED IN EMOTION, ATTENTION, AND ASSESSING SIGNIFICANCE. SUCH ACTIVITY CAN CREATE THE PAIN EXPERIENCE IN THE ABSENCE OF A CAUSE.

PATHWAY OF PAIN

Pain signals are transmitted to several areas of the cortex, where they activate neurons that monitor the state of the body. Two such areas are the somatosensory cortex, which lets the brain know the part of the body the pain stems from, and the insular cortex – the deep fold that divides the temporal and frontal lobes. The other cortical site associated with pain experience is the anterior (front) of the cingulate cortex (ACC), which lies in the groove between the hemispheres. The ACC seems to be particularly concerned with the emotional significance of pain and with determining how much attention an injury should command.

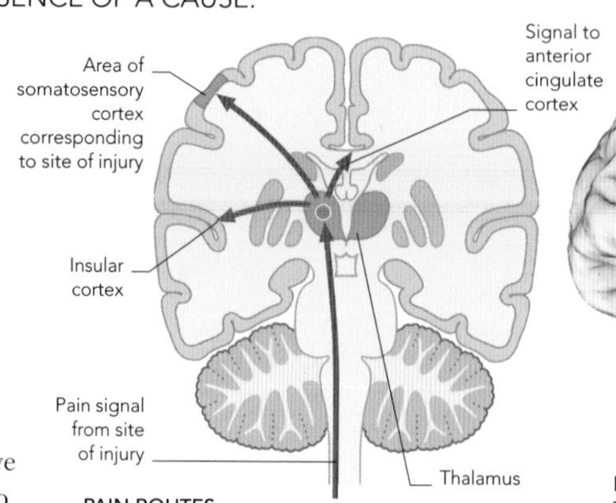

PAIN ROUTES
Pain signals from the body ascend to the brain via the spinal cord, then rise through the brainstem to the thalamus. Thereafter, they are distributed to various cortical areas for processing.

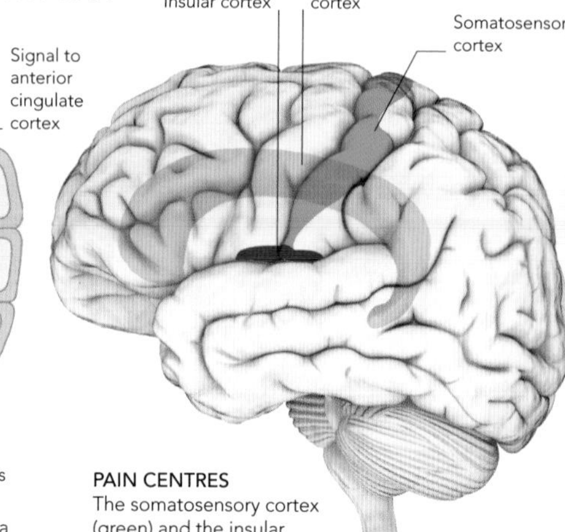

PAIN CENTRES
The somatosensory cortex (green) and the insular cortex (red) are responsible for pinpointing the exact site of the pain stimulus.

A WHOLE-BRAIN AFFAIR

Pain is so important to our survival that it may involve practically every part of the brain. Three main "pain areas" (see above) register and assess pain signals, and pinpoint the site of their source, but other areas also come into play. The supplementary motor and motor cortices may plan and execute movement aimed at escaping the pain stimulus. Parts of the parietal cortex may direct attention to the threat, and several parts of the frontal cortex may be involved in working out the significance of the pain and what to do about it.

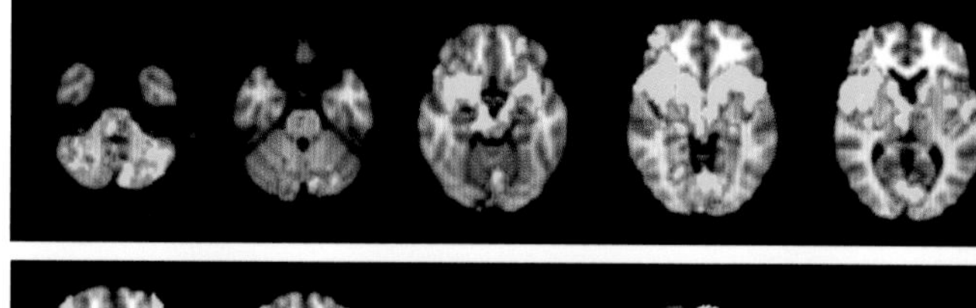

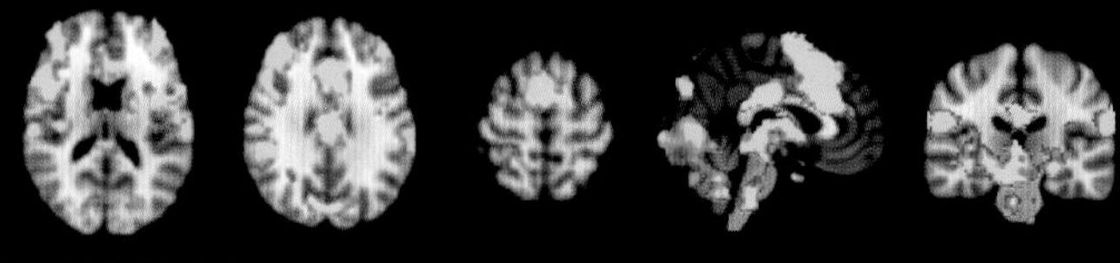

PAIN STUDY
The fMRI scans above show various "slices" through the brain of a healthy person who is being subjected to a painful stimulus on the arm. The regions highlighted in yellow show areas of neural activity in response to the stimulus, revealing how widespread the effects of pain are on the brain.

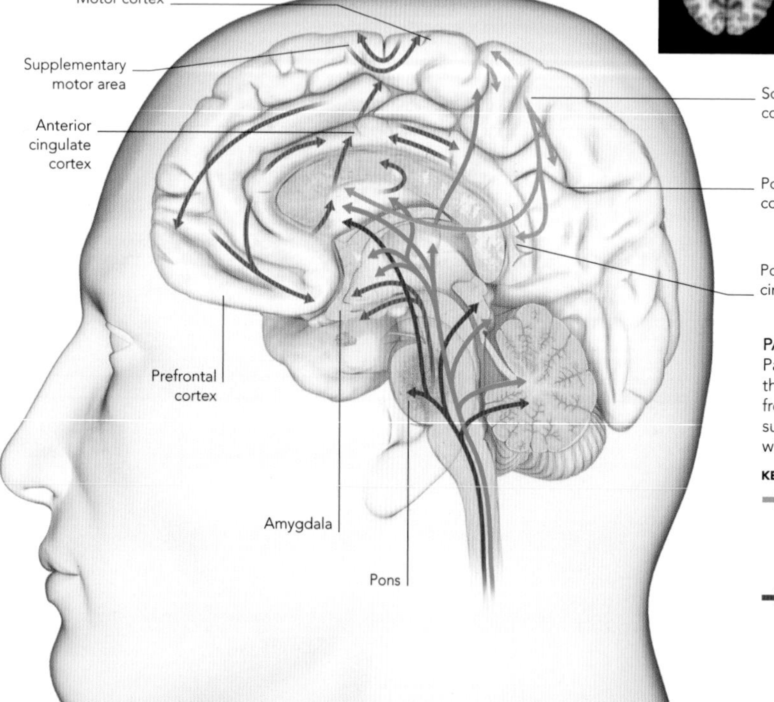

PAIN CIRCUITS
Pain signals travel along many different neural circuits to hit their targets. Some follow the paths of nerves that ascend from areas of the body, while others stem from brain nuclei, such as those in the hypothalamus, which are concerned with combating the effects of the pain stimulus.

KEY
- **DIRECT SPINAL INPUT** to areas that monitor the state of the body, direct attention, and prioritize response.
- **DIRECT SPINAL INPUT** to areas involved in automatic response to pain, such as arousal and movement.
- **CIRCUIT THROUGH** cortical and limbic areas involved in evaluation and monitoring of pain.
- **CIRCUIT THROUGH** cortical and limbic areas that affect pain, including intensity, emotion, and pain memory.

BRAIN OVER PAIN

Part of the role of higher brain areas is to modify pain. Nerve signals that travel from the brain into the body interrupt pain signals travelling up from the site of the injury before they reach the brain. This reduces the number of pain signals reaching the brain and, therefore, the amount of pain felt. Also, our thoughts, expectations, and emotions can all have a profound effect on the degree to which a person is "pained" by pain. People can affect pain consciously by directing attention away from it, or imagining that they are pain-free. An intensely imagined experience generates almost identical brain activity to the equivalent "real" experience, so an imagined state of physical ease may be achieved even as pain fibres in the body are being stimulated.

PLACEBO AND NOCEBO

Pain may be exacerbated or reduced as a result of the way in which we think about it. Believing that pain is being alleviated, by surgical intervention or a drug, for example, can help to ease the pain. This is known as the placebo effect. Expecting pain to be intractable or bad does the opposite, known as the nocebo effect.

FREEZING OUT PAIN

The cingulate cortex is an area of the brain that is partly concerned with determining how much attention to give to a pain stimulus. People can develop the ability to tone down activity in this region by learning to shift attention away from the pain stimulus, creating an analgesic effect. Using virtual reality as a focus point has been found to help distract attention away from pain.

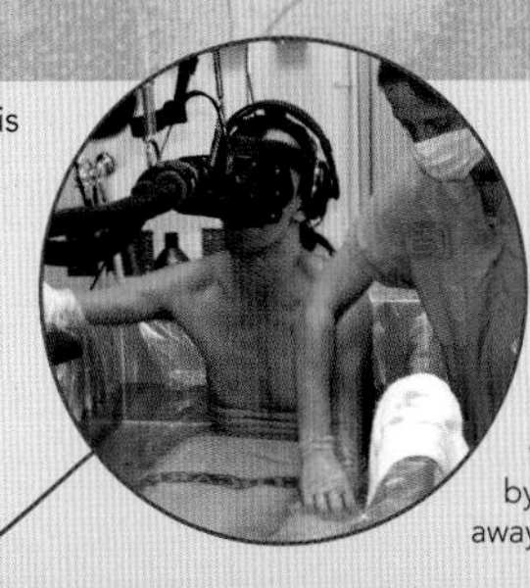

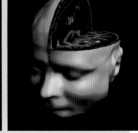

DISTRACTING ATTENTION
Burns victims have been found to experience pain relief when immersed in a cooling virtual environment, which is thought to work by distracting attention away from pain.

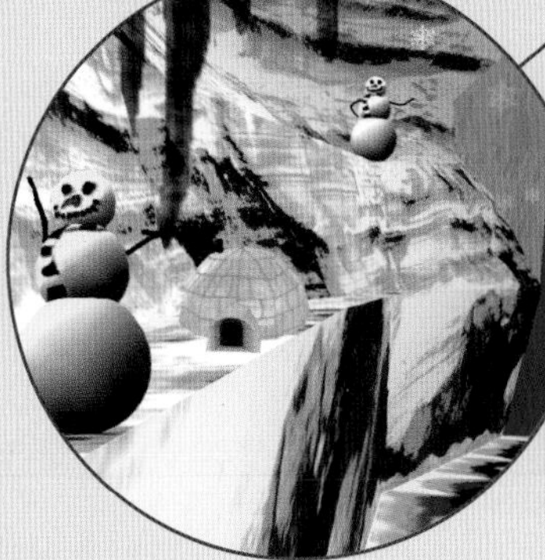

VIRTUAL ENVIRONMENT
Virtual reality is so distracting, it leaves less attentional resources available for the brain to process pain signals.

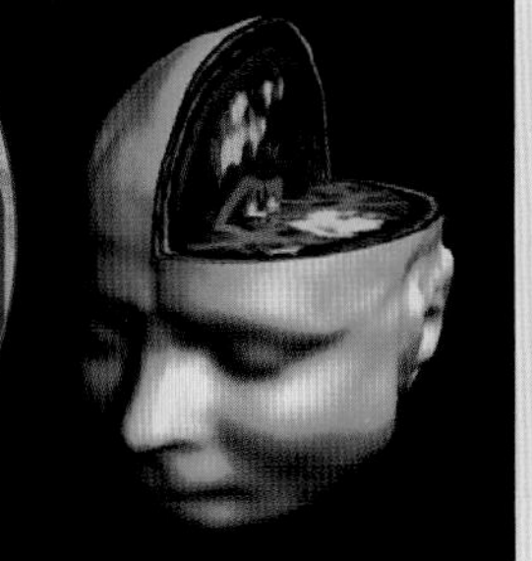

NO VIRTUAL REALITY

USING VIRTUAL REALITY

PAIN-RELATED BRAIN ACTIVITY
The areas coloured yellow in these images show activity related to pain. The distraction provided by virtual reality significantly reduces activity in these areas (right).

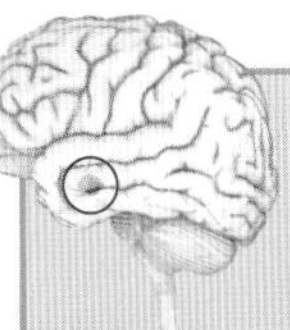

Anxiety signals from the amygdala – pain-related or otherwise – spark brain activity in a way that is associated with the experience of pain.

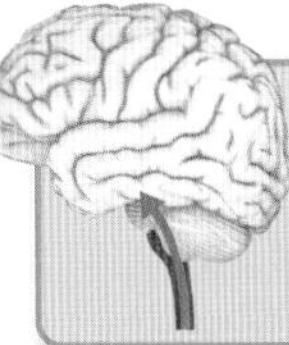

Pain stimulus arrives in the brain via the spinal cord, causing levels of anxiety to become increased.

PAIN

Nocebo effect
Anxiety plus pain input from the body produces a pain-related experience that is more intense than if either factor occurred alone. Anxiety is therefore an example of the nocebo effect – an intensification of pain due to the effects of negative thoughts, beliefs, or expectations.

Placebo effect
The belief that an intervention such as a drug or a medical procedure will alleviate pain is itself able to reduce pain experience. This is because experience is subjective so, if you think you do not feel pain, you don't. The process by which belief becomes fact is known as the placebo effect.

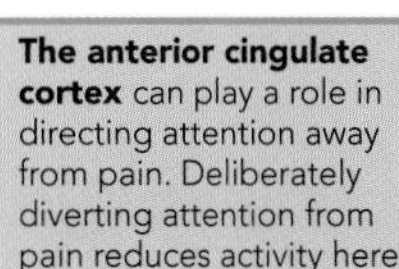

Descending signals from the prefrontal cortex of the brain can interrupt incoming pain signals. This can be unconscious or consciously controlled.

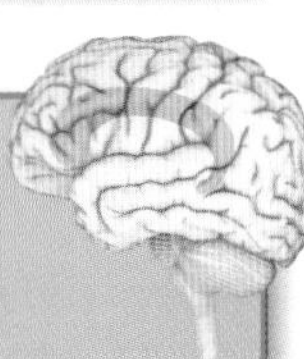

The anterior cingulate cortex can play a role in directing attention away from pain. Deliberately diverting attention from pain reduces activity here.

PAIN AND THE BRAIN

Although the brain is responsible for the experience of pain, it does not feel pain itself because it contains no pain receptors. This fact becomes very useful during brain surgery, because it allows surgeons to operate while the patient is conscious. The patient can report their experiences when different areas of the brain are stimulated and, therefore, help the surgeons recognize areas of the brain that have crucial functions. In this way, surgeons can carefully work their way towards, say, a brain tumour without damaging important and healthy brain tissue.

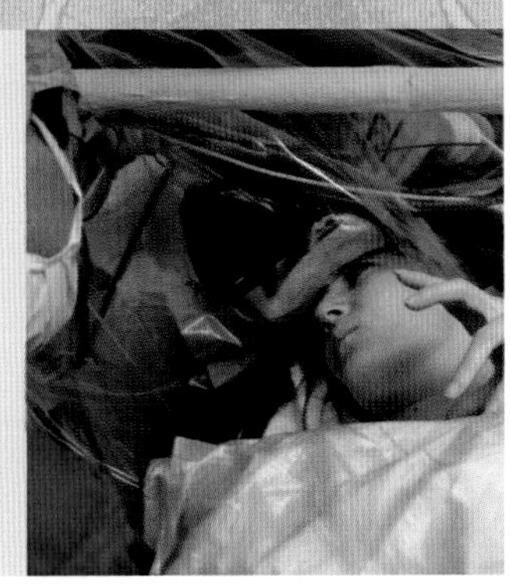

BRAIN SURGERY
Patients who remain conscious during brain operations can tell surgeons when the scalpel is close to a crucial area by responding to questions.

LIFE WITHOUT PAIN

A very few people – probably about one in 125 million – are born without the ability to feel pain. The condition is caused by a genetic disorder, congenital analgesia, that results in a lack of pain-sensitive nerve endings in the body. Some people with this condition are able to feel touch or pressure, which relies on different types of nerves. Although the idea of not feeling any pain may, at first, sound rather desirable, the effect is disastrous. Pain normally warns people that they are in danger and forces them to take action to protect themselves. Without it, physical perils are likely to be unnoticed or ignored, leading to lethal injuries and often to premature death.

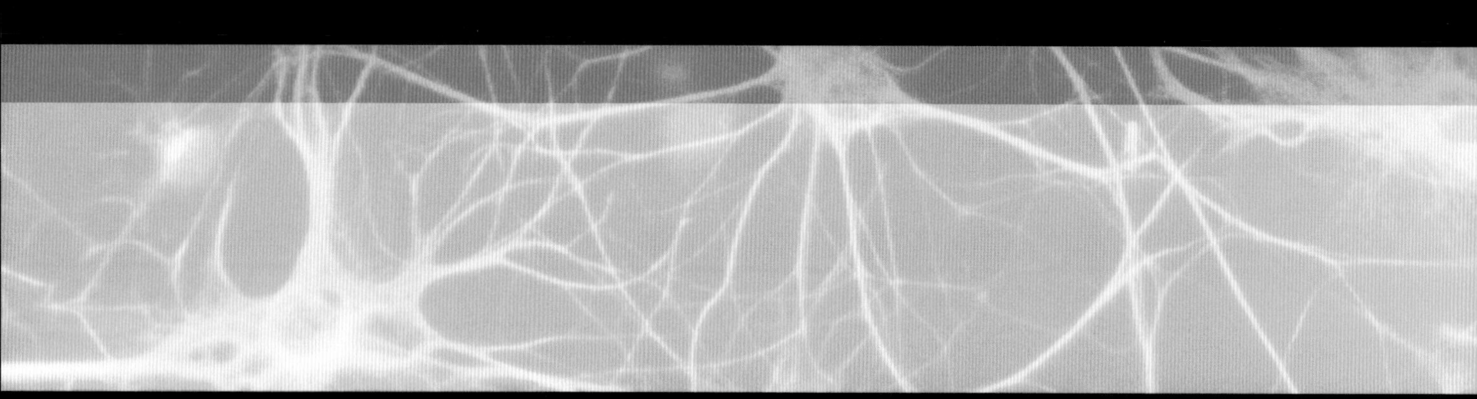

THE BRAIN IS IN CONSTANT COMMUNICATION WITH THE REST OF THE BODY, CONTROLLING EVEN ITS MOST BASIC PROCESSES. IN DOING SO, IT INITIATES MANY MOVEMENTS THAT WE ARE NOT AWARE OF, SUCH AS SPEEDING UP OR SLOWING DOWN OUR RATE OF BREATHING. SOME OTHER MOVEMENTS ARE MADE AS REFLEX ACTIONS, WITHOUT ANY SIGNALS REACHING THE BRAIN AT ALL. SUCH UNCONSCIOUS ACTION LEAVES THE CONSCIOUS BRAIN FREE TO DIRECT ITS ATTENTION TO OTHER THINGS, INCLUDING MOVEMENTS THAT REQUIRE GREAT CONCENTRATION, AS WELL AS CAREFUL PLANNING.

MOVEMENT AND CONTROL

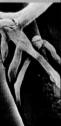

REGULATION

THE BODY'S BASIC FUNCTIONS ARE CAREFULLY CONTROLLED IN ORDER TO MAINTAIN A STABLE INTERNAL ENVIRONMENT. THE HYPOTHALAMUS AND BRAINSTEM WORK WITH CHEMICAL MESSENGERS CALLED HORMONES TO KEEP THE BODY TICKING OVER – MOSTLY WITHOUT US BEING AWARE OF IT.

THE RETICULAR FORMATION

The reticular formation is located in the brainstem and is made up of a series of long nerve pathways that modulate sensory inputs and carry information to and from the cerebral cortex. It also plays an important role in regulating the autonomic nervous system (ANS), which is responsible for maintaining a balanced internal environment. The reticular formation contains neuronal centres that manage various functions, such as controlling the heart rate and rate of respiration. It is also involved in regulating other basic functions such as digestion, salivation, perspiration, urination, and sexual arousal. The reticular formation and its connections constitute the reticular activating system (RAS), an arousal mechanism that keeps the brain alert and awake.

Activating signals Various areas of cerebral cortex receive signals from RAS via thalamus

Thalamus

Cerebral cortex

Medulla

Excitatory area of reticular formation (transmits and amplifies signals)

Inhibitory area of reticular formation (suppresses unwanted signals)

Reticular formation

Impulses from spinal cord

THE RETICULAR ACTIVATING SYSTEM
The RAS receives incoming sensory information and transfers it to the cortex to keep it alert and primed for environmental changes.

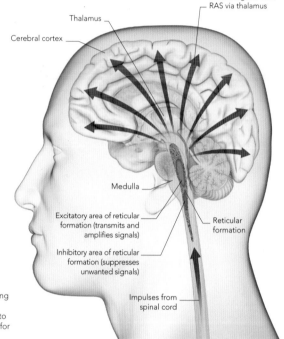

GENERAL ANAESTHETICS

A cornerstone of modern medicine, general anaesthetics allow surgeons to carry out operations that were previously unfeasible. Yet in which an anaesthetic causes loss of consciousness in a controlled and reversible way is still not fully understood. Ether, chloroform, and halothane act on neurons in the reticular activating system, suppressing alertness and awareness, and also on neurons in the hippocampus, temporarily wiping out memories. These substances also affect the nuclei in the thalamus, by interrupting the flow of sensory information from the body to the brain. Together, the actions of anaesthetics on the brain produce an experience of deep oblivion.

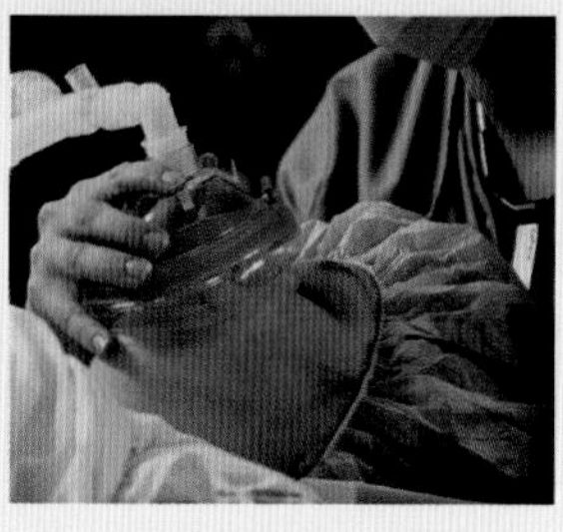

REGULATION OF HEART RATE

The heart rate is regulated by the hormonal action of the ANS, which, in turn, is regulated by the reticular formation. The sympathetic branch of the ANS speeds up the heart rate and the parasympathetic branch slows it down. The medulla in the brainstem contains a hub of neurons that constitute the cardioregulatory centre, which, in response to information from the ANS, sends signals to the sinoatrial node and the atrioventricular node in the heart. These signals set the heartbeat according to the body's need for oxygen.

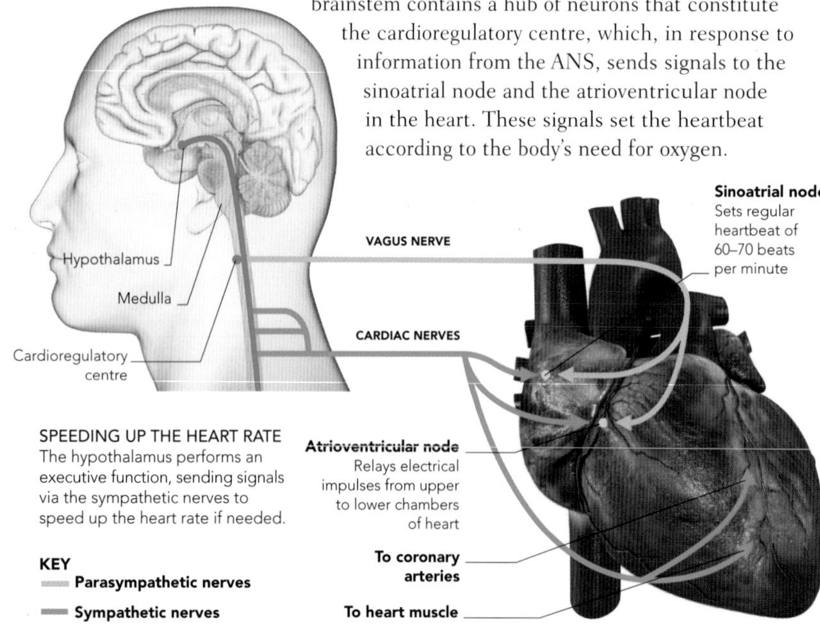

SPEEDING UP THE HEART RATE
The hypothalamus performs an executive function, sending signals via the sympathetic nerves to speed up the heart rate if needed.

REGULATION OF BREATHING

The rate of breathing in and out is regulated by collections of neurons in the reticular formation, called the dorsal and ventral respiratory groups. These respond to levels of oxygen and carbon dioxide in the blood and regulate the breathing rate accordingly to maintain constant levels. The basal rate of breathing can also be adjusted (in response to increased activity or metabolism) through electrical impulses sent by the pontine respiratory centre.

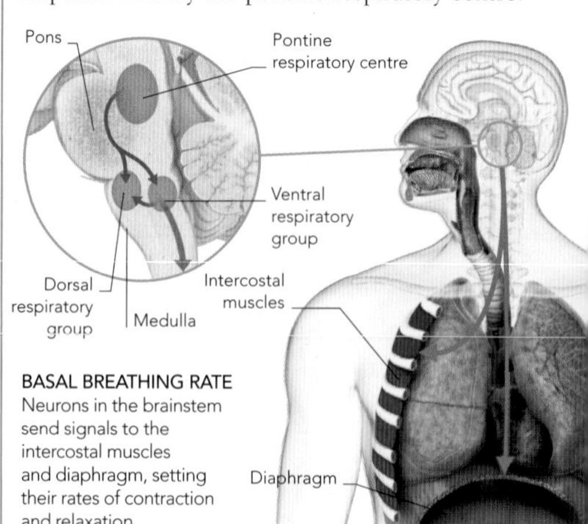

BASAL BREATHING RATE
Neurons in the brainstem send signals to the intercostal muscles and diaphragm, setting their rates of contraction and relaxation.

FUNCTIONS OF THE HYPOTHALAMUS

The hypothalamus contains many minute clusters of neurons, called nuclei, which perform specific functions, including controlling body temperature, feeding and drinking behaviour, water balance, hormonal levels, and sleep-wake cycles. Among other things, the hypothalamus is regarded as the major co-ordinating centre of the limbic system, and it has extensive connections with the pituitary gland and autonomic nervous system. Through these connections, it produces vital responses to body conditions and initiates feelings such as hunger, anger, and fear. The hypothalamus's functions are essential to life, so even subtle damage can have dramatic effects on behaviour and survival.

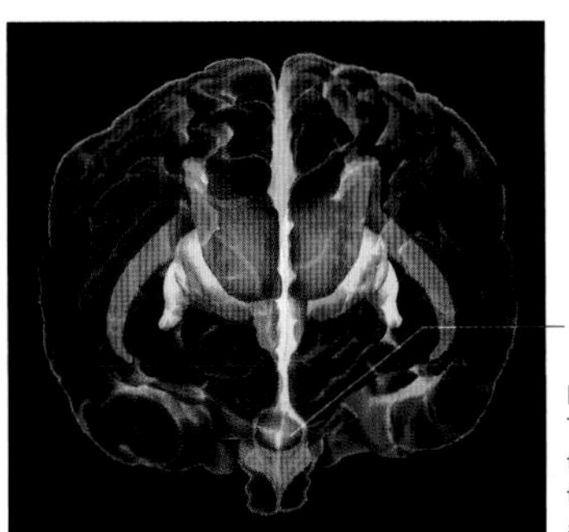

Hypothalamus

HYPOTHALAMUS
This illustration shows the location of the hypothalamus. It lies beneath the thalamus, near the brainstem, and is about the size of a sugar cube.

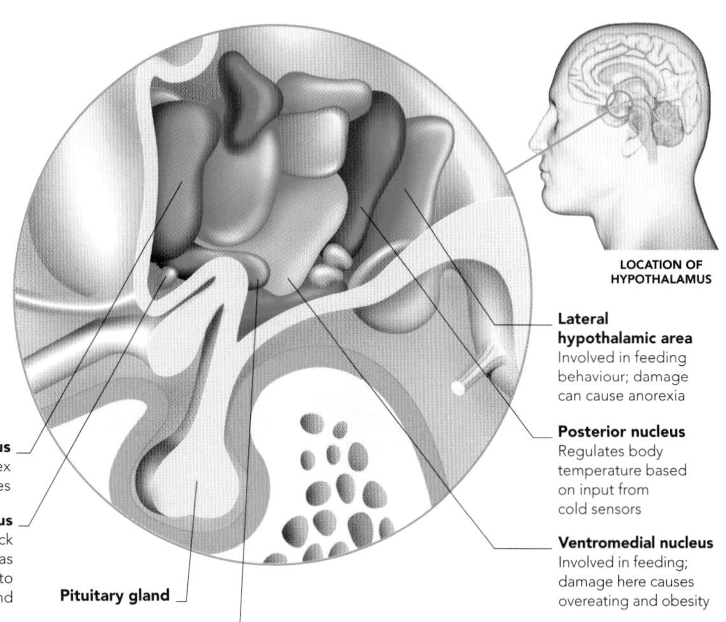

Medial preoptic nucleus Regulates production of sex hormones

Suprachiasmatic nucleus Helps regulate body clock and circadian rhythms; has numerous connections to pituitary gland

Pituitary gland

Anterior nucleus Neurons in this region are concerned with temperature control and process data from body's heat sensors

Lateral hypothalamic area Involved in feeding behaviour; damage can cause anorexia

Posterior nucleus Regulates body temperature based on input from cold sensors

Ventromedial nucleus Involved in feeding; damage here causes overeating and obesity

HYPOTHALAMIC NUCLEI
Groups of neurons (nuclei) within the hypothalamus have specialized roles in controlling specific responses and regulating the body's systems. Their complete range of functions is not fully known, but some functions have been identified and isolated to specific regions.

THE BODY'S THERMOSTAT

The skin has a number of thermoreceptors that convey information to the hypothalamus about the surrounding temperature. There are six types of receptor, each responding to a specific temperature range; some are sensitive to ranges of heat, others to ranges of cold, but none is sensitive to both. Information from these receptors travels via the spinal cord to the hypothalamus, where specialized nuclei receive the information and initiate various responses to bring the core temperature back to around 37°C (99°F). Some of the thermoregulatory responses are voluntary, arising as a result of conscious activity in the cerebral cortex, while others are involuntarily triggered by the autonomic nervous system.

THE BODY'S RESPONSE TO COLD
When the hypothalamus detects a drop in skin temperature, it responds by triggering heat production and conservation measures.

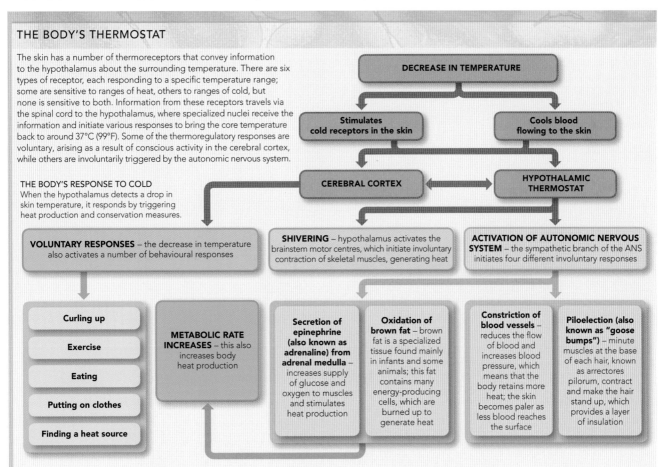

DECREASE IN TEMPERATURE

Stimulates cold receptors in the skin

Cools blood flowing to the skin

CEREBRAL CORTEX

HYPOTHALAMIC THERMOSTAT

VOLUNTARY RESPONSES – the decrease in temperature also activates a number of behavioural responses

- **Curling up**
- **Exercise**
- **Eating**
- **Putting on clothes**
- **Finding a heat source**

SHIVERING – hypothalamus activates the brainstem motor centres, which initiate involuntary contraction of skeletal muscles, generating heat

ACTIVATION OF AUTONOMIC NERVOUS SYSTEM – the sympathetic branch of the ANS initiates four different involuntary responses

Secretion of epinephrine (also known as adrenaline) from adrenal medulla – increases supply of glucose and oxygen to muscles and stimulates heat production

Oxidation of brown fat – brown fat is a specialized tissue found mainly in infants and some animals; this fat contains many energy-producing cells, which are burned up to generate heat

METABOLIC RATE INCREASES – this also increases body heat production

Constriction of blood vessels – reduces the flow of blood and increases blood pressure, which means that the body retains more heat; the skin becomes paler as less blood reaches the surface

Piloelection (also known as "goose bumps") – minute muscles at the base of each hair, known as arrectores pilorum, contract and make the hair stand up, which provides a layer of insulation

THE NEUROENDOCRINE SYSTEM

THE BRAIN MAINTAINS THE BODY'S STABLE INTERNAL STATE, KNOWN AS HOMEOSTASIS, THROUGH THE ACTION OF HORMONES. NEURAL-CONTROL CENTRES IN THE BRAIN INFLUENCE THE BODY'S GLANDS TO PRODUCE AND RELEASE THE HORMONES NEEDED TO MAINTAIN THIS VITAL BALANCE.

HORMONE SYNTHESIS AND CONTROL

Glands are organs that respond to imbalances in the body in order to regulate internal activities, such as the absorption of nutrients, and influence activities such as the intake of food or water. They react by increasing or decreasing their production of hormones, which then travel to a target organ, where they lock onto specialized receptors on the surface of cells. This binding triggers a physiological change that restores homeostasis. The hypothalamus is the crucial link between the nervous system and endocrine system, releasing hormones that, in turn, trigger the pituitary gland to either stop or start secreting its hormones.

HORMONES RELEASED BY THE PITUITARY GLAND	
Melanocyte-stimulating hormone (MSH)	Stimulates the production and release of melanin, the determinant of skin and hair colour
Adrenocorticotropic hormone (ACTH)	Triggers the adrenals to produce steroid hormones that control stress response
Thyroid-stimulating hormone (TSH)	Increases the activity of thyroid gland, which controls metabolism
Growth hormone (GH)	Acts on whole body, but especially important for growth and development in children
Luteinizing and follicle- stimulating hormone	Triggers the sex glands in males and females to make their own hormones
Oxytocin	Causes contractions during labour; also involved in the release of milk from the mammary glands
Prolactin	Stimulates the production of milk from the mammary glands
Antidiuretic hormone (ADH)	Controls amount of water removed from the blood by microfilters in the kidneys

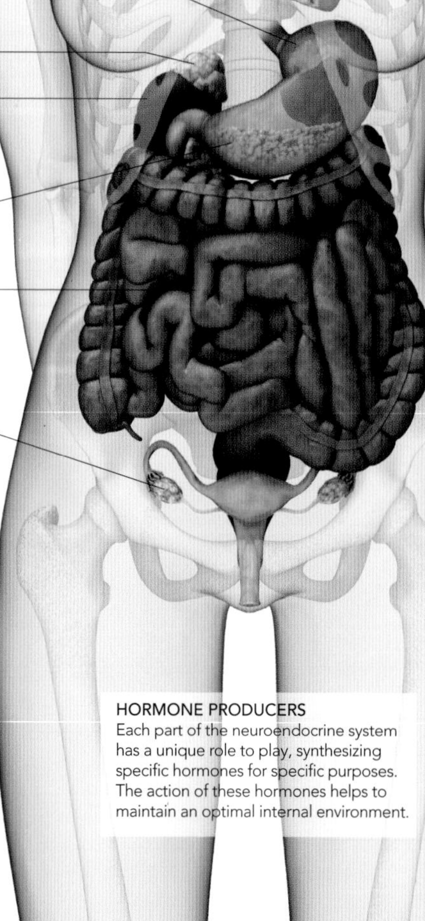

Pineal gl
Pea-sized
that make
melatonin
a hormon
crucially
involved
with the s
wake cycl

Hypothala
The vital lin
between th
nervous sy
and endoc
system; pr
two of its c
hormones

Pituitary gland
Known as the "master gland", as it controls many other endocrine glands; manufactures eight hormones on site, and receives two hormones directly from hypothalamus

Thyroid gland
Controls metabolic and heart rates; can store hormones, unlike the other glands

Thymus gland
Produces hormones involved in development of white blood cells

Heart
Produces hormone atriopeptin, which reduces blood volume and pressure

Stomach
Makes hormones that stimulate production or release of enzymes that aid digestion

Adrenal gland
Produces hormones that regulate metabolism of glucose, sodium, and potassium; also makes adrenaline

Kidney
Secretes erythropoietin, which stimulates production of red blood cells in bone marrow

Pancreas
Produces insulin and glucagon, which raise and lower blood glucose levels

Intestines
Manufactures hormones that stimulate production or release of enzymes that aid digestion

Ovary
Produces female sex hormones oestrogen and progesterone

HORMONE PRODUCERS
Each part of the neuroendocrine system has a unique role to play, synthesizing specific hormones for specific purposes. The action of these hormones helps to maintain an optimal internal environment.

FEEDBACK MECHANISMS

Imbalances in the body are detected and corrected using feedback mechanisms, or loops. Levels of a hormone within the bloodstream are gauged and the information is sent to the control unit in charge of that hormone, which in most cases is the hypothalamus-pituitary unit. If the level of a hormone is high, the control unit responds by reducing the production of that hormone to achieve balance. If the level is low, the control unit initiates an increase in production. Feedback mechanisms are also used to trigger rare homeostatic functions, such as contractions during labour.

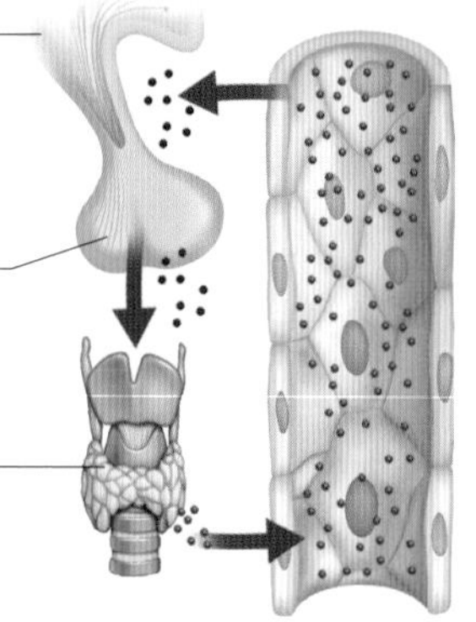

Hypothalamus
Detects rising blood glucose levels; produces fewer hormones for pituitary gland

Pituitary gland
Reacts to drop in hormone levels by releasing fewer hormones for thyroid

Thyroid gland
Produces fewer hormones that stimulate glucose production

NEGATIVE FEEDBACK
In response to a rise in blood glucose, the hypothalamus triggers a chain reaction of reduced hormone production that results in a fall in glucose levels, which restores balance.

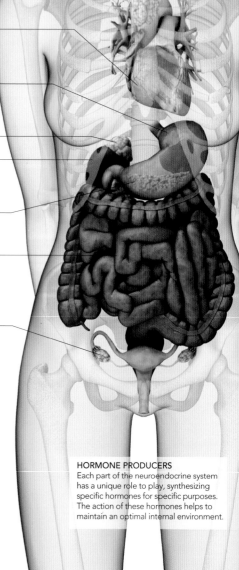

HUNGER

The body maintains its weight at a set point by using hormones to trigger the sensations of either hunger or satiety. To stimulate the appetite, the stomach produces the hormone ghrelin, while fat tissues decrease their production of leptin and insulin. These changes signal to specific neurons (referred to as neuron type B on the chart below) to start producing more neuropeptide (NPY) and agouti-related peptide (AgRP), which stimulate eating. The production of these peptides also causes other neurons (referred to below as neuron type A) to inhibit the production of the hormone melanocortin, which usually works to suppress the appetite. These signals are transmitted to the lateral hypothalamic nucleus (via other neurons), which generates the sensation of hunger. To suppress the appetite, the body's fat tissues increase production of leptin and insulin. These hormones signal to neuron type B to inhibit production of NPY and AgRP. At the same time, the increased leptin and insulin trigger neuron type A to produce melanocortin. These signals reach the ventromedial nucleus in the hypothalamus, which creates the feeling of satiety.

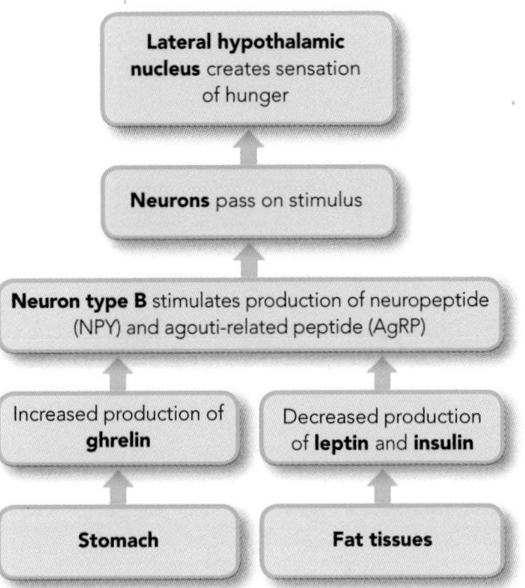
Lateral hypothalamic nucleus creates sensation of hunger
Neurons pass on stimulus
Neuron type A inhibits production of melanocortin
Neuron type B stimulates production of neuropeptide (NPY) and agouti-related peptide (AgRP)
Increased production of **ghrelin**
Decreased production of **leptin** and **insulin**
Stomach
Fat tissues
KEY
INHIBITS
STIMULATES

THE SENSATION OF HUNGER
Feeling hungry is caused by a chain reaction that begins in fat tissues, which reduce the production of leptin and insulin, and in the stomach, which increases production of the hormone ghrelin.

SUGAR ADDICTION

As a "reward" for performing functions essential for the survival of both the individual and the species, such as eating or reproducing, the brain releases opiates, which create sensations of pleasure. Sugar-rich diets generate heightened reward signals, so that the more sugar you have, the more you want. This can override self-control mechanisms and lead to addiction.

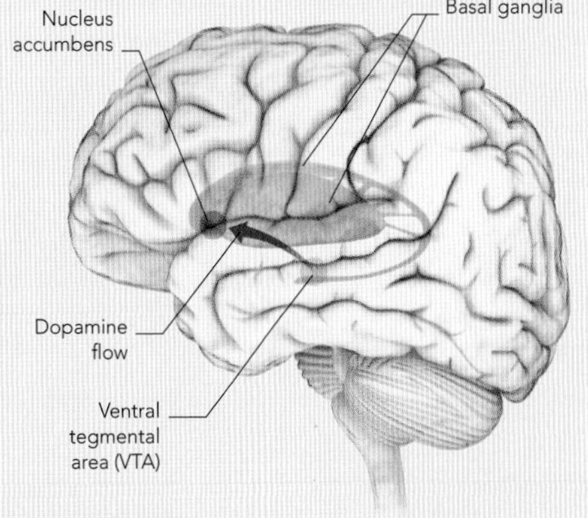
Nucleus accumbens
Basal ganglia
Dopamine flow
Ventral tegmental area (VTA)

REWARD SYSTEM
The VTA in the midbrain processes information about how well various needs are being met and transfers this data to the nucleus accumbens in the basal ganglia, via the neurotransmitter dopamine. The more dopamine, the greater the pleasure, and the more likely the action will be repeated in the future.

THIRST

When the body's water levels fall, salt concentration increases and blood volume decreases. Pressure receptors in the cardiovascular system and salt-concentration-sensitive cells in the hypothalamus detect these changes. In response, the pituitary gland releases antidiuretic hormone (ADH), which acts on the kidneys to retain water and produce less urine. The kidneys secrete the enzyme renin into the blood which, via a series of reactions, forms the hormone angiotensin II. This is detected by the subfornical organ, which is connected to the hypothalamus, which in turn activates more ADH-producing cells and creates the sensation of thirst, leading to drinking.

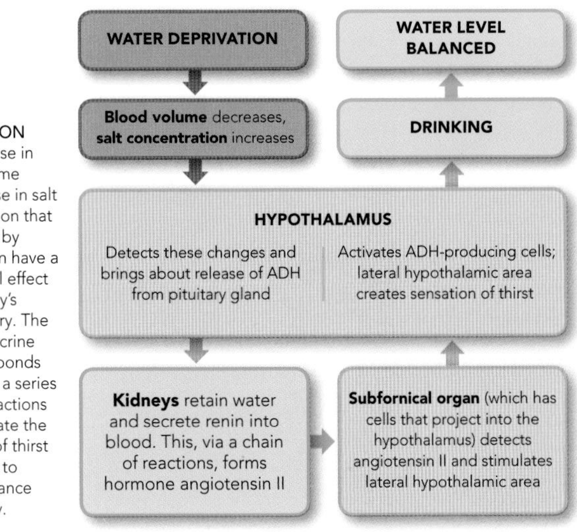
WATER DEPRIVATION
Blood volume decreases, **salt concentration** increases
HYPOTHALAMUS
Detects these changes and brings about release of ADH from pituitary gland
Activates ADH-producing cells; lateral hypothalamic area creates sensation of thirst
Kidneys retain water and secrete renin into blood. This, via a chain of reactions, forms hormone angiotensin II
Subfornical organ (which has cells that project into the hypothalamus) detects angiotensin II and stimulates lateral hypothalamic area
DRINKING
WATER LEVEL BALANCED

WATER DEPRIVATION
The decrease in blood volume and increase in salt concentration that are caused by dehydration have a detrimental effect on the body's biochemistry. The neuroendocrine system responds swiftly with a series of chain reactions that stimulate the sensation of thirst in an effort to restore balance in the body.

SLEEP–WAKE CYCLES

The suprachiasmatic nucleus (SCN) in the hypothalamus plays a key role in sleep–wake cycles. Light levels are sensed by the retina, and this information is relayed to the SCN, which then sends a signal to the pineal gland. This triggers the release of melatonin, the hormone that tells the body when to sleep. At this point, the brain becomes less alert and tiredness starts to take over. When melatonin levels fall in response to increased light, the waking part of the cycle begins.

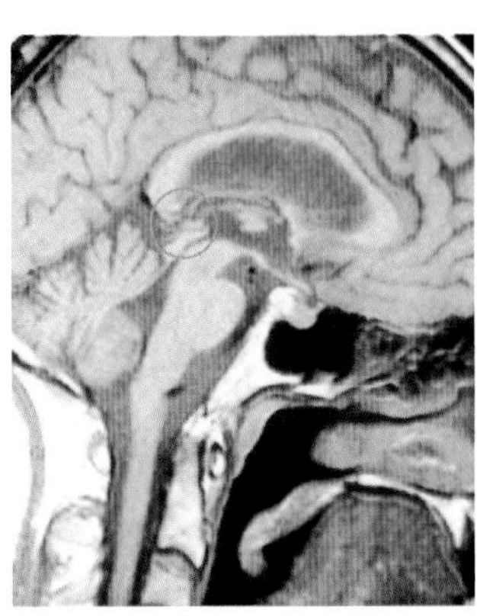

PINEAL GLAND
The circle on this lateral MRI scan of the brain pinpoints the pineal gland, a pea-sized gland located beneath the thalamus. It is responsible for the secretion of melatonin.

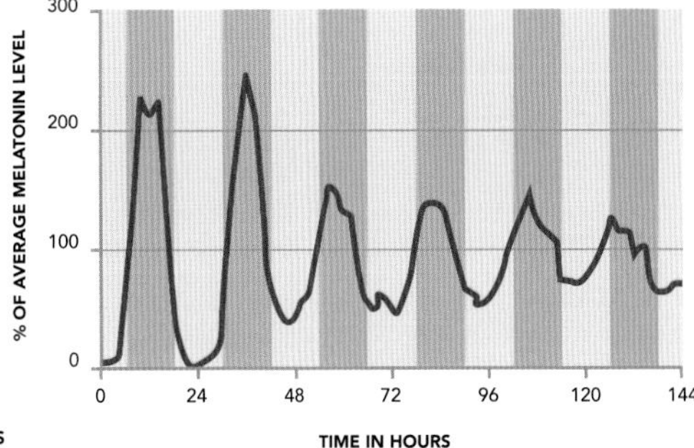
% OF AVERAGE MELATONIN LEVEL
300
200
100
0
0
24
48
72
96
120
144
TIME IN HOURS
KEY
NIGHT
DAY
MELATONIN LEVELS

MELATONIN
Falling levels of light trigger the production of melatonin, which forms a link between the external environment and the brain's sleep-wake cycles.

PLANNING A MOVEMENT

MOVEMENTS MAY BE PLANNED EITHER CONSCIOUSLY OR UNCONSCIOUSLY, AND BOTH TYPES MAY PRODUCE COMPLEX ACTIONS THAT LOOK VERY MUCH ALIKE. ALL PLANNED MOVEMENTS INVOLVE THE BRAIN, ALTHOUGH CONSCIOUS MOVEMENTS ARE HATCHED IN A DIFFERENT AREA FROM UNCONSCIOUS MOVEMENTS. THE MORE SKILLED WE ARE AT MAKING A PARTICULAR MOVEMENT, THE LESS LIKELY IT IS TO REQUIRE CONSCIOUS PLANNING.

CONSCIOUS AND UNCONSCIOUS MOVEMENT

Many of our actions are conscious – thinking about picking up an object, for example, and then actually picking it up. However, there are many actions that take place without our awareness, such as blinking. Some unconscious actions may be triggered directly by environmental stimuli – the sight of food may trigger an automatic reaching movement, for example. Whether a complex movement is conscious or unconscious depends largely on the individual's level of skill. As an action becomes increasingly familiar, it can become "automatic". However, these movements can also be performed consciously if the individual turns attention to them.

SKILLED DRIVER familiar route	SKILLED DRIVER unfamiliar route	LEARNER DRIVER
SEEKING THE TURNING	SEEKING THE TURNING	SEEKING THE TURNING
CHECK MIRROR	CHECK MIRROR	CHECK MIRROR
CHANGE GEAR	CHANGE GEAR	CHANGE GEAR
TURN WHEEL	TURN WHEEL	TURN WHEEL

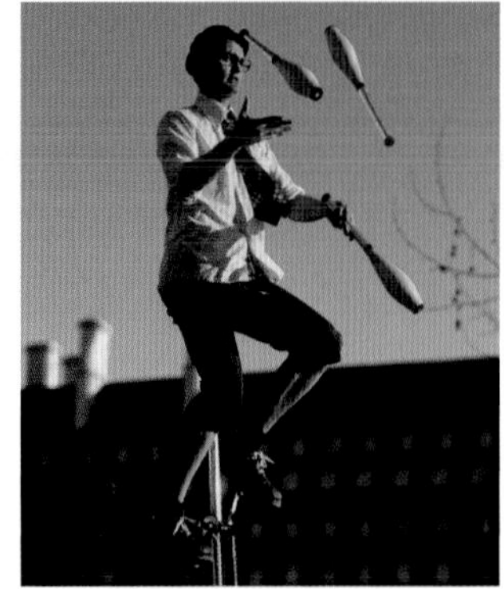

COMPLICATED ACTIONS
Even advanced movements, such as juggling and unicycling simultaneously, can be performed unconsciously.

SKILL AND FAMILIARITY
The chart to the left shows that a skilled driver on a familiar route will carry out all of the individual actions involved with turning the car unconsciously, while a learner will be conscious of all the actions. A skilled driver on an unfamiliar route will only be conscious of seeking out the turning.

KEY
CONSCIOUS
UNCONSCIOUS

REFLEX ACTIONS

Reflex actions are motor actions that are programmed into the spinal cord. The brain is not involved, and the actions cannot be consciously controlled. Most reflex actions protect the body by producing rapid reactions to escape from potentially damaging stimuli. In each case, the stimulus causes sensory nerve endings to fire; these signals pass through the nerve fibres to the spine, and trigger firing in the adjacent motor neurons, which then feed back to the relevant area and cause it to move.

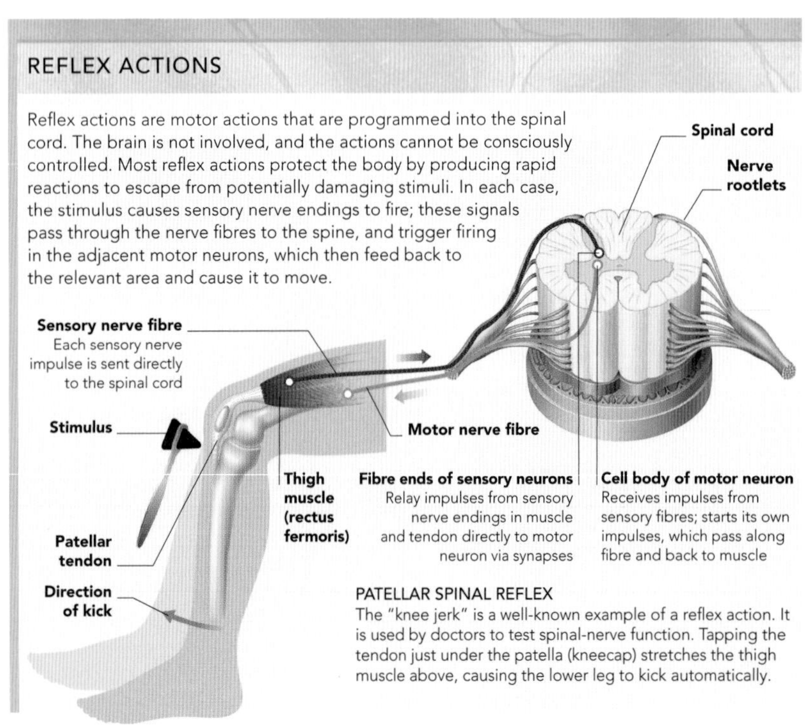
Spinal cord
Nerve rootlets
Sensory nerve fibre
Each sensory nerve impulse is sent directly to the spinal cord
Stimulus
Motor nerve fibre
Thigh muscle (rectus fermoris)
Fibre ends of sensory neurons
Relay impulses from sensory nerve endings in muscle and tendon directly to motor neuron via synapses
Cell body of motor neuron
Receives impulses from sensory fibres; starts its own impulses, which pass along fibre and back to muscle
Patellar tendon
Direction of kick

PATELLAR SPINAL REFLEX
The "knee jerk" is a well-known example of a reflex action. It is used by doctors to test spinal-nerve function. Tapping the tendon just under the patella (kneecap) stretches the thigh muscle above, causing the lower leg to kick automatically.

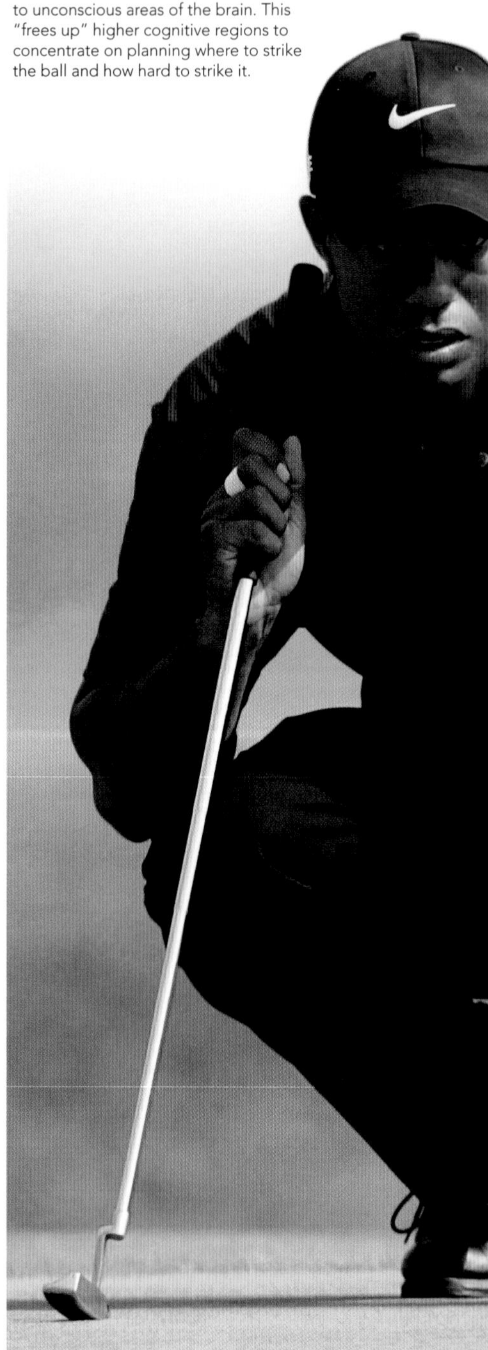

COMPLEX PLANNING
Some actions require lengthy conscious deliberation. If a person is highly skilled at doing something – a professional golfer putting a ball, for example – the execution of the action will be relegated to unconscious areas of the brain. This "frees up" higher cognitive regions to concentrate on planning where to strike the ball and how hard to strike it.

BRAIN AREAS AND MOVEMENTS

Both conscious and unconscious actions involve the primary motor cortex, which sends the "go" signals that contract the muscles (via the spinal cord and motor nerves). However, while unconscious movements are planned by areas in the parietal lobe, conscious actions involve "higher" frontal brain areas, including the premotor and supplementary motor cortices. They may also involve prefrontal areas, such as the dorsolateral prefrontal cortex, where actions are consciously assessed. It may feel as though conscious actions result from a decision. In fact, unconscious areas of the brain plan and start to execute movements before we consciously decide to do them. The "decision" may, therefore, merely be the conscious recognition of what the unconscious mind is planning to do.

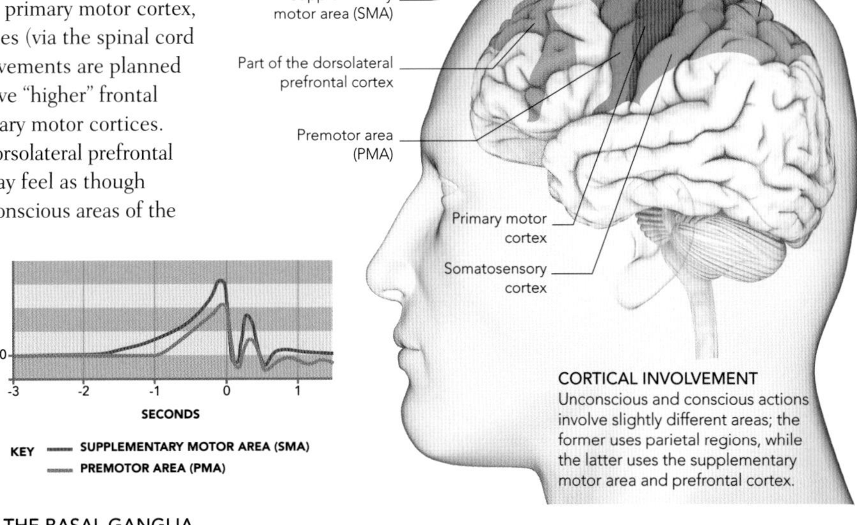

READINESS POTENTIAL
Unconscious activity in the SMA and PMA starts two seconds before an action. The conscious "decision" to act occurs only a fraction of a second before the action.

CORTICAL INVOLVEMENT
Unconscious and conscious actions involve slightly different areas; the former uses parietal regions, while the latter uses the supplementary motor area and prefrontal cortex.

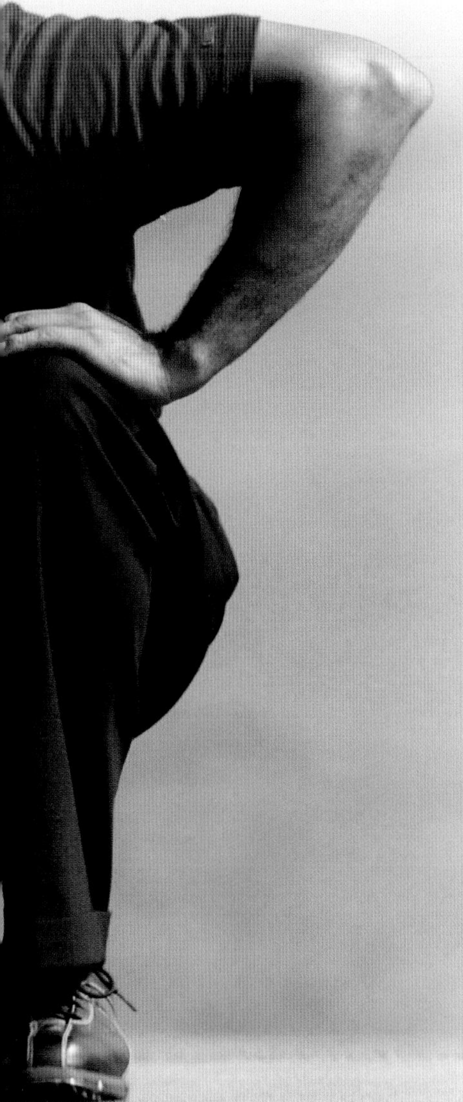

THE BASAL GANGLIA

Action plans that are made in the parietal and frontal brain areas are fed down to the basal ganglia and then routed, via the thalamus, back up to the SMA and PMA before execution. The basal ganglia are thought to act as a filter, blocking plans that are inappropriate, for example, inhibiting automatic, environment-triggered responses, such as grasping food.

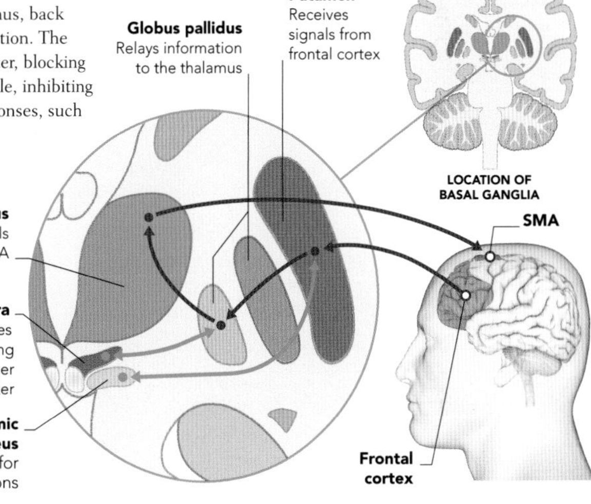

RESPONSE CONTROL
As action plans are routed around the basal ganglia, the information is made more or less potent – and thus likely to be executed – by the action of various neurotransmitters.

KEY
BASAL GANGLIA LOOP
MODULATING CIRCUITS

THE CEREBELLUM

For the body to make any complex movement, the sequence and duration of each of its elements must be co-ordinated very precisely. This is controlled by the cerebellum, via a circuit that connects it to the motor cortex. It also modulates the signals that the motor cortex subsequently sends to the motor neurons. The cerebellum ensures that when one set of muscles initiates a movement, the opposing set acts as a brake, so that the body part in question arrives accurately at its target.

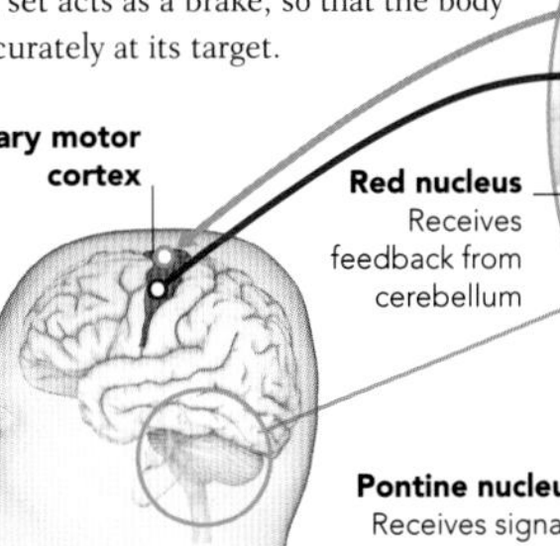

PRECISE TIMING
The cerebellar circuits include a system that measures time. It feeds its calculations to the primary motor cortex, which sends the signals to the muscles.

KEY
SIGNALS FROM CEREBELLUM
SIGNALS TO CEREBELLUM

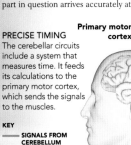

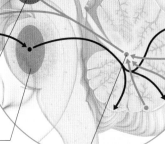

Red nucleus
Receives feedback from cerebellum

Pontine nucleus
Receives signals about impending movement and sends them to cerebellum

Dentate nucleus
Sends signals back to motor cortex

Cerebellar cortex
Motor programmes are stored here

EXECUTING A MOVEMENT

ONCE A MOVEMENT HAS BEEN PLANNED, THE BRAIN AREAS RESPONSIBLE SEND SIGNALS TO THE MUSCLES TO EXECUTE THE ACTION. SOME OF THESE SIGNALS ARE SENT FIRST TO THE MOTOR CORTEX, AND THEN ONWARDS THROUGH THE SPINAL CORD. OTHERS TRAVEL VIA MORE DIRECT ROUTES. MOVEMENT OCCURS WHEN THE SIGNALS REACH THE MUSCLE FIBRES, CAUSING THEM TO CONTRACT.

SPINAL TRACTS

Action plans generated in the supplementary, premotor, and parietal cortices are forwarded to the motor cortex for execution. The motor cortex is made up of about one million neurons, which send long axons down the spinal cord. These are bundled together, along with axons that come directly from the somatosensory cortex, to form the lateral corticospinal tract. Just before entering the spinal cord, the nerves from each hemisphere of the brain separate and cross over, so the fibres from the left hemisphere of the cortex go down the right side of the spinal cord, and vice versa. The rubrospinal tract originates from the red nucleus in the midbrain, and helps to produce fine movements. The vestibulospinal and reticulospinal tracts start lower down in the brainstem and help control balance and orientation.

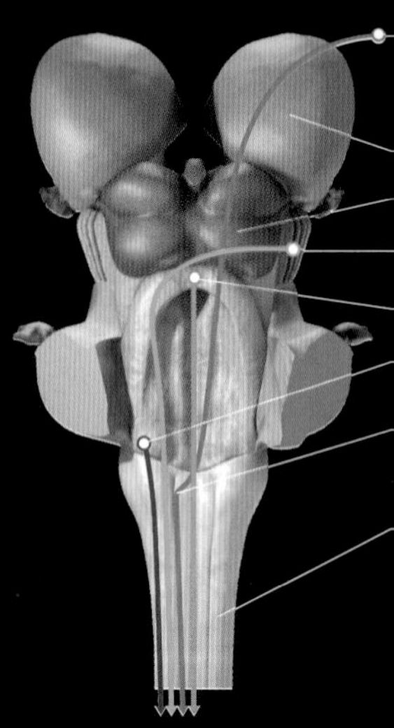

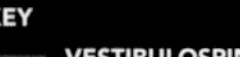

LIMB CONTROL
The lateral corticospinal tract is the only spinal tract to originate in the cerebral cortex and is mostly responsible for controlling limb movements.

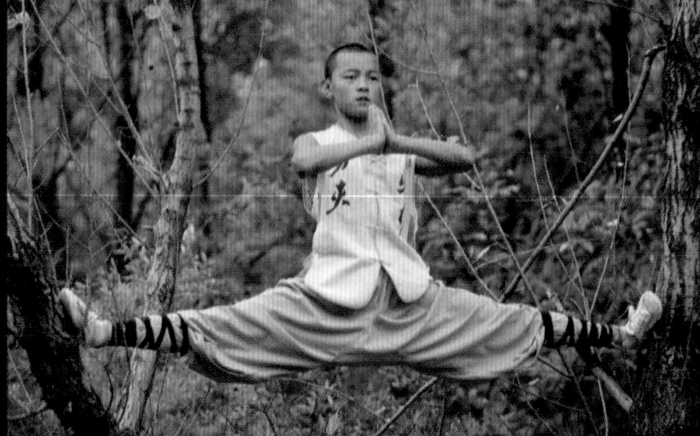

BALANCING ACT
The reticulospinal and vestibulospinal tracts help control balance and orientation, and neutralize the effects of gravity.

SPINE TO MUSCLE

The axons of the motor neurons, which receive signals from the spinal tracts, emerge from between the vertebrae and travel to the muscles. The nerve endings infiltrate the muscle fibres at neuromuscular junctions, and when they fire they release the neurotransmitter acetylcholine. This diffuses across the narrow "synaptic cleft" connecting the muscle to the nerve and binds to acetylcholine receptors in the muscle cell membrane, which, via a series of reactions, makes the specific muscle contract. Muscles required to carry out fine movements have correspondingly higher numbers of neurons than those required to perform gross movements.

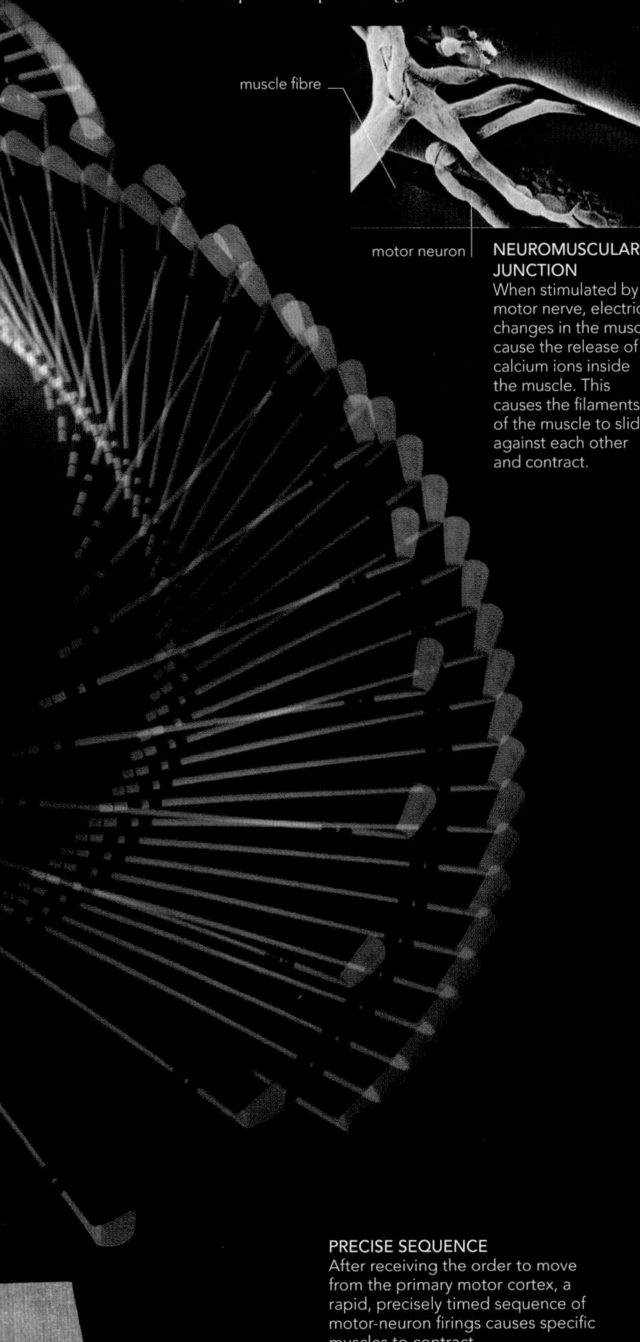
muscle fibre
motor neuron

NEUROMUSCULAR JUNCTION
When stimulated by a motor nerve, electrical changes in the muscle cause the release of calcium ions inside the muscle. This causes the filaments of the muscle to slide against each other and contract.

PRECISE SEQUENCE
After receiving the order to move from the primary motor cortex, a rapid, precisely timed sequence of motor-neuron firings causes specific muscles to contract.

MOTOR DISORDERS

Motor disorders can be divided into two principal groups: hyperkinesia (overactivity) and hypokinesia (too little movement). The former includes a wide range of motor disorders, from involuntary, slow shaking of various body parts to tics, which are uncontrollable, rapid, disjointed movements and/or sounds. Sudden, shock-like muscle contractions are symptoms of myoclonus, while quick, random, usually jerky limb movements are caused by chorea and ballism. Hyperkinesia disorders include: general slowness of movement (bradykinesia); "freezing" or inability to begin a movement or involuntary arrest of a movement; rigidity – an increase in muscle tension when a limb encounters force; and postural instability, which is the loss of ability to maintain an upright posture.

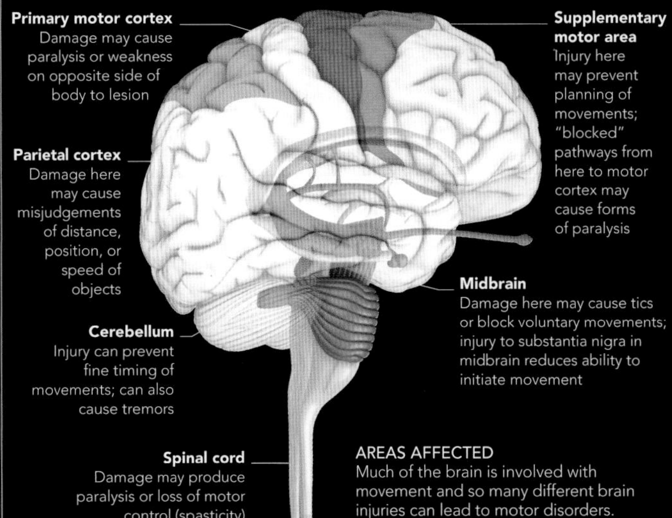
Primary motor cortex
Damage may cause paralysis or weakness on opposite side of body to lesion
Supplementary motor area
Injury here may prevent planning of movements; "blocked" pathways from here to motor cortex may cause forms of paralysis
Parietal cortex
Damage here may cause misjudgements of distance, position, or speed of objects
Midbrain
Damage here may cause tics or block voluntary movements; injury to substantia nigra in midbrain reduces ability to initiate movement
Cerebellum
Injury can prevent fine timing of movements; can also cause tremors
Spinal cord
Damage may produce paralysis or loss of motor control (spasticity)

AREAS AFFECTED
Much of the brain is involved with movement and so many different brain injuries can lead to motor disorders.

MOTOR RECOVERY

Movement disorders may result from damage to many different areas of the brain, and it is very common for one of these to follow a stroke. Damage to the motor cortex, for example, may cause whole or partial paralysis of the opposite side of the body, and strokes in sub-cortical areas may lead to loss of control of voluntary movements. The affected neural pathways can, however, rebuild to a certain extent, reducing the long-term effect of the damage. Studies show that damaged midbrain-cortical motor pathways form new connections in as little as three months after remedial therapy.

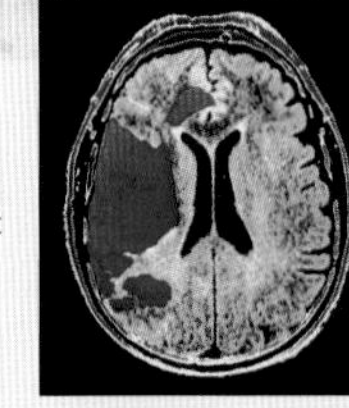

STROKE
This CT scan shows the extent of internal bleeding in the brain caused by a stroke.

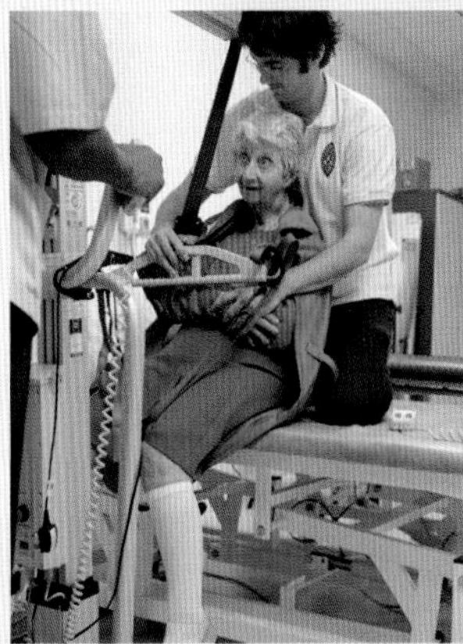

STROKE REHABILITATION
The neural pathways damaged by a stroke do rebuild themselves to a limited degree. Physiotherapy encourages the rewiring of motor circuits, and recovery is often directly related to the intensity of the therapy.

UNCONSCIOUS ACTION

THE BRAIN REGISTERS EVENTS VIA THE SENSE ORGANS ALMOST IMMEDIATELY, BUT IT TAKES UP TO HALF A SECOND TO BECOME CONSCIOUS OF THEM. IN ORDER TO GENERATE EFFECTIVE RESPONSES IN A FAST-CHANGING ENVIRONMENT, THE BRAIN THEREFORE PLANS AND EXECUTES MOMENT-BY-MOMENT ACTIONS UNCONSCIOUSLY.

REACTION PATHWAYS

It takes up to 400 milliseconds (ms) for the brain to process incoming information to the stage where it may become conscious. It takes a similar length of time to prepare the body for action. So if we waited to be conscious of a sight or sound before starting to respond to it, our behaviour would lag almost a second behind the events to which we are responding. By the time we leapt out of the path of a speeding car, it is likely to have run us over. The brain speeds up our physical responses by fast-tracking sensory information to the

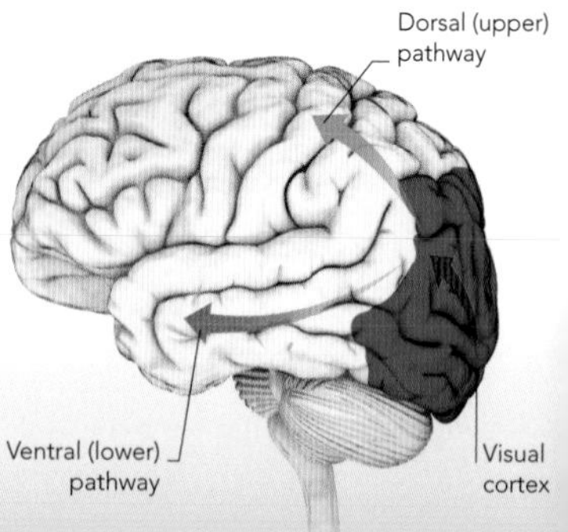

DORSAL AND VENTRAL ROUTES
Visual stimuli are processed along parallel pathways. The unconscious dorsal route generates physical responses while the ventral route creates conscious perception.

RETURNING A SERVE

Professional tennis players can plan and initiate the complex moves required to return a fast service before they are consciously aware that the ball is on its way. Unlike novice players, they do not have to think consciously about each muscle movement because practice has turned the relevant action sequences into automated motor programmes that are stored and run unconsciously. Familiarity with their opponents' body language also allows them to make well-informed unconscious predictions about where the ball will land.

EVENTS IN RECEIVER'S BRAIN

0ms Attention

The player's brain prepares for action by focusing attention on his opponent. This prevents the brain from responding to irrelevant stimuli and amplifies information coming from the part of the visual field containing the target of attention. If the player is familiar with the opponent's playing style, his brain will register the movements made by the opponent as he serves and compare them with previous observations to help predict where the ball will land. Attention to such cues may speed up reactions by 20–30 milliseconds.

Frontal lobes
Thalamus

LOCKING ON
The thalamus directs attention to the target, while the frontal lobes inhibit distracting thoughts.

70ms Body memory

The ball is not yet consciously visible to the player, but unconsciously his brain is already planning the actions he must make to return it. At this stage he is mainly using information about his opponent's movements to decide how his own body should move. A skilled player processes fewer visual cues than an inexperienced one because their brain identifies irrelevant signals at a very early stage and ignores them. The visual information from his opponent's movements activates the player's parietal cortex, which in turn calls up relevant procedural memories. These are learned actions – such as how to return a serve – that have become encoded as automatic motor programmes. They are stored in an unconscious brain module called the putamen that replays them as the situation demands.

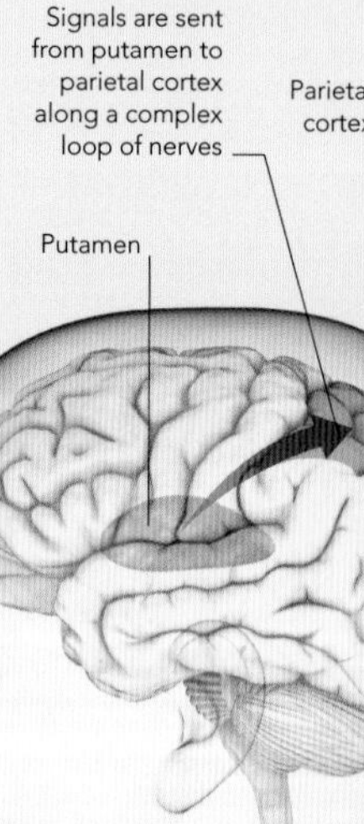

MOVEMENT MEMORY
Part of the basal ganglia, the putamen acts as a store of memories about deeply ingrained habits of movement. Signals from the putamen are passed to the parietal cortex.

SERVER

motor-planning areas along an unconscious pathway. A visual stimulus such as a moving object prompts neural activity that works out where it is in relation to the body. Various parts of the occipital and parietal cortex, between them, calculate the object's shape, size, relative motion, and trajectory. This information is then brought together and used to form an action plan. This might involve hitting (swatting a fly, for example), avoidance (ducking or jumping out of the way of a missile), or grabbing (a falling fruit or a stumbling child). The chosen response is largely learned; for example, a skilled ball-game player is likely to catch or hit a speeding ball while an unpractised player might duck it.

TENNIS PLAYERS UNDER OBSERVATION

Tennis players watching a video of another player serving a ball imagine themselves making the action. These fMRI images show that watching a moving ball (left) activates areas of the brain that track visual objects, but watching someone serve a ball (right) activates visual areas plus large parts of the parietal cortex. The additional activation shows the viewer's brain is "acting out" the moves seen in the video. This information helps the viewer predict where the ball will go.

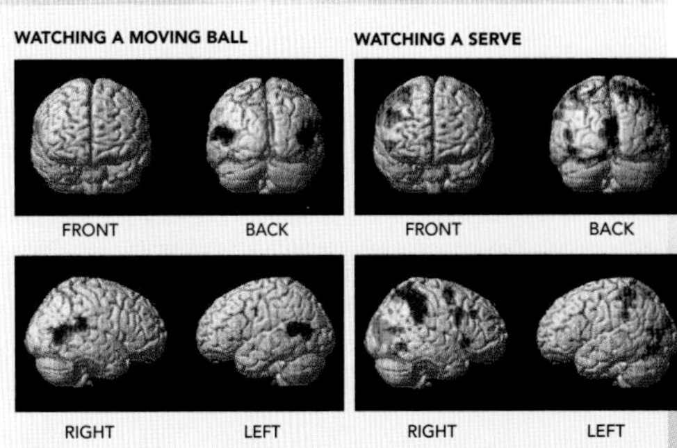

250ms Action plan

The receiving player's brain brings together the information that has been registered so far to construct a response to the fast-approaching ball. The plan is informed by information gathered from the opponent's body movements, the (still unconscious) knowledge of the ball's speed and trajectory, and the procedural memories triggered by these stimuli. The plan is held in the premotor area, which lies just in front of the motor cortex. This is like a rehearsal stage, allowing action to be played out as a pattern of neuronal activity without affecting the muscles.

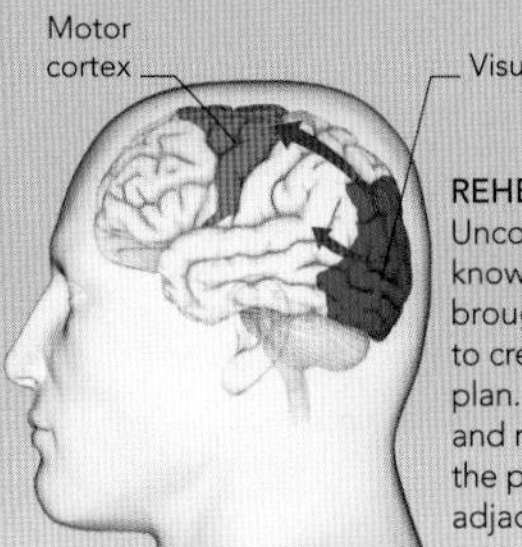

REHEARSAL Unconscious knowledge is brought together to create an action plan. This is formed and rehearsed in the premotor area, adjacent to the motor cortex.

355ms Sending signals

The action plan held in the premotor cortex is transmitted to the neighbouring motor cortex. The neurons in this strip of brain connect via the spine to skeletal muscles, and when they fire they cause the muscles to contract. In this case, the firing of neurons about halfway down the right side of the motor strip move the player's left arm and hand to position the racket to connect with the ball. Other neurons control the rest of the body. The sequence in which these neurons fire – and therefore the sequence of limb movement – is controlled by the cerebellum.

Motor cortex

Cerebellum

Signal from motor cortex travels to player's hand

INSTRUCTION TO MOVE Neural signals from the motor cortex are sent along the spine, causing muscles to contract and leading to overt movement.

500ms Conscious act

If the player's conscious perception of the ball's trajectory differs markedly from his earlier, unconscious, prediction he may veto the earlier action plan and start to construct an alternative, or try to adjust the current plan to take into account the new information. It takes another 200-300ms, however, to incorporate the new, conscious, information into a revised action plan and by then the ball has travelled too far for any player to return.

The situation is similar to that which occurs when a person steps forward onto what their brain predicted was flat ground, but which is actually a downward step. The resultant physical catastrophe, in both cases, triggers a further cascade of signals that may generate a wide range of emotions, including anger, embarrassment, and a feeling of failure.

285ms Conscious thought starts

The player's brain becomes consciously aware – belatedly – of the ball moving away from the opponent's racket. But his brain has already (unconsciously) predicted its real-time position, and – providing the two information streams do not clash – the player is likely to think he sees the ball where it really is.

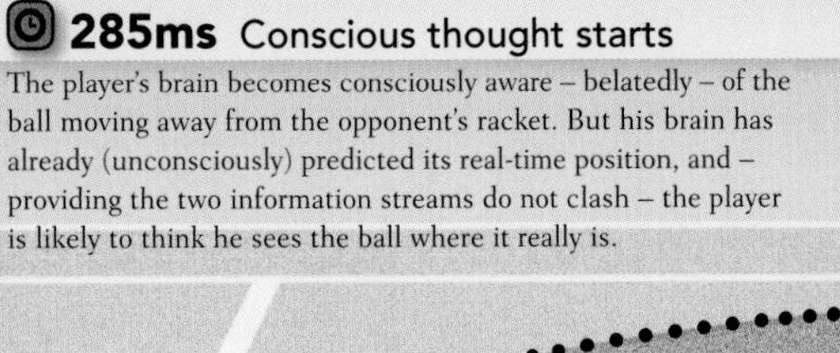

Ball comes into conscious view

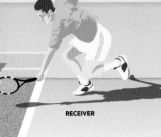

RECEIVER

MIRROR NEURONS

CERTAIN NEURONS ARE ACTIVATED WHEN YOU MOVE, AND ALSO WHEN YOU SEE SOMEONE ELSE MOVING. THIS MEANS WE UNCONSCIOUSLY MIMIC THE ACTIONS OF OTHERS, AND THUS SHARE, TO SOME EXTENT, THEIR EXPERIENCE. MIRROR NEURONS ALSO ALLOW US TO KNOW WHAT ANOTHER PERSON IS FEELING, WITHOUT HAVING TO THINK ABOUT IT. THESE FINDINGS ARE AMONG THE MOST SIGNIFICANT NEUORSCIENTIFIC DISCOVERIES IN RECENT YEARS.

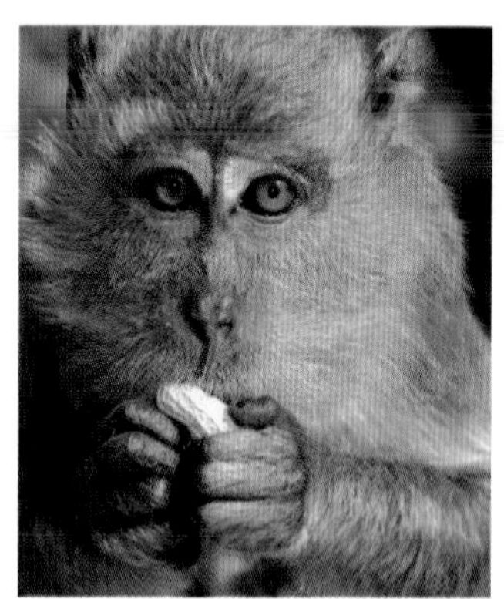

HOW THEY WERE DISCOVERED
Mirror neurons were discovered in a monkey whose brain was wired up to show which nerve cells lit up as it reached out to grasp food. When laboratory staff made the same movement while the monkeys sat and watched, the same neurons lit up.

WHAT ARE THEY?

Mirror neurons were first discovered in the motor-planning area in the brains of macaques (a species of monkey) and subsequent brain-imaging studies suggest that they exist in humans too. The human mirror system seems to be broader in scope than that of monkeys, in that mirror neurons exist not only in movement areas, but also in areas concerned with emotions, sensations, and even intentions. They provide people with immediate knowledge of what is going on in another's mind; this ability to know what another person is feeling or doing is thought to be the basis of mimicry.

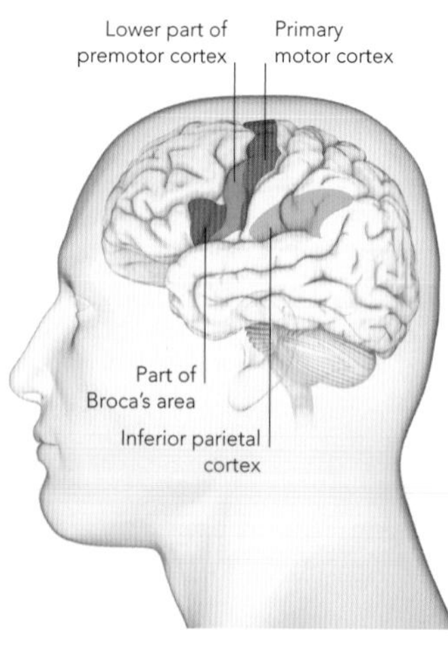
Lower part of premotor cortex
Primary motor cortex
Part of Broca's area
Inferior parietal cortex

WHERE THEY ARE
In humans, mirror neurons seem to extend into the areas of the frontal lobe that are concerned with intentions, such as part of the premotor cortex. They are also found in the parietal lobe, which is involved with sensations. However, the full extent of these neurons is still being researched.

MIRRORING TOUCH

Mirror neurons also seem to operate in the somatosensory cortex – the area of the brain that registers touch. In one study, subjects' brains were scanned, first while their leg was brushed, and then while they watched a video of someone else's leg being touched. Activity in their brains revealed that some parts of the somatosensory areas are activated only by direct touch and others are activated by the sight of another being touched. A third group of neurons, however, are activated both by direct touch and by seeing others being touched. These mirror neurons – shown in white on the scans below – were limited to the left hemisphere in this study, though in other experiments they have been detected in both hemispheres.

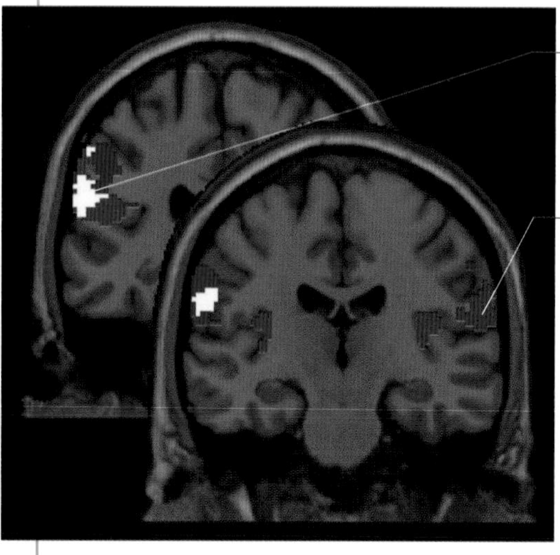
Somatosensory areas in left hemisphere activated by both touch and vision-of-touch
Activity only arises in the right hemisphere from direct touch, but mirror neurons have been detected here in similar experiments.
KEY
AREAS ACTIVATED BY TOUCH
AREAS ACTIVATED BY VISION-OF-TOUCH
AREAS ACTIVATED BY BOTH

ACTIVATED AREAS
These MRI scans are coronal sections taken from the same brain. They show the areas stimulated by touch, watching another being touched, and the overlap between the two.

MIRRORING SPEECH

Mirror neurons may help people communicate by "syncing" their brains when they talk together. Partners in a conversation unconsciously imitate one another, adopting a similar rate of speaking and the same sort of grammatical structures. This helps one person predict what the other is going to say next, making communication quicker and smoother. Speech is combined with body movements and facial expressions to convey full meaning, and these tiny movements amplify the perception of another's voice. Watching a speaker's face is equivalent in effect to turning up the volume by 15 decibels.

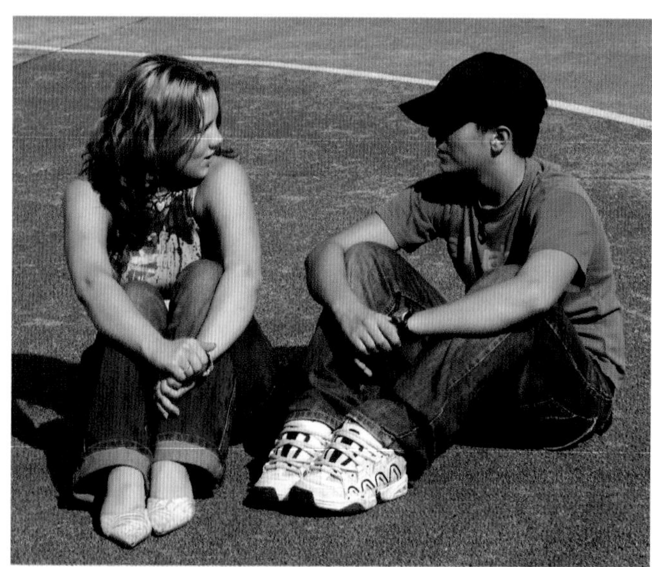

BODY LANGUAGE
As well as mirroring speech patterns and speed, people unconsciously adapt their body language to match whoever they are speaking to. Partners in a conversation focus on each other's faces, picking up minute movements that help express meaning.

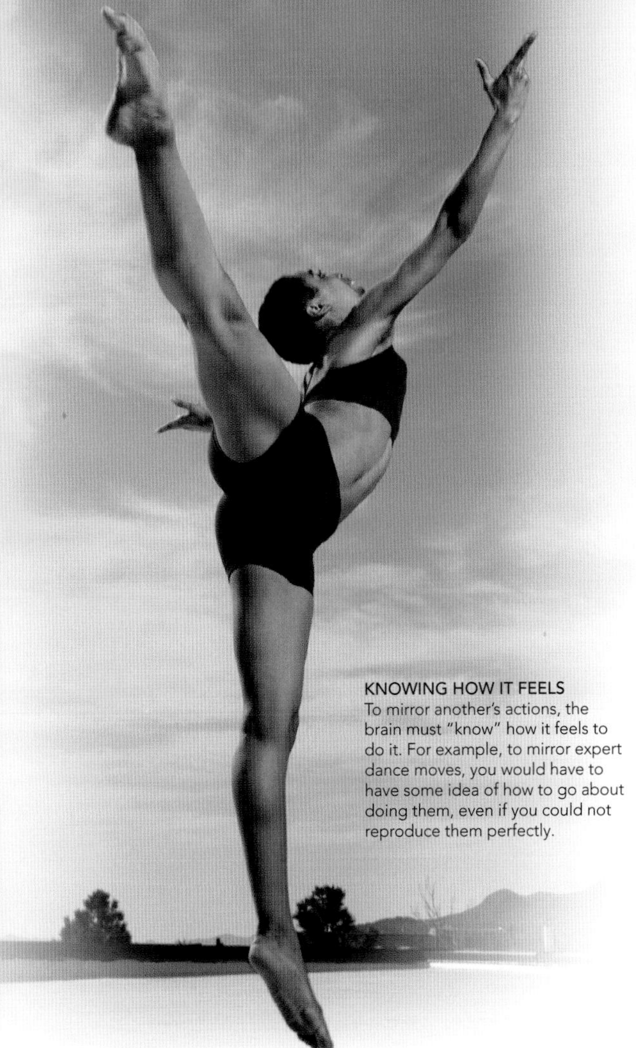

KNOWING HOW IT FEELS
To mirror another's actions, the brain must "know" how it feels to do it. For example, to mirror expert dance moves, you would have to have some idea of how to go about doing them, even if you could not reproduce them perfectly.

MIRRORING MOVEMENT

Recent studies have found that a certain, as yet unknown, proportion of mirror neurons are active both when moving and when watching movement. Neurons in the premotor cortex concerned with planning to move the legs are activated when you watch a person running, for example. In other words, when you see someone doing something, in your brain you do it too. However, in order to mirror another's action, the sight of the action must "resonate" with a motor programme that the brain has already learned.

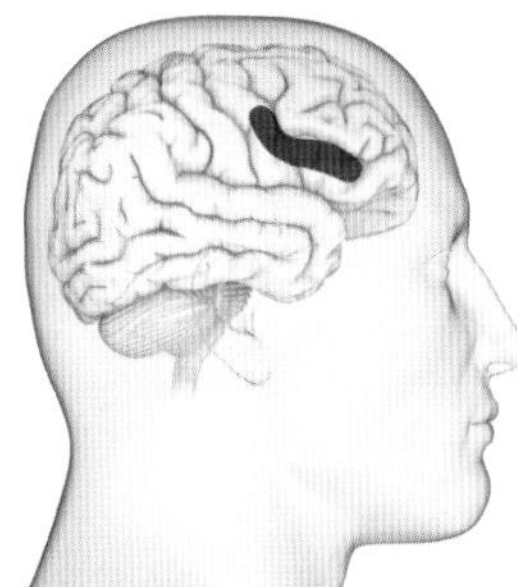

WATCHING CHEWING
Simply watching another person chewing shows activity in both the premotor cortex and the part of the primary motor cortex concerned with mouth and jaw movements.

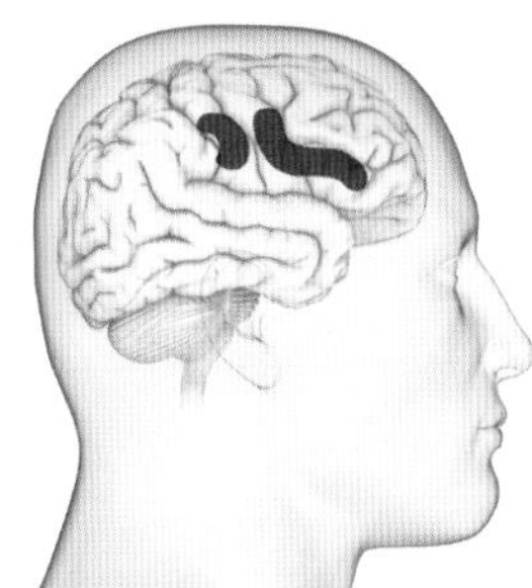

ACTING ON AN OBJECT
When the movement involves acting on an object – biting an apple, for example, rather than just simply chewing – areas of the parietal cortex also light up.

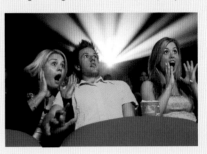

MIRRORING EMOTIONS

When one person sees another expressing an emotion, the areas of the brain that are associated with feeling that emotion are activated, making emotions transmittable. In one study, volunteers inhaled a disgusting smell, and later, watched a video of someone else smelling something and expressing disgust. Both produced neuronal activity in the area of the brain associated with feeling disgust. Emotion mirroring is thought to be the basis of empathy. Autistic people, who tend to lack empathy, have been found to show less mirror-neuron activity.

HORROR MOVIE
Seeing someone else looking frightened makes you feel scared yourself. Mirror neurons, therefore, help to whip up emotion in audiences.

MIRRORING INTENTIONS

Two movements may be identical, but may signal very different things in different contexts. Human mirror neurons seem to take this into account. When one person sees another picking up a cup in order to drink from it, a different set of neurons are activated from those that light up at the sight of a person making the identical movement but in a context that suggests they are clearing the cup away. Hence, the observer's brain does not just generate a faint idea of what the other person is doing with their body, but also an echo of their intention in doing it. This allows us to get a glimpse of another individual's plans and thought processes without us consciously having to work it out.

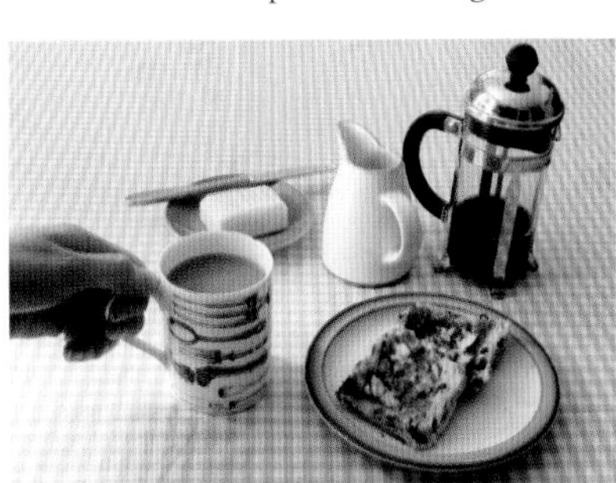

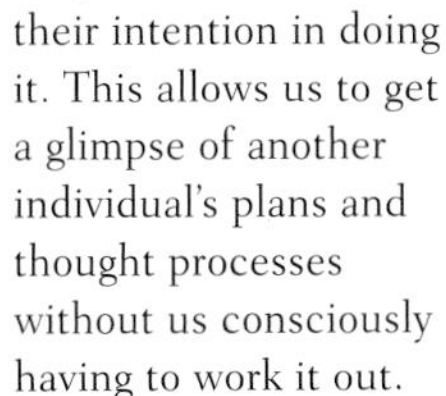

DRINKING AND CLEANING UP
The top image shows a table set for breakfast, while the image at the bottom shows the table after the meal has been finished. The action of grasping the cup can be exactly the same in both, but our brains take into account the difference in contexts and therefore we automatically "know" that each one signals a different intention.

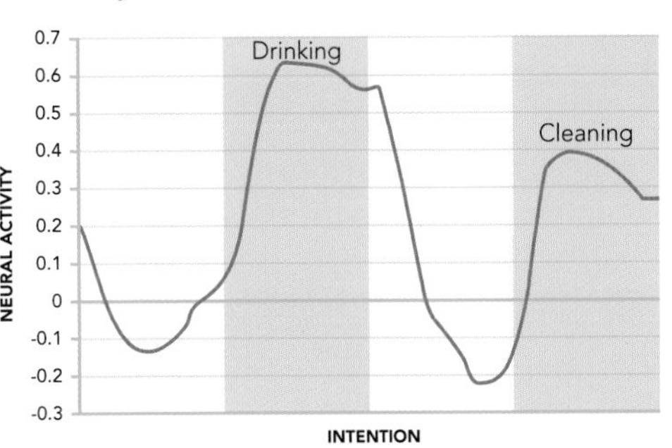

LEVEL OF ACTIVITY
The increased activity associated with watching the intention to drink is thought to be because it is more commonly practised than the intention to clear up.

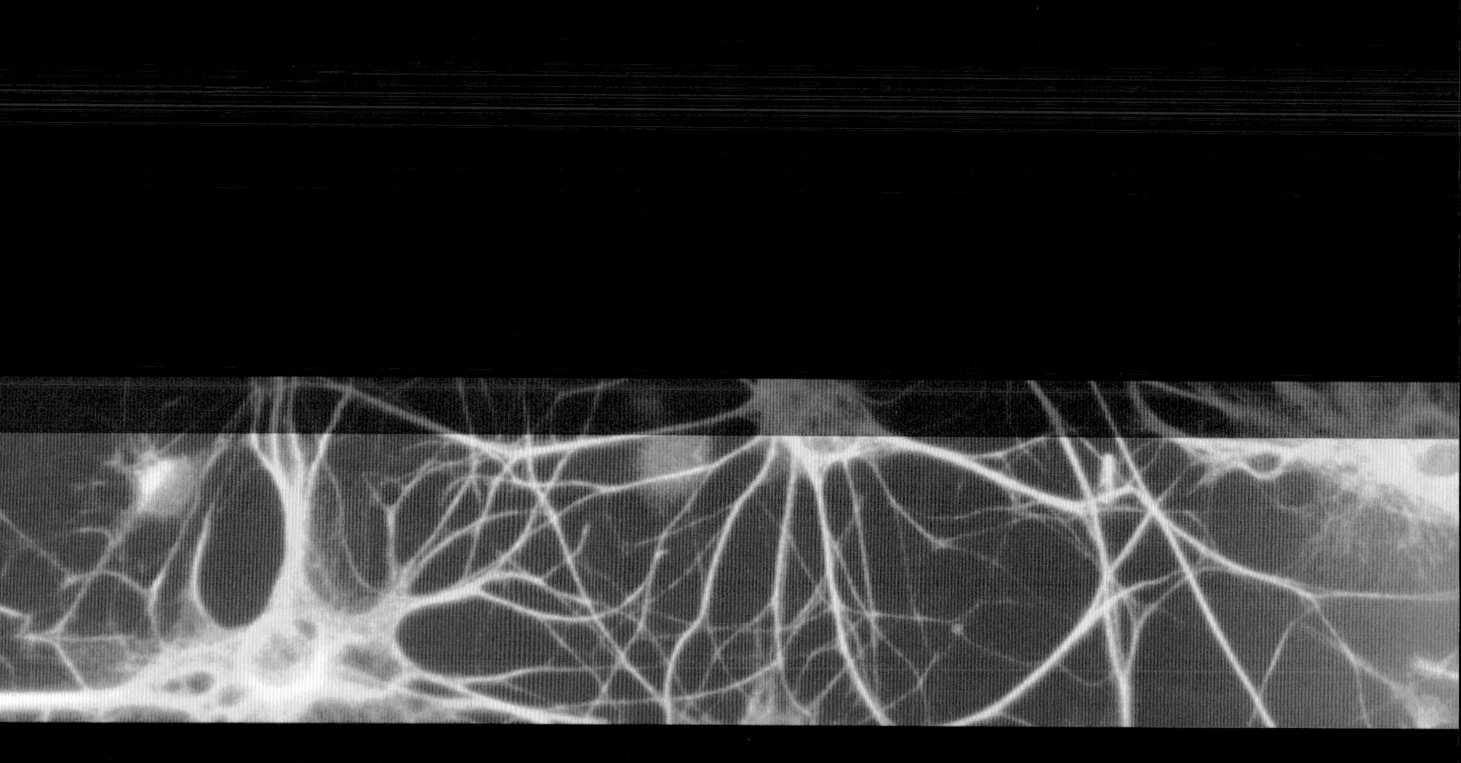

EMOTIONS CAN BE THOUGHT OF AS BODILY CHANGES THAT PROMPT US TO ACT. THEY HAVE EVOLVED TO GET US TO DO WHAT WE HAVE TO IN ORDER TO SURVIVE AND PASS OUR GENES ON TO THE NEXT GENERATION. TO REINFORCE THEIR EFFECTIVENESS, EMOTIONALLY TRIGGERED ACTIONS ARE ASSOCIATED WITH PLEASANT OR UNPLEASANT CONSCIOUS FEELINGS. EMOTIONS TEND TO BE SHORT-LIVED, LASTING A FEW HOURS AT MOST, BUT THEY CAN LEAD TO MORE PERSISTENT CONDITIONS CALLED MOODS.

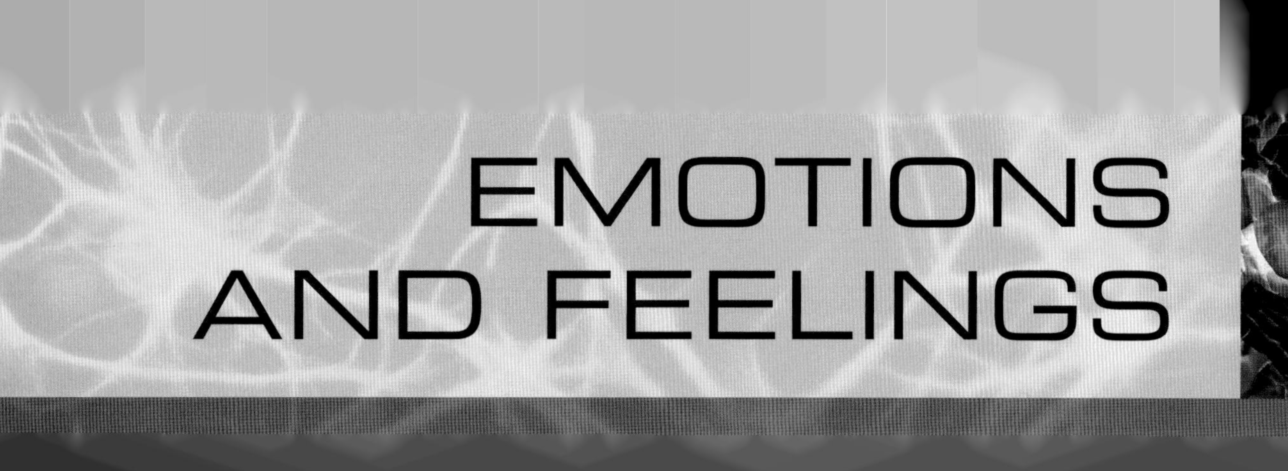

EMOTIONS AND FEELINGS

others feel and reacting to their emotions.

of the sex to which they are changing.

system than passing signals back down.

Olfactory complex
The olfactory bulbs carry messages about smell straight to the limbic areas – unlike the pathways serving the other senses, which pass signals via the thalamus to the cortex for processing. This is why scents create such an intense, instant emotional response. The olfactory complex is thought to be the brain's original "emotional" centre, and probably evolved before sight and hearing.

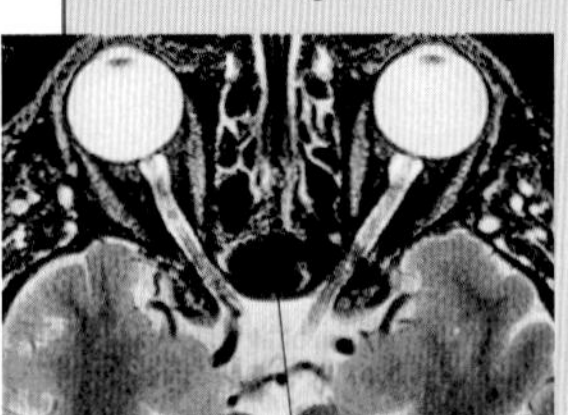

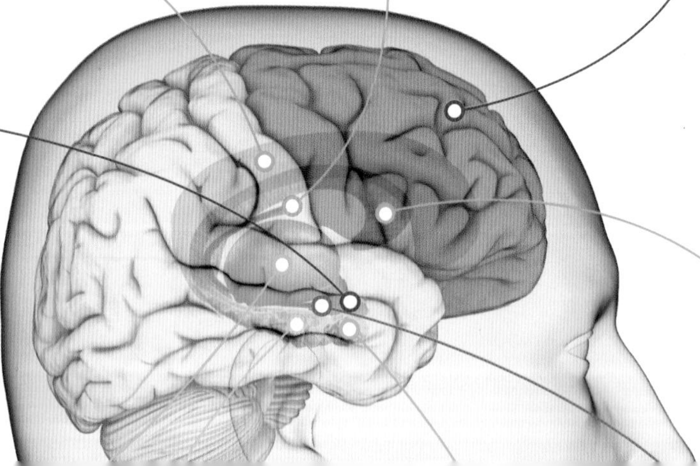

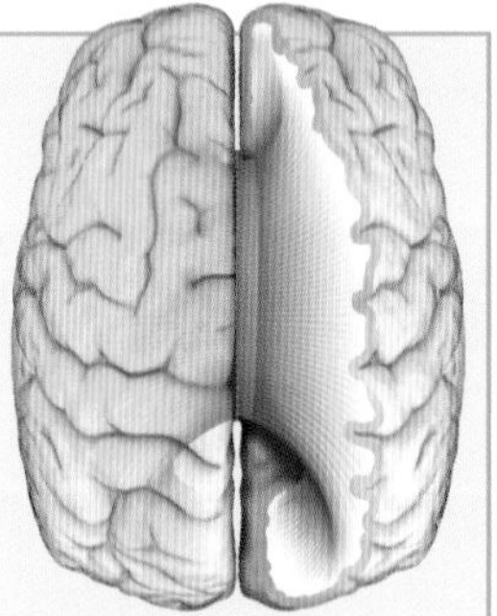

Corpus callosum
The corpus callosum (CC) plays an important role in transmitting emotions between the left and right hemispheres. Women, on average, have a greater density of fibres in the CC than men; this may account for some differences between the sexes

AMYGDALA

The amygdala "tastes" all stimuli and signals other areas to produce appropriate emotional reactions. It contains distinct regions called nuclei, which generate different kinds of responses to fear. The central nucleus generates the fear response of freezing, while the basal nucleus generates the fear response of flight. The nuclei are affected by sex hormones, and are therefore different in men and women. Activation of the amygdala can be modulated by the hypothalamus (see right).

MEDIATING AMYGDALA RESPONSE

The amygdala is activated by frightening stimuli (right). The hormone oxytocin, secreted by the hippocampus, damps down amygdala activity (below right) and with it the feeling of fright.

FEAR RESPONSE

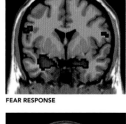

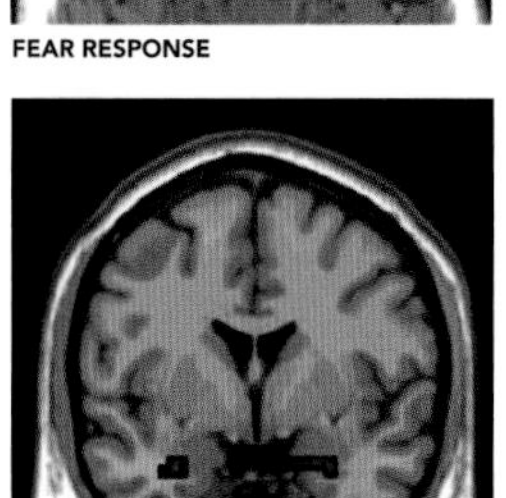

WITH OXYTOCIN

CORE OF EMOTION

Emotions engage widespread areas of the brain but the "core" network is centred on the red parts shown here – the amygdala and the dorsomedial and orbitofrontal cortices.

core limbic areas

POSITIVE EMOTION

Limbic system structures next to the amygdala are involved in feelings of pleasure, mainly by reducing activity in the amygdala and in cortical areas concerned with anxiety. Anticipation and pleasure-seeking are influenced by the "reward" circuit. This acts on the hypothalamus and amygdala: it secretes dopamine, which provides anticipation and drive, and GABA, which inhibits neurons from firing.

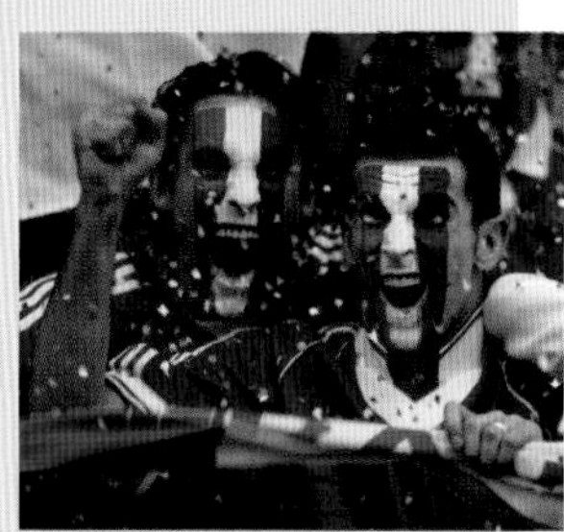

PLEASURE AND THE BRAIN

Pleasurable stimuli, such as watching your football team score a goal, activate brain areas close to the limbic system.

FEELING FEAR

The amygdala acts as a store for good and bad memories, especially emotional traumas. It is also "hard-wired" to fear certain stimuli, such as low-flying birds, spiders, and snakes. For a phobia to develop, however, there also needs to be an environmental trigger, such as a nasty encounter with a "hard-wired" stimulus, or the sight of someone else being frightened by it. It is often very hard to get rid of a phobia because the amygdala is not under conscious control. It can, however, "learn" to reduce its reaction to the stimulus.

PANIC RESPONSES

The autonomic nervous system, responsible for automatic body functions, produces the physical responses felt in a phobic reaction.

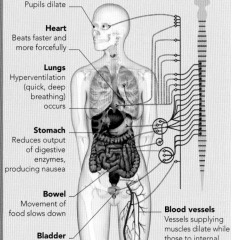

Eyes Pupils dilate

Heart Beats faster and more forcefully

Lungs Hyperventilation (quick, deep breathing) occurs

Stomach Reduces output of digestive enzymes, producing nausea

Bowel Movement of food slows down

Bladder Sphincter muscle constricts

Blood vessels Vessels supplying muscles dilate while those to internal organs narrow; blood pressure rises

UNCONSCIOUS EMOTION

We have evolved a conscious emotional system, but we retain the primitive, automatic responses at the heart of emotion. A frightening sight or sound, for example, registers in the amygdala before we are even conscious of it. While the sensory information is sent to the cortex to be made conscious, the amygdala sends messages to the hypothalamus, which triggers changes that ready the body for flight, fight, or appeasement. This "quick and dirty" route allows us to take instant action to save ourselves. When we "start" at a loud noise, then relax on realizing that it is harmless, we are experiencing both stages – unconscious reaction and conscious response.

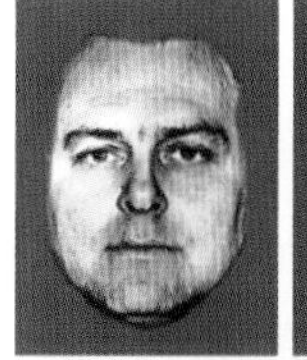
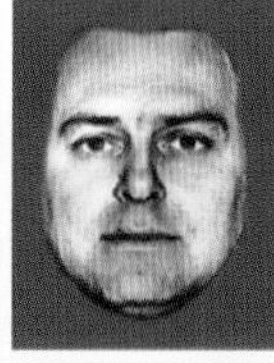
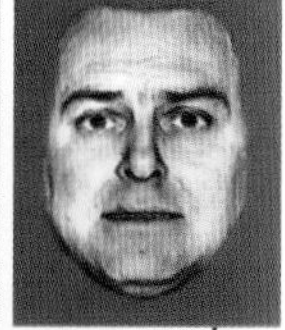
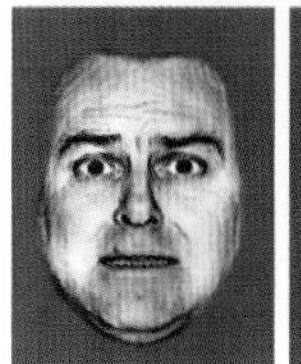
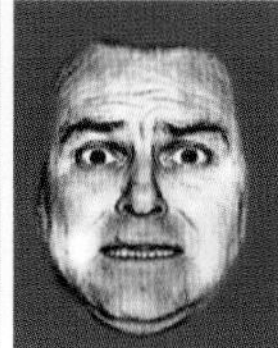
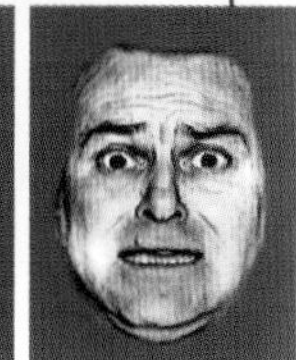

FACES OF FEAR

This series of images shows the onset of fear. The amygdala registers the emotional facial expressions of others, and produces a reaction before we even know we have seen them.

CONSCIOUS AND UNCONSCIOUS ROUTES

The amygdala picks up on emotional stimuli before we are also aware of them. This allows the body to react very quickly to threat or reward. Emotional stimuli are processed along a second route that does not involve the amygdala. This takes the information through cortical areas that produce conscious awareness and a more thoughtful response.

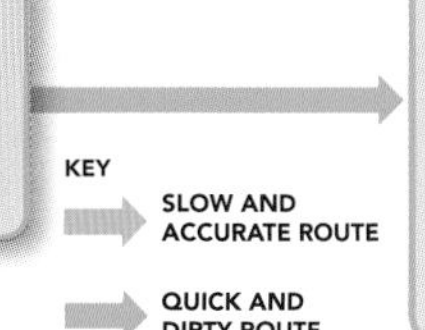

Thalamus
Sensory information is directed to the amygdala for quick assessment and action, and also to cortical areas for processing to conscious awareness.

Sensory cortex
Sensory information is transmitted along this route to the sensory cortex for recognition. More information is extracted along this path, but it takes longer.

Hippocampus
Information that is consciously perceived is encoded in the hippocampus to form memories. The hippocampus also feeds back stored information confirming or modifying the initial response.

Amygdala
The amygdala instantly assesses incoming information for emotional content, and sends signals to other areas for immediate bodily action. It operates unconsciously, and is thus liable to produce errors.

Hypothalamus
Signals from the amygdala are used to trigger hormonal changes that make the body ready for taking action in response to emotional stimuli; these responses include muscle contraction and an increase in heart rate.

KEY
SLOW AND ACCURATE ROUTE
QUICK AND DIRTY ROUTE

CONSCIOUS EMOTION

EMOTIONS ARE GENERATED IN THE LIMBIC SYSTEM, WHICH DOES NOT SUPPORT CONSCIOUSNESS ITSELF. INTENSE EMOTIONS CREATE "KNOCK-ON" ACTIVITY IN THE CORTEX, ESPECIALLY IN THE FRONTAL LOBES, WHICH WE EXPERIENCE AS A CONSCIOUS "FEELING" OR MOOD. SOMETIMES, AN EMOTION IS CLEARLY LINKED TO AN EXPERIENCE. AT OTHER TIMES, THE CAUSE IS NOT OBVIOUS, BUT BEING AWARE OF THE EMOTION MAKES IT EASIER TO UNDERSTAND WHAT IS HAPPENING TO US.

FEELING EMOTION

Emotions are primarily unconscious physical reactions to threat or opportunity. The sight of a snake, for example, automatically prepares the body for flight. In humans, emotions are consciously experienced as powerful "feelings" that give our lives meaning and value. The unconscious physiological component of emotion is generated in deep brain areas as signals that are then sent to the body to prepare it for action. Some signals travel upwards to activate cortical areas, and this activation produces the feeling of emotion. The type of emotion experienced depends on which parts of the cortical areas are activated.

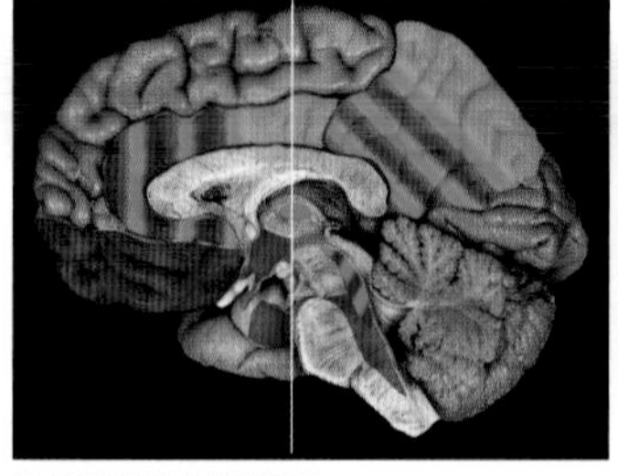

EMOTIONS INITIATED
Emotions arise in the amygdala, brainstem, and hypothalamus (blue). Conscious feelings (red) involve the orbitofrontal and cingulate cortex.

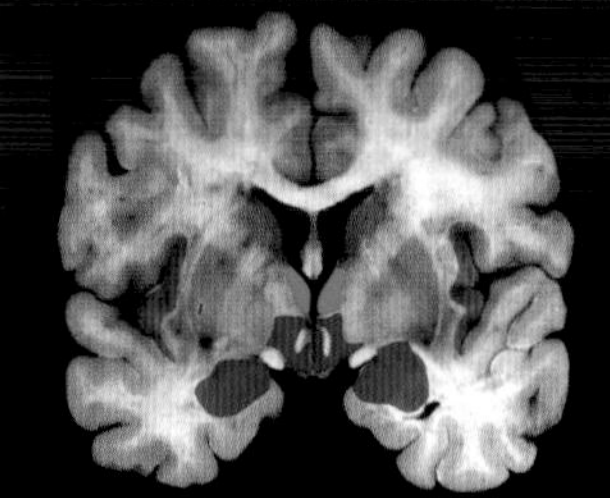

CONSCIOUS EXPRESSION
The amygdala and hypothalamus (blue) are active in expressing emotion, while the thalamus (green) maintains consciousness.

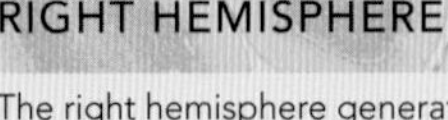

RIGHT HEMISPHERE

The right hemisphere generates more negative emotions than the left, and recognition and consciousness of sadness and fear depend on signals from the right hemisphere being received and processed by the left hemisphere. If the signals do not get through, a person may remain unconscious of their emotions, even though their behaviour may be affected by them.

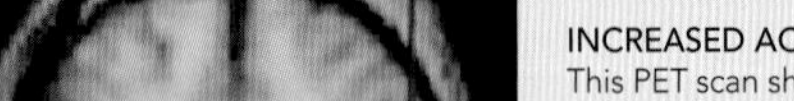

INCREASED ACTIVITY
This PET scan shows brain activity in a volunteer who is watching a person display various emotional facial expressions and gestures. These stimulate far more activity in the right frontal cortex (targeted) than in the same area in the left hemisphere.

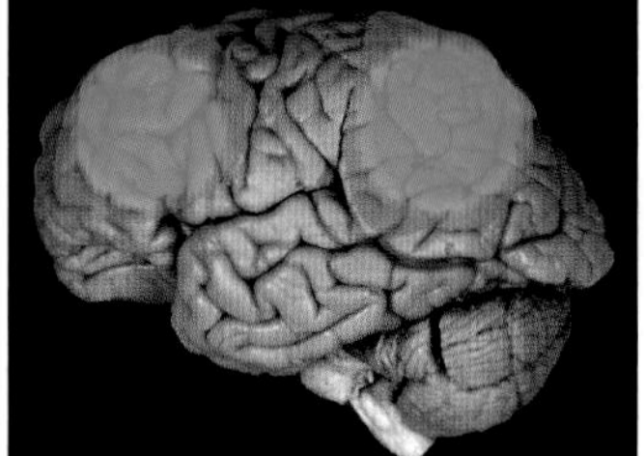

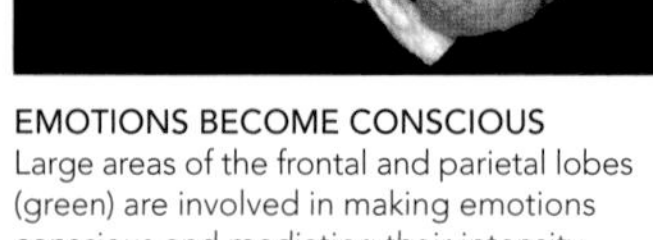

EMOTIONS BECOME CONSCIOUS
Large areas of the frontal and parietal lobes (green) are involved in making emotions conscious and mediating their intensity.

DISGUST
This cutaway shows the insula (red – also in top scan), part of which is active during the generation of emotion, particularly disgust.

EMOTION CIRCUITS

Information from the environment, and from the rest of the body, is constantly "tasted" for emotional content. The main emotion "sensor" is the amygdala, which is particularly sensitive to threat and loss. The amygdala takes in information both directly from the sense organs, and via the sensory cortices, and connects to the cortex and also to the hypothalamus, creating a circuit. When the amygdala is activated, it sends signals around this circuit. These trigger bodily changes as they pass through the hypothalamus, and create conscious recognition of the emotion as they pass through the frontal lobe. Positive emotions are passed along a slightly separate circuit, which takes in an area of the brainstem that produces the mood-lifting neurotransmitter dopamine.

PROCESSING EMOTION
Information about the identification and orientation of emotion travels from the thalamus, ventral striatum, and amygdala to the rostral (lower) anterior cingulate cortex. Regulatory signals travel from areas of the frontal and prefrontal cortices to meet them.

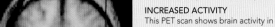

FEELING HATRED

Each emotion sparks a slightly different pattern of activity in certain brain areas. Hatred, for example, activates the amygdala (which responds to all negative emotion), the insula (which is associated with disgust and rejection), and also areas of the brain concerned with action and calculation.

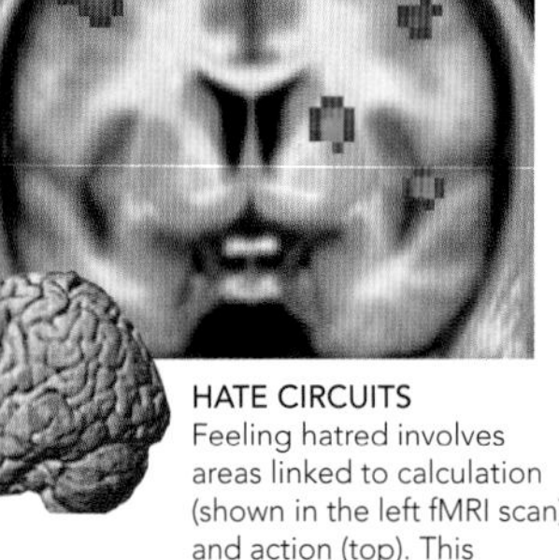

HATE CIRCUITS
Feeling hatred involves areas linked to calculation (shown in the left fMRI scan) and action (top). This pattern may reflect plotting, followed by attack.

TIMING EMOTION

Things that we find emotionally moving grab attention rapidly (see illustrations, right) compared with things that we do not. The sight of something that poses a threat, for example, is brought to conscious awareness faster than a non-emotional stimulus. This may be because the amygdala unconsciously picks up the threat and primes the conscious brain to "expect" an important perception. Good things also attract attention fast. Research shows that people react as quickly to an image of a smiling baby as they do to one of an angry face – both elicit quicker reactions than non-emotional stimuli.

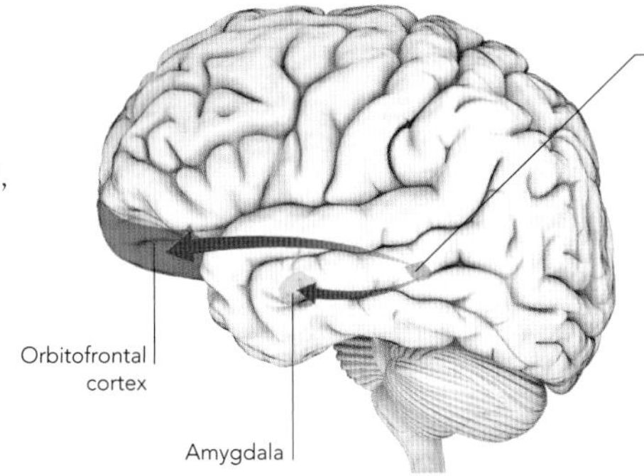

Less than 100ms

Initial awareness

Responses to emotional visual stimuli can travel in less than one-tenth of a second from the superior colliculus in the brainstem to the frontal cortex, where the emotion is consciously experienced.

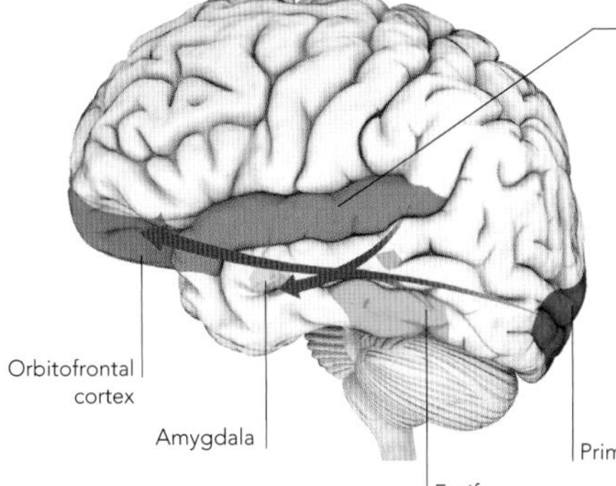

100–200ms

Further information

A little later, information comes in from the sensory corticesand association areas – such as the face-recognition area in the fusiform gyrus – providing more detailed input to emotion-inducing parts of the brain, such as the amygdala.

Insula

Superior temporal colliculus

Orbitofrontal cortex

Amygdala

Response signal from body

Primary visual cortex

Fusiform gyrus

350ms

Full awareness

After about 350 milliseconds, the emotional meaning of a stimulus has been evaluated by the brain. Signals from the amygdala trigger a conscious response in the body, which in turn feeds back to areas such as the insula.

WEARING YOUR EMOTIONS

Scientists have developed clothing that can project the emotion of the wearer. Biometric sensors that pick up minute changes or detect EEG signals are being incorporated into garments next to the skin. The clothes then change colour according to the information received. This futuristic dress developed by Philips shines bright white when the wearer is happy but turns blue when she is sad. It has a corset layer containing sensors that send information to an outer skirt layer causing it to change colour.

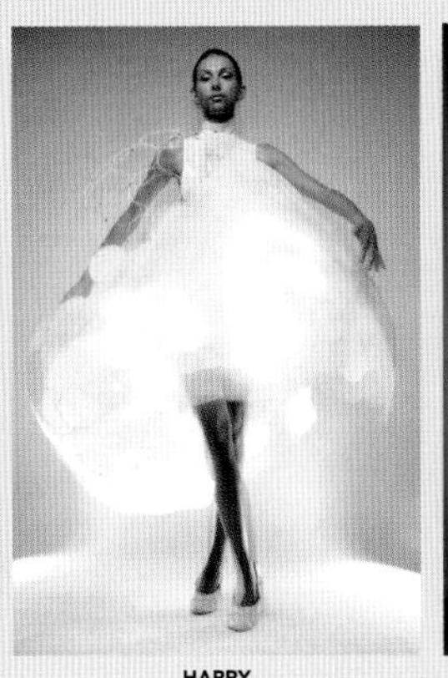

HAPPY

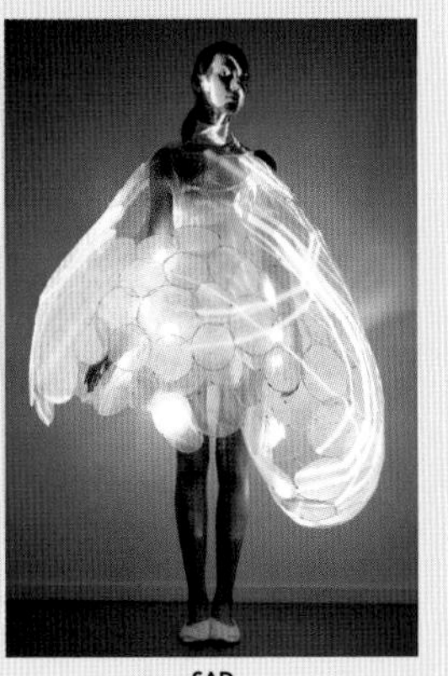

SAD

EMOTIONS AND MOODS

An emotion is usually transient and arises in response to the thoughts, activities, and social situations of the day. Emotions act as cues that prompt adaptive behaviour (see table, right). Moods, in contrast, may last for hours, days, or even months, in the case of some illnesses. Thus, the emotional state of distress, when extended over time, is called sadness; if it persists, unrelenting, for a period of weeks, it is referred to as depression (see p.239). Moods can be initiated very quickly by things that we are not even aware of. One study, for instance, found that flashing pictures of a disgusting nature for a split second – too fast to be seen consciously – made those who were subjected to them more sensitive to other stimuli of a similar nature afterwards. The feelings elicited by these unconscious stimuli were described by the volunteers as "moods" rather than emotions.

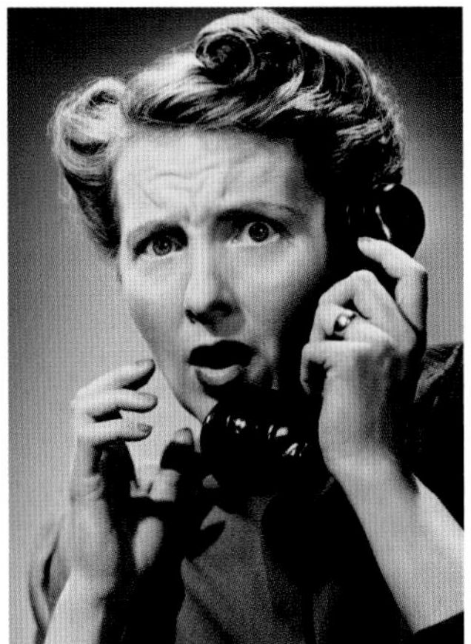

TELLING THE DIFFERENCE
Emotions are sudden, intense reactions to events, such as unexpected bad news, whereas moods are more diffuse and tend to last longer.

ADAPTIVE BEHAVIOURS

EMOTION OR FEELING	POSSIBLE STIMULUS	ADAPTIVE BEHAVIOUR
Anger	Challenging behaviour from another person	"Fight" reaction prompts dominant and threatening stance or action
Fear	Threat from stronger or dominant person	Flight, to avoid the threat, or appeasement, to show a lack of challenge to the dominant person
Sadness	Loss of loved one	Backward-looking state of mind and passivity, to avoid additional challenge
Disgust	Unwholesome object (e.g. rotting food or unclean surroundings)	Aversion behaviour – remove oneself from the unhealthy environment
Surprise	Novel or unexpected event	Focus attention on the object of surprise, ensuring maximum information input to guide further actions

DESIRE AND REWARD

DESIRE IS HARD TO DEFINE PRECISELY, BUT IT CAN BEST BE DESCRIBED AS WANTING OR YEARNING FOR SOMETHING THAT YOU FEEL WILL BRING PLEASURE OR SATISFACTION ONCE YOU OBTAIN IT. THERE ARE SPECIFIC BRAIN CIRCUITS LINKED TO DESIRE AND REWARD (PLEASURE). DESIRE FOR FOOD AND SEX HAS A SURVIVAL VALUE, BUT DESIRE CAN ALSO BE DESTRUCTIVE IF IT FUELS AN ADDICTION.

DESIRE

Desire is a complex drive that strongly reflects personal preferences. It is made up of two different components – liking and wanting. Put simply, liking is linked to getting pleasure, while wanting is linked to an actual need for something. With some activities, such as eating, sleeping, and sexual activity, liking and wanting overlap, and the resulting desire has survival value. However, an individual with an addiction may want and "need" a drug, but not particularly like or enjoy it, so the resulting pleasure is tainted with destruction. Liking and wanting seem to use somewhat different brain circuits, although dopamine is the most important neurotransmitter in both cases.

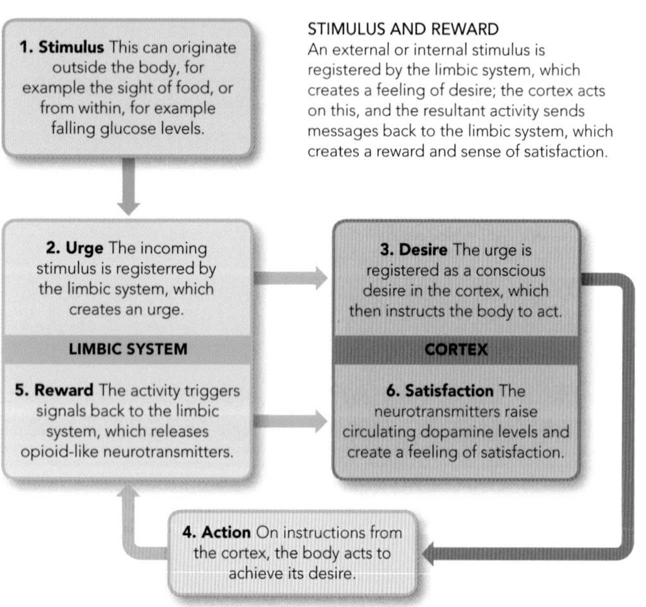

1. Stimulus This can originate outside the body, for example the sight of food, or from within, for example falling glucose levels.
2. Urge The incoming stimulus is registered by the limbic system, which creates an urge.
3. Desire The urge is registered as a conscious desire in the cortex, which then instructs the body to act.
LIMBIC SYSTEM
CORTEX
5. Reward The activity triggers signals back to the limbic system, which releases opioid-like neurotransmitters.
6. Satisfaction The neurotransmitters raise circulating dopamine levels and create a feeling of satisfaction.
4. Action On instructions from the cortex, the body acts to achieve its desire.

STIMULUS AND REWARD
An external or internal stimulus is registered by the limbic system, which creates a feeling of desire; the cortex acts on this, and the resultant activity sends messages back to the limbic system, which creates a reward and sense of satisfaction.

ANTICIPATION

Learning and memory clearly play an important role in shaping desires and preferences. This leads to the possibility of anticipation, which is the expectation of a reward. Anticipation has been studied by researchers using a game of chance. In the anticipation phase, where participants were told they might win money, fMRI scans showed that cerebral blood flow in the amygdala and orbitofrontal cortex increased, indicating activity in the nucleus accumbens and the hypothalamus – all rich in dopamine receptors. The bigger the potential reward, the greater the brain activity.

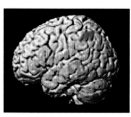

LEFT INTRAPARIETAL CORTEX

REWARD ANTICIPATION
This fMRI scan shows activity in the left intraparietal cortex. Activity in the anterior cingulate cortex and intraparietal cortex show that greater attention is paid to a task when a person is anticipating a reward.

COMPLICATED GRIEF

Losing a loved one is hard, but most people do recover in time. For about 10 to 20 per cent of bereaved people, grief endures and is referred to as "complicated". In one fMRI study, it was revealed that in such people, reminders of the deceased activate a brain area associated with reward processing, pleasure, and addiction. A group of women were shown pictures and words linked to a loved one lost to breast cancer. Brain networks associated with social pain became activated in all women, but in those with complicated grief, the reminders also excited the nucleus accumbens, suggesting that grief was linked, somehow, with pleasure.

PLEASURE-SEEKING AND ADDICTION

Addictive substances can activate the dopamine reward system, providing pleasure, even though the substances are not essential to survival. Chronic exposure to drugs leads to the suppression of reward circuits, increasing the amounts needed to generate the same effect. The opiate system is involved in pain and anxiety relief. Heroin and morphine lock onto the opiate receptors, creating a sense of euphoria. The cholinergic circuits – where nicotine acts – are involved in memory and learning. Cocaine acts at the noradrenergic receptors, which are involved in stress responses and anxiety.

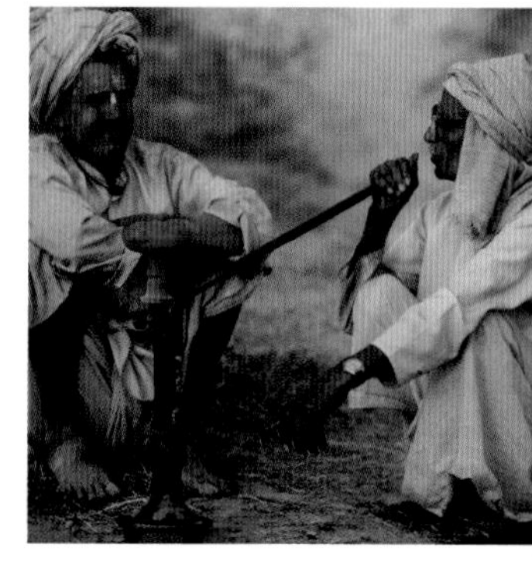

CULTURAL EXPOSURE
Smoking is regarded as a highly social activity in many cultures. Prolonged exposure to addictive substances may lead to increasing dependence, drug-seeking behaviour, and withdrawal problems.

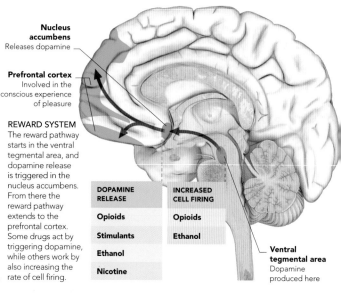

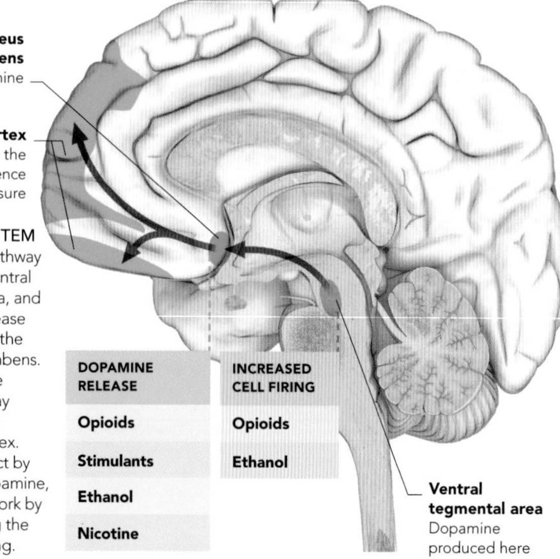

DOPAMINE RELEASE	INCREASED CELL FIRING
Opioids	Opioids
Stimulants	Ethanol
Ethanol	
Nicotine	

REWARD SYSTEM
The reward pathway starts in the ventral tegmental area, and dopamine release is triggered in the nucleus accumbens. From there the reward pathway extends to the prefrontal cortex. Some drugs act by triggering dopamine, while others work by also increasing the rate of cell firing.

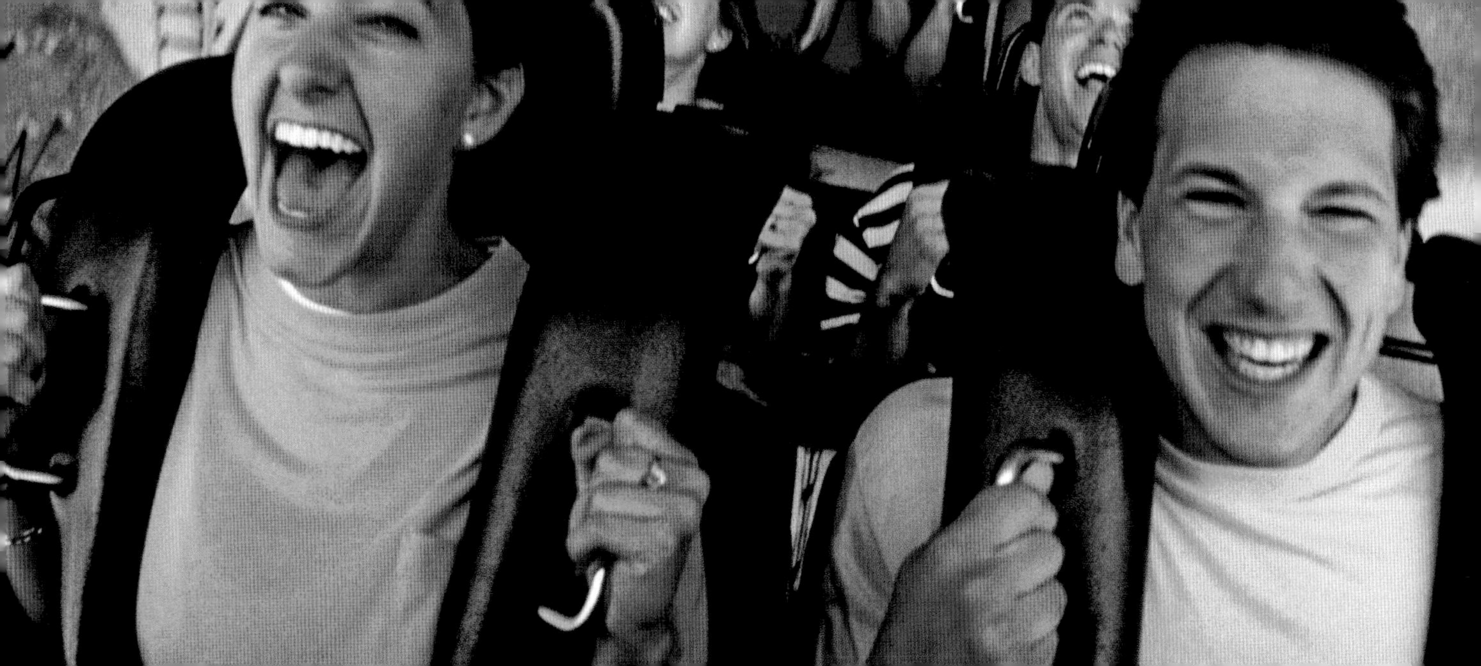

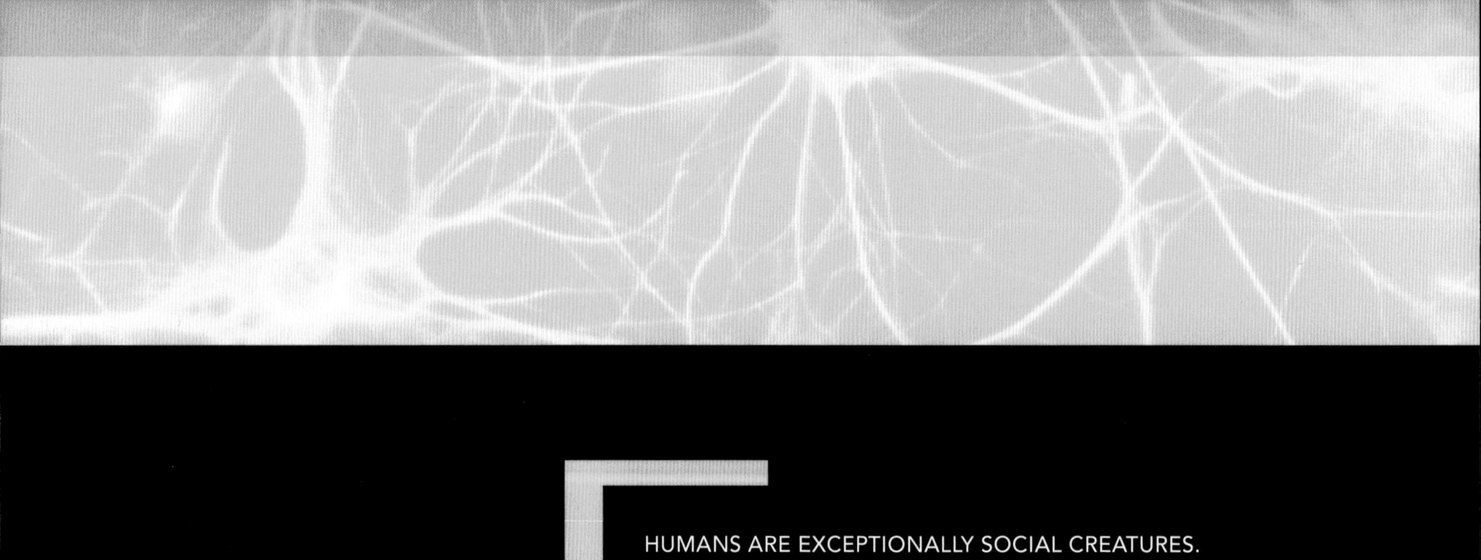

HUMANS ARE EXCEPTIONALLY SOCIAL CREATURES. WE NEED EACH OTHER, FOR MUTUAL SUPPORT AND PROTECTION, AND TO THIS END WE HAVE EVOLVED BRAINS THAT ARE EXQUISITELY SENSITIVE TO OTHERS OF OUR KIND

THE SOCIAL BRAIN

SEX, LOVE, AND SURVIVAL

SEX HAS SURVIVAL VALUE IN THAT IT DRIVES REPRODUCTION. SEXUAL ACTIVITY STIMULATES THE BRAIN'S REWARD SYSTEM – IF IT DID NOT, PEOPLE MIGHT NOT BOTHER WITH IT AND HUMANITY WOULD DIE OUT. RECENT RESEARCH HAS SHED LIGHT ON THE BRAIN CIRCUITS INVOLVED IN SEX AND LOVE. ROMANTIC LOVE, WHICH BRINGS COUPLES TOGETHER, AND MATERNAL LOVE, WHICH BINDS MOTHER AND CHILD, ALSO HAVE SURVIVAL VALUE.

DIFFERENT TYPES OF LOVE

Love is a complex phenomenon, encompassing sex, friendship, intimacy, and commitment. Not only does it have a survival value for the individual as well as the species, it also adds greatly to quality of life. As far as sex is concerned, humans engage in it whenever they wish, unlike most other species who undertake sex only when the female is ready to conceive. Therefore, sex has become disconnected from reproduction in humans. Romantic love, which is what many people mean by "love", has a survival advantage as it promotes pair bonding – an ideal setting for the care and protection of young children. Friendship and social networks are also important for promoting health and wellbeing. We know a little about the neurotransmitters involved in "falling in love", but not much about corresponding brain circuits. Phenylethylamine and dopamine are involved in the initial euphoria, which probably act in the pathways between the limbic system (concerned largely with emotions) and cortical areas (concerned with reason).

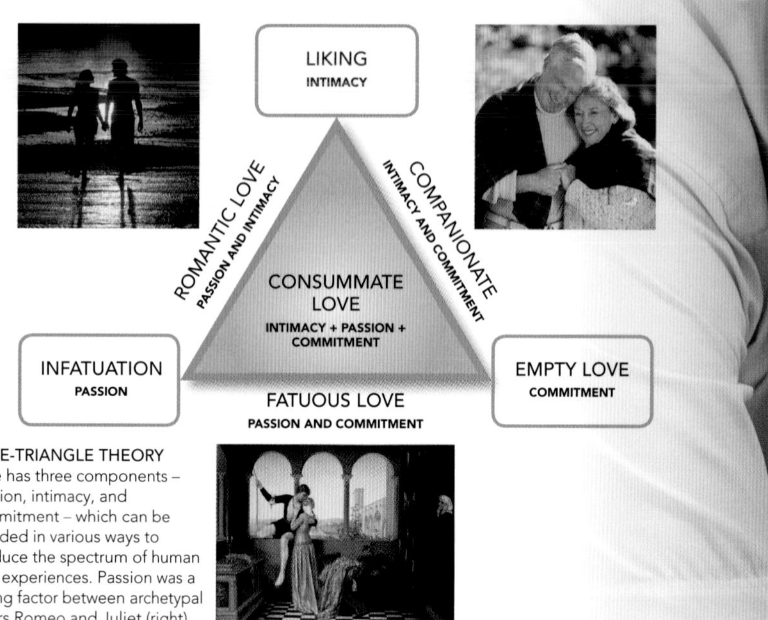

LOVE-TRIANGLE THEORY
Love has three components – passion, intimacy, and commitment – which can be blended in various ways to produce the spectrum of human love experiences. Passion was a strong factor between archetypal lovers Romeo and Juliet (right).

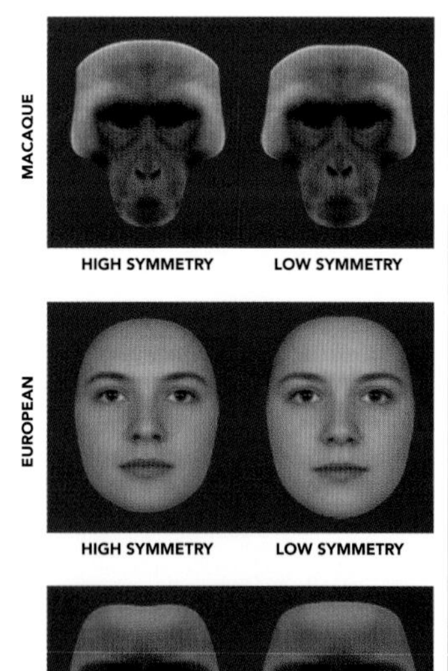

MALE

HIGH SYMMETRY LOW SYMMETRY

HIGH SYMMETRY LOW SYMMETRY

HIGH SYMMETRY LOW SYMMETRY

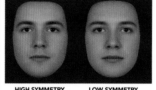

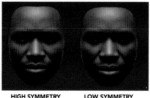

GENDER AND SYMMETRY
These composite faces, from photos of individuals from three groups, represent high- and low-symmetry faces for each group. High-symmetry faces are often selected as most gender typical.

SEXUAL ATTRACTION

An individual's face is an important element in how attractive they appear to others and whether they are instinctively considered a good mating prospect. The degree of symmetry, which is linked to how masculine or feminine they appear, has been shown to be an important aspect of facial attractiveness. A recent study shows that these properties are involved in sexual pairings in groups of Europeans, African hunter-gatherers, and one group of non-human primates (see below and left). Because the relationship is common to two human groups and one primate group, it may be universal. It seems, therefore, that symmetry and how masculine or feminine a face appears are linked to an underlying biological mechanism that could advertise a person's level of attractiveness and genetic fitness as a mate.

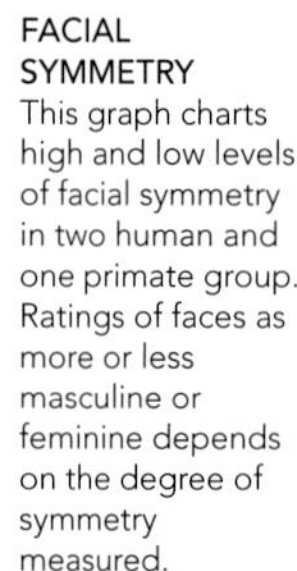

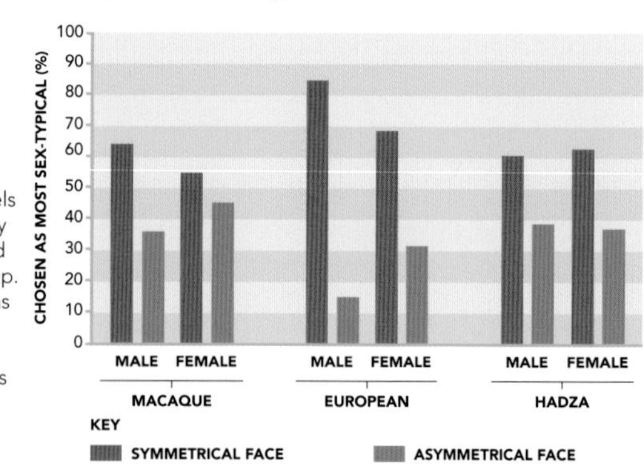

FACIAL SYMMETRY
This graph charts high and low levels of facial symmetry in two human and one primate group. Ratings of faces as more or less masculine or feminine depends on the degree of symmetry measured.

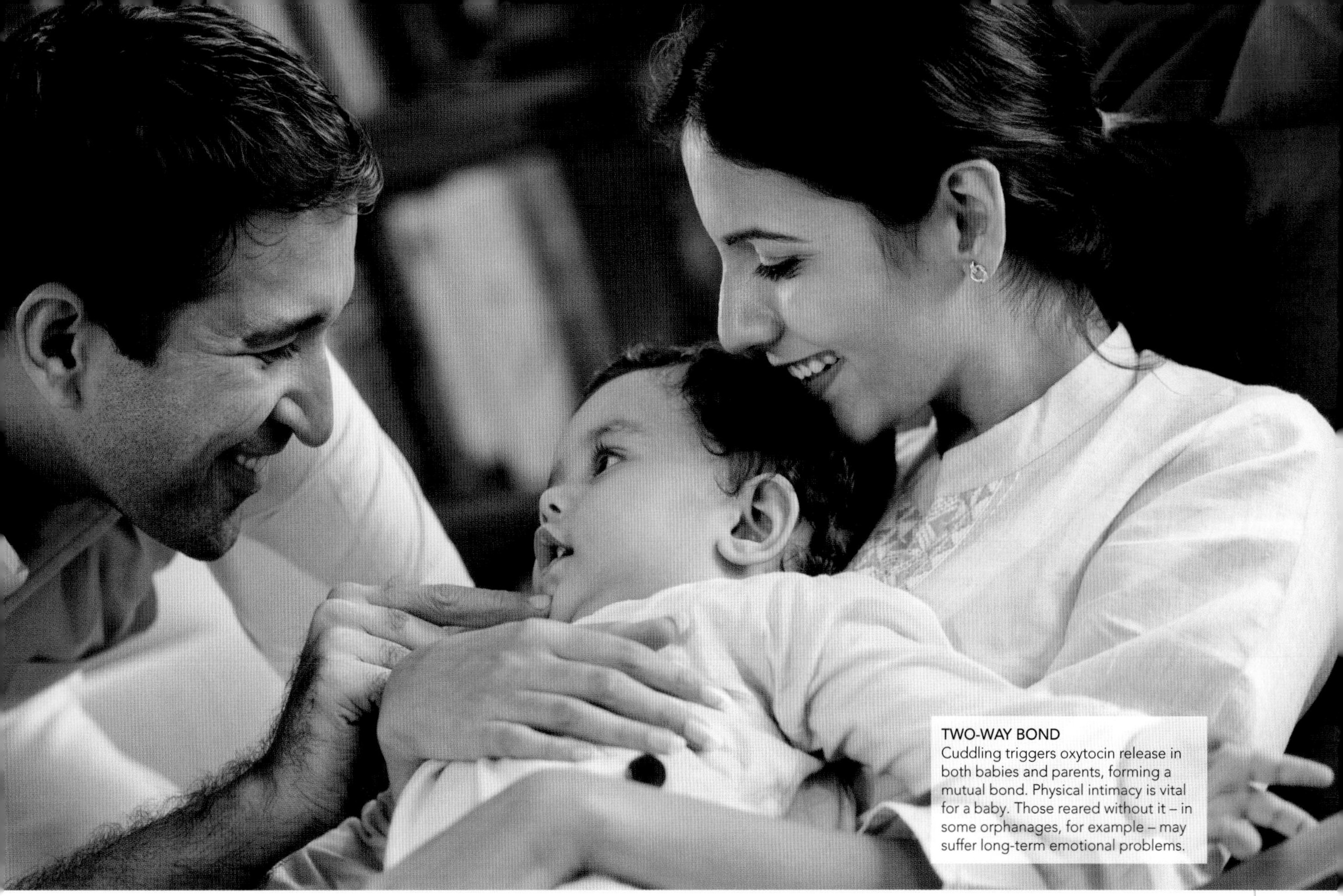

TWO-WAY BOND
Cuddling triggers oxytocin release in both babies and parents, forming a mutual bond. Physical intimacy is vital for a baby. Those reared without it – in some orphanages, for example – may suffer long-term emotional problems.

OXYTOCIN – THE FEEL-GOOD FACTOR

Oxytocin is a hormone produced by the hypothalamus and released by stimulation of the sex and reproductive organs, during orgasm and in the final stages of childbirth. It produces a pleasurable feeling that promotes bonding. This could be because, like the closely related hormone vassopressin, oxytocin helps the processing of social cues involved in the recognition of individuals, and may play a role in laying down shared memories. It is possible that oxytocin has a somewhat "addictive" effect, like dopamine. This may explain why people feel anguish at being parted from loved ones – they miss the oxytocin "rush" involved in being with them.

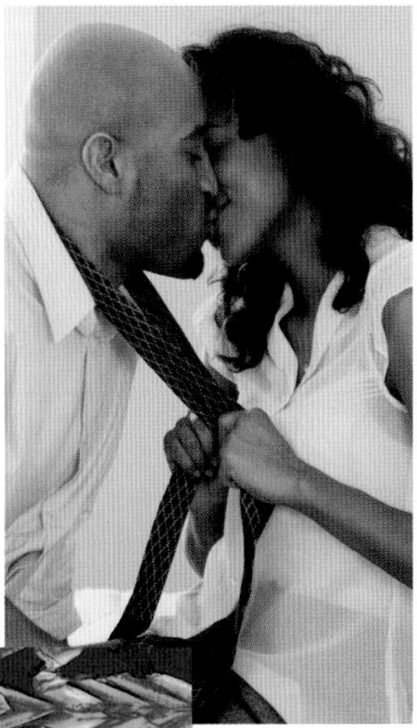

FEELING CLOSE
Kissing and cuddling trigger the release of oxytocin into the bloodstream. This may help to heighten feelings of closeness and strengthen the bond between partners.

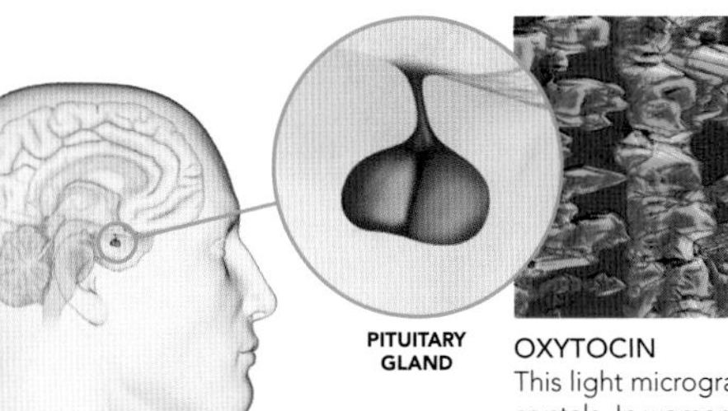

OXYTOCIN
This light micrograph shows oxytocin crystals. In women, this hormone is secreted naturally by the pituitary gland during childbirth, breastfeeding, and sex.

THE DARK SIDE OF OXYTOCIN

Oxytocin creates trust and kindness among "bonded" individuals, but it amplifies distrust and aggression towards those outside a bonded group. Experiments show that volunteers who are given a dose of oxytocin before playing a trading game are more generous than others to those players who "play fair", but more punitive to others who try to cheat. And one effect of military "bonding sessions" – in which oxytocin is probably engaged – is to make teams of soldiers fight enemies more fiercely.

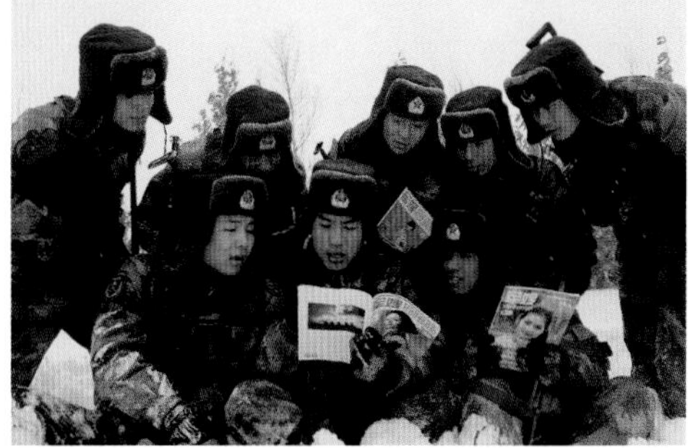

BONDING SESSION
Soliders who train together form a tight social bond, which is likely to engage oxytocin. This helps forge trust among the unit but also increases aggression towards perceived outsiders.

EXPRESSION

HUMANS ARE HIGHLY INTERDEPENDENT – WHAT ONE DOES INVARIABLY AFFECTS WHAT HAPPENS TO OTHERS. IT IS THEREFORE VERY USEFUL FOR US TO BE ABLE TO READ EACH OTHERS' EMOTIONS IN ORDER TO PREDICT WHAT SOMEONE MIGHT DO NEXT. WE ALSO NEED TO SIGNAL OUR OWN EMOTIONS IN ORDER TO NUDGE OTHERS TO DO WHAT WE WANT.

EXPRESSING EMOTION

Expressions are more than just signals – they are an extension of the emotion itself. When we feel something, the neural activation pattern associated with the emotion includes the firing of neurons which, if not inhibited, cause face and body muscles to contract in characteristic ways. There are six basic, or universal, emotions (see bottom). Recent studies have looked at the range of expressions used by people who have been blind since birth and found that they are similar or identical to those displayed by sighted people. This suggests that learning plays quite a small part in expression.

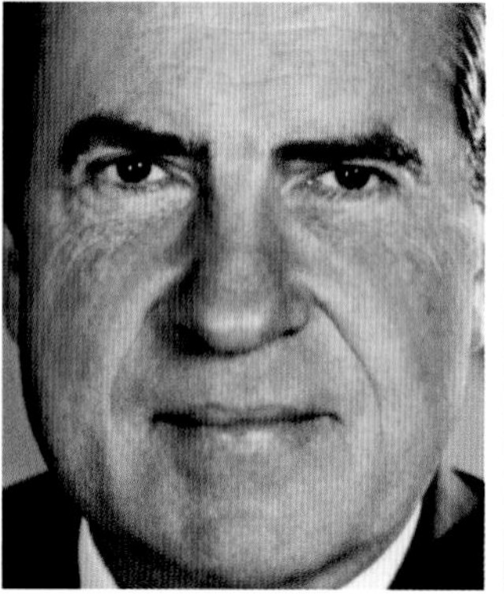

TRUE EXPRESSION?
The left hemisphere controls movement on the right side of the face, while the more emotional right brain controls the left side.

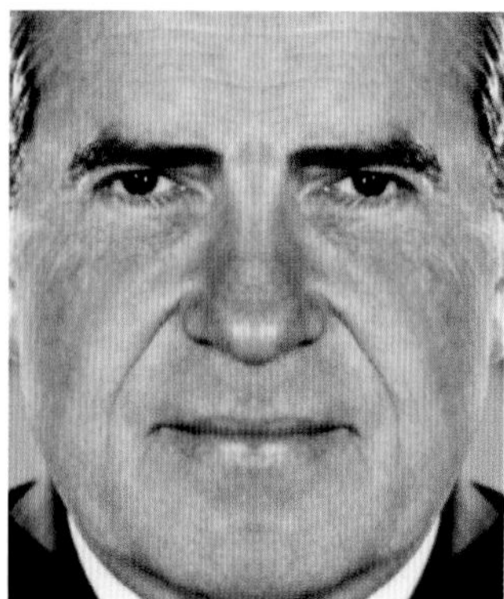

RIGHT AND RIGHT
The two right sides of former US president Richard Nixon's face hint at his unconscious feelings. Here the eyes appear less engaging.

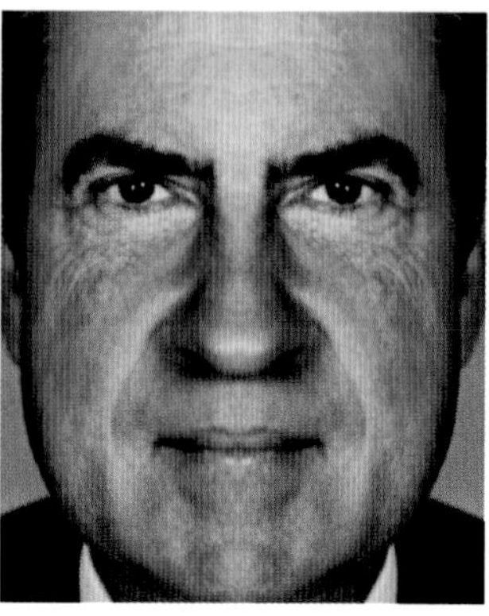

LEFT AND LEFT
The two left halves together give a clearer picture of the intended or "social" facial expression that looks more eager to please.

MICROEXPRESSIONS

As well as making the obvious "macro" expressions, people make facial changes that are tiny or momentary (or both), and which they can't easily control and are probably unaware of. These "micro" and "subtle" expressions occur when people are trying not to show what they are thinking or feeling. It is easy to miss these fleeting giveaways, but when you know what to look for you can learn to spot and decode them. Microexpressions come and go in a fraction of a second, while subtle expressions may last throughout a conversation, but the muscular changes may be so slight as to be barely visible.

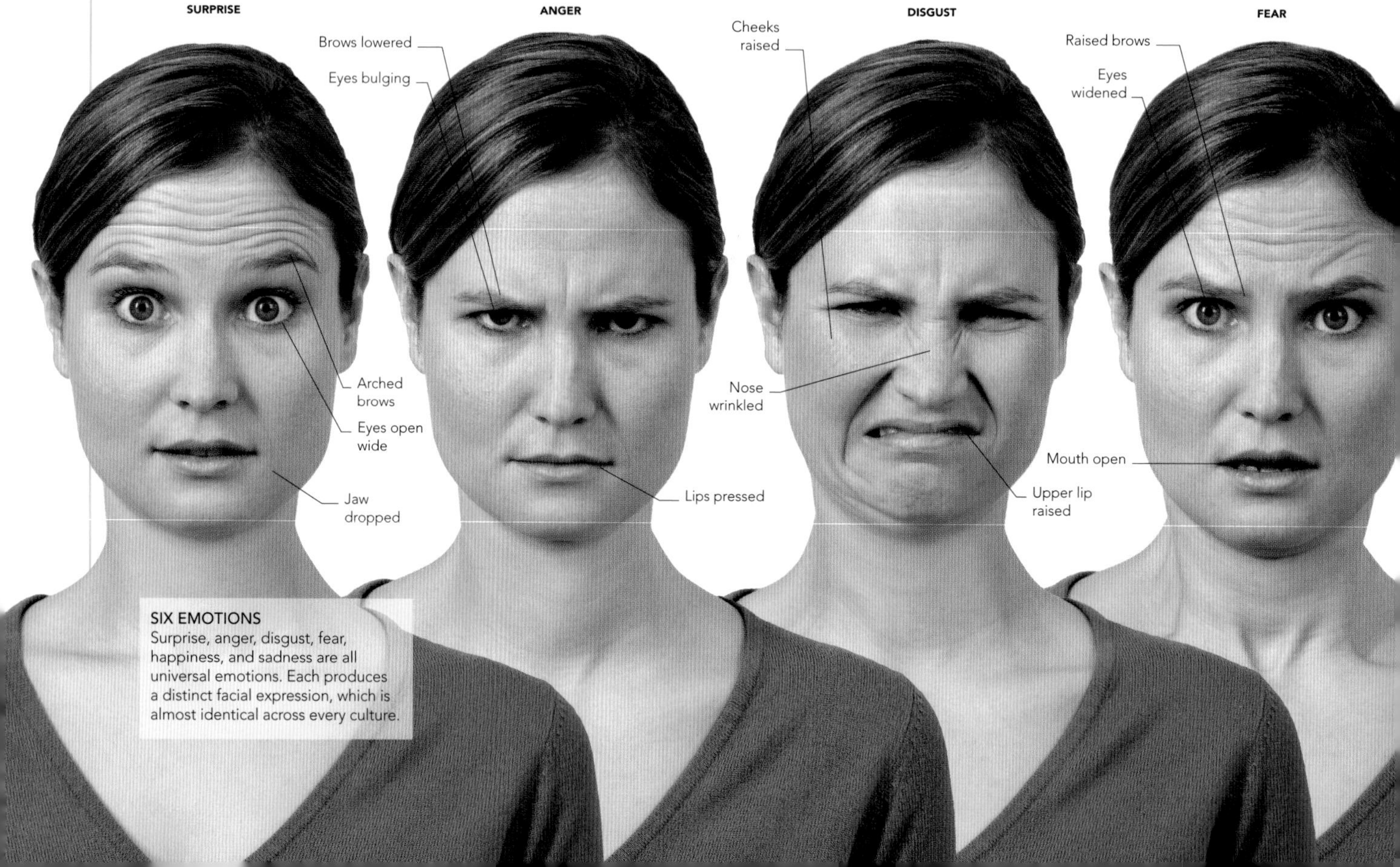

SURPRISE
Arched brows
Eyes open wide
Jaw dropped

ANGER
Brows lowered
Eyes bulging
Lips pressed

DISGUST
Cheeks raised
Nose wrinkled
Upper lip raised

FEAR
Raised brows
Eyes widened
Mouth open

SIX EMOTIONS
Surprise, anger, disgust, fear, happiness, and sadness are all universal emotions. Each produces a distinct facial expression, which is almost identical across every culture.

ANATOMY OF A SMILE

There are two fairly distinct types of human smile: the conscious "social" smile, and the genuine "Duchenne" smile, which is named after the French neurologist Guillame Duchenne who first described it. The first involves consciously activating the muscles that stretch the mouth sideways. The second involves an additional set of muscles, which are mainly controlled by unconscious brain processes. These muscles make the lower lids of the eyes swell and the edges crinkle into "crows' feet". Expressions not only show what a person is feeling, they can also actually bring about the feeling that they are associated with. In laboratory tests, consciously producing a smile was found to produce a weak, but detectable, sense of happiness in those who displayed it. So, even producing a "fake" social smile can promote a faint but real sensation of happiness in the person expressing it.

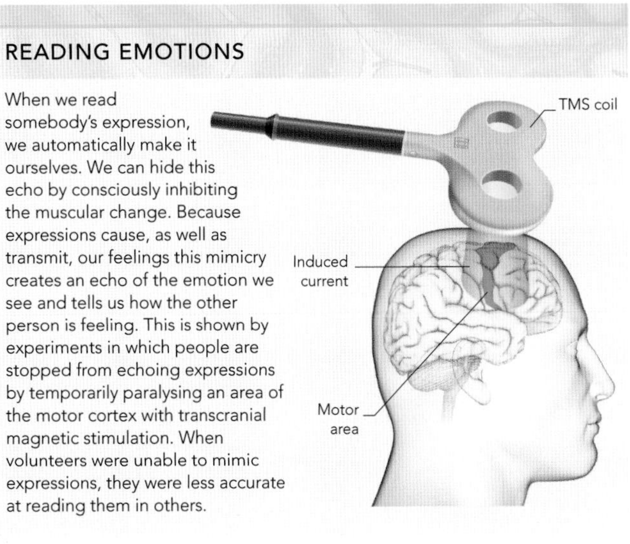
TMS coil
Induced current
Motor area

READING EMOTIONS

When we read somebody's expression, we automatically make it ourselves. We can hide this echo by consciously inhibiting the muscular change. Because expressions cause, as well as transmit, our feelings this mimicry creates an echo of the emotion we see and tells us how the other person is feeling. This is shown by experiments in which people are stopped from echoing expressions by temporarily paralysing an area of the motor cortex with transcranial magnetic stimulation. When volunteers were unable to mimic expressions, they were less accurate at reading them in others.

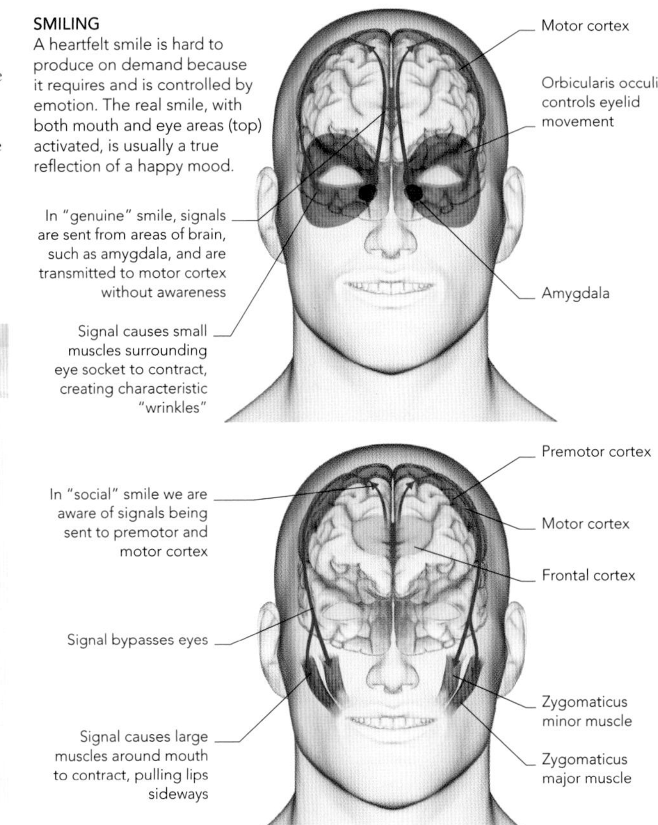
Motor cortex
Orbicularis occuli, controls eyelid movement
In "genuine" smile, signals are sent from areas of brain, such as amygdala, and are transmitted to motor cortex without awareness
Amygdala
Signal causes small muscles surrounding eye socket to contract, creating characteristic "wrinkles"
Premotor cortex
In "social" smile we are aware of signals being sent to premotor and motor cortex
Motor cortex
Frontal cortex
Signal bypasses eyes
Zygomaticus minor muscle
Signal causes large muscles around mouth to contract, pulling lips sideways
Zygomaticus major muscle

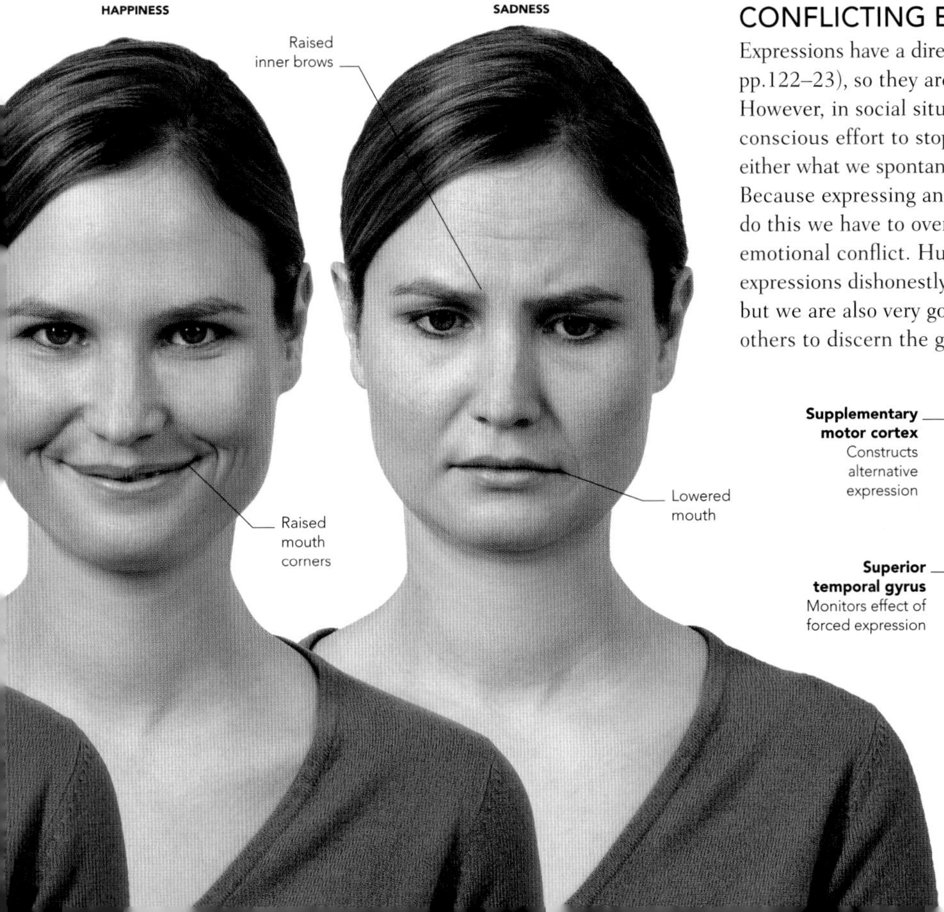

SMILING
A heartfelt smile is hard to produce on demand because it requires and is controlled by emotion. The real smile, with both mouth and eye areas (top) activated, is usually a true reflection of a happy mood.

HAPPINESS

SADNESS

Raised inner brows

Raised mouth corners

Lowered mouth

CONFLICTING EMOTIONS

Expressions have a direct effect on those who see them (see pp.122–23), so they are useful to get others to serve our needs. However, in social situations we sometimes have to make a conscious effort to stop making the expression that matches either what we spontaneously feel or what we see in others. Because expressing an emotion creates that emotion, when we do this we have to override one emotion with another, creating emotional conflict. Humans are probably unique in using facial expressions dishonestly, and we have become experts at doing so, but we are also very good at scrutinizing the expressions of others to discern the genuine from the fake.

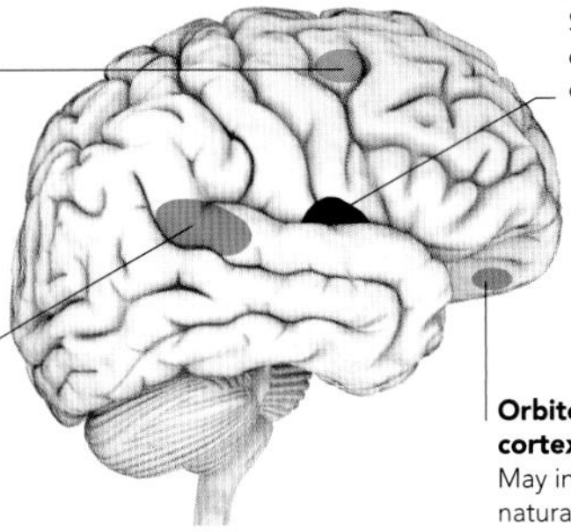

Supplementary motor cortex Constructs alternative expression

Insula Suggests emotional effort

Superior temporal gyrus Monitors effect of forced expression

Orbito-frontal cortex May inhibit natural mimicry

AREAS OF CONFLICT
Trying to override natural mimicry of an emotion by expressing a conflicting one engages various brain areas.

THE SELF AND OTHERS

THE HUMAN ANIMAL IS AN INTENSELY SOCIAL SPECIES, AND OUR SURVIVAL DEPENDS LARGELY ON SUCCESSFUL INTERACTIONS WITH OUR NEIGHBOURS. AS WITH OTHER SOCIAL ANIMALS, WE HAVE EVOLVED DISTINCT BRAIN CIRCUITS DEDICATED TO BONDING, CO-OPERATION, AND PREDICTING THE ACTIONS OF OTHERS. WE CAN ALSO RECOGNIZE THAT OTHER PEOPLE HAVE THEIR OWN THOUGHTS AND FEELINGS.

MADE TO BE SOCIABLE

One of the most distinctive features of the human brain is the large area of neocortex, its relatively recently developed outer layer. The frontal cortex (the part of the neocortex surrounding the frontal lobe) is responsible for abstract reasoning, conscious thought and emotion, planning, and organization, and is highly developed in humans. One reason for the substantial growth of the neocortex may be that humans adapted this way in response to the demands of living in large, close-knit groups. Social living requires moderating one's own behaviour in order to accommodate others, competing subtly for reproductive rights, and predicting how others will behave, all of which need neocortical activity. Spending time in social activity also seems to grow the areas of the brain responsible for understanding and dealing with others. People who have large numbers of friends on social networking sites have correspondingly large social brain regions.

AVERAGE GROUP SIZE (1, 2, 4, 6, 8, 10, 20, 40, 60, 80, 100)
NEOCORTEX RATIO (1, 2, 3, 4, 5, 6)
KEY
● MONKEYS
○ APES

GROUP SIZE MATTERS
In primates, the size of the neocortex relative to other brain areas increases in almost direct proportion to the average size of the social group.

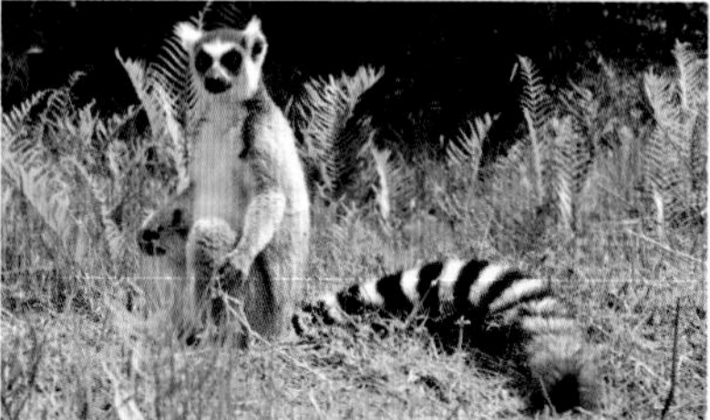

SOCIAL ANIMAL
Animals that live in large groups are socially smarter than those that don't. A study found that ring-tailed lemurs, which live in big groups, learned to steal food from people only when they were not looking. Other animals with comparable intelligence failed to do this.

CONTAGIOUS YAWNING

Social behaviours can be deliberate or unconscious. For example, it is thought that "catching" a yawn is an unconscious way of synchronizing group behaviour. One theory about yawning is that, when one person does it, it signals that it is time for the entire group to sleep. By mimicking the yawn, other members implicitly agree. Another theory is that yawning keeps the brain alert. Its contagious nature ensures that each member of the group sharpens up.

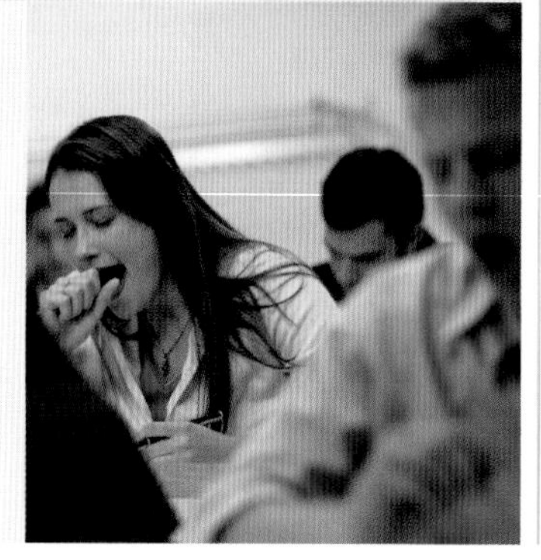

SOCIAL AWARENESS

Social awareness covers a wide range of cognition that generates a sense of a "self" as well as of that self in a social context. For example, we adapt our behaviour to co-operate with others, we predict what other people are likely to do and their reasons for doing it, we understand that others may hold different ideas and beliefs from our own, we are able to imagine how other people see us, and we can scrutinize our own minds. The range and diversity of skills required means that several areas of the brain are involved.

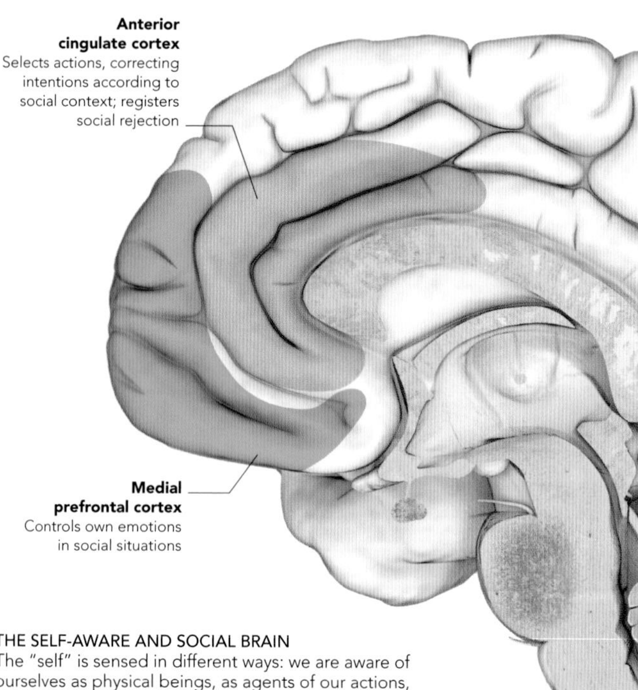
Anterior cingulate cortex
Selects actions, correcting intentions according to social context; registers social rejection
Medial prefrontal cortex
Controls own emotions in social situations

THE SELF-AWARE AND SOCIAL BRAIN
The "self" is sensed in different ways: we are aware of ourselves as physical beings, as agents of our actions, as objects in the world, and as components of a social system. Each type of self-awareness is generated by activity in different areas, and the information is combined to decide on socially appropriate actions.

THE INSULA

The insula may be responsible for humans experiencing the feeling of a "self" and having a sense of the boundary of that self, allowing for the distinction between "me" and "you". According to a school of thought known as "embodied cognition", which proposes that rational thought cannot be separated from emotions and their impact on the body, the insula detects bodily states that are induced by emotions as part of a process that brings our emotional experiences into our consciousness.

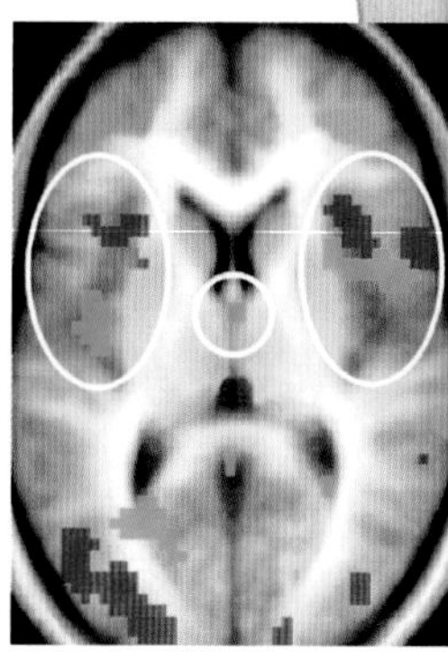

OBSERVING PAIN
Tests using fMRI scans show insula activity (green) in participants watching a person in pain, suggesting that the insula triggers empathic feelings.

THE PAIN OF REJECTION

In one study, fMRI scans were conducted on people playing a virtual ball game from which they were progressively excluded. Upon awareness of rejection, the anterior cingulate cortex (ACC) was activated, an area that also registers body pain, suggesting that the emotional impact of the two is similar. Part of the prefrontal cortex that helps control emotions was also activated, which seemed to reduce feelings of rejection.

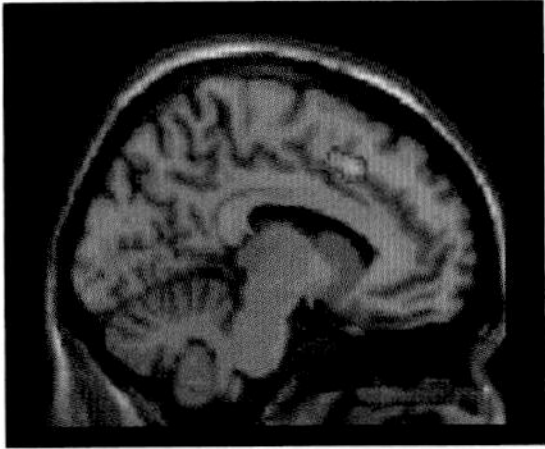

ANTERIOR CINGULATE CORTEX
Social rejection causes the same type of activity in the anterior cingulate cortex (ACC) as physical pain.

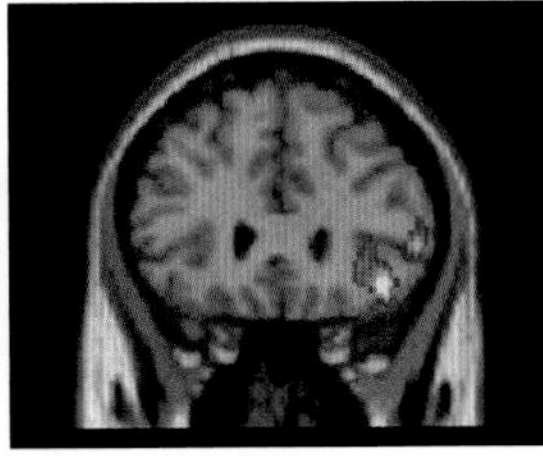

PREFRONTAL CORTEX
The ventral prefrontal cortex then interacts with the ACC, which seems to reduce the pain of social rejection.

CONGRUENCE

Our brains are highly sensitive to the movements of other animals, especially other humans. The mirror neuron system (see pp.122–23) automatically makes us mirror the actions of others. The effect is so strong that when one person notices another not mirroring their own actions, it often makes them falter in their own actions. This "interference effect" applies only to biological motion – when participants observe a robot, no such interference occurs, even if the actions are human-like.

MIRRORING
A person is discomfited if someone fails to mirror their actions, but whether or not a robot does so has no effect.

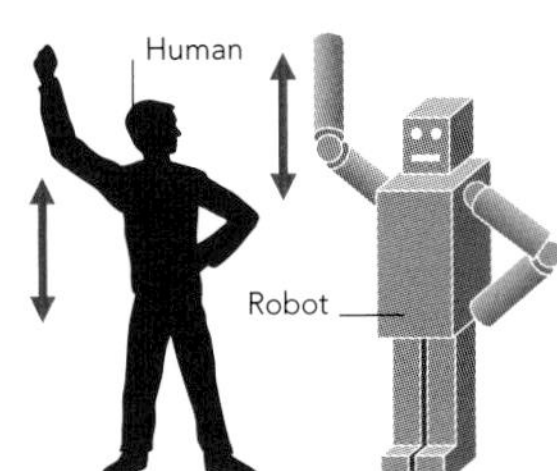

THEORY OF MIND

Theory of mind (ToM) refers to the instinctive "knowledge" that other people may hold different beliefs from one's own, and that it is those beliefs, not the facts of a situation, that inform and determine their behaviour. One way to test for ToM is the Sally-Ann test (see diagram, below). Recent studies have shown that infants as young as 10 months may "pass" the Sally-Ann test.

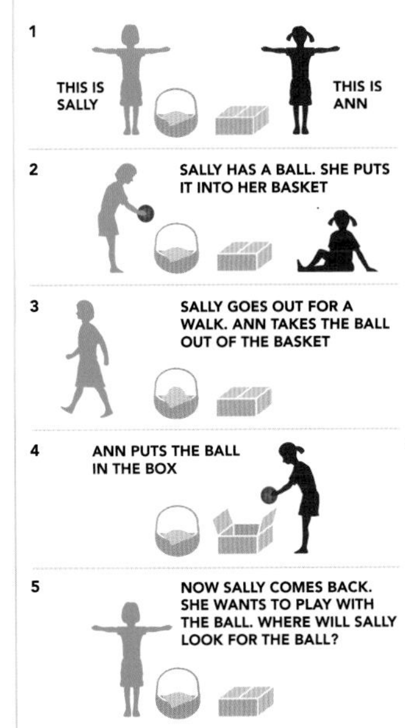
1
THIS IS SALLY
THIS IS ANN
2
SALLY HAS A BALL. SHE PUTS IT INTO HER BASKET
3
SALLY GOES OUT FOR A WALK. ANN TAKES THE BALL OUT OF THE BASKET
4
ANN PUTS THE BALL IN THE BOX
5
NOW SALLY COMES BACK. SHE WANTS TO PLAY WITH THE BALL. WHERE WILL SALLY LOOK FOR THE BALL?

SALLY-ANN TEST
If children indicate that, on her return, Sally will look in the place she expects the ball to be (in the basket), they appear to have ToM.

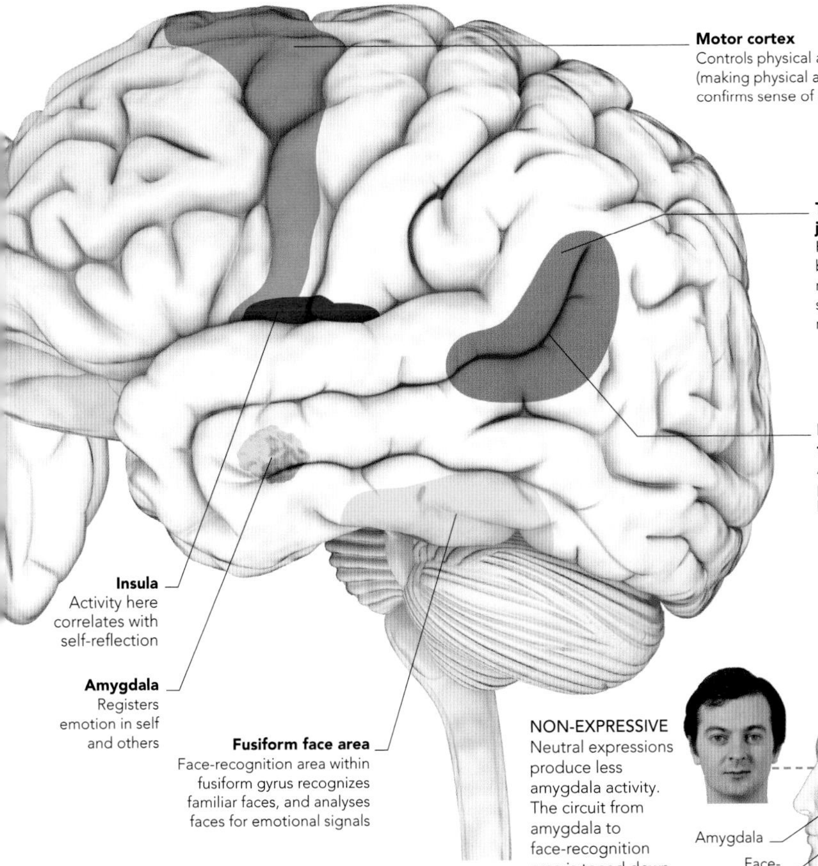

Motor cortex
Controls physical actions (making physical actions confirms sense of self)

Temperoparietal junction
Holds a "map" of body and constantly monitors physical self in relation to rest of world

Posterior temporal sulcus
A sense of one's own presence is triggered by activity here

Insula
Activity here correlates with self-reflection

Amygdala
Registers emotion in self and others

Fusiform face area
Face-recognition area within fusiform gyrus recognizes familiar faces, and analyses faces for emotional signals

NON-EXPRESSIVE
Neutral expressions produce less amygdala activity. The circuit from amygdala to face-recognition area is toned down and the brain takes in less information.

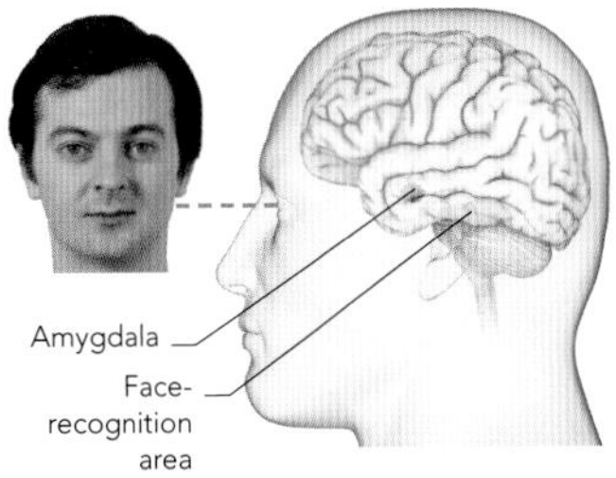

Amygdala
Face-recognition area

EXPRESSIVE
The amygdala reacts to facial expressions by "mirroring" the emotion. A smile, for example, triggers signals that begin the process of smiling back.

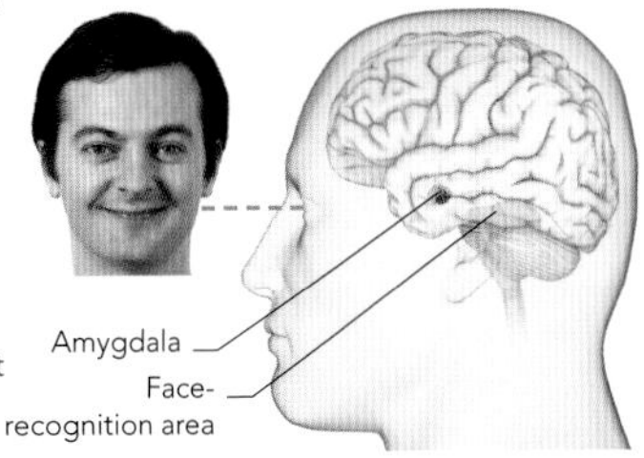

Amygdala
Face-recognition area

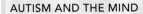

RESPONDING TO EMOTION

Facial expression is a signal – of intention and state of mind – and also a means of achieving empathy between people. Expressions are initially processed unconsciously by the amygdala, which monitors incoming data for emotional content. It responds by generating the emotion that has been observed. A fearful expression, for example, produces amygdala activation that triggers fear in the observer. Soon after the amygdala activation, the expression registers in the face-recognition area situated in the fusiform gyrus. Studies suggest that if a face expresses emotion, the amygdala signals this area to scrutinize it for meaning.

AUTISM AND THE MIND

Autism is marked by the absence of ToM. Rather than just "knowing" why Sally acts according to a false belief, people with Asperger's syndrome (a form of autism) consciously "work out" what is happening using part of the brain (yellow) that is thought to be more recently evolved than the area that generates ToM (red).

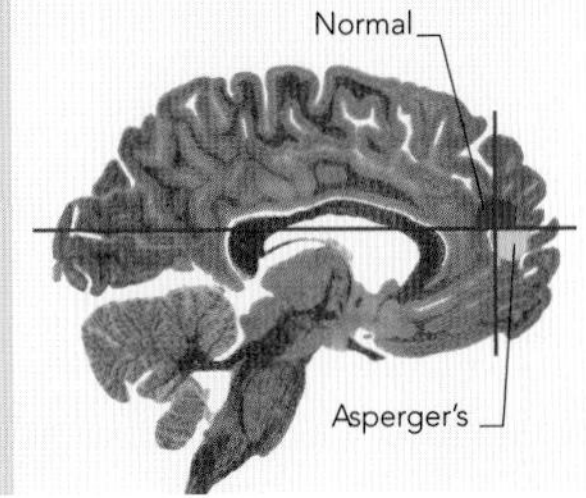

THE MORAL BRAIN

NORMAL PEOPLE BROUGHT UP IN A NORMAL ENVIRONMENT DEVELOP AN INSTINCTIVE SENSE OF RIGHT AND WRONG THAT SEEMS TO BE, AT LEAST IN PART, "HARD-WIRED" INTO THE BRAIN. THIS NATURAL "MORALITY" IS NOT NECESSARILY RATIONAL OR FAIR, AND PROBABLY EVOLVED BECAUSE BEHAVIOUR PROMOTING SOCIAL COHESION ALSO, INDIRECTLY, AIDS SELF-SURVIVAL.

EMPATHY AND SYMPATHY

"Feeling" for another person – experiencing a faint version of their sorrow or flinching when you see them hurt – seems to be largely instinctive. It depends partly on theory of mind (see pp.138–39), which ensures that we "know" what is likely to be going on in other people's minds. Empathy goes a step further, in that it also involves "echoing" the emotions of another person. When a person is told a story about someone experiencing emotional trauma, the activated areas in the listener's brain come into play when they themselves are in such a situation.

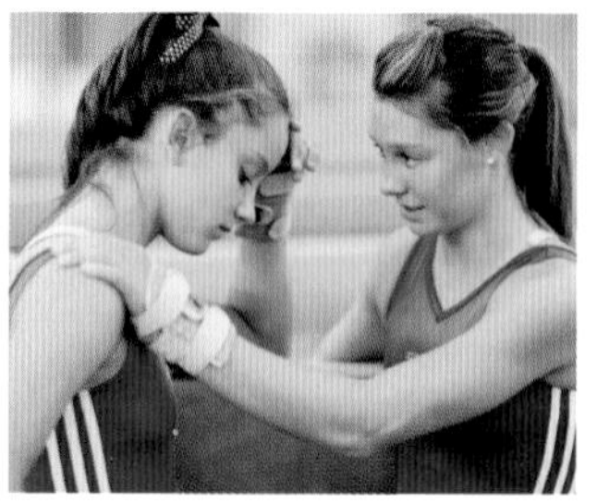

SYMPATHETIC STANCE
Being able to put yourself into someone else's situation, to experience an echo of what they feel, and sympathize with them appears to be an instinctive human trait.

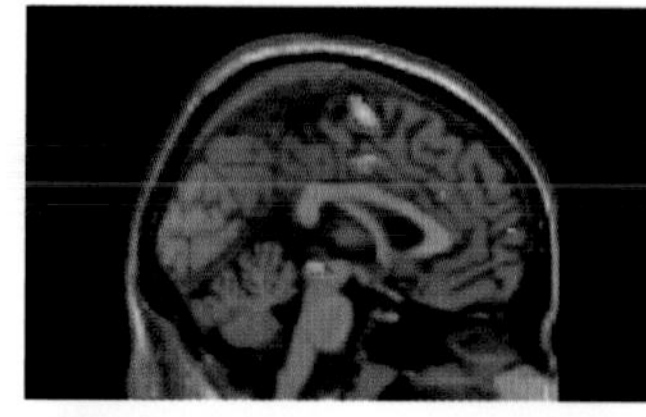

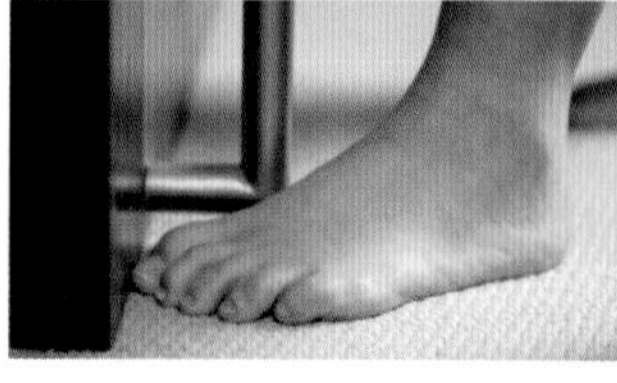

WITNESSING ACCIDENTAL PAIN
This fMRI scan shows that seeing someone hurt by accident produces similar brain activity as if the viewer was accidentally hurt.

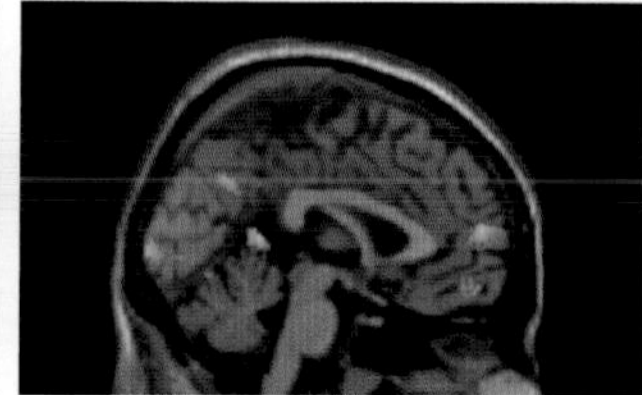

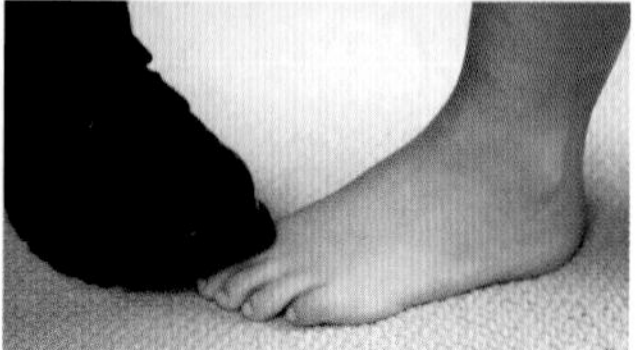

WITNESSING INTENTIONAL INJURY
When witnessing someone hurt intentionally, brain areas concerned with judgements and moral reasoning (above) are also activated.

MORALITY

Our sense of right and wrong permeates all our social perceptions and interactions. Moral decision-making is partly learned, but it also depends on emotions, which give "value" to actions and experiences. When making moral judgements, two overlapping but distinct brain circuits come into play. One is a "rational" circuit, which weighs up the pros and cons of an action objectively. The other circuit is emotional. It generates a fast and instinctive sense of what is right and wrong. The two circuits do not always arrive at the same conclusion, because emotions are biased towards self-survival and/or protecting those who are loved or related to oneself. Emotional bias in moral judgements seems to rely on activity in the ventromedial and orbitofrontal prefrontal cortex. Studies of people with damage to this area have found that their moral judgements are more rational than those of others, suggesting that human "morality" is hard-wired into the brain, and evolved more to protect ourselves than to "do good".

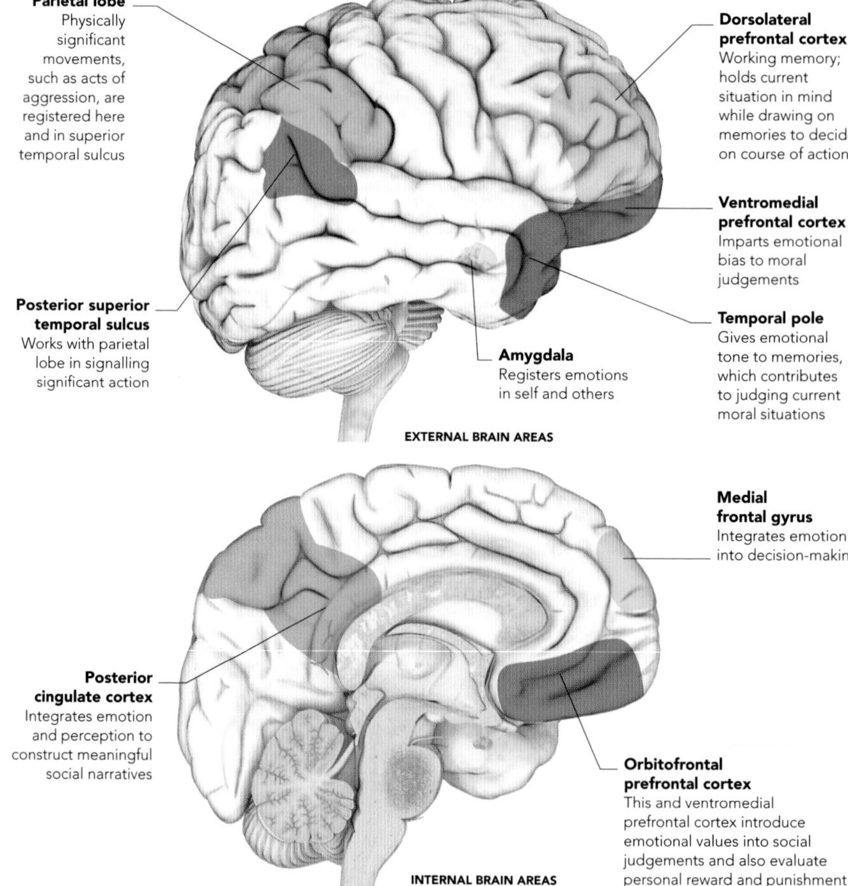
Parietal lobe
Physically significant movements, such as acts of aggression, are registered here and in superior temporal sulcus
Dorsolateral prefrontal cortex
Working memory; holds current situation in mind while drawing on memories to decide on course of action
Ventromedial prefrontal cortex
Imparts emotional bias to moral judgements
Temporal pole
Gives emotional tone to memories, which contributes to judging current moral situations
Posterior superior temporal sulcus
Works with parietal lobe in signalling significant action
Amygdala
Registers emotions in self and others
EXTERNAL BRAIN AREAS
Medial frontal gyrus
Integrates emotion into decision-making
Posterior cingulate cortex
Integrates emotion and perception to construct meaningful social narratives
Orbitofrontal prefrontal cortex
This and ventromedial prefrontal cortex introduce emotional values into social judgements and also evaluate personal reward and punishment
INTERNAL BRAIN AREAS

MORAL JUDGEMENT CIRCUITS
Emotions play a crucial role in moral decision-making (see p.169). In order to arrive at moral decisions, areas of the brain associated with emotional experience work alongside those that register facts and consider possible actions and outcomes.

ALTRUSIM

The notion of altruism assumes that people can do things for others with no motivation of a direct reward for themselves. However, brain scans show that doing "good" things is personally rewarding. One fMRI study was conducted while participants made or withheld donations to real charities. The participants could keep any donations they refused to make. The result showed that both keeping the money and giving it away activated the brain's "reward" pathways. Giving away money also enhanced activity in areas concerned with belonging and group bonding.

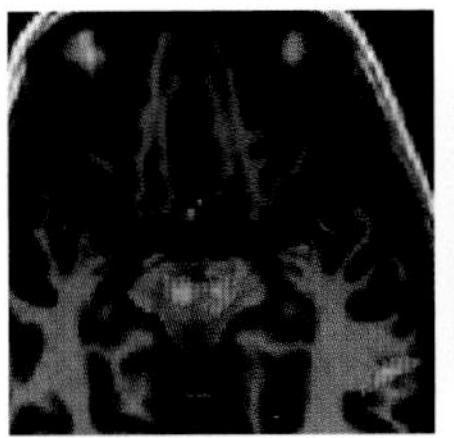

RECEIVING

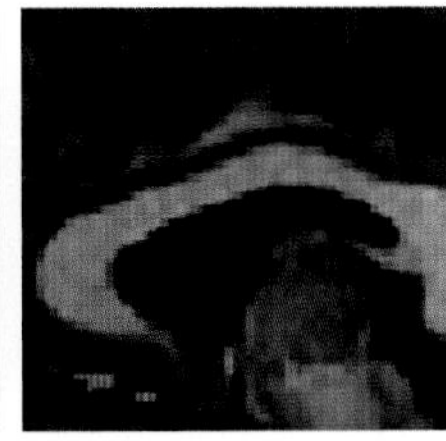

GIVING

REWARD AREAS
Giving and receiving activate areas linked to pleasure and satisfaction. Areas linked to bonding and social cohesion are active when giving.

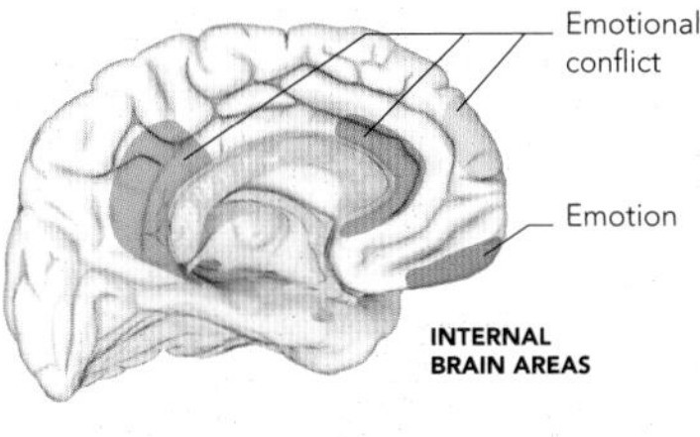

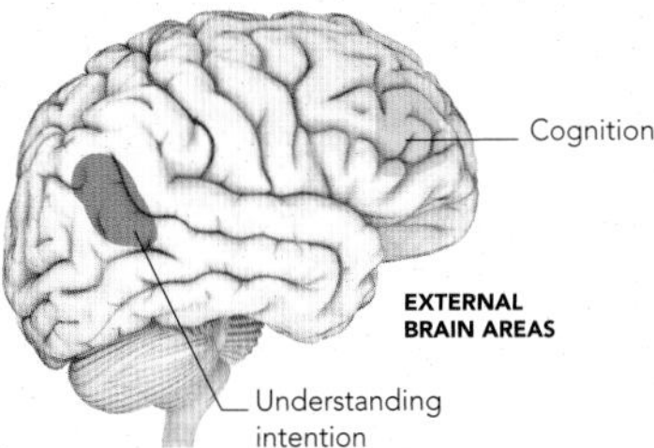

BRAIN DAMAGE AFFECTS MORALS
Damage to any one of several brain areas can affect moral judgement. They include: areas involved in feeling emotion and assessing emotional intent and conflict; the frontal areas involved in thinking about current situations and assessing action; and the area at the junction of the parietal and temporal lobes, which allows for understanding others' intentions.

PHINEAS GAGE

The idea that our moral sense may have a biological basis in the brain arose largely as a result of a freak accident in 1848. A railway worker called Phineas Gage blew a hole in the front of his brain with a tamping rod. He survived with little damage to most of his faculties but his behaviour changed dramatically. From being polite and thoughtful, Gage was described by his doctor as: "fitful, irreverent, indulging at times in the grossest profanity (which was not previously his custom), manifesting but little deference for his fellows, impatient of restraint of advice when it conflicts with his desires, at times pertinaciously obstinent, yet capricious and vacillating... his mind was radically changed, so decidedly that his friends and acquaintances said he was 'no longer Gage'."

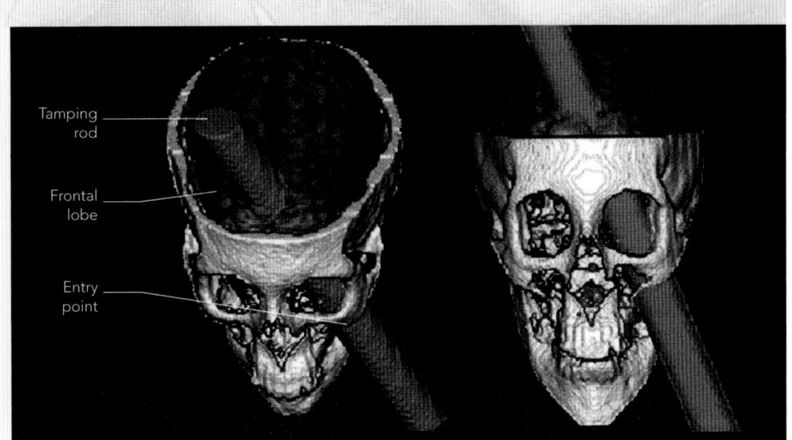

RECONSTRUCTION
Computer-generated images reveal the exact location of the damage to Phineas Gage's brain. Apart from going blind in one eye, he suffered few physical effects, but his behaviour changed dramatically.

PSYCHOPATHY

Psychopaths are marked by an abnormal lack of empathy, to the extent that some even enjoy seeing others suffer. They may, however, be charming, intelligent, and capable of mimicking normal emotions so well that they are difficult to spot. Psychopathic behaviour is linked to risk-taking, irresponsible, and generally selfish behaviour, but those with high intelligence can curb these tendencies and become very successful. A large number of leading businesspeople show psychopathic tendencies, as well as a large proportion of criminals. The brains of people who have psychopathic tendencies show less emotional response to images of people being hurt, and the emotional parts of their brains have fewer connections with the frontal areas that consciously "feel" for others.

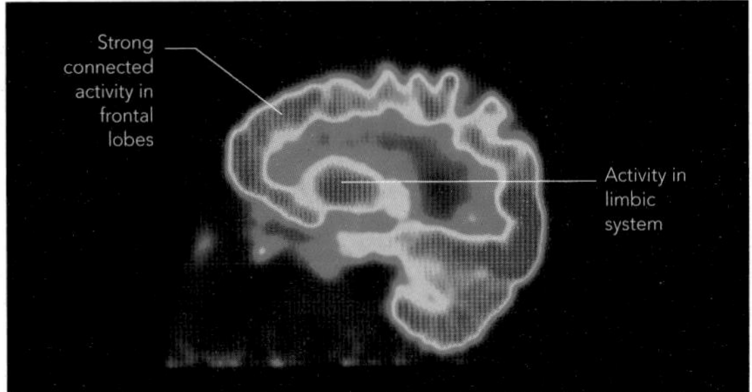

NORMAL BRAIN

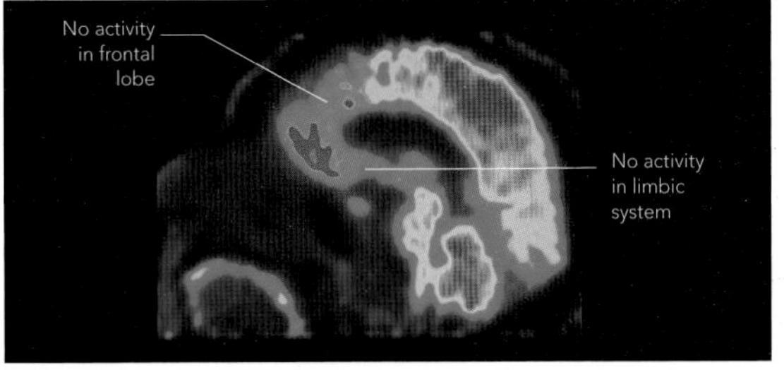

PSYCHOPATHIC BRAIN

PSYCHOPATHIC BRAINS
Psychologist James Fallon studied psychopathic prisoners and scanned their brains (bottom right) as they viewed emotional images. Professor Fallon found that his own brain has psychopathic markers, which he acknowledges reflects his lack of empathy. His intelligence and insight allow him to overcome his emotional dysfunctions.

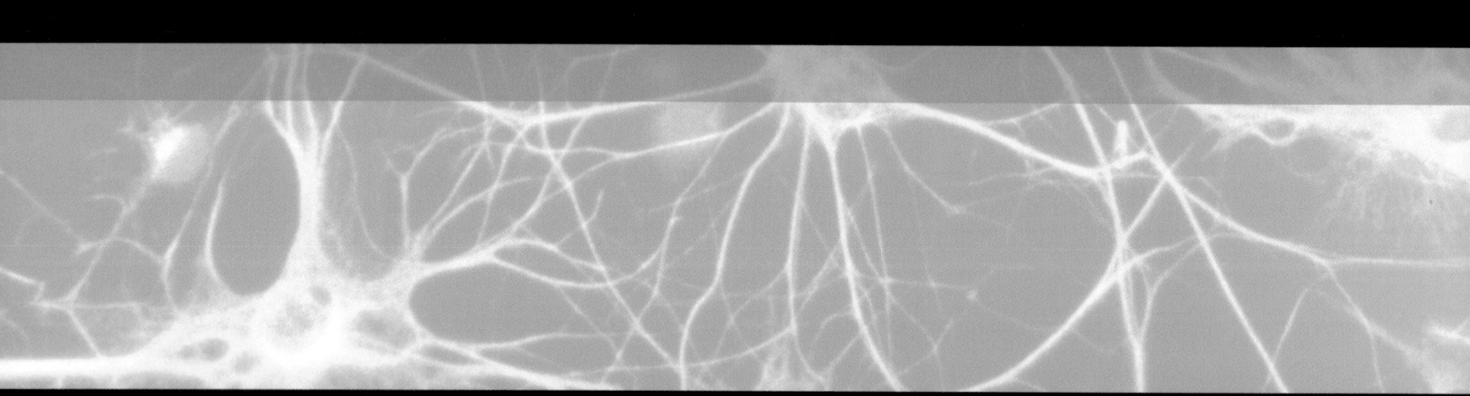

WE SIGNAL OUR INTENTIONS TO EACH OTHER IN VARIOUS WAYS. A SURPRISINGLY LARGE AMOUNT OF INFORMATION CAN BE TRANSMITTED BY GESTURES AND BODY LANGUAGE. THIS IS AN ABILITY THAT HUMANS SHARE WITH MANY OTHER ANIMALS, BUT WE CAN ALSO COMMUNICATE IN WAYS THAT ARE UNIQUE TO OUR SPECIES. ONLY THE HUMAN BRAIN HAS AREAS DEDICATED TO LANGUAGE. WE USE THESE TO SPEAK AND TO READ AND WRITE. ALTHOUGH READING AND WRITING HAVE TO BE LEARNED, WE SEEM TO BE BORN WITH THE ABILITY TO SPEAK AND TO USE COMPLEX RULES OF GRAMMAR.

LANGUAGE AND COMMUNICATION

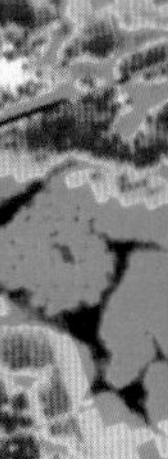

GESTURES AND BODY LANGUAGE

WE SIGNAL OUR THOUGHTS, FEELINGS, AND INTENTIONS BY GESTURE AND BODY LANGUAGE AS WELL AS BY SPEECH. HALF OF OUR COMMUNICATION IS TYPICALLY NON-VERBAL, AND WHEN THEY CONFLICT, GESTURES "SPEAK" LOUDER THAN WORDS.

EYE TALK

Human eyes convey information through facial expression and movement. Unlike in most species, the visible white of the human eye makes it easy to see in which direction a person is looking and thus where their attention is directed. People have a strong instinct to follow another's eye gaze, and this simple mechanism ensures that when someone is in sight of another person, they can manipulate each other's attention and share information without even having to communicate with words.

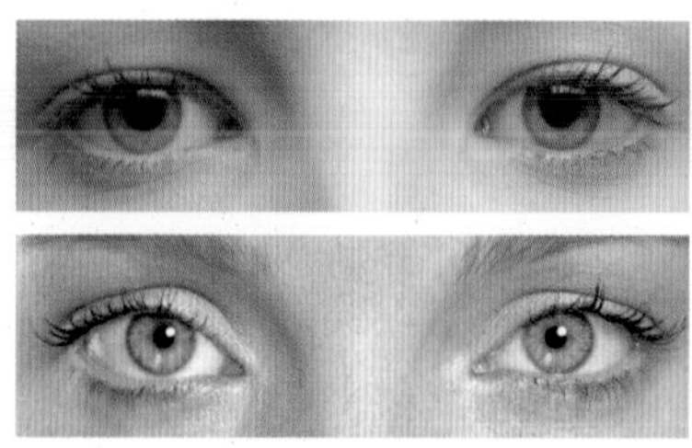

STRONG SIGNALLERS
Pupils dilate when a person has an emotional reaction. Some drugs have a similar effect – belladonna was once used by women to send signals of sexual excitement.

MIRRORING PARENTS

By three months old, babies have the ability to follow another person's eye gaze, and they are quick to pick up any emotion contained in a look. Experiments show that if a parent looks towards something and displays fear, for example, by widening their eyes, the child is very likely to mirror this reaction and be scared too, even if the object is clearly harmless.

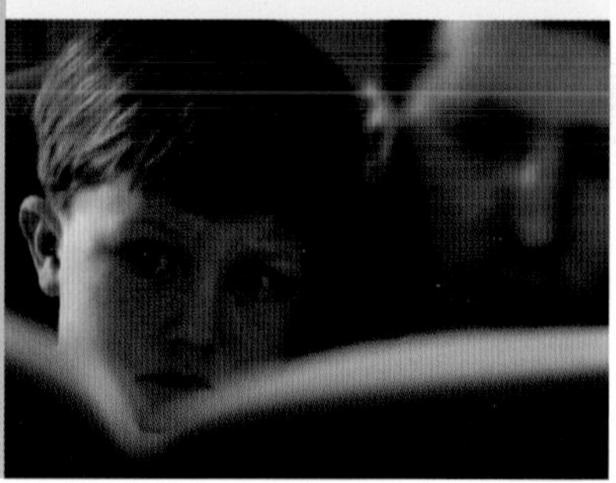

BODY LANGUAGE

Body language is mostly instinctive, consisting largely of unconscious "breakthrough" acts. Some of these are remnants of primitive reflexes, when other living things were often seen primarily as either predator or prey. These ancient reflexes programme us to approach small, soft stimuli, which suggest prey, and to withdraw from strong, hard stimuli, which suggest a predator. Aggression is usually shown through tensed muscles and an upright or forward-leaning stance, indicating that a predator is ready to pounce. Fear is displayed by a softer body contour and backward stance, indicating that the prey is preparing to flee. When emotions are mixed, a person may take up a midway stance from which they can shift quickly from one posture to another.

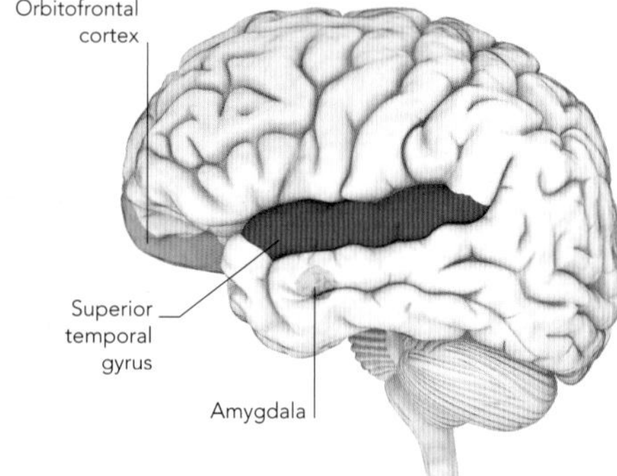

BRAIN PROCESSES
Giveaway eye, mouth, hand, and body movements, as well as deliberate gestures are registered in the superior temporal sulcus, a brain area concerned with the self in relation to others. The amygdala notes the emotional content, and the orbitofrontal cortex analyses it.

EXPRESSION AND BODY LANGUAGE STUDY
When body language and facial expression do not match each other, we are biased towards the emotion signalled by the body, rather than the expression on the face.

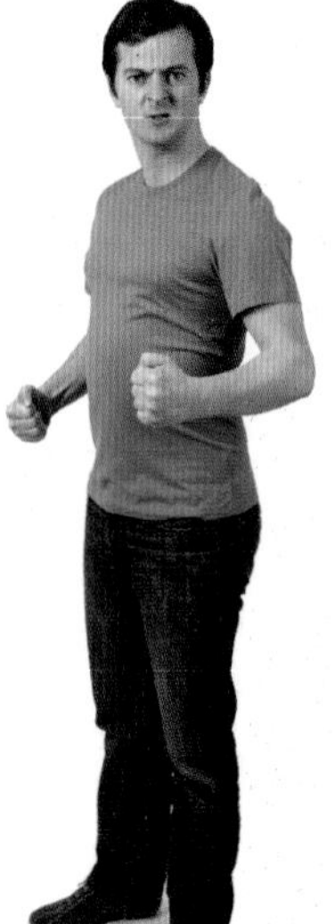

ANGRY EXPRESSION; ANGRY BODY LANGUAGE

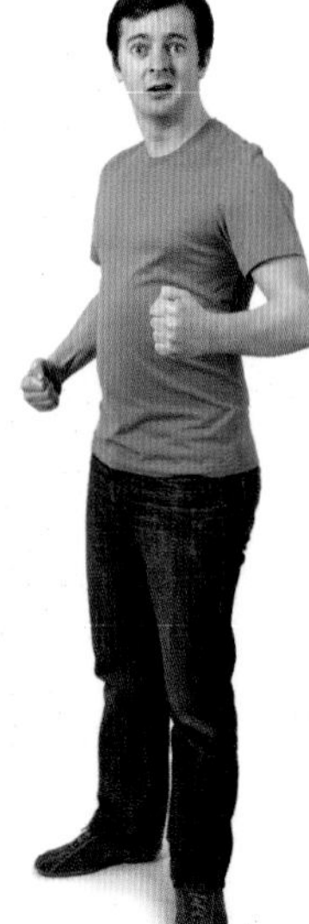

FEARFUL EXPRESSION; ANGRY BODY LANGUAGE

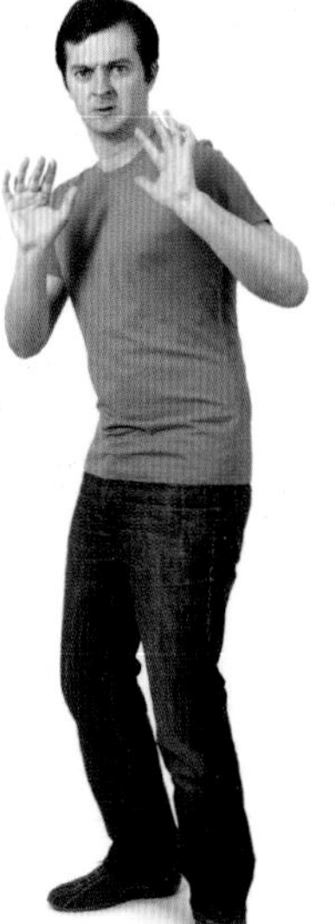

ANGRY EXPRESSION; FEARFUL BODY LANGUAGE

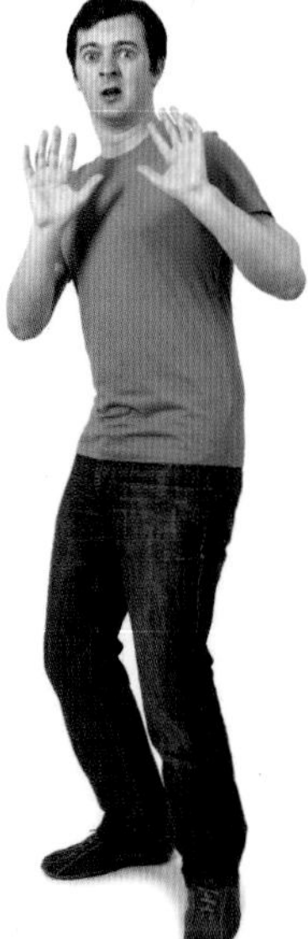

FEARFUL EXPRESSION; FEARFUL BODY LANGUAGE

REACTING TO BODY LANGUAGE

Body language showing fear or anger sparks activity in brain areas involved in movement, while that expressing happiness stirs activity in the visual cortex. In one study, subjects' brains were scanned while they were shown images of actors with blurred faces in fearful, happy, or neutral poses. Happy gestures, such as arms spread in welcome, spurred activity in the visual cortex. Fearful ones, like cowering, caused activity in emotional centres and in areas involved in movement. This might explain how fear spreads in a crowd and prepares the body to flee.

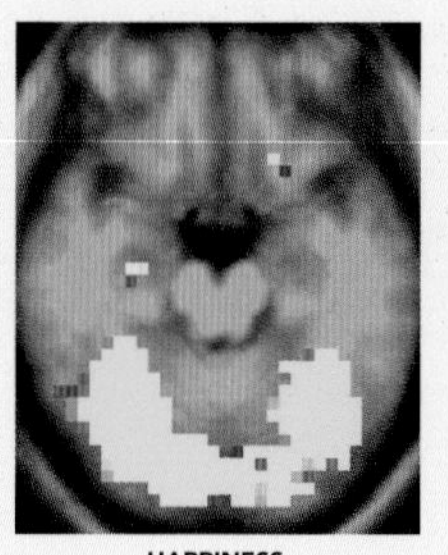

HAPPINESS **FEAR**

GESTURES

Although body language is mostly unconsciously performed, we have a greater degree of conscious control over its more refined form – gestures. Many parts of the body can be involved with making gestures, but most tend to include hand and finger movements, which can display complex spatial relations, issue directions, and show the shape of imagined objects. They can help convey emotions and thoughts, insults, and invitations. Gestures are used throughout the world, although they by no means have universal meanings. Even simple gestures, such as pointing at a person, which is commonly used in many parts of the world, can be highly offensive in parts of Asia.

THREE MAIN CATEGORIES

"Natural" gestures tend to be used for three main purposes: to tell a story, to convey a feeling or idea, or to emphasize a spoken statement. Invented gestures, such as the Masonic handshake, may be completely arbitrary or developed from natural body language.

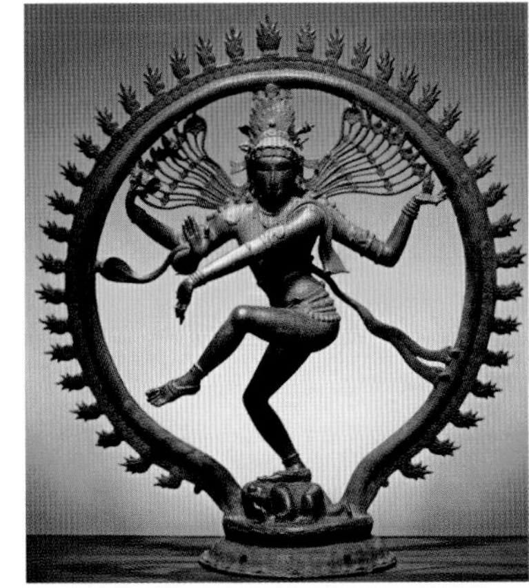

INTRICATE GESTURES
Statues of Hindu deities often convey symbolic meanings through the specific positioning of their hands. With his outward-facing palm, the god Shiva is assuring protection.

THE GRAMMAR OF GESTURE

Unlike the rules of speech, which vary from language to language, gesturing seems to have a universal "grammar". Asked to communicate a simple statement using words of their native languages, English, Chinese, and Spanish speakers started with the subject, then the verb and finally the object, whereas Turkish speakers used the subject, object, then the verb. However, when just using gestures, speakers of all of these languages placed the subject, object, and verb in that order.

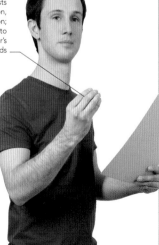

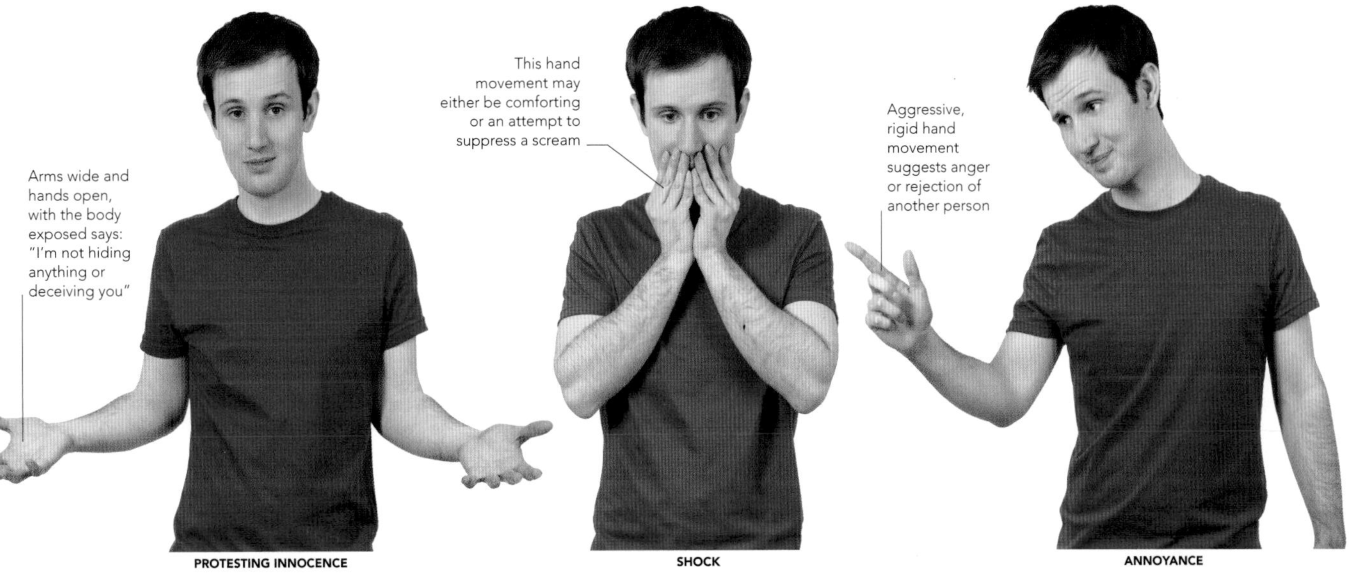

PROTESTING INNOCENCE

SHOCK

ANNOYANCE

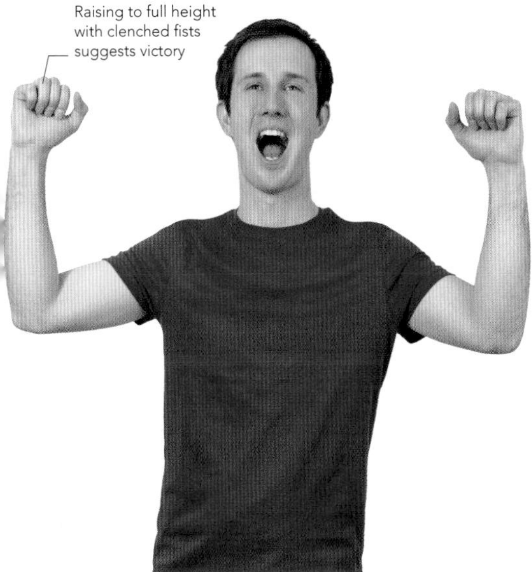
Raising to full height with clenched fists suggests victory

JUBILATION

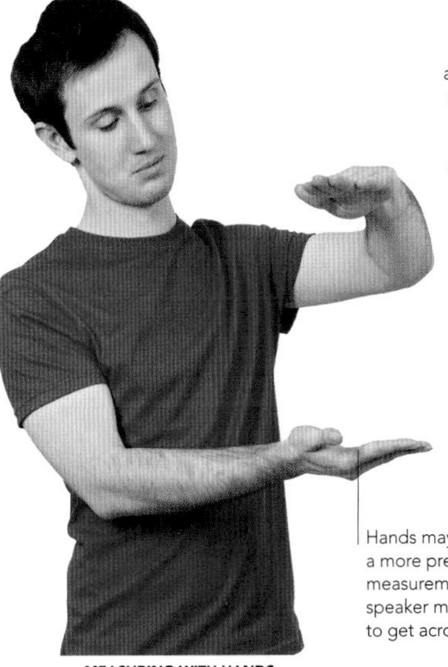
Hands may convey a more precise measurement than the speaker might be able to get across verbally

MEASURING WITH HANDS

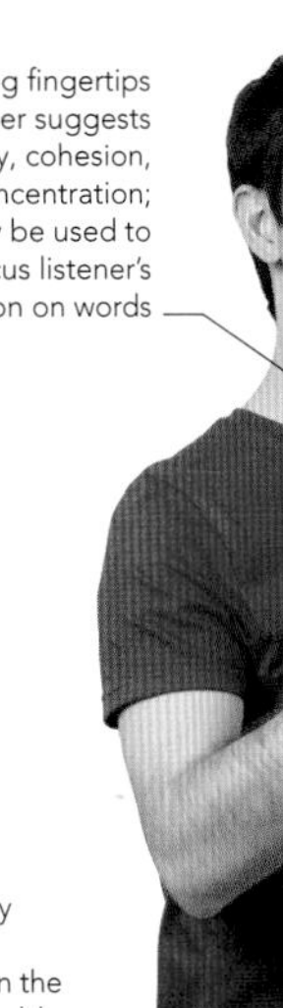
Pulling fingertips together suggests accuracy, cohesion, and concentration; may be used to focus listener's attention on words

REINFORCING A POINT

THE ORIGINS OF LANGUAGE

HUMANS HAVE AN INNATE CAPACITY FOR LANGUAGE – A FACULTY THAT SEEMS TO RELY ON ONE OR MORE GENES THAT ARE UNIQUE TO OUR SPECIES. IT IS NOT KNOWN, THOUGH, WHETHER LANGUAGE AROSE AS A DIRECT RESULT OF GENETIC MUTATION, OR AS A RESULT OF THE INTERACTION BETWEEN SUBTLE BIOLOGICAL CHANGES AND ENVIRONMENTAL PRESSURES.

HEMISPHERE SPECIALIZATION

Compared to the brains of other species, human brains are less symmetrical in terms of functions. Language is the most obvious example of this lopsidedness, and the vast majority of people have the main language areas on the left side of the brain, although a few seem to have language functions distributed on both sides, and some have it only on the right. Generally, language is associated with the "dominant" side of the brain – that is, the one that controls the most competent hand. Language is thought by some to be the mechanism that elevates the brain to full consciousness, and before language evolved it is possible that our ancestors were not consciously aware of themselves. Because language is so important, disruptions have awful consequences, so brain surgeons have to be very careful to avoid damaging the language areas. This is one of the reasons for the Wada test.

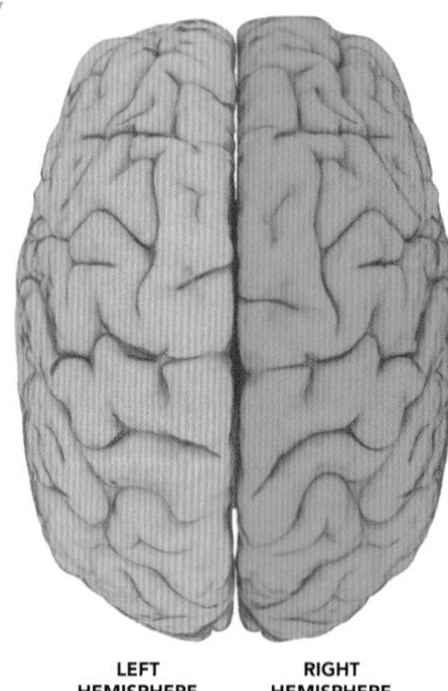

LANGUAGE FUNCTIONS

The three principal language areas are usually found in the left hemisphere, while four other important language areas are located in the right hemisphere.

HEMISPHERE	FUNCTION
Left	Articulating language
Left	Comprehending language
Left	Word recognition
Right	Recognizing tone
Right	Rhythm, stress, and intonation
Right	Recognizing the speaker
Right	Recognizing gestures

AREAS INVOLVED
The main language skills of recognizing, understanding, and generating speech are situated in the left hemisphere in most people. The right hemisphere, however, processes aspects of language that are needed to obtain "full" comprehension.

THE WADA TEST

The Wada test, named after neurologist Juhn Wada, involves anaesthetizing one hemisphere of the brain while leaving the other fully active. This is possible because each hemisphere of the brain has its own blood supply. If the patient is able to speak when one brain hemisphere is asleep, the principal language areas must be on the conscious side. This information is vital for surgeons to plan operations. The Wada test will be replaced by advanced scanning techniques.

Left internal carotid artery

Right internal carotid artery

CAROTID ARTERIES
This coloured magnetic resonance angiogram (MRA) shows the arteries that supply the brain. The Wada test involves injecting one of the internal carotid arteries to put one brain hemisphere to sleep.

SILBO LANGUAGE

Most languages use words – that is, noises made by exercising muscles in the throat and mouth that chop up (articulate) and vary the sound of the passage of air from the lungs. Silbo, however, is a language made up entirely of whistles, used by the inhabitants of La Gomera in the Canary Islands. Brain-imaging studies show that Silbo-users process the whistles in the main language areas of their brains, whereas those who do not know the language process the whistles simply as a collection of sounds, which are registered in other areas of the brain.

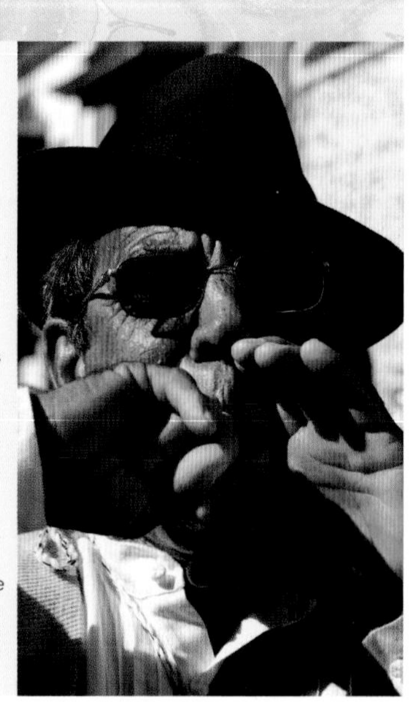

WHISTLE WHILE YOU WORK
Silbo developed among islanders who needed to communicate in a landscape where deep ravines made shouting impractical – their whistles carry further than words and with less distortion.

WHAT IS LANGUAGE?

Language is not just a matter of stringing symbols together to convey meaning. Language is governed by a complex set of rules, known as grammar. The details of these rules differ from language to language, but they share a similar type of complexity. Simple, word-like sounds do not engage language areas in the same way that words that form part of a language do – the brain just treats them as noises. Some theorists believe that the overarching rules of language – the structure that is common to them all – is embedded in the human brain and is instinctive rather than learned. Although primates have learned how to link visual symbols on keyboards to objects, and some can understand sign language, it has not been possible to teach another species spoken language.

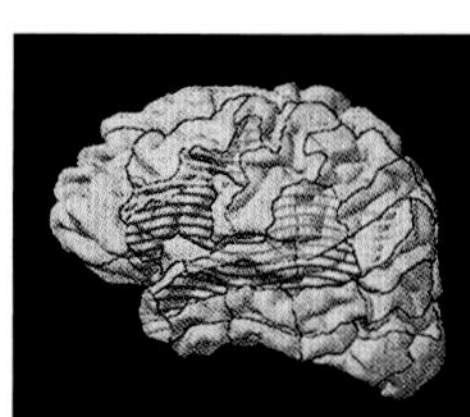
LEFT HEMISPHERE

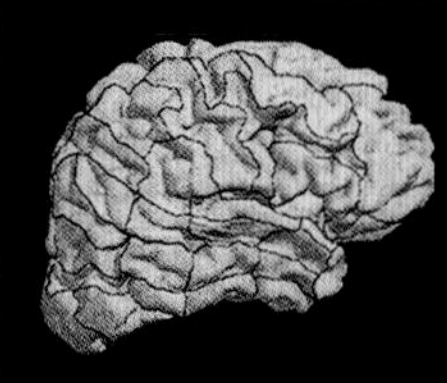
RIGHT HEMISPHERE

SENTENCES AND CONSONANT STRINGS
Several areas in the brain's left hemisphere become active when people hear a familiar language spoken to them, compared to a small area of the right hemisphere that is active when they hear strings of consonants that do not make any sense.

THE EVOLUTION OF LANGUAGE

Spoken language leaves no traces in the historic record, so we shall probably never know how or even exactly when it originated. The ability to generate speech and understand language is something only humans possess, although some primates' brains have regions that may function as primitive language areas. An important factor in the evolution of language took place in the throat and larynx, around the time that our ancestors started walking upright. These changes affected the variety and intricacy of the sounds they could produce. This improved ability to communicate probably increased the chances of survival of those who used it most effectively and therefore the chances of it being passed on to subsequent generations.

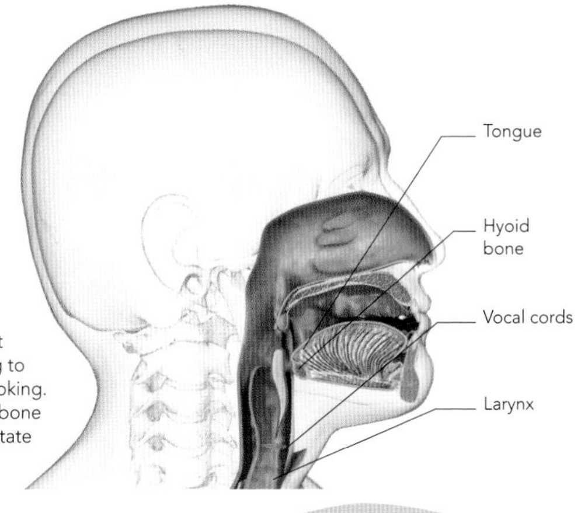

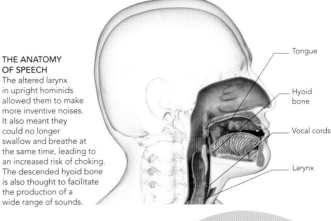

THE ANATOMY OF SPEECH
The altered larynx in upright hominids allowed them to make more inventive noises. It also meant they could no longer swallow and breathe at the same time, leading to an increased risk of choking. The descended hyoid bone is also thought to facilitate the production of a wide range of sounds.

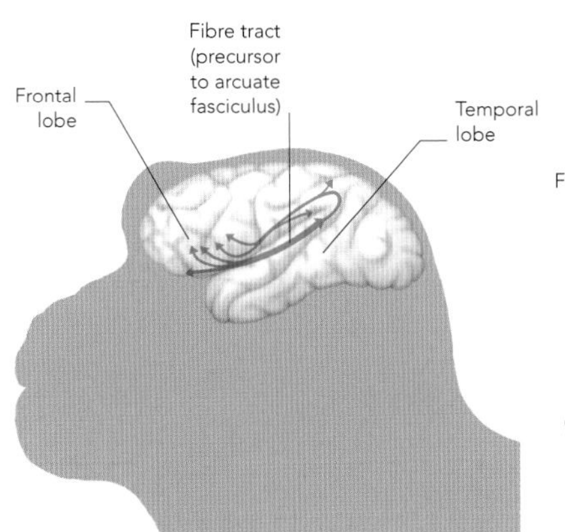

MACAQUE FIBRE TRACT
Macaques have simple language areas. A crucial part of this region is a thick bundle of fibres, which links the areas associated with understanding language in the temporal lobe with the areas that generate it, in the frontal lobe.

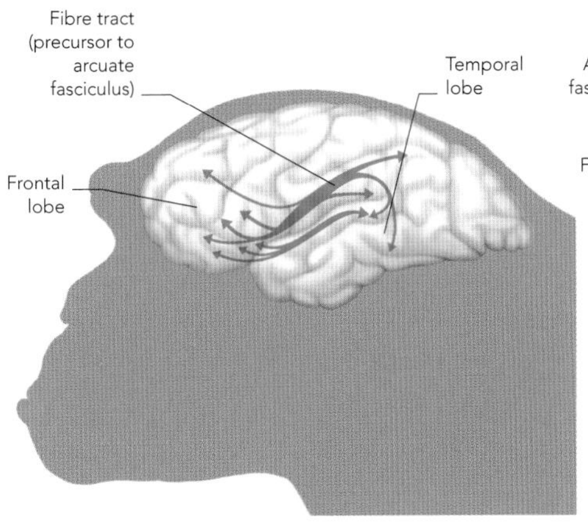

CHIMPANZEE FIBRE TRACT
The connections between the frontal lobe and the temporal lobe are more advanced than in macaques, allowing for improved cognitive abilities, but unlike humans, they do not have prominent temporal-lobe projections of this tract.

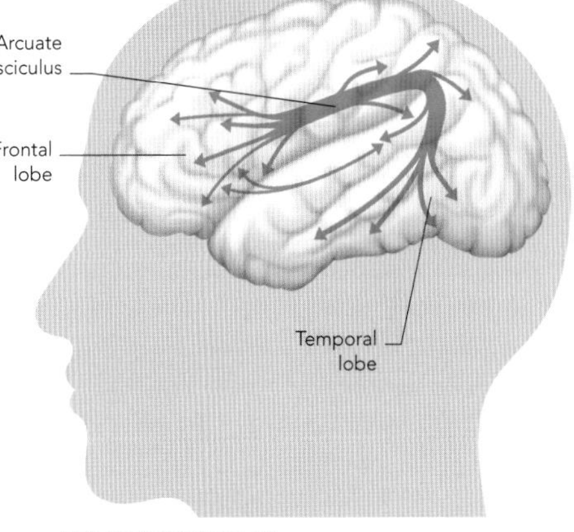

HUMAN FIBRE TRACT
In the human brain, the tract is known as the arcuate fasciculus, connecting areas crucial for speech and comprehension. It is one of the specializations that is thought to have led to the evolution of language.

LANGUAGE GENES

Hundreds of genes combine to make language possible, but one gene in particular is associated with the normal development of speech and language. FOXP2 is a gene that helps to connect the many brain areas that work together to produce fluent speech. People with a particular mutation on this gene have a condition known as childhood apraxia of speech. Those affected have problems producing words, and in some cases may also have difficulty understanding speech. Animals that communicate through sound, including songbirds, mice, whales, and other primates, also have the FOXP2 gene. However, in humans it is thought to have evolved further and faster, resulting in the formation of more complex connections in the brain. Certain mutations to the FOXP2 gene – in both the human and animal versions – may produce comparable problems, however. In mice, for instance, a particular change in the gene makes them "stutter" in their squeaking "songs", just as it does in people.

LANGUAGE AND PERCEPTION

Language is much more than just a way of signalling things to one another – evidence shows that it shapes the way we perceive the world. If your language makes a distinction between blue and green, for example, you will be less likely to confuse a blue colour chip with a green one when recalling them, because you will have been able to attach a mental label to each of them. If a language does not distinguish between colours in the same way, it will be more difficult to recall them. Similarly, the Amazonian Piraha tribe do not have words for numbers above two, and are unable to reliably tell the difference between four and five objects placed in a row.

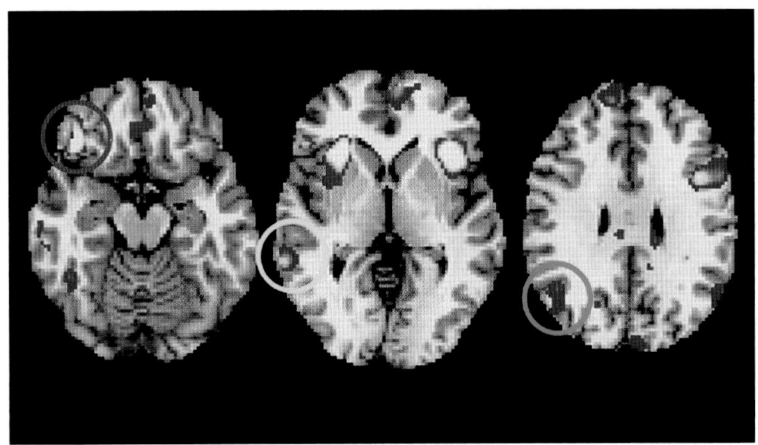

COLOUR STUDY
Areas of the brain involved in recognition and word retrieval (circled, left) are engaged more when people distinguish between colours that have different names than between colours that share the name, even if they are visually distinctive.

THE LANGUAGE AREAS

THE HUMAN BRAIN DIFFERS FROM THAT OF OTHER SPECIES, IN THAT IT HAS A REGION THAT IS DEDICATED TO LANGUAGE ALONE. IN THE VAST MAJORITY OF PEOPLE, THIS IS SITUATED IN THE LEFT HEMISPHERE, BUT IN ABOUT 20 PER CENT OF LEFT-HANDED PEOPLE, IT IS IN THE RIGHT HEMISPHERE.

MAIN LANGUAGE AREAS

Language processing occurs mainly in Broca's and Wernicke's areas. Broadly speaking, words are comprehended by Wernicke's area and articulated by Broca's. A thick band of tissue called the arcuate fasciculus connects these two areas. Wernicke's area is surrounded by an area known as Geschwind's territory. When a person hears words spoken, Wernicke's area matches the sounds to their meaning, and special neurons in Geschwind's territory are thought to assist by combining the many different properties of words (sound, sight, and meaning) to provide full comprehension. When a person speaks, the process happens in reverse – Wernicke's area finds the correct words to match the thought that is to be expressed. The chosen words then pass to Broca's area via the arcuate fasciculus (or, possibly, via a more circuitous route through Geschwind's territory). Broca's area then turns the words into sounds by moving the tongue, mouth, and jaw into the required position and by activating the larynx.

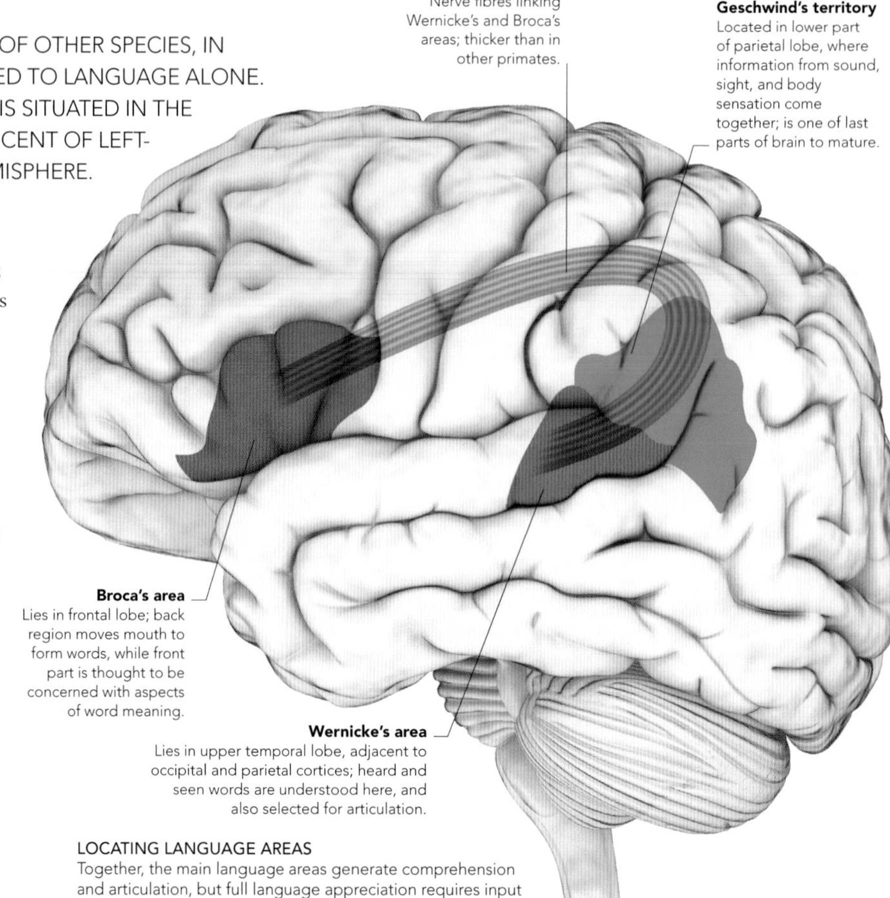
Arcuate fasciculus
Nerve fibres linking Wernicke's and Broca's areas; thicker than in other primates.
Geschwind's territory
Located in lower part of parietal lobe, where information from sound, sight, and body sensation come together; is one of last parts of brain to mature.
Broca's area
Lies in frontal lobe; back region moves mouth to form words, while front part is thought to be concerned with aspects of word meaning.
Wernicke's area
Lies in upper temporal lobe, adjacent to occipital and parietal cortices; heard and seen words are understood here, and also selected for articulation.

LOCATING LANGUAGE AREAS
Together, the main language areas generate comprehension and articulation, but full language appreciation requires input from areas concerned with tone, emotion, and rhythm.

Part of visual cortex

Part of Broca's area

Wernicke's area

Geschwind's territory

SEEING WORDS PASSIVELY

LISTENING TO WORDS

AREAS ACTIVATED IN DIFFERENT TASKS
These fMRI scans show distinct patterns of activity in the three main language areas, depending on if the person undertaking the task is listening to speech or pronouncing words. Simply looking at words passively does not involve much activity in the language areas.

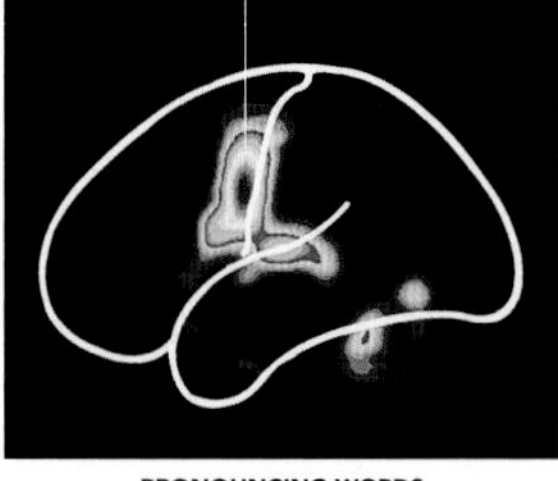
Area activated includes part of Broca's area

PRONOUNCING WORDS

LANGUAGE TASKS

Different types of language tasks activate a number of different areas of the brain. However, the key language areas only become active when language is turned into meaning. So merely looking at words as marks on a page involves areas of the brain such as the visual cortex, which is responsible for processing incoming visual information, whereas listening to spoken words triggers activity in Wernicke's area and Geschwinds's territory, signifying that the sounds are being turned into meaningful information. Broca's area is significantly involved in listening, too, because understanding words involves, to some extent, articulating them "in your head" (also referred to as "sounding out"). Broca's area is strongly activated when the task involves pronouncing words, while generating words involves both Wernicke's and Broca's areas, as well as Geschwind's territory.

SHIFTING GROUND

Wernicke's and Broca's areas are now well defined, but immediately around them lie large regions of the cortex that become active during a variety of different language studies. Their precise functions remain unclear, and their shapes and locations differ from person to person. Even with a single individual, the peripheral areas engaged in language may shift over the course of that person's life.

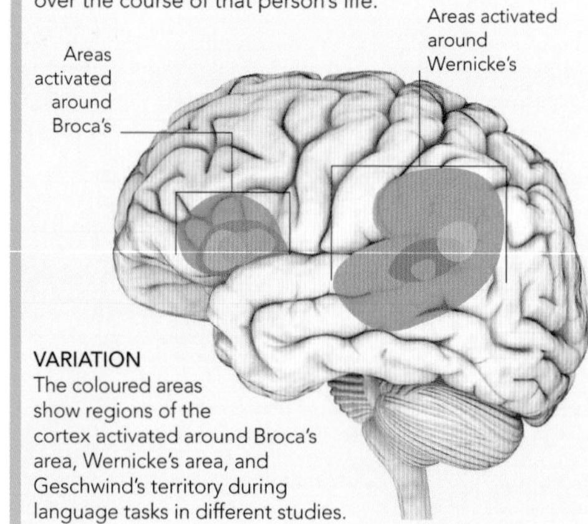
Areas activated around Broca's
Areas activated around Wernicke's

VARIATION
The coloured areas show regions of the cortex activated around Broca's area, Wernicke's area, and Geschwind's territory during language tasks in different studies.

THE MULTILINGUAL BRAIN

Being fluent in two languages, particularly from early childhood, enhances various cognitive skills and might also protect against the onset of dementia and other age-related cognitive decline. One reason for this may be that speaking a second language builds more connections between neurons. Studies show that bilingual adults have denser grey matter, especially in the inferior frontal cortex of the brain's left hemisphere, where most language and communication skills are controlled. The increased density was most pronounced in people who learned a second language before the age of five.

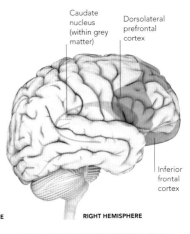

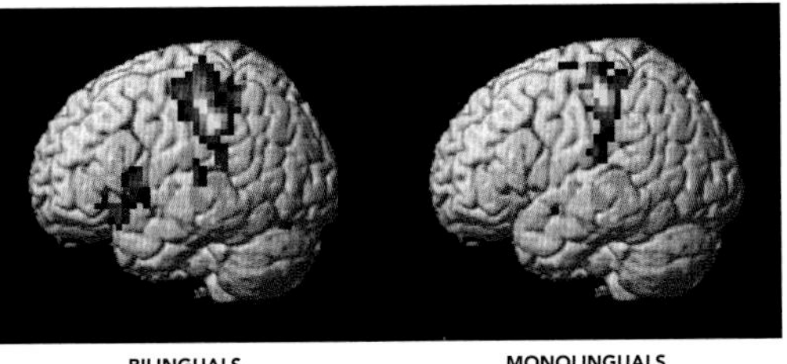

CONTRASTING ACTIVATION
These scans show the brains of bilingual and monolingual individuals when hearing the same language.

Dorsolateral prefrontal cortex
Broca's area
Inferior frontal cortex
Caudate nucleus (within grey matter)
LEFT HEMISPHERE

Caudate nucleus (within grey matter)
Dorsolateral prefrontal cortex
Inferior frontal cortex
RIGHT HEMISPHERE

KEY
- Areas used when speaking one language
- Areas activated in bilinguals when switching languages

NEURAL SIGNATURE OF BILINGUALISM
The purple area is used by both mono- and bilingual individuals when speaking one language; areas in green are activated when bilingual speakers switch languages. The caudate nucleus is also activated during the switch.

LANGUAGE PROBLEMS

There are a wide range of speech and language problems that can arise from a correspondingly varied number of injuries and impairments. Some problems only affect comprehension, whereas others specifically hinder expression; learning disabilities, such as dyslexia (see p.153) and specific language impairment (see p.248), can affect both. Traumatic brain injuries and strokes can lead to aphasia, which is the loss of the ability to produce and/or comprehend language. By contrast, dysphasia is the partial loss of the ability to communicate, although these terms are often incorrectly used interchangeably.

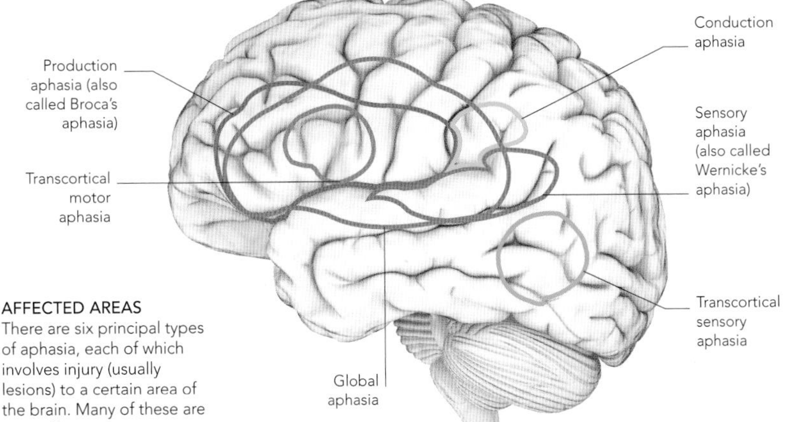

AFFECTED AREAS
There are six principal types of aphasia, each of which involves injury (usually lesions) to a certain area of the brain. Many of these are caused by strokes.

STUTTERING

About 1 per cent of people (75 per cent of them men) stutter. In most cases, stuttering (also known as stammering) begins between the ages of two and six. Imaging studies have shown that the brains of stutterers behave differently to those of non-stutterers when processing speech, in that many more areas of the brain are activated during speech production. It may be that these interfere with one another and cause the stuttering, or it may be the result of stuttering.

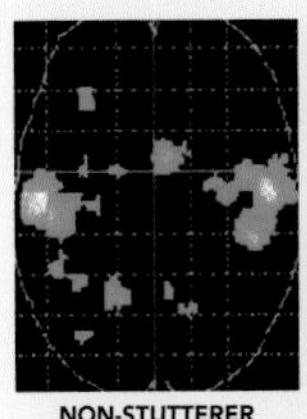
NON-STUTTERER

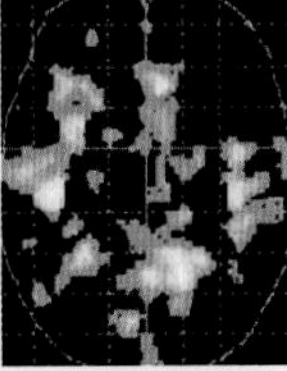
STUTTERER BEFORE TREATMENT

TREATMENT FOR STUTTERING
Speech therapy is often successful as these PET scans show. As treatment progresses, brain activity during speech dies down to near normal.

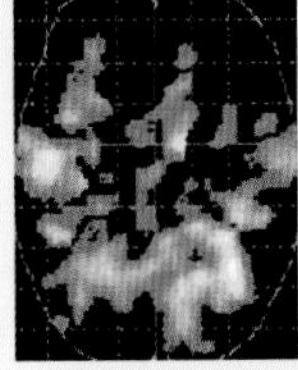
EARLY STAGE OF TREATMENT

LATER STAGE OF TREATMENT

TYPES OF APHASIA

Aphasia is usually associated with a brain injury (such as a stroke), which affects the brain's language areas. Depending on the type of damage, the area affected (see right), and the extent of damage, someone suffering from aphasia may be able to speak, yet have little or no comprehension of what they or others are saying. Or they may be able to understand language, yet be unable to speak. Sometimes, sufferers can sing but not speak, or write but not read.

Production aphasia (damage to Broca's area) Inability to articulate words or string them together; if words can be uttered, they tend to be verbs or nouns, with abnormal tone and rhythm.

Global aphasia (widespread damage) General deficits in comprehension, repetition, naming, and speech production; automatic phrases (e.g. reeling off numbers) may be spared.

Transcortical motor aphasia (damage around Broca's) Good comprehension but non-fluent speech, often limited to two words at a time. Sufferers retain the ability to repeat words and phrases.

Conduction aphasia (damage to link between Wernicke's and Broca's areas) Speech errors include substituting sounds, but good comprehension and fluent speech production.

Transcortical sensory aphasia (damage to temporal-occipital-parietal junction) Inability to comprehend, name, read, or write, but with normal ability to recite previously learned passages.

Sensory aphasia (damage to Wernicke's area) Inability to understand language, often combined with general comprehension problems and lack of awareness of own deficiency.

A CONVERSATION

CONVERSATION COMES NATURALLY TO MOST OF US, BUT IN TERMS OF BRAIN FUNCTION IT IS ONE OF THE MOST COMPLICATED CEREBRAL ACTIVITIES WE ENGAGE IN. BOTH SPEAKING AND LISTENING INVOLVE WIDESPREAD AREAS OF THE BRAIN, REFLECTING MANY DIFFERENT TYPES AND LEVELS OF COGNITION.

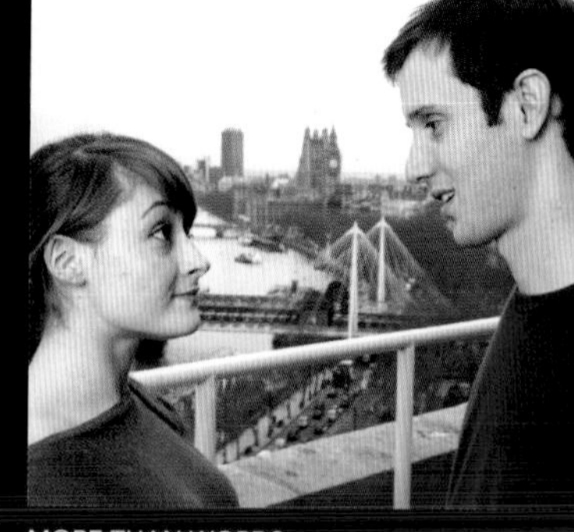

MORE THAN WORDS
Face-to-face conversations involve more than just decoding words – tone and body language are also part of "understanding".

LISTENING

The sound of spoken words take a short time – about 150 milliseconds – to pass from the speaker's mouth to the listener's ear, for the ear to turn this stimulus into electrical signals, and for this to be processed as sound by the auditory cortex. Words are decoded in Wernicke's area in the left hemisphere, but other areas are also at work to provide full comprehension, including parts of the right hemisphere concerned with tone, body language, and rhythm. If any of these areas are damaged, a person may be left with an incomplete understanding of what is being communicated.

1 50–150 MS
AFTER WORDS ARE SPOKEN SOUND REGISTERED
Sound from the speaker registers in the auditory cortex and is distributed to areas concerned with decoding the words and other areas of the brain involved with emotion, tone, and rhythm.

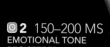

2 150–200 MS
EMOTIONAL TONE REGISTERED
The amygdala is quick to pick up on the emotional tone of the speech and subsequently produces an appropriate emotional reaction.

3 250–350 MS
STRUCTURE OF WORD STREAM ANALYSED AND MEANING OF WORDS EXTRACTED
Speech is decoded in Wernicke's area (orange, below right) in the left hemisphere. Then, the anterior temporal lobe (brown, below left) and inferior frontal cortex (purple, below left) in both hemispheres start to extract the meaning of the words.

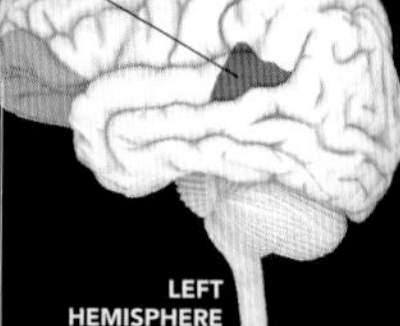

4 400–550 MS
MEANING CONSCIOUSLY COMPREHENDED
Turning the sound of speech into a stream of meaning requires more than just decoding the words – they also have to be associated with memories to give full comprehension. This takes place in part of the frontal lobe.

THE LISTENER
The illustration above highlights the areas of the brain involved in listening. Zero represents the time at which the words are spoken. The rest of the times are measured in milliseconds (ms) after that. It takes just over half a second for the brain to comprehend the meaning of the words.

SPEAKING

The speech process starts about a quarter of a second before words are actually uttered. This is when the brain starts to select the words that are to convey whatever the person wants to say. The words then have to be turned into sounds, and are finally articulated. Most of this complicated activity occurs in specific language areas, which in most people are on the left side of the brain. However, in a minority of people they are situated in the right, or spread between both hemispheres. Right-hemisphere language dominance is more prevalent among left-handers (see p.199).

SHIFTING FUNCTIONS

Speech and comprehension problems often result from strokes, which damage the language areas. If the damage happens early in life, the speech functions may shift to the opposite hemisphere. In older people, this is less likely to be successful, but undamaged areas can still take on some functions of the damaged areas.

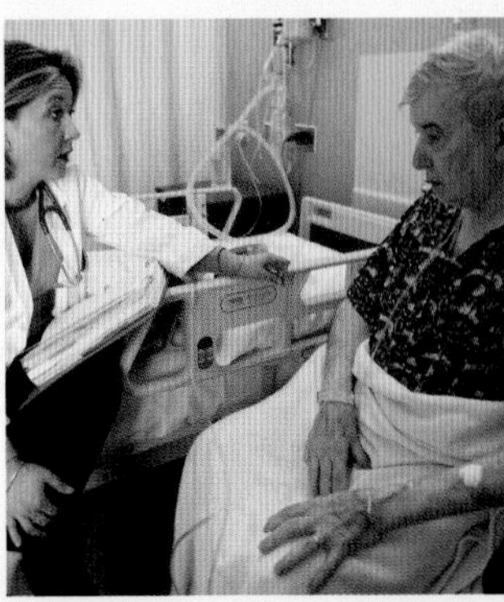

SPEECH AND LANGUAGE THERAPY
It is possible for people who suffer from aphasia as a result of a stroke to recover some language functions through intense speech and language therapy.

CRUCIAL PATHWAY
"Prepared" words are transmitted to Broca's area via a bundle of nerve fibres called the arcuate fasciculus. It is much thicker and better developed in humans than in other species, and is thought to be key to the development of language.

2 –200 MS
WORDS TO PHONOLOGY
Shortly after they have been retrieved from memory, the words are matched to the sounds in Wernicke's area, which is adjacent to the auditory cortex, where sounds are distinguished.

3 –150 MS
PHONOLOGY TO SYLLABLES
Broca's area is the part of the brain most closely associated with speech. It matches the sounds of words to the specific mouth, tongue, and throat movements required to actually voice them.

4 –100 MS
ARTICULATION
The mouth, tongue, and throat movements needed to articulate the selected words are directed by the part of the motor cortex that controls these parts of the body.

1 –250 MS
BEFORE SPEAKING
CONCEPTS TO WORDS
Words are attached to memories and ideas and act as "handles" by which the brain can grasp the correct ones to express an idea. The matching of words to concepts happens in the temporal lobe.

5 UNDER 100 MS
FINE CONTROL OF ARTICULATION
The cerebellum is concerned with orchestrating the timing of speech production. The right cerebellar hemisphere connects to the left cerebral hemisphere, and this shows greatest activation during speech, whereas the left cerebellar hemisphere is more active during singing.

THE SPEAKER
The illustration above highlights the six crucial brain areas that are activated immediately before speaking. Zero is the point on the timescale when words are actually uttered; the timings of the stages before this are therefore indicated by negative values.

READING AND WRITING

OUR ABILITY TO SPEAK AND TO UNDERSTAND THE SPOKEN WORD HAS EVOLVED SO THAT OUR BRAINS ARE WIRED FOR SPEECH. READING AND WRITING, HOWEVER, DO NOT NATURALLY COME TO US IN THE SAME WAY. IN ORDER TO LEARN TO READ AND WRITE, EACH INDIVIDUAL HAS TO TRAIN THEIR BRAIN TO DEVELOP THE NECESSARY SKILLS.

LEARNING TO READ AND WRITE

To learn how to read and write, a child has to translate the shapes of letters on the page into the sounds they make if they are spoken aloud. The word "cat", for instance, must be broken down into its phonological components – "kuh", "aah", and "tuh". Only when the word on the page is translated into the sound that is heard when the word is spoken, can the child match it to its meaning. Learning to write uses even more of the brain. As well as the language areas concerned with comprehension, and the visual areas concerned with decoding text, writing involves integrating the activity in these areas with those concerned with manual dexterity, including the cerebellum, which is involved with intricate hand movements.

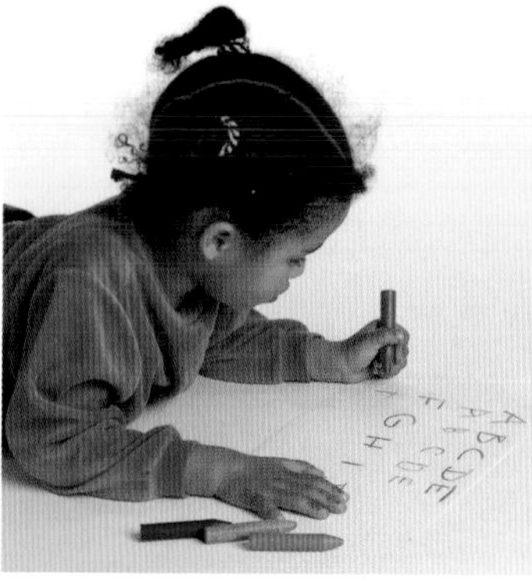

VISUAL DISTINCTIONS
Distinguishing between written letters uses a part of the brain that evolved to make detailed visual distinctions between natural objects. This may be why many letters resemble shapes seen in nature.

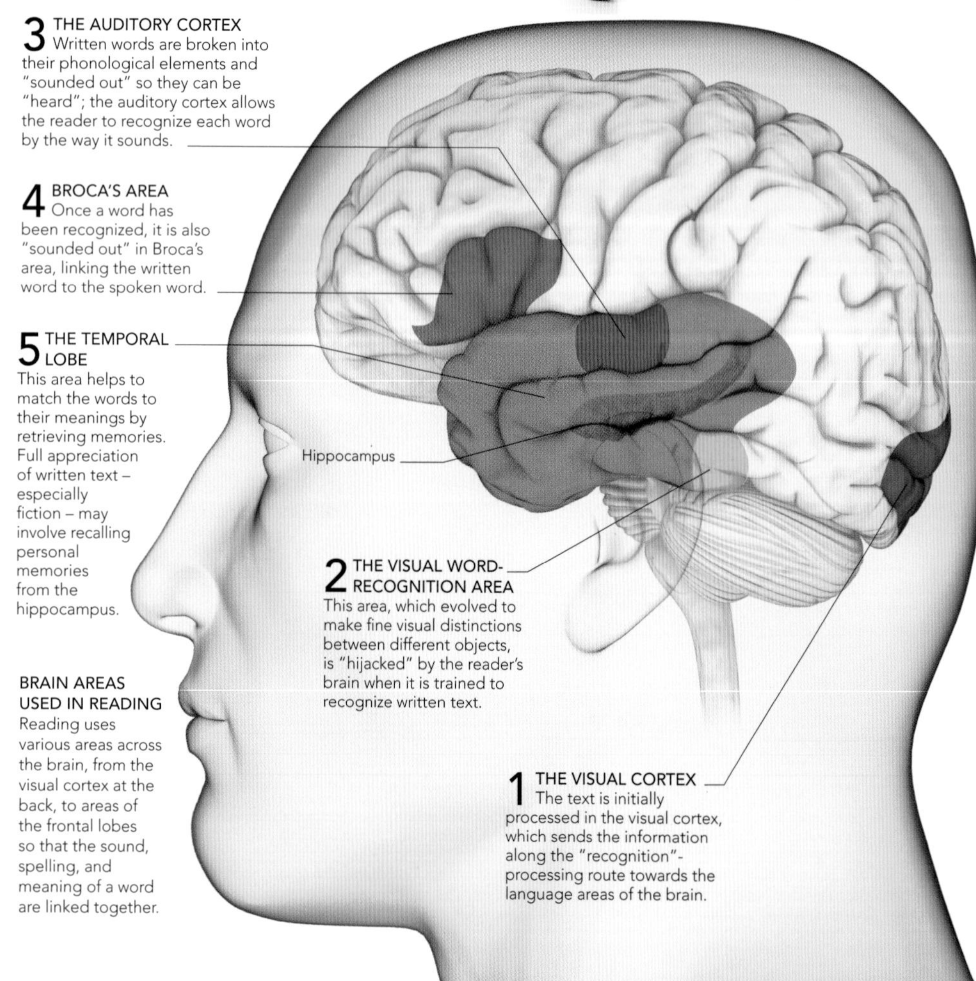

3 THE AUDITORY CORTEX
Written words are broken into their phonological elements and "sounded out" so they can be "heard"; the auditory cortex allows the reader to recognize each word by the way it sounds.

4 BROCA'S AREA
Once a word has been recognized, it is also "sounded out" in Broca's area, linking the written word to the spoken word.

5 THE TEMPORAL LOBE
This area helps to match the words to their meanings by retrieving memories. Full appreciation of written text – especially fiction – may involve recalling personal memories from the hippocampus.

2 THE VISUAL WORD-RECOGNITION AREA
This area, which evolved to make fine visual distinctions between different objects, is "hijacked" by the reader's brain when it is trained to recognize written text.

1 THE VISUAL CORTEX
The text is initially processed in the visual cortex, which sends the information along the "recognition"-processing route towards the language areas of the brain.

BRAIN AREAS USED IN READING
Reading uses various areas across the brain, from the visual cortex at the back, to areas of the frontal lobes so that the sound, spelling, and meaning of a word are linked together.

SKILLED READERS

While we are learning to read, our brains have to work very hard to translate the symbols on the page into sounds. This activates an area in the upper rear of the temporal lobe, in which sounds and vision are brought together. This process becomes automatic with practice, and the brain becomes more concerned with the meaning of the words. Hence, the areas concerned with meaning are more active in a skilled reader's brain (usually an adult's) during reading.

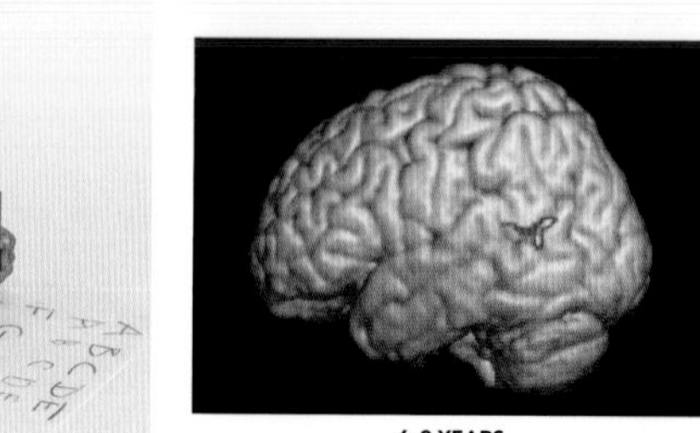

6–9 YEARS

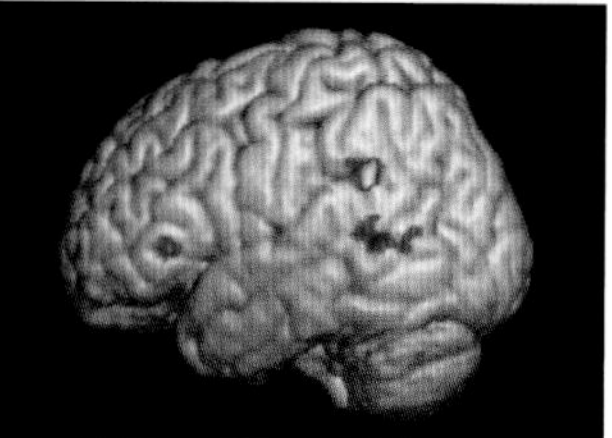

9–18 YEARS

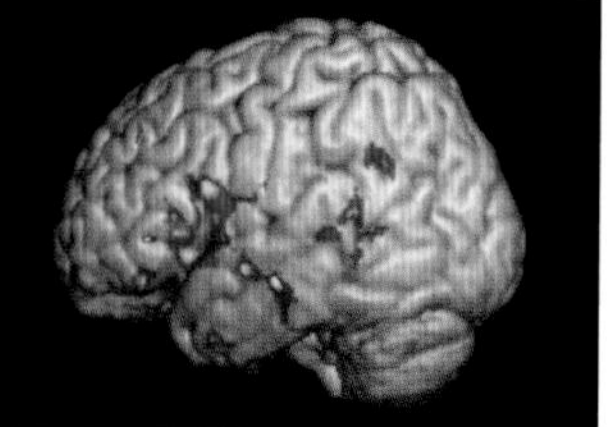

20–23 YEARS

READING DEVELOPMENT
These fMRI scans show that children learning to read rely on a brain area that matches written symbols to sounds (top). As skill develops, areas involving meaning (middle and bottom) become more active.

HOW LITERACY AFFECTS THE BRAIN

Learning to read and write involves building complex new neural connections in many different parts of the brain. This improves a person's ability to distinguish speech sounds and encourages more and wider mental connections, effectively increasing imagination. Reading people-based fiction has also been found to improve the capacity for empathy.

DYSLEXIA

Dyslexia is a language-development disorder with a genetic basis. It may affect 5 per cent of the population, and is most obvious when a language, such as English, has a complex mapping system between speech sounds and letters of the alphabet. One explanation for dyslexia, known as the phonological deficit hypothesis, is that dyslexics cannot analyse and remember the sounds contained in words. This slows down the learning of spoken language and makes it very difficult to map sounds to their corresponding letters of the alphabet when learning to read.

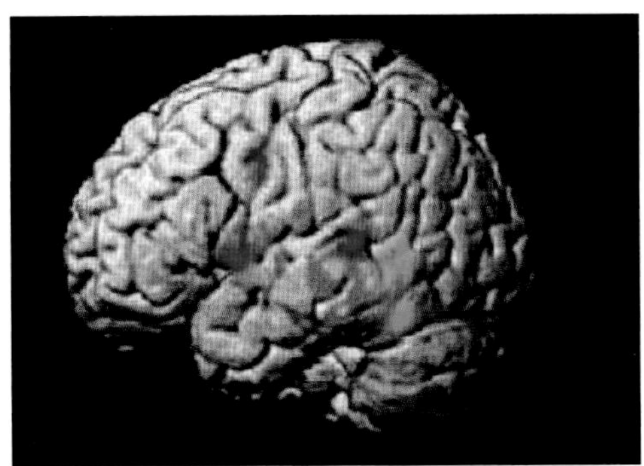

HOW DYSLEXICS DIFFER
Dyslexics differ mostly in the brain area in which words are translated from visual symbols into sounds (shown in green on this fMRI scan). Research has found that dyslexics have more grey matter in this area than non-dyslexics, but the significance of this finding is not fully understood.

TREATING DYSLEXIA?

There is no cure for dyslexia, but dyslexics can improve reading skills through compensatory learning, using the help of specialist teachers to find ways to remember spellings. While reading is likely to remain slow and spelling error-prone, audio books, spell checkers, and voice-recognition programs can help to circumvent the problems of dyslexia.

VISUAL TECHNIQUES
Some cases of dyslexia are thought to be improved by using coloured spectacles or by wearing a patch over one eye.

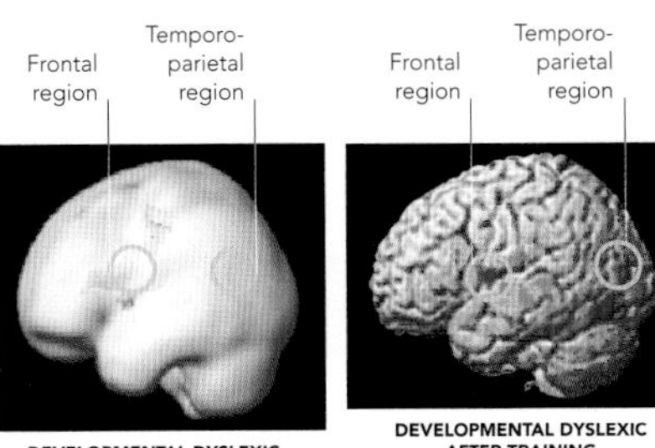

DEVELOPMENTAL DYSLEXIC

DEVELOPMENTAL DYSLEXIC AFTER TRAINING

REMEDIATION
Early studies suggest that a process of listening to slowed-down sounds can aid dyslexics. The circles in the left-hand scan show inactivity in crucial reading areas of a dyslexic's brain; the more detailed right-hand scan shows greater activity in reading areas after training.

HYPERLEXIA

Hyperlexic children exhibit extremely advanced reading and writing skills, but may experience difficulty in understanding spoken words. They often have problems with social interaction and may have symptoms of autism. Some hyperlexics learn to spell fairly long words before the age of two, and to read sentences by three. Brain scans of one such child suggest that hyperlexia is neurologically opposite to dyslexia in that, when the child was reading, brain areas that are sluggish in dyslexic children were overactive.

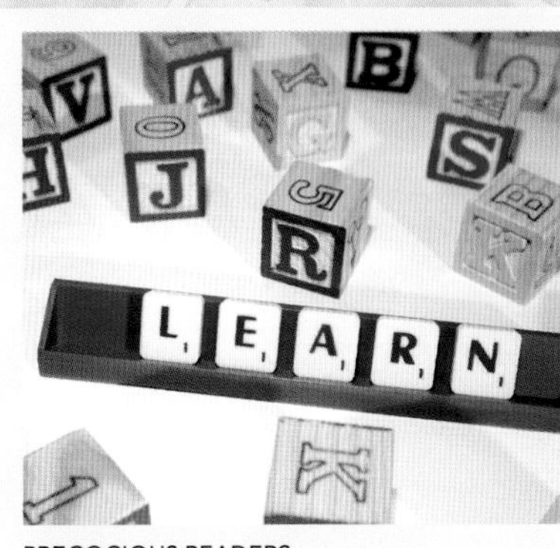

PRECOCIOUS READERS
Hyperlexic children are fascinated by letters and numbers and learn how to read from an early age, but sometimes find it hard to understand spoken language.

LANGUAGE DIFFERENCES

English speakers have a particularly hard time learning to read. English spelling rules are notoriously difficult to master, and skilled readers know that they cannot rely on letter-to-sound decoding rules, as there are too many exceptions – for example, "i" is pronounced differently in "ice" and "ink". For dyslexics, these exceptions are difficult to master, and learning to read and spell takes years longer than it does for non-dyslexics.

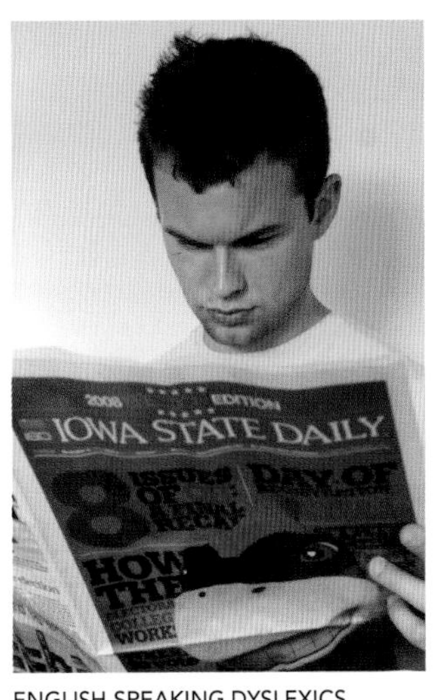

ENGLISH-SPEAKING DYSLEXICS
Learning to read English can be challenging for dyslexics due to the number of words that do not follow standard spelling rules.

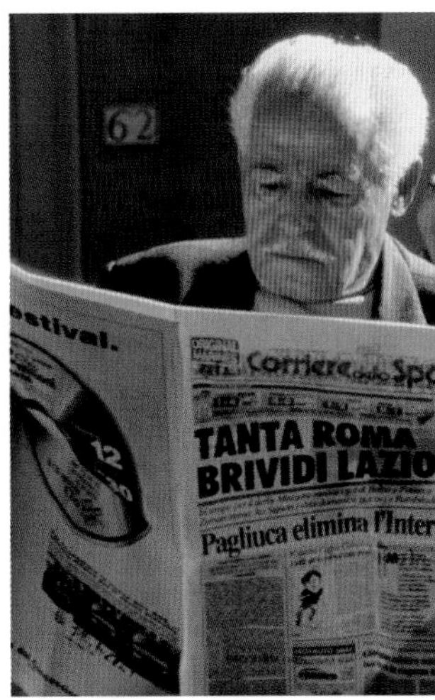

ITALIAN-SPEAKING DYSLEXICS
Italian dyslexics are more accurate at word recognition than their English counterparts, as Italian spelling rules are less complex.

DYSGRAPHIA

Some people have great difficulty writing, even though they may read well. Known as dysgraphia, this may be either language- or motor-based. The first is due to difficulty turning sounds into visual marks, while the second is a problem making the fine movements needed to write or difficulty flowing from one such movement to another. Both show up as wobbly, indistinct, or mangled handwriting – far worse than normal. Some letter reversal is normal in young children but usually it disappears well before adulthood.

This is what mirror writing looks like!

MIRROR-WRITING
Fluent mirror-writing, in which all the letters are reversed, is very rare and extremely difficult for normal writers to do. It may reflect an abnormal layout of language areas in the brain.

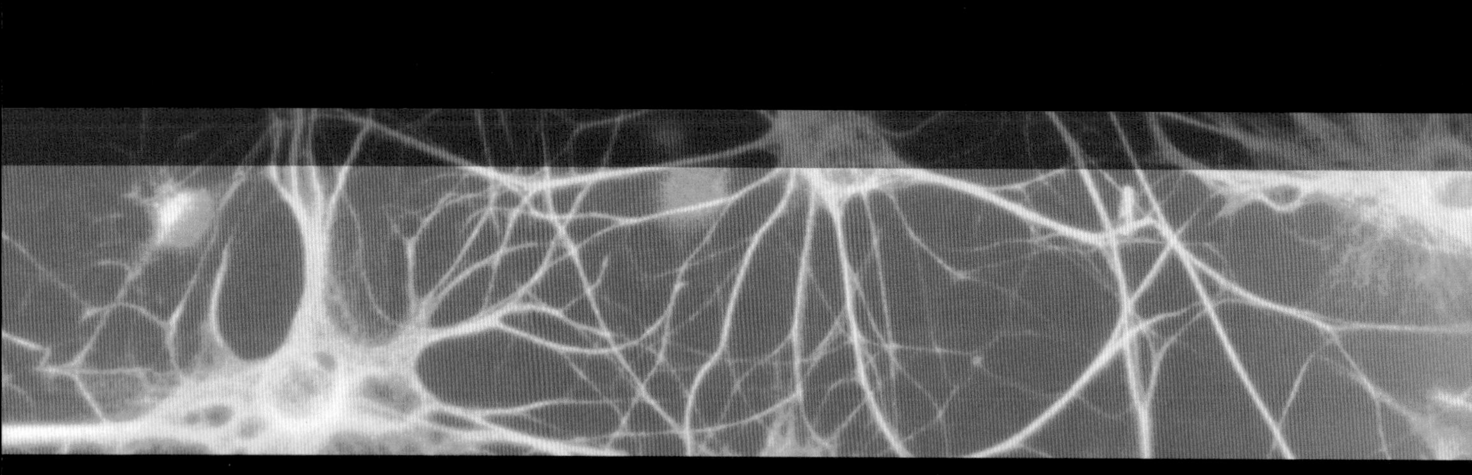

MOST OF OUR MOMENT-BY-MOMENT EXPERIENCES PASS RAPIDLY INTO OBLIVION, BUT A TINY FEW ARE ENCODED IN THE BRAIN AS MEMORIES. WHEN WE REMEMBER AN EVENT, THE NEURONS INVOLVED IN GENERATING THE ORIGINAL EXPERIENCE ARE REACTIVATED. HOWEVER, RECOLLECTIONS ARE NOT REPLAYS OF THE PAST, BUT RECONSTRUCTIONS OF IT. THE PRIMARY PURPOSE OF MEMORY IS TO PROVIDE INFORMATION TO GUIDE OUR ACTIONS IN THE PRESENT, AND TO DO THIS EFFICIENTLY WE GENERALLY RETAIN ONLY THOSE EXPERIENCES THAT ARE IN SOME WAY USEFUL. OUR RECALL OF THE PAST IS THEREFORE SELECTIVE AND UNRELIABLE.

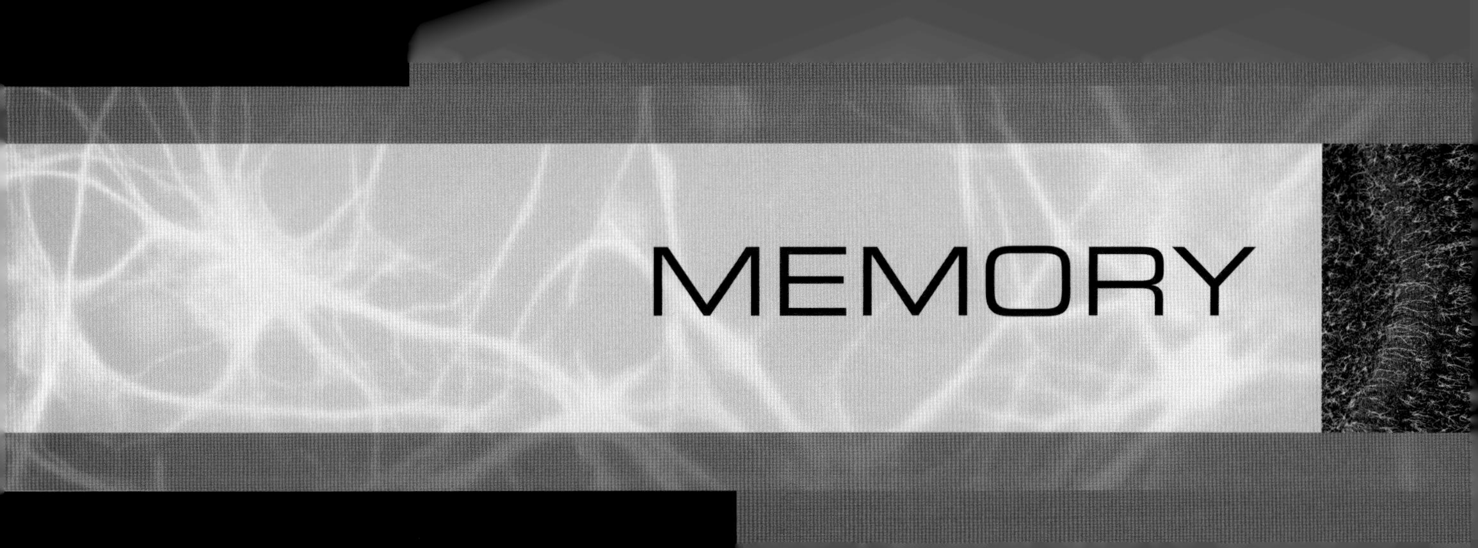

MEMORY

produce a particular experience are altered so that they have a tendency to fire together again. The subsequent combined firing of the neurons reconstructs the original experience, producing a "recollection" of it. The act of recollecting makes the neurons involved even more likely to fire again in the future, so repeatedly reconstructing an event makes it increasingly easy to recall.

	new information.	
Forgetting	Items start to be forgotten as soon as they have been registered, unless they are regularly refreshed. Unnecessary information is deleted.	Important or useful information is forgotten. Alternatively, unnecessary or even damaging memories are not.

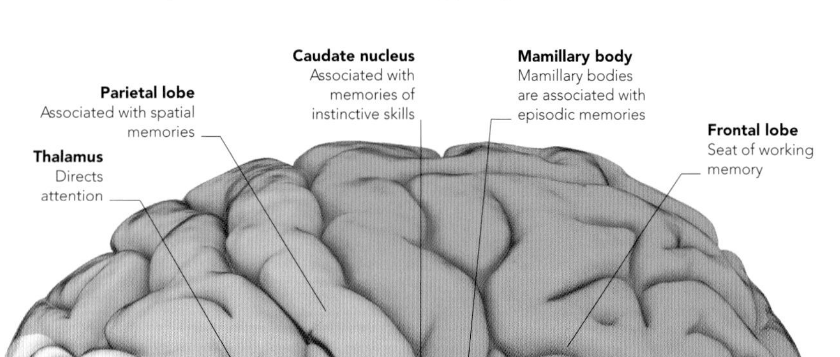

Caudate nucleus
Associated with memories of instinctive skills
Mamillary body
Mamillary bodies are associated with episodic memories
Parietal lobe
Associated with spatial memories
Thalamus
Directs attention
Frontal lobe
Seat of working memory

SHORT- AND LONG-TERM MEMORY

Short-term memories generally stay with us only so long as we need them. A telephone number you use just once is an example. Short-term memories are held in the mind by a process of "working" memory (see opposite page). Long-term memories, in contrast, can be recalled years or even decades later. The address of your childhood home may be such a memory. In between these extremes, we have many medium-term memories, which may last for months or years and finally fade away.

TYPES OF MEMORY

We have five different types of memory, for particular purposes. Episodic memory comprises reconstructions of past experiences, including sensations and emotions; these usually unfold like a movie and are experienced from one's own point of view. Semantic memory is non-personal, factual knowledge that "stands alone". Working memory is the capacity to hold information in mind for just long enough to use it. Procedural "body" memories comprise learned actions, such as walking, swimming, or riding a bicycle. Implicit memories are those we don't know we have. They affect our actions in subtle ways; for example, you might take an inexplicable dislike to a new person because they remind you of someone nasty.

LEARNING IS GOOD FOR YOU

Learning involves making new connections between clusters of neurons in different parts of the brain. This builds up the brain, making it fitter. For example, practising spatial skills such as finding your way around a city has been shown to increase the size of the rear hippocampus. The more connections you create, the better you can use what you learn and the longer it takes you to forget it.

ENLARGED AREAS
This image shows areas to do with implicit learning (red) and explicit skills (yellow) that have grown denser with practice.

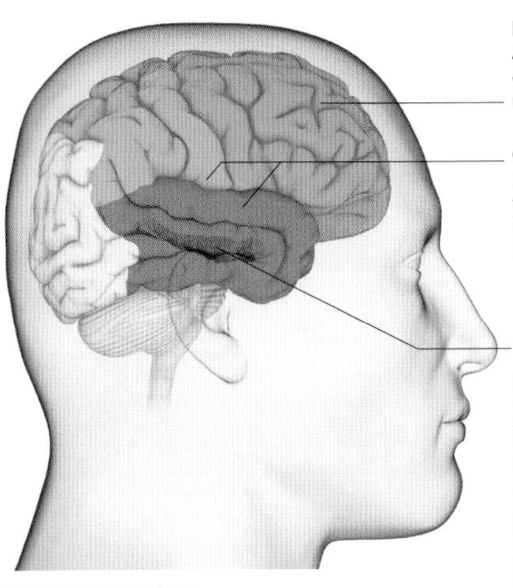

Frontal lobe
Activity here ensures that episodic memories are not mistaken for real life

Cortical areas
Episodic memories activate the areas originally involved in the experience that is being recalled

Hippocampus
Events are turned into memories here

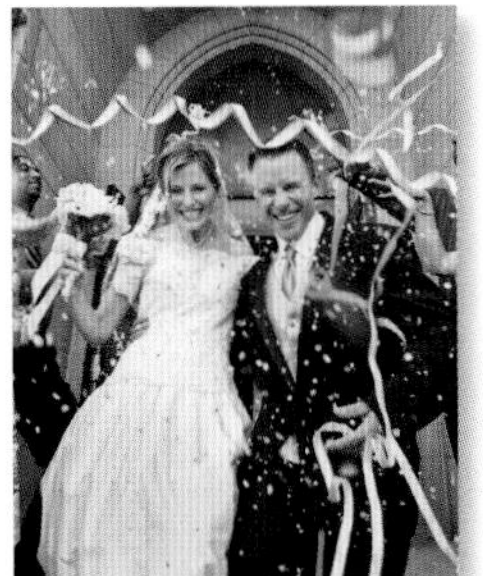

EPISODIC MEMORY
The parts of the brain involved in episodic memories depend on the content of the original experience. Highly visual experiences, for example, will activate visual areas of the brain, while remembering a person's voice will activate the auditory cortex.

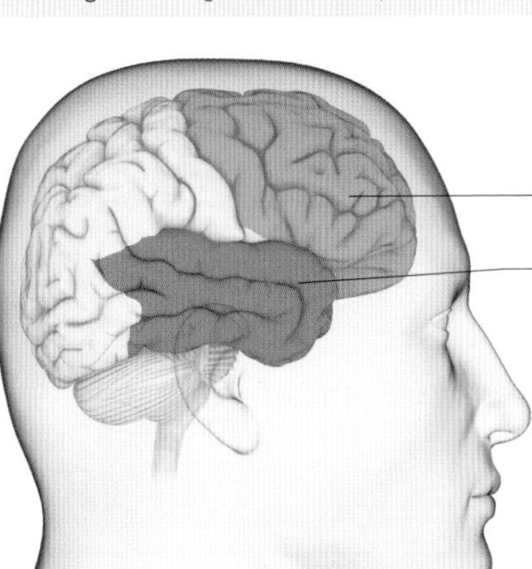

Frontal lobe
Semantic memories are activated by frontal lobe areas that draw on stored knowledge to guide current behaviour

Temporal lobe
The temporal lobes encode factual information, and activity here is a marker of facts being recalled

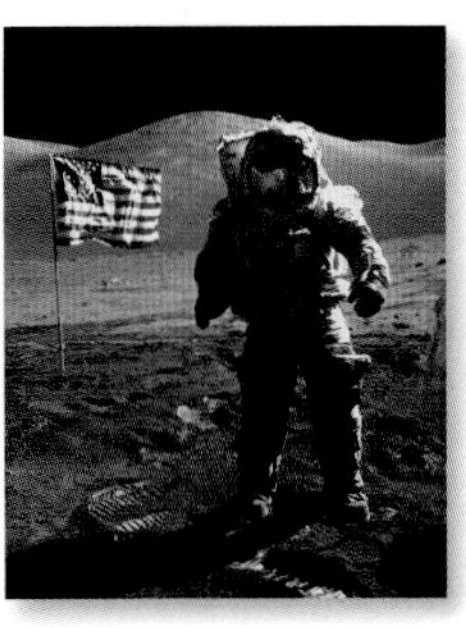

SEMANTIC MEMORY
Semantic memories are facts that may once have had a personal context but now stand as simple knowledge. The fact that a man once walked on the Moon, for example, may once have been part of your personal experience, but now it is just "knowledge".

ntral executive
olds entire plan, luding language component

Language scratch pad
Uses Broca's area as "inner voice" that repeats information

Visual scratch pad
Maintains an image of what needs to be done, by activating areas near visual cortex

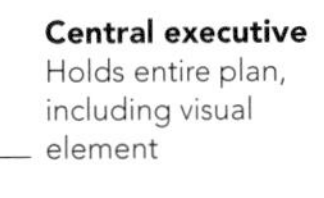

Central executive
Holds entire plan, including visual element

Phonological loop
"Inner ear" where the sounds of words are kept in mind

Visual cortex

LEFT SIDE

RIGHT SIDE

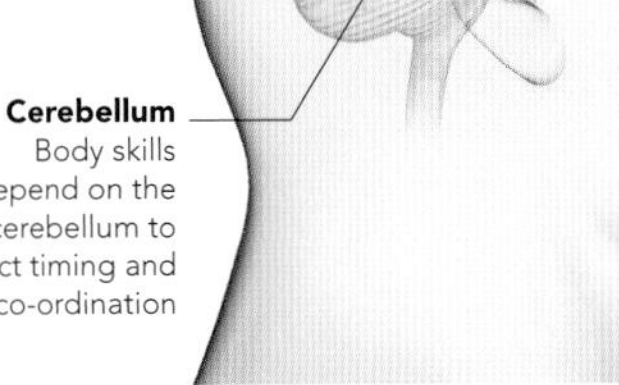

WORKING MEMORY
One part of the frontal lobes, the central executive, holds a plan of action while calling up items from the rest of the brain. There are also two neural loops, for visual data and for language; these act as scratch pads, temporarily holding data until it is erased by the next job.

Caudate nucleus
Instinctive actions such as grooming are stored here

Putamen
Learned skills such as riding a bike are stored here

Cerebellum
Body skills depend on the cerebellum to direct timing and co-ordination

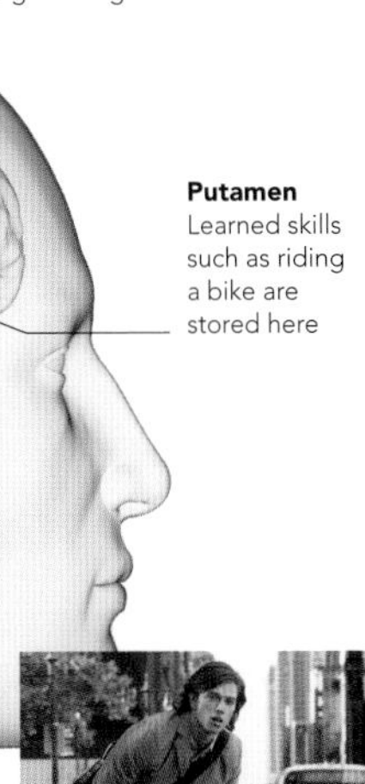

PROCEDURAL MEMORY
"Body" memories allow us to carry out ordinary motor actions automatically, once we have learned them. Such skills are stored in brain areas that lie beneath the cortex. They can be recalled to mind, but usually remain unconscious.

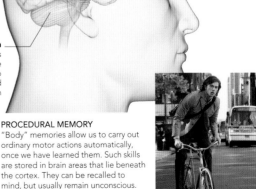

THE MEMORY WEB

MEMORIES ARE STORED IN FRAGMENTS THROUGHOUT THE BRAIN. ONE WAY TO ENVISAGE THE PATTERN OF MEMORIES IN THE BRAIN IS AS A COMPLEX WEB, IN WHICH THE THREADS SYMBOLIZE THE VARIOUS ELEMENTS OF A MEMORY THAT JOIN AT THE NODES, OR INTERSECTION POINTS, TO FORM A WHOLE, ROUNDED MEMORY OF AN OBJECT, PERSON, OR EVENT.

BRAIN–WIDE WEB

"Declarative" memories – episodes and facts you can bring to mind consciously – are laid down and accessed by the hippocampus, but are stored throughout the brain. Each element of a memory – the sight, sound, word, or emotion that it consists of – is encoded in the same part of the brain that originally created that fragment. When you recall the experience, you recreate it in essence by reactivating the neural patterns that were generated during the original experience that was encoded to memory. Take, for example, the memory of a dog you once owned. Your recall of his colour is created by the "colour" area of the visual cortex; the recollection of walking with him is reconstructed (in part at least) by the motor area of your brain; his name is stored in the language area, and so on.

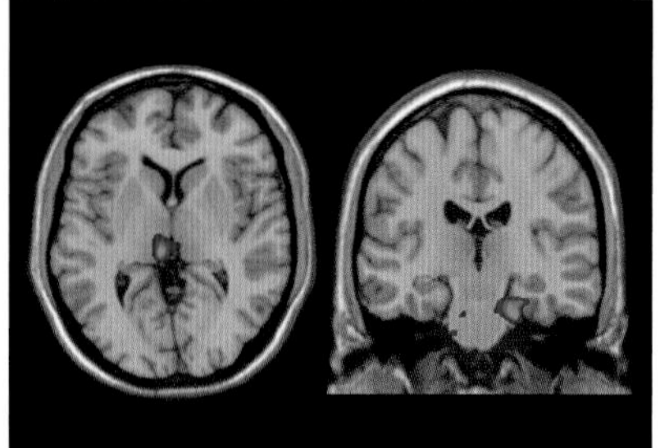

RECALLING MEMORY
The fMRI scan to the left shows activity in the pulvinar – the sensory area of the thalamus – when sensory aspects of a memory are recalled. The scan to the right shows activity in the hippocampus, which plays a central role in memory management and is strongly activated here as the person consciously tries to recall a memory.

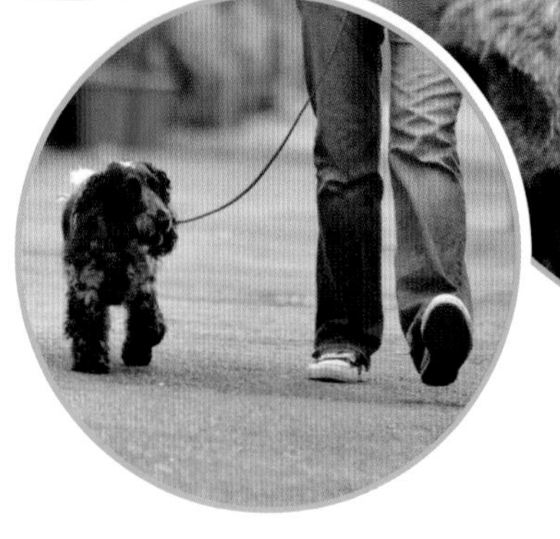

FACETS OF A MEMORY
Once a memory is sparked off, the hippocampus triggers various aspects of it in unison. If you remember a pet dog, different brain areas recall a variety of memories of the dog and peripheral items such as dog bowls, as well as memories of things connected to the idea of "dog".

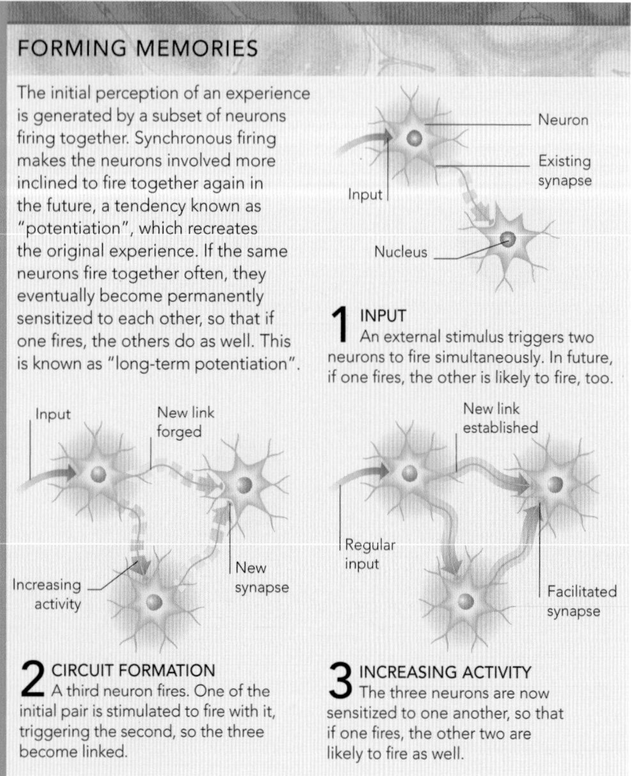

FORMING MEMORIES

The initial perception of an experience is generated by a subset of neurons firing together. Synchronous firing makes the neurons involved more inclined to fire together again in the future, a tendency known as "potentiation", which recreates the original experience. If the same neurons fire together often, they eventually become permanently sensitized to each other, so that if one fires, the others do as well. This is known as "long-term potentiation".

1 INPUT An external stimulus triggers two neurons to fire simultaneously. In future, if one fires, the other is likely to fire, too.

2 CIRCUIT FORMATION A third neuron fires. One of the initial pair is stimulated to fire with it, triggering the second, so the three become linked.

3 INCREASING ACTIVITY The three neurons are now sensitized to one another, so that if one fires, the other two are likely to fire as well.

DISTRIBUTED MEMORIES

Our memories are distributed throughout the brain, so even if one part of an experience is lost, many others will remain. One benefit of such a distributed storage system is that it makes long-term memories more or less indestructible. If they were held in a single brain area, damage to that place – for example, from a stroke or head injury – would eradicate the memory completely. As it is, brain trauma and degeneration may nibble away at memories but rarely destroy them entirely. You may lose a person's name, for example, but not the memory of their face. Some studies have found that memories persist even when the synapses encoding them are broken. This suggests that neurons themselves may also store certain aspects of memory. One theory is that dendrites – the branches on neurons that receive information from other cells – change sensitivity if they are repeatedly stimulated.

Neighbouring neuron
Circuit joins network of neurons
Input
New neuron assimilated

EXPANDING WEB
The memory web spreads through the brain as existing neurons make connections with new neurons by firing together.

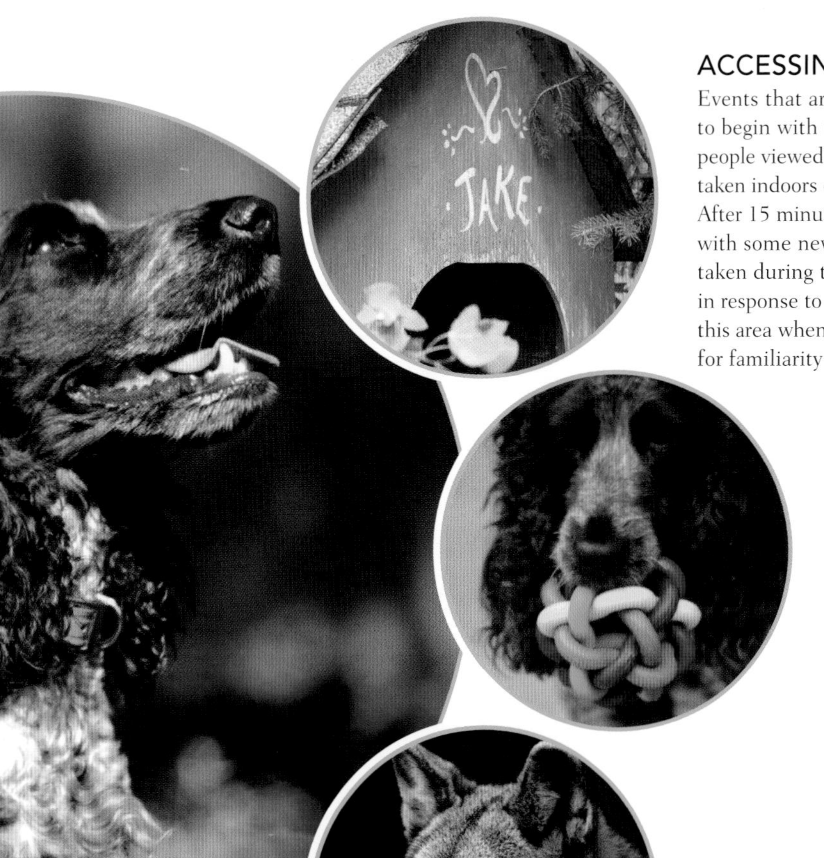

ACCESSING MEMORIES

Events that are destined to be recalled are more strongly encoded to begin with than events that are later forgotten. In one study, 16 people viewed 120 photographs and answered which pictures were taken indoors or outdoors. Each image was then shown once again. After 15 minutes, the subjects were shown the photos again, along with some new ones, and asked if they remembered them. Scans taken during the test show strong activation of the hippocampus in response to recalled photos at the first viewing, but less activity in this area when the photos were repeated. This pattern is a "marker" for familiarity (see below).

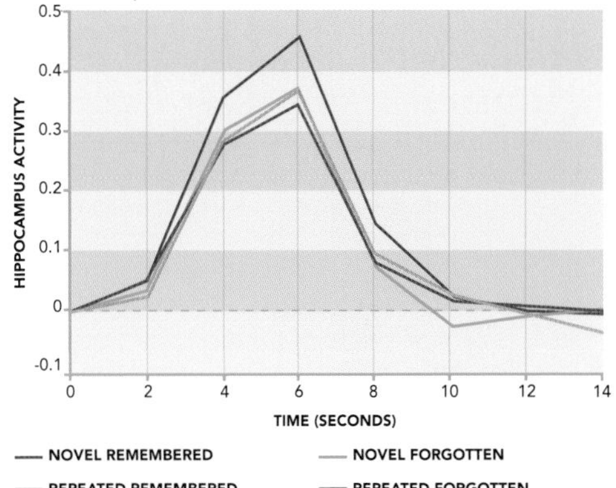

HIPPOCAMPAL ACTIVITY AND MEMORY FORMATION

Things that get remembered are marked by high activity in the hippocampus when they are first experienced but less activity when they are seen a second time. This distinguishes the recalled scenes from those that are new or forgotten.

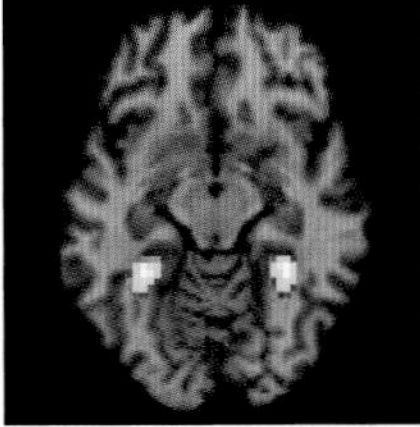

PARAHIPPOCAMPAL ACTIVITY

When you recall an episode from your life, the hippocampus and the area around it (shown in yellow on this fMRI scan) are activated. During memory recall, the hippocampus is busy pulling together the various facets of the memory from widely distributed areas of the brain.

INABILITY TO STORE

In 1953 surgery was performed on a patient known as HM to relieve the symptoms of severe epileptic seizures. The operation involved removing a large part of the hippocampus. This controlled the seizures, but it also produced a severe memory deficit. From the time HM woke up from the operation he was unable to lay down conscious memories. Day-to-day events remained in his mind for only a few seconds or minutes. When he met someone, even a person he had seen many times a day, year after year, he did not recognize them. HM believed himself to be a young man right into his eighties, because the years since his operation did not, effectively, exist for him. His case shows how essential the hippocampus is for memory storage.

THE MISSING PIECE

The hippocampus is embedded deep in the temporal lobes. Experiences "flow through it" constantly, and some of them are encoded in memory through a process of long-term potentiation. Thereafter, the hippocampus is involved in retrieving most types of memory.

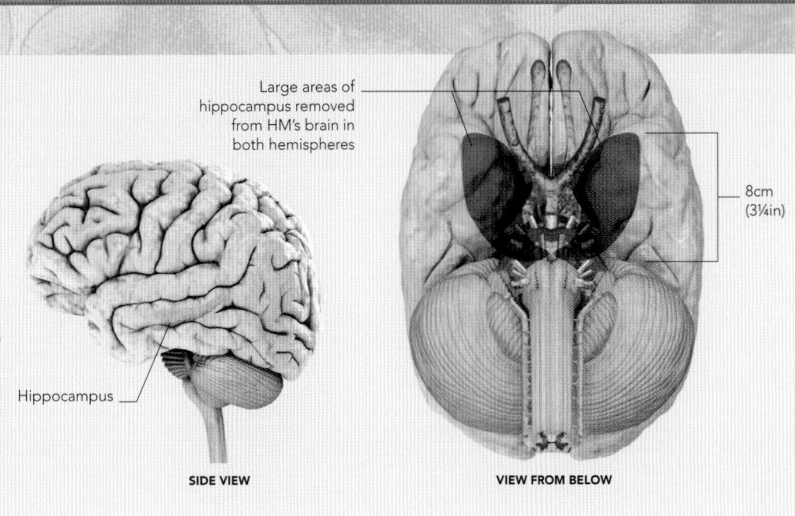

LAYING DOWN A MEMORY

MOST EXPERIENCES LEAVE NO PERMANENT TRACE. A FEW, THOUGH, ARE SO STRIKING THAT THEY ALTER THE STRUCTURE OF THE BRAIN BY FORGING NEW CONNECTIONS BETWEEN NEURONS. THESE CHANGES MAKE IT POSSIBLE FOR THE NEURAL ACTIVITY THAT GENERATED THE INITIAL EXPERIENCE TO BE RECONSTRUCTED, OR "RECOLLECTED", AT A LATER DATE.

THE ANATOMY OF MEMORY

Only experiences giving rise to unusually prolonged and/or intense neural activity become encoded as memories. It takes up to two years to consolidate the changes that create a long-term memory (see sequence below) but, once encoded, that memory may remain available for life. Long-term memories include events from a person's own life (episodic memories) and impersonal facts (semantic memories). Together, these are termed "declarative memories", as they can be recalled consciously ("declared"). Procedural (body) memories and implicit (unconscious) memories may also be stored long-term.

Somatosensory cortex

Gustatory association cortex

Visual association cortex

Auditory association cortex

Hippocampus The hippocampus encodes new memories, and helps to recall some others

Amygdala

Olfactory cortex

MEMORY MAKERS
Experiences that become memories are usually prolonged or emotionally charged, and register strongly in the sensory cortices and hippocampus.

FORMING A LONG-TERM MEMORY

0.2 seconds Attention

The brain can only absorb a finite amount of sensory input at any point. It can sample a little input about several events at once, or focus attention on one event and extract lots of information from that alone. Attention causes the neurons that register the event to fire more frequently. Such activity makes the experience more intense; it also increases the likelihood that the event will be encoded as a memory. This is because the more a neuron fires, the stronger connections it makes with other brain cells.

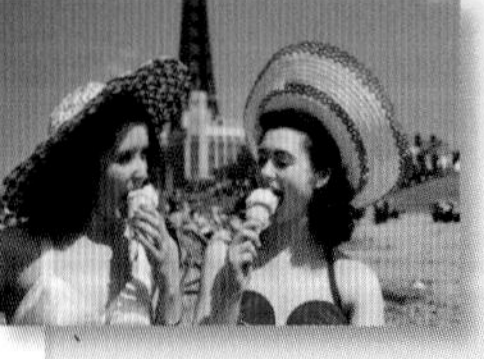

MEMORABLE EVENT
Zooming in on an event helps to capture it as a memory, rather like a camera taking a snap.

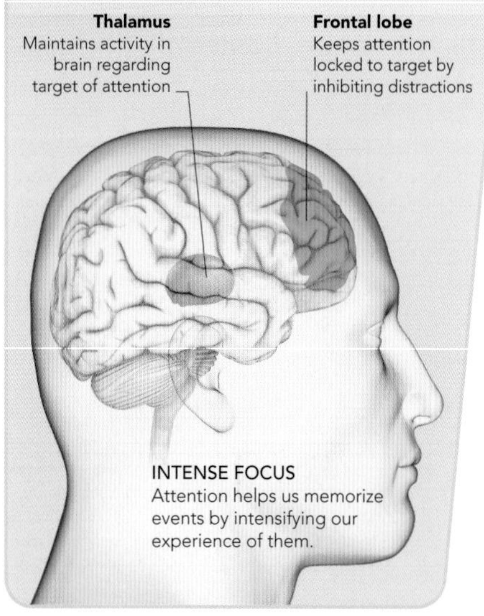
Thalamus
Maintains activity in brain regarding target of attention
Frontal lobe
Keeps attention locked to target by inhibiting distractions

INTENSE FOCUS
Attention helps us memorize events by intensifying our experience of them.

0.25 seconds Emotion

Intensely emotional experiences, such as the birth of a child, are more likely to be laid down in memory because emotion increases attention. The emotional information from a stimulus is processed initially along an unconscious pathway that leads to the amygdala; this can produce an emotional response even before the person knows what they are reacting to, as in the "fight or flight" response. Some traumatic events may be permanently stored in the amygdala.

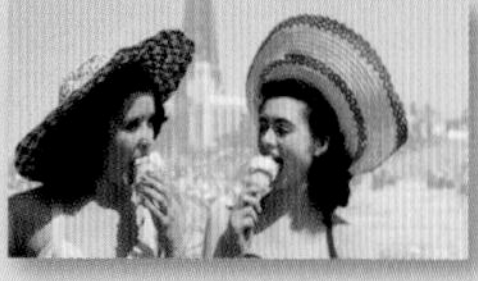

EMOTIONAL EVENTS
Personal interactions and other emotional events "grab" attention, so are more likely to be stored.

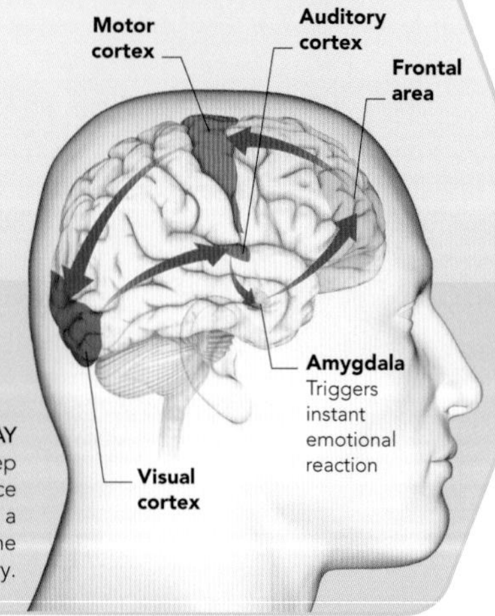
Motor cortex
Auditory cortex
Frontal area
Amygdala
Triggers instant emotional reaction
Visual cortex

EMOTION PATHWAY
The amygdala helps keep an emotional experience "live" by replaying it in a loop, which begins the encoding of a memory.

0.2–0.5 seconds Sensation

Most memories derive from events that included sights, sounds, and other sensory experiences. The more intense the sensations, the more likely it is that the experience is remembered. The sensational parts of such "episodic" memories may later be forgotten, leaving only a residue of factual knowledge. For example, a person's first experience of seeing the Blackpool Tower may be reduced to the simple "fact" of what the tower looks like. When the tower is recalled, it triggers a ghost of a visual image, encoded in the sight area of the brain.

TASTE
Sensory perceptions, such as taste, sight, or smell, form the raw material of memories.

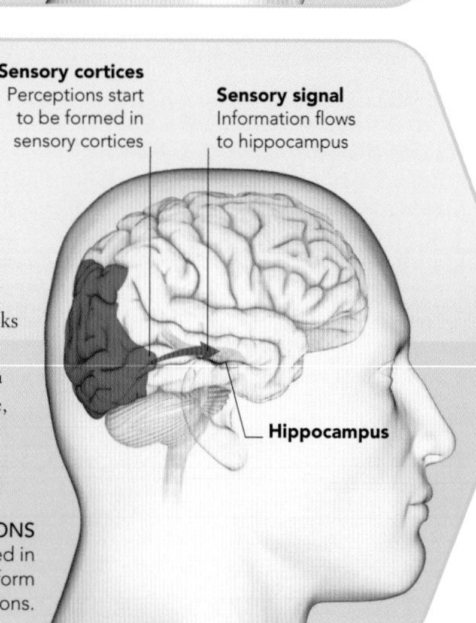
Sensory cortices
Perceptions start to be formed in sensory cortices
Sensory signal
Information flows to hippocampus
Hippocampus

FORMING PERCEPTIONS
Sensations are combined in association areas, to form conscious perceptions.

HIPPOCAMPUS REPLACEMENT

Neuroscientists from the University of Southern California, in Los Angeles, have developed an artificial hippocampus that may one day help people with dementia to halt memory loss. A small pilot study in which people were fitted with the implant showed that their memory for images improved over their previous performance by nearly 40 per cent. The researchers first devised a model of how the hippocampus performs by observing its input–output patterns. Then they built the model into a silicon chip designed to interface with the brain, taking the place of damaged tissue. One side of the chip records the electrical activity coming in from the rest of the brain, while the other sends appropriate electrical instructions back out to the brain.

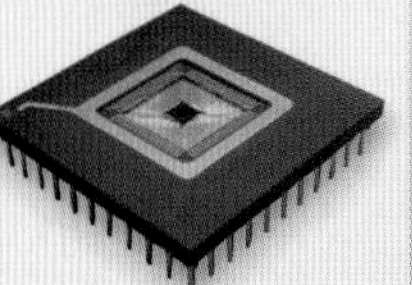

MEMORY CHIP
The chip is designed to be spliced into the hippocampus and communicate with the brain through electrodes placed on either side of the damaged area.

THE LOCATION OF MEMORIES

After consolidation, long-term memories are stored throughout the brain as groups of neurons that are primed to fire together in the same pattern that created the original experience. "Whole" memories are divided into their components (sensations, emotions, thoughts, and so on); each component is stored in the brain area that initiated it. Groups of neurons in the visual cortex, for instance, will encode a sight, and neurons in the amygdala will store an emotion. The simultaneous firing of all these groups constructs the memory in its entirety.

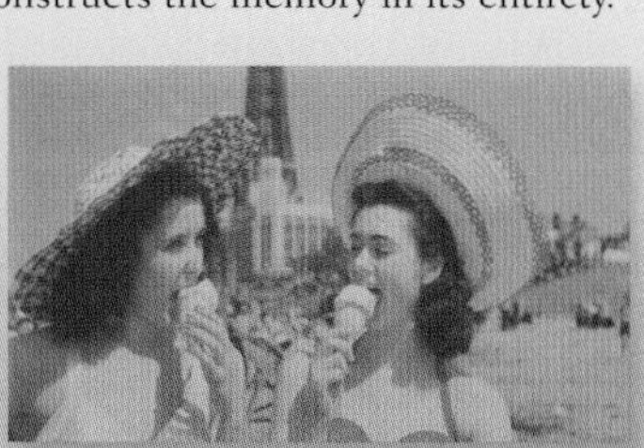

LASTING IMPRESSION
Some memories seem to be cast in stone. In fact, no recollection is ever perfectly sharp or complete.

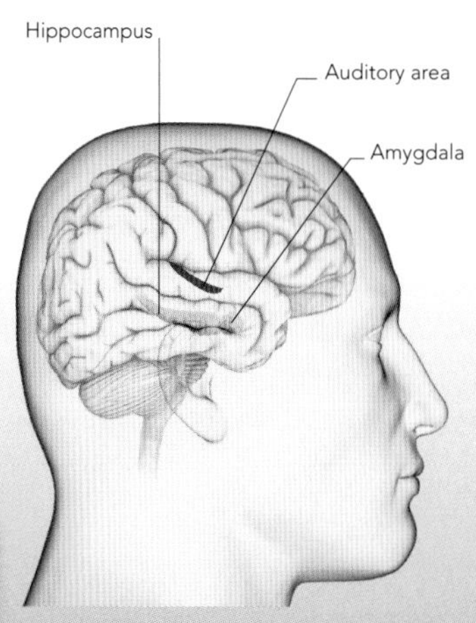

MEMORY STORE
Memories are encoded in the neurons that created them: for example, sounds in the auditory cortex and emotions in the amygdala. The hippocampus pulls them together.

0.5 seconds–10 minutes
Working memory

Short-term, or "working", memory is like text on a whiteboard that is constantly refreshed. It begins with an experience, and continues as that experience is "held in mind" by repetition. A telephone number, for example, may be repeated for as long as it takes to dial. Working memory is thought to involve two neural circuits (see p.157) around which the information is kept alive for as long as it is needed. One circuit is for visual and spatial information, and the other for sound. The routes of the circuits encompass the sensory cortices, where the experience is registered, and the frontal lobes, where it is consciously noted. The flow of information into and around these circuits is controlled by neurons in the prefrontal cortex.

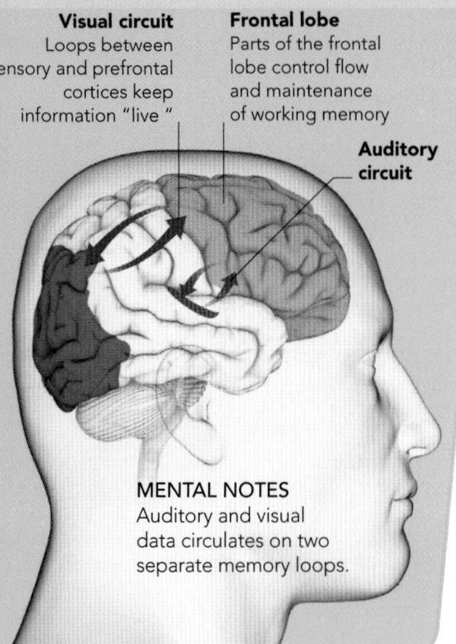

MENTAL NOTES
Auditory and visual data circulates on two separate memory loops.

10 minutes–2 years
Hippocampal processing

Particularly striking experiences "break out" from working memory and travel to the hippocampus, where they undergo further processing. They cause neural activity that loops around coiled layers of tissue; the hippocampal neurons start to encode this information permanently by a process called long-term potentiation (see p.158). The strongest information "plays back" to the parts of the brain that first registered it. A sight, for example, returns to the visual cortex, where it is replayed as an echo of the original event.

Hippocampus
Information circulates here, then returns to brain areas where it originated

Entorhinal cortex
Collects information from many different areas of brain

One-way system
Information follows a one-way path as it is encoded

PREPARATION FOR STORAGE
This activity in the hippocampus begins to turn short-term memories into those that might remain for life.

2 years onwards
Consolidation

It takes up to two years for a memory to become firmly consolidated in the brain, and even after that it may be altered or lost. During this time, the neural firing patterns that encode an experience are played back and forth between the hippocampus and the cortex. This prolonged, repetitive "dialogue" causes the pattern to be shifted from the hippocampus to the cortex; this may happen in order to free up hippocampal processing space for new information. The dialogue takes place largely during sleep. The "quiet" or slow-wave phase of sleep is thought to be more important to this process than rapid eye movement sleep (see p.188).

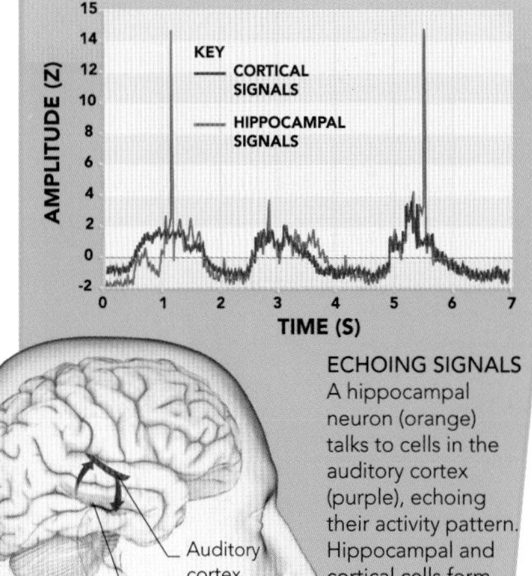

ECHOING SIGNALS
A hippocampal neuron (orange) talks to cells in the auditory cortex (purple), echoing their activity pattern. Hippocampal and cortical cells form almost identical copies of the same experience.

RECALL AND RECOGNITION

MEMORIES OCCUR WHEN THE BRAIN "REPLAYS" A PATTERN OF NEURAL ACTIVITY THAT WAS ORIGINALLY GENERATED IN RESPONSE TO A PARTICULAR EVENT. SO SIMILAR IS THE PATTERN TO THE ORIGINAL THAT THE MEMORY ECHOES THE BRAIN'S PERCEPTION OF THE REAL EVENT. BUT THESE REPLAYS ARE NEVER IDENTICAL TO THE ORIGINAL – IF THEY WERE, WE WOULD NOT KNOW THE DIFFERENCE BETWEEN THE GENUINE EXPERIENCE AND THE MEMORY.

THE NATURE OF MEMORIES

When we recall an event, we re-experience it – but only up to a point. Even when "lost" in reminiscence, we maintain some awareness of the present moment, so the neural activity is not identical to the one that produced the remembered event. Rather, the experience is that of the original mixed with an awareness of the current situation. This experience of remembering "overwrites" the memory, so each time an event is brought to mind it is really a recollection of the last time we remembered it. Hence, memories gradually change over the years, until eventually they might bear very little resemblance to the original event.

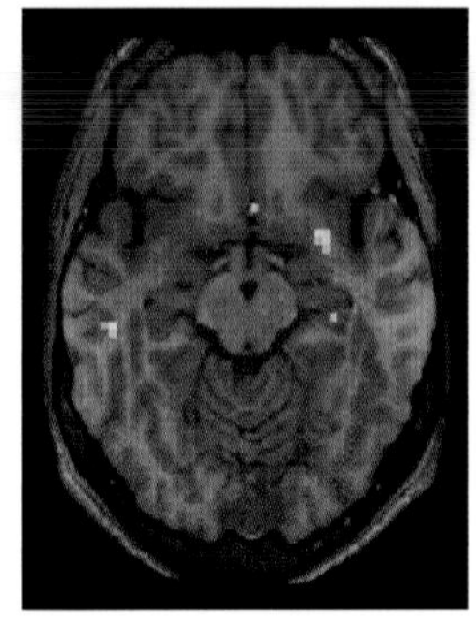
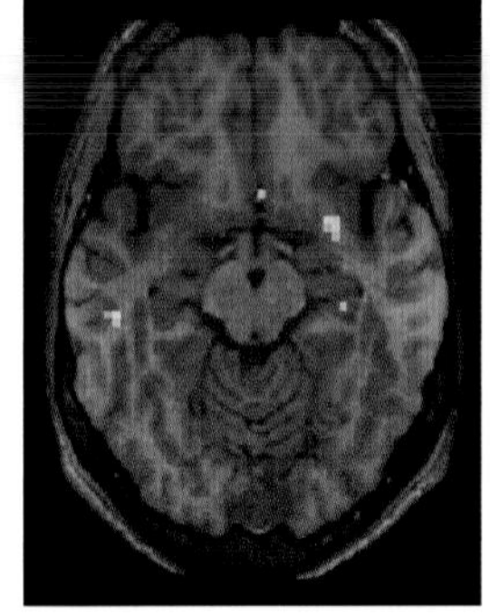

SENSORY MEMORY
Tests using fMRI scans show that objects we associate with specific smells spark activity in the olfactory cortex (largest yellow area). In this way, cues trigger all senses, conjuring detailed memories.

STATE-DEPENDENT MEMORY

If you learn or experience something when in a certain state of mind or while concurrently experiencing a particular sensation, you will subsequently recall it more readily when you are again in that state. For example, if you read a book on a sunny beach during a holiday, you may appear to forget it completely when you get home. But years later, on another sunny beach, the plot may come flooding back. Similarly, certain behaviours may be learned when in a particular situation or state of mind, and subsequently displayed only when in the same situation or state of mind, and "forgotten" at other times, giving the impression that the person has more than one personality.

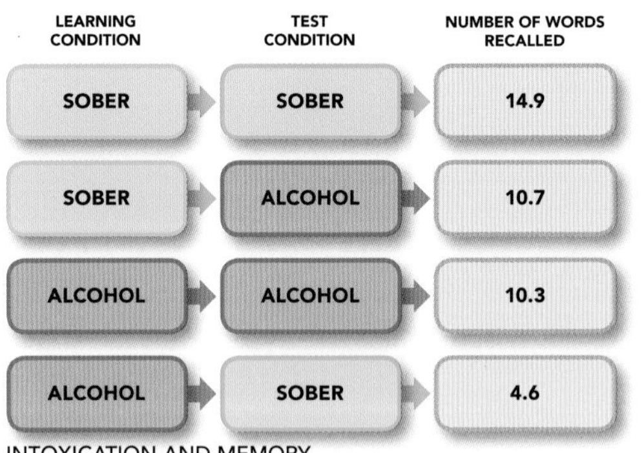

LEARNING CONDITION	TEST CONDITION	NUMBER OF WORDS RECALLED
SOBER	SOBER	14.9
SOBER	ALCOHOL	10.7
ALCOHOL	ALCOHOL	10.3
ALCOHOL	SOBER	4.6

INTOXICATION AND MEMORY
Subjects drank a nonalcoholic or alcoholic beverage prior to studying a list of words, later recalling them while sober or intoxicated. Those intoxicated in both phases recalled more words than those intoxicated in the study phase only.

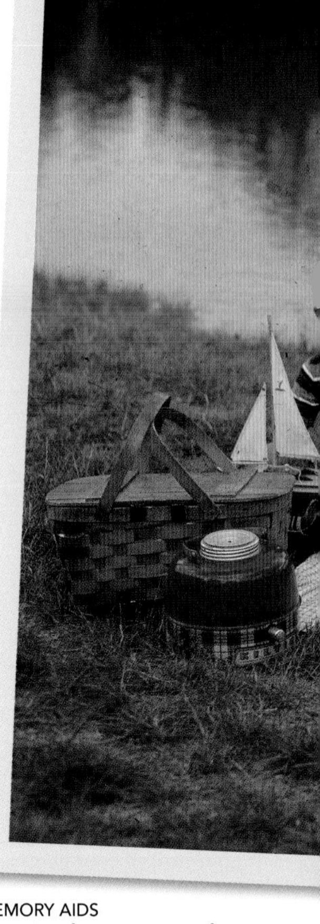

MEMORY AIDS
Memories of past events are often "jogged" into consciousness when we re-encounter some of the sensations involved in the original experience. Photographs and similar memory aids work in this way. Even if the sensations they trigger are not identical to the original ones, they are likely to be similar enough to jog memories of the same period.

SPATIAL MEMORY

The structure of the human brain reveals just how important spatial orientation and memory are for our species. The whole parietal lobe of the brain – the area under the crown of the skull – is given over to "maps" of our bodies and of our position in space. Also, a sizeable part of the hippocampus is concerned with registering the landscape through which we travel and laying down memory maps. Damage to either of these areas can seriously affect a person's ability to find their way around. If the "navigation" area of the hippocampus is affected by stroke or injury, for instance, a person may lose the ability to remember new routes.

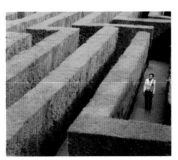

MAZE-MINDED
People who can find their way out of mazes use the hippocampus in both hemispheres. Those who remain lost use one side only.

THE KNOWLEDGE

Some people have better memories for places than others. In part, this is a matter of habit and training – those whose lives depend on their ability to find their way around vast tracts of land naturally attend more closely to landmarks. London taxi drivers, for example, are famously adept at finding their way around the city's labyrinthine streets. Their skill is developed during a two-year training, known as "the knowledge", during which time they "exercise" the part of the hippocampus responsible for spatial memory. The training seems to increase the size of the hippocampus, much as a muscle is enlarged by weight training.

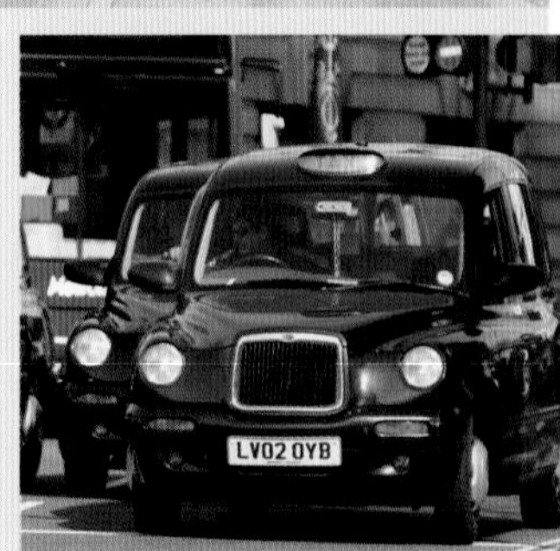

NATURAL NAVIGATORS
A brain-scanning study found that the rear hippocampus, which encodes spatial memories, is larger in taxi drivers.

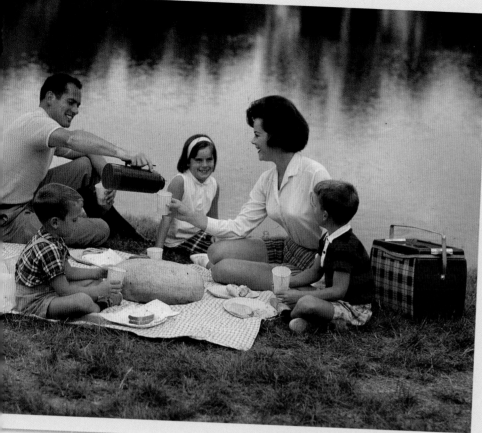

DÉJÀ VU AND JAMAIS VU

Déjà vu is characterized by a sudden, intense feeling of familiarity and the sense that you have experienced the same moment before. One explanation for this is that the new situation triggers a memory of a similar experience in the past, but the recollection is confused with the present as it is recalled, creating a sense of recognition without bringing to mind the previous event. Research suggests that déjà vu occurs when a new situation is mistakenly "marked" as familiar when processed in the limbic system. Jamais vu, by contrast, occurs when one is in a situation that should be familiar, but which seems strange. You might suddenly find your own home to be unfamiliar, for instance. Jamais vu is thought to be a glitch in recognition, whereby the emotional input that usually accompanies familiar experiences fails to occur.

RECOGNITION

Recognizing a person fully involves collating a huge number of memories. They include different types of facts about the person – I know him/he owns a dog/he walked right past me the last time I saw him/his name is Bill. At the same time, you have an emotional reaction to the person based on memories, which produces the feeling of familiarity. Most or all of this happens unconsciously – you see the person and immediately "know" who it is.

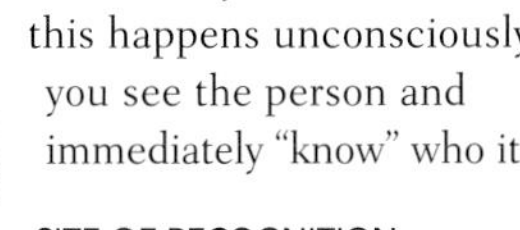

SITE OF RECOGNITION
This area processes the sight of a face (see p.84) by extracting information about expression and familiarity.

EMOTIONAL RECOGNITION

When you spot someone you know, the information is first processed by the visual cortex, and is then shunted through the brain along different pathways (see pp.84–85) as shown on this diagram (right). One path travels through the limbic areas that generate a sense of familiarity – separate from conscious recognition – when a familiar person is seen. If this route is blocked, a person may recognize consciously that they know a person, but feel strangely detached from them. Without this input, even one's nearest relatives would feel like strangers.

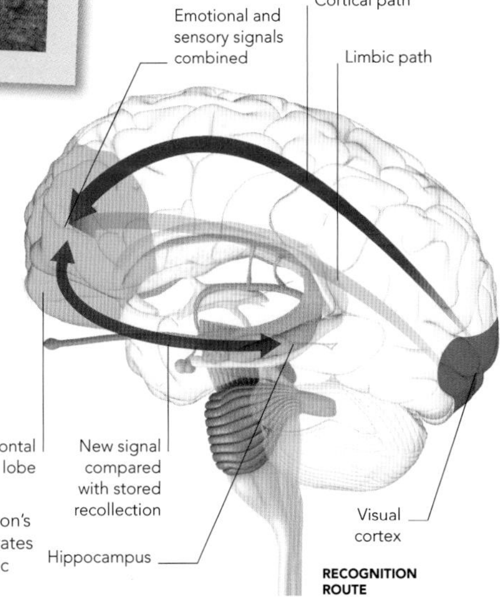

RECOGNITION PATHWAYS
The cortical path (red) processes data about a person's movements and intentions. Another (purple) generates conscious knowledge of who a person is. The limbic path (yellow) generates a sense of familiarity.

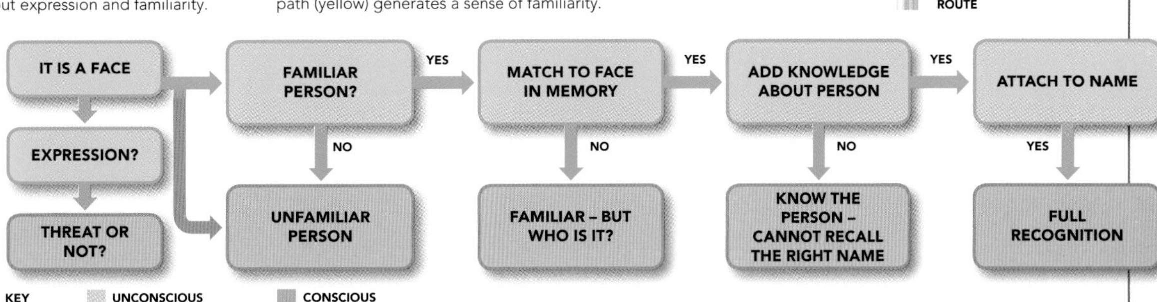

RECOGNIZING A PERSON
Recognizing a person and assigning them their correct name is a complicated process. When it works properly, it seems easy, because it happens unconsciously and apparently instantly. But if the process fails at any stage, recognition is incomplete.

UNUSUAL MEMORY

"BAD" MEMORY USUALLY MEANS FORGETTING. BUT THERE ARE MANY OTHER TYPES OF MEMORY PROBLEM: CLEAR BUT FALSE RECOLLECTION, BLURRED MEMORIES, AND INTRUSIVE FLASHBACK MEMORIES OF TRAUMATIC EVENTS. IT IS EVEN POSSIBLE TO REMEMBER THINGS TOO CLEARLY.

FORGETTING

The purpose of human memory is to use past events to guide future actions, and keeping a perfect and complete record of the past is not a useful way to achieve this. It is more important to be able to generalize from experience. When you first drive a car, for example, you learn the pedal positions of the first vehicle you use. Subsequently, when you get in any car, you assume that the pedal positions are the same. The specific memory of the layout of one particular car is lost while the general knowledge, the position of the pedals, is retained. Forgetting specifics is not a fault – it is essential.

FALSE MEMORY

Our brains sometimes lay down memories that are false from the start. This usually happens because an event is misinterpreted. For example, if you expect to see a particular thing something similar may easily be mistaken for it. The memory will be of what was assumed to be there, rather than what really was. False memories can also be created during, what seems like, recall. If a person is persuaded that a given thing happened to them they may "patch together" the event from scraps of other memories and then experience it as a "real" recollection.

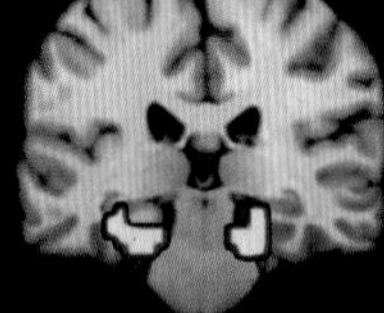

HIPPOCAMPAL ACTIVITY

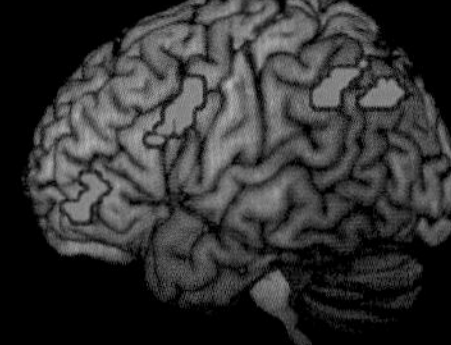

FRONTAL AND PARIETAL ACTIVITY

CONFIDENT RECALL
True memory (left) sparks activity in the hippocampus, which "lays down" memory. Confident recall of false memory (right) activates frontal areas associated with familiarity rather than precise recollections.

TRAUMATIC MEMORY

Post Traumatic Stress Disorder (PTSD) is a condition in which people have vivid "flashback" memories of a traumatic experience (see p.241). Such memories can ambush a person out of the blue – the sound of a car back-firing, for example, may plunge a soldier back into the middle of a gunfight, complete with the emotions they experienced at the time. Emotionally traumatic experiences are by their nature more likely to be remembered because emotion amplifies experience. Yet there is also a strong incentive to put such events "out of mind" and it seems the brain has a mechanism that can make this possible. Experts have found that the brain is able to block memories at will (see below).

SUPERMEMORY

Some people have extraordinarily clear memories for events that happened to them or that were of particular interest to them. For example, an American woman can recount details of every TV programme she has seen, and an Australian woman recalls every birthday she's had since she was one. The condition is called hyperthymesia, and brain scans of people who display it often show markers suggestive of synaesthesia or obsessive-compulsive disorder. It is also associated with autism, though not exclusively.

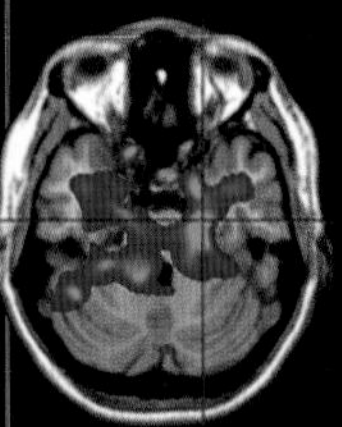

ACTIVE SUPPRESSION

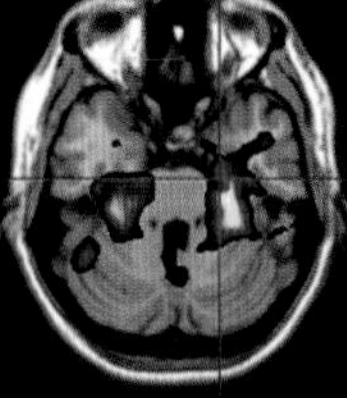

ACTIVE RECALL

ACTIVE MEMORY
Emotional memory recall activates the hippocampus and amygdala (emotion). If the memory is suppressed there is less activity in these areas and in brain areas that recreate the sensations associated with the recalled event.

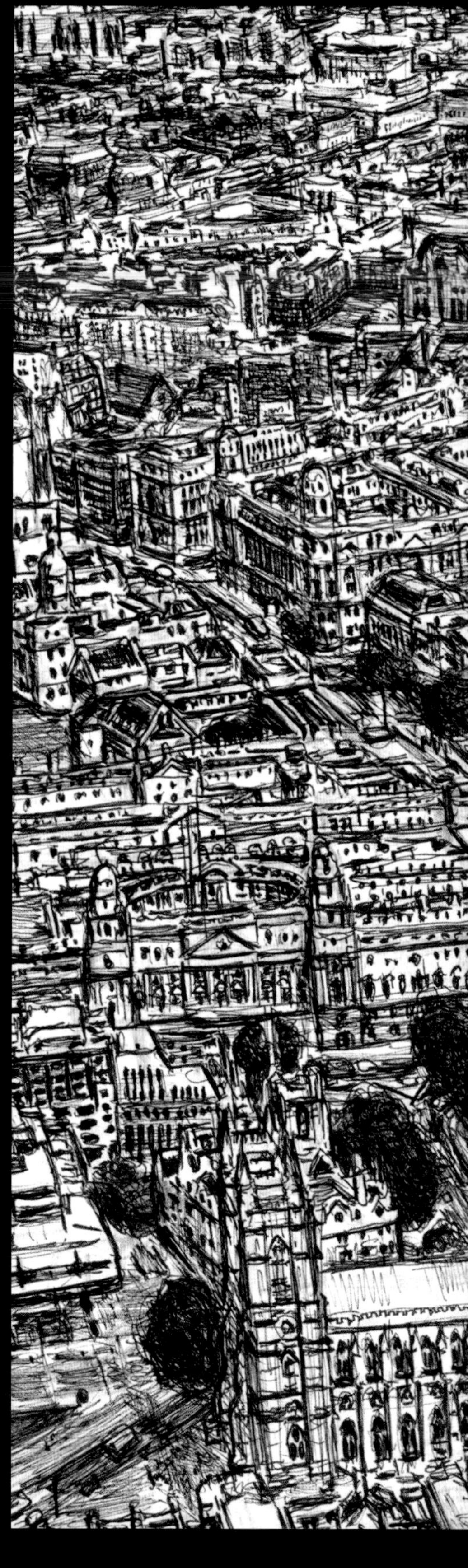

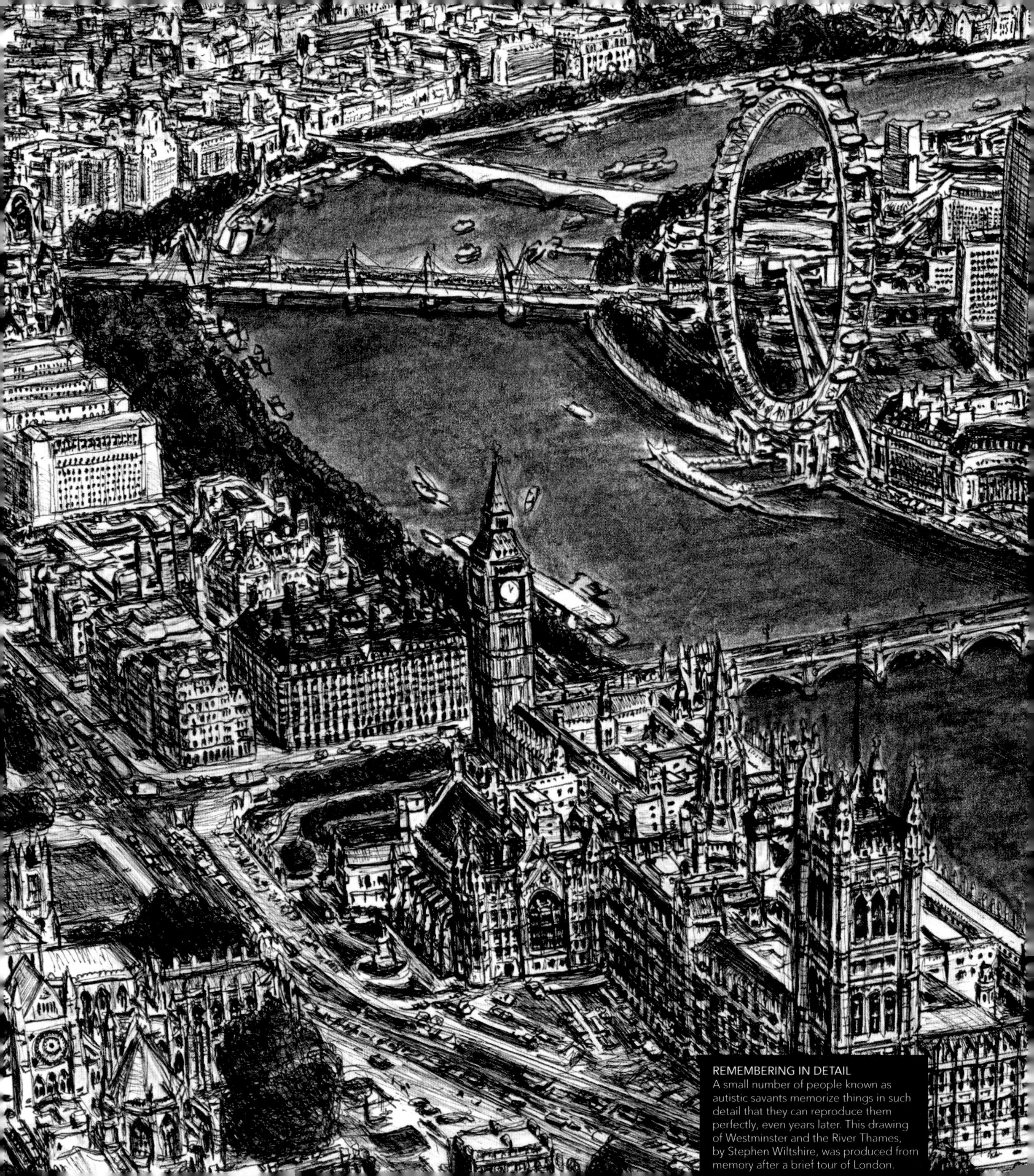

REMEMBERING IN DETAIL
A small number of people known as autistic savants memorize things in such detail that they can reproduce them perfectly, even years later. This drawing of Westminster and the River Thames, by Stephen Wiltshire, was produced from memory after a brief tour of London.

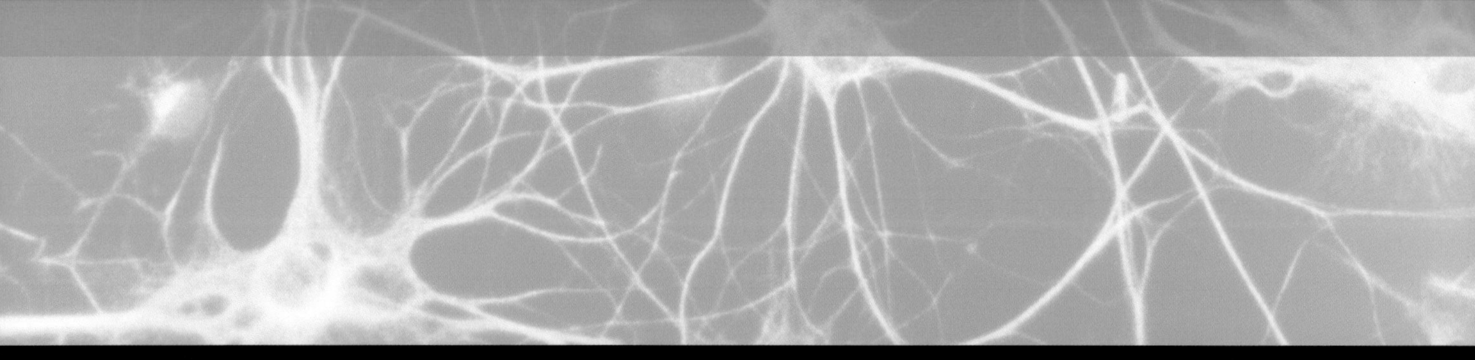

DECIDING WHAT TO DO IN A COMPLEX WORLD TAKES THOUGHT. BY THINKING WE CAN EXPLORE THE POTENTIAL CONSEQUENCES OF OUR ACTIONS IN OUR IMAGINATION. THIS, IN TURN, INVOLVES HOLDING ONE OR MORE IDEAS IN MIND AND MANIPULATING THEM. THINKING IS AN ACTIVE, CONSCIOUS, ATTENTION-DEMANDING PROCESS THAT USUALLY DRAWS ON SEVERAL AREAS OF THE BRAIN. THINKING UNDERPINS SOME PARTICULARLY HUMAN ABILITIES AND TENDENCIES, INCLUDING CREATIVITY AND THE CONSTRUCTION OF IMAGINATIVE EXPLANATIONS

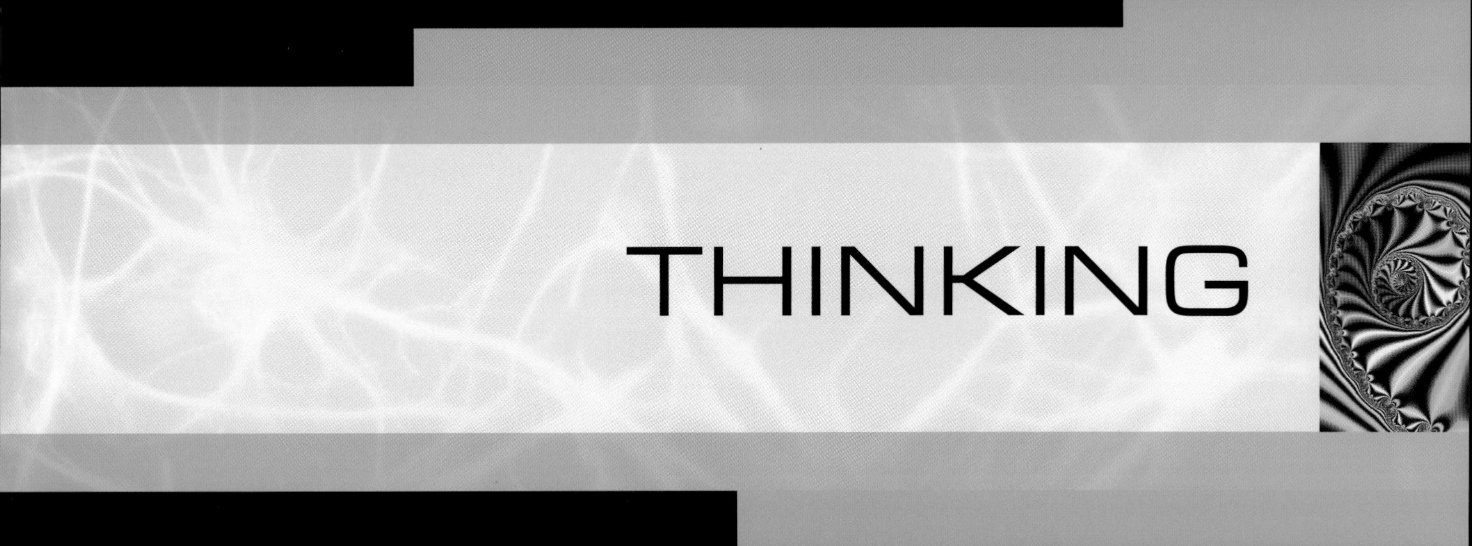

THINKING

INTELLIGENCE

"INTELLIGENCE" REFERS TO THE ABILITY TO LEARN ABOUT, LEARN FROM, UNDERSTAND, AND INTERACT WITH ONE'S ENVIRONMENT. IT EMBRACES MANY DIFFERENT TYPES OF SKILL SUCH AS PHYSICAL DEXTERITY, VERBAL FLUENCY, CONCRETE AND ABSTRACT REASONING, SENSORY DISCRIMINATION, EMOTIONAL SENSITIVITY, NUMERACY, AND ALSO THE ABILITY TO FUNCTION WELL IN SOCIETY.

THE BRAIN'S SUPERHIGHWAY

The frontal lobes are thought to be the seat of intelligence, as damage to these areas affects the ability to concentrate, make sound judgements, and so on. Yet frontal-lobe damage does not always affect a person's IQ ("intelligence quotient", measured by testing spatial, verbal, and mathematical dexterity), so other brain areas must also be involved. Research suggests that intelligence relies on a neural "superhighway" linking the frontal lobes, which plan and organize, with the parietal lobes, which integrate sensory information. The speed at which the frontal lobes receive ready-to-use data via this route may affect IQ, as does the extent to which frontal-lobe activity is enhanced by education.

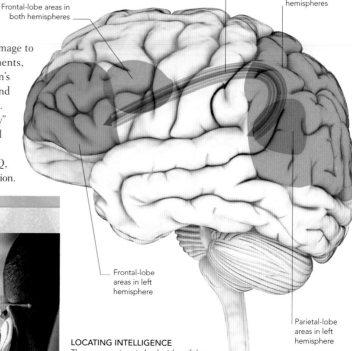

Pathway of data from parietal lobe to frontal lobe

Parietal-lobe areas in both hemispheres

Frontal-lobe areas in both hemispheres

Frontal-lobe areas in left hemisphere

Parietal-lobe areas in left hemisphere

LOCATING INTELLIGENCE
There are regions in both sides of the brain (orange) as well as areas in the left hemisphere only (blue) that are strongly associated with intelligence and reasoning. The arcuate fasciculus (green), a thick bundle of nerve fibres, provides a neural link between the parietal and frontal lobes.

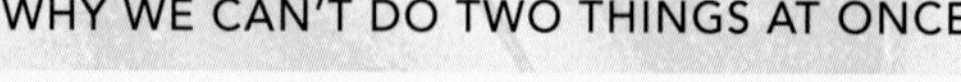

WHY WE CAN'T DO TWO THINGS AT ONCE

If you try to do something while still working on a previous task, your brain stalls. This may be because the prefrontal cortex, which disengages attention from one task and switches it to another, cannot do so instantly, resulting in a short "processing gap". The brain is also unable to do two similar things simultaneously as the tasks compete for the same neurons. For example, listening to speech while reading words activates overlapping brain areas, so is difficult to achieve, but listening to speech while looking at a landscape is easy.

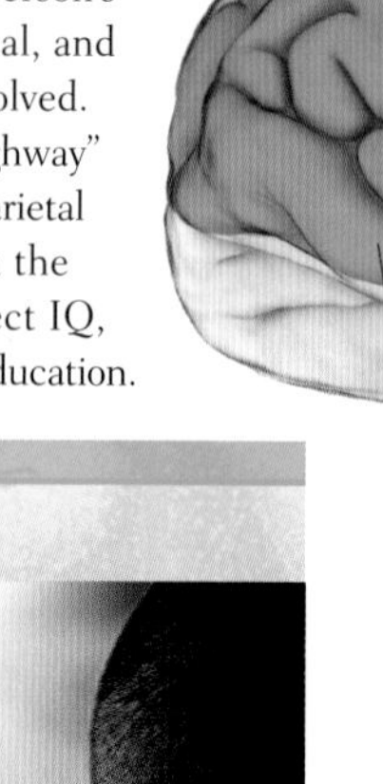

JUGGLING TASKS
The brain needs a minimum of 300 milliseconds to switch from one distinct task to the next. This "processing gap" makes a task combination such as talking on a phone while driving potentially lethal.

THE DARK SIDE OF BEING BRIGHT

Having a high IQ is generally advantageous, but it is associated with mental ill health. A study of members of MENSA, a club for people with high IQ, found a disproportionate number suffered mental problems. The reason for the link is not clear – it might be because intelligence often coincides with creativity, which is associated with abstract thoughts rather than practical matters. Grappling with big ideas may create stress, which triggers some conditions. Studies suggest high IQ is a sign of hyper brain activity, which also manifests as mental instability.

SUPER-CHARGED
Some researchers think high IQ may signify a hyperactive brain, within a hyperactive body. This may result in vulnerability to a range of conditions.

KEY
AVERAGE IQ, DISORDER DIAGNOSED
HIGH IQ, DISORDER DIAGNOSED

HIGH IQ, DISORDER DIAGNOSED AND SELF-DIAGNOSED

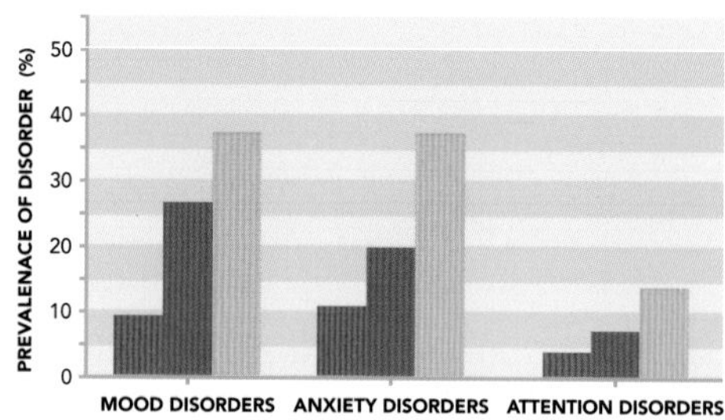

WHAT CONTRIBUTES TO INTELLIGENCE?

Tests for IQ measure general intelligence rather than quantity of knowledge or the level of a specific skill. A score of 100 is average, and the vast majority of people fall in the range of 80–120. High scores are correlated with a number of both social and physical factors.

FACTOR	EFFECT
Genes	There are thought to be about 50 different genes related directly to IQ, but so far very few have been identified. Identical twins raised apart typically have very similar IQs, even when raised in strikingly different environments.
Brain size	Those with bigger brains compared to other members of the same sex seem to have a slight intelligence advantage. Overall size, however, may be less important than the size, or neural density, of areas concerned with reasoning.
Signalling efficiency	The smoothness and speed of neural signalling may determine how much information is available for action and how well it can be integrated into plans. Depression, tiredness, and some types of illness reduce efficiency.
Environment	A stimulating, social environment in infancy is essential for normal brain development and continues to be important throughout childhood. Verbal interaction seems to be especially useful for IQ.

MAKING DECISIONS

Intelligence is largely the ability to make sensible decisions, which involves calculating pros and cons. First, the brain assesses the "goal value" – the reward expected as a result of the decision. Next, it calculates the "decision value" – the net outcome, or the reward minus the cost. Finally, the brain makes a prediction of how likely it is that the decision will deliver the reward envisaged, which can be compared with the actual outcome, giving a "prediction error". The more complex the problem, the more the frontal areas of the brain are involved.

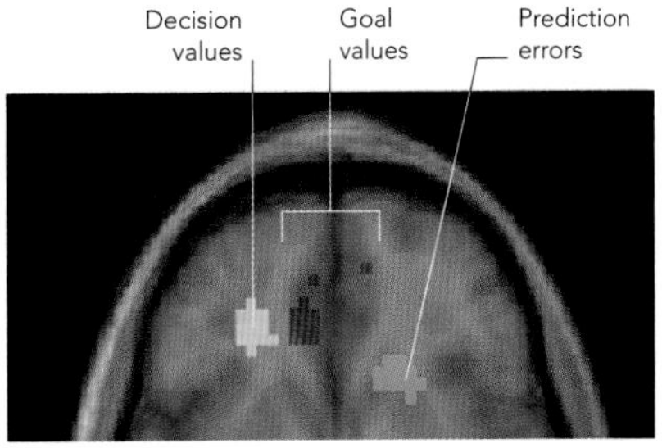

ACTIVATION MAP

Activity in the medial orbitofrontal cortex correlates with goal values (red), activity in the central orbitofrontal cortex (yellow) correlates with decision values, and activity in the ventral striatum, part of the caudate nucleus and putamen, correlates with prediction errors (green).

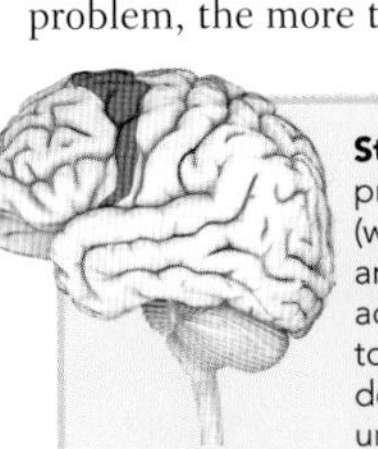

Step 1 The premotor cortex (where actions are prepared) is activated first, to make basic decisions about unconscious physical movements.

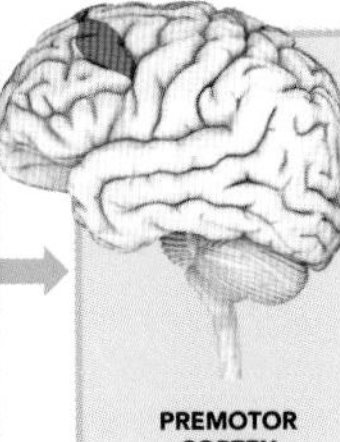

Step 2 If more than a simple physical action is needed, an area of cortex slightly further forward is brought in, to plan and refine a course of action.

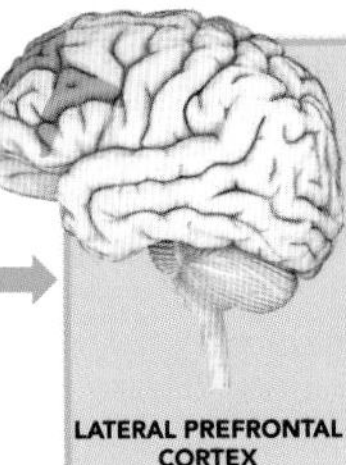

Step 3 If the decision is made in a complicated context, prefrontal areas concerned with comparing past and present situations are activated.

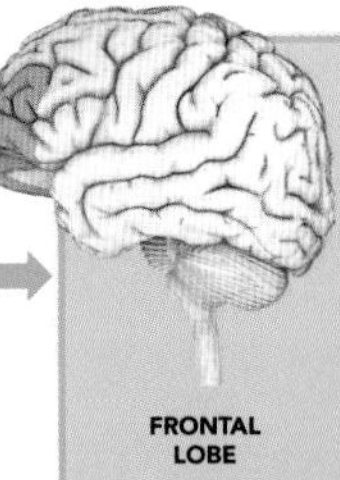

Step 4 Finally, the most frontal area of the brain kicks in, combining all the information gathered so far into a single, fully integrated plan.

THE ROLE OF EMOTIONS

Decision-making and judgement are profoundly affected by emotions. This is because emotion "drives" action – without it, the brain is like a car with steering but no power. Moods may have a profound effect on the outcome of decision-making. Being in a pleasant, anxious, or neutral mood, or experiencing extreme emotion, can have a significant short-term influence on areas of the brain that are critical for reasoning, intelligence, and other types of higher cognition.

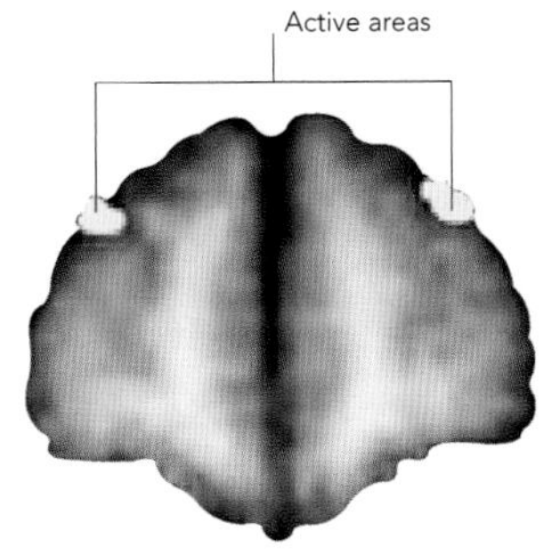

MOODS

The ventrolateral prefrontal cortex is shown in fMRI scans to work harder if a person is in the "wrong" mood for a task, perhaps by stifling emotions.

DECISION – OR PREDICTION?

When we make a conscious "decision", it feels as though we could have chosen something else instead – we seem to be exercising free will. Experiments show, however, that the conscious decision to do a voluntary act arises after the brain has unconsciously computed what to do and sent the appropriate instructions to the muscles (see p.193). This suggests that a "decision" marks the moment at which we know what we are about to do – a prediction rather than a choice.

THE NUMERICAL BRAIN

Number sense seems "hard-wired" into the human brain. Babies as young as six months can spot the difference between one and two. One study recorded electrical activity from babies' brains while they watched a pair of soft toys. The toys were then momentarily screened and one was removed, then the screen was lifted to reveal just one toy. The babies' brains registered the "error" by activating the same circuit known to mark error detection in adults, suggesting that even very young babies are able to recognize such discrepancies.

TESTING BABIES

When two toys in this test "become" one, the brains of babies register an error, showing they can discriminate between one and two.

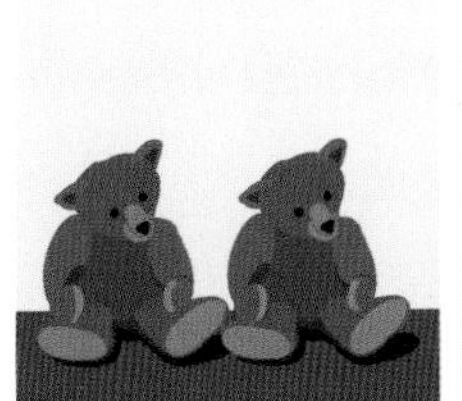

TWO STUFFED TOYS DISPLAYED

TOYS SCREENED MOMENTARILY

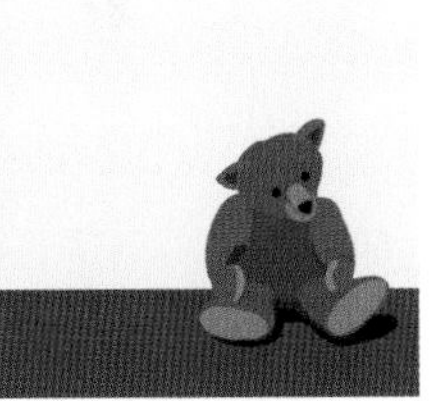

ONLY ONE TOY IS REVEALED WHEN SCREEN IS REMOVED

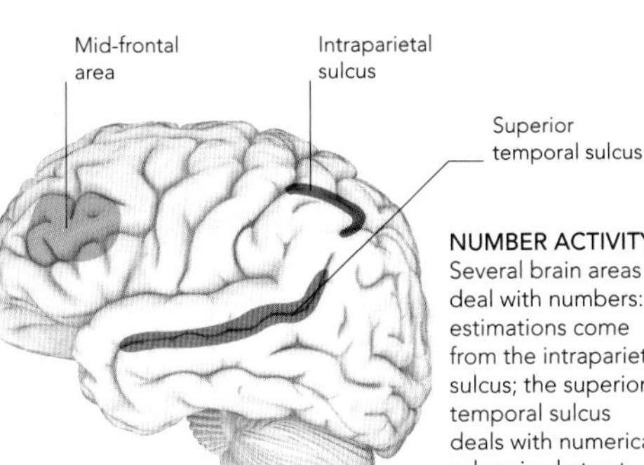

NUMBER ACTIVITY

Several brain areas deal with numbers: estimations come from the intraparietal sulcus; the superior temporal sulcus deals with numerical values in abstract form; and the mid-frontal area notes when numbers seem wrong.

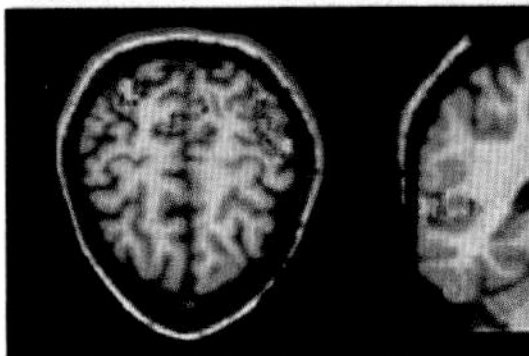
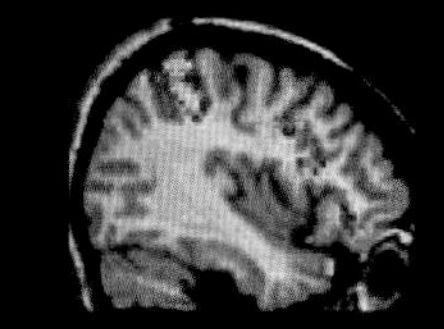

FMRI SCANS OF ADULT BRAINS

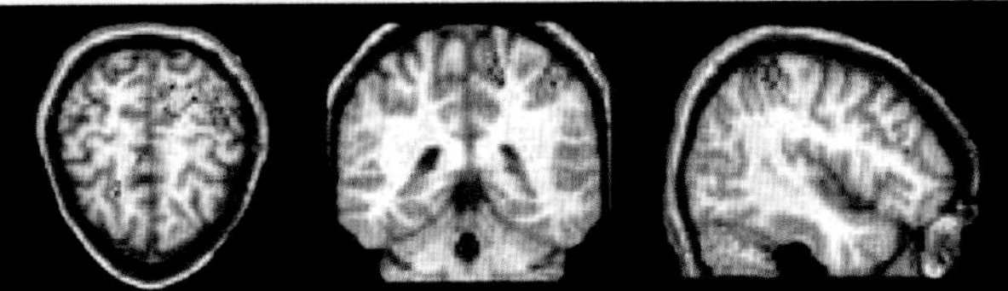

FMRI SCANS OF CHILDREN'S BRAINS

NUMBER DEVIATION

When confronted with a numerical "error", such as the number of items on view unexpectedly changing, children's brains register the change in an area that estimates quantities of what is seen. Adults engage both this area and one concerned with abstract numbers. This suggests that the ability to "guesstimate" develops earlier than the ability to think of numbers in the abstract, and also that, as numeracy develops, our brains deal with numbers in different ways.

CREATIVITY AND HUMOUR

CREATIVITY IS THE ABILITY TO RECONFIGURE WHAT YOU KNOW, OFTEN IN THE LIGHT OF NEW INFORMATION, AND COME UP WITH AN ORIGINAL CONCEPT OR IDEA. IN ORDER TO BE CREATIVE, A PERSON MUST BE CRITICAL, SELECTIVE, AND GENERALLY INTELLIGENT.

THE CREATIVE PROCESS

Our brains are bombarded with stimuli, much of which is filtered out before it reaches consciousness. Focusing on immediate tasks is vital in day-to-day life, but to be creative it is necessary to open our minds to new inputs and memories that may not seem useful. This process allows us to connect things that otherwise stay apart. The brain state most conducive to kindling new ideas is relaxed attentiveness, or the resting state (see p.184), characterized by alpha waves (see p.181). Being creative involves connecting information and reconfiguring it to make something new. The resting state allows information to flow around the brain. The "Eureka moment" that occurs when several thoughts combine into a new idea is marked by a change in brain activity involving a shift to the temporal lobe and anterior cingulate cortex. A period of critical assessment may follow, marked by a switch from the resting state to a task-oriented pattern centred on frontal lobe activity.

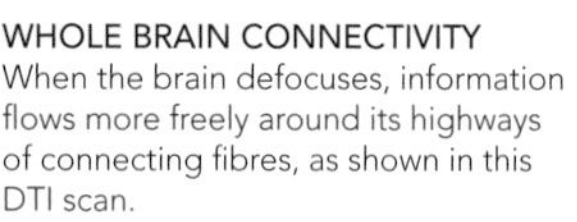

WHOLE BRAIN CONNECTIVITY
When the brain defocuses, information flows more freely around its highways of connecting fibres, as shown in this DTI scan.

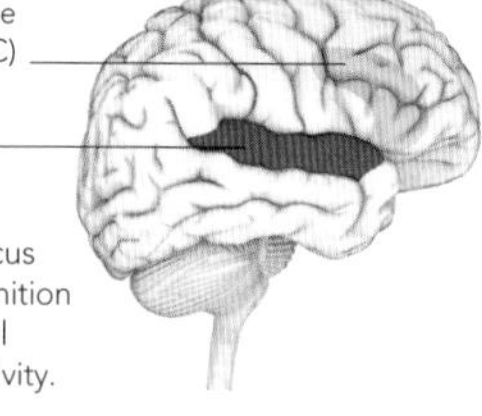

"EUREKA MOMENT" AREAS
Activity in the superior temporal sulcus in "eureka" moments signifies recognition of a new association of ideas. Critical analysis of new ideas sparks ACC activity.

CREATIVE INDIVIDUALS

Everyone is creative, but those who can put their brains into "idle" on demand are more likely to open up their minds to new possibilities and generate original ideas. This process only works, however, if the brain is already "primed" with knowledge that can be combined with the new material. Artists who have mastered the basics of their discipline, for instance, have a foundation of knowledge onto which improvements and changes can be fused. Their expertise allows this process to operate unconsciously, leaving greater resources available for processing new stimuli. Creative people also have relatively high IQs (see p.168), plus the ability to snap back to alertness when a new idea is hatched, and to subject that idea to rigorous scrutiny and criticism. Ideas that survive this second creative thought process are likely to be valuable and therefore judged as genuinely new.

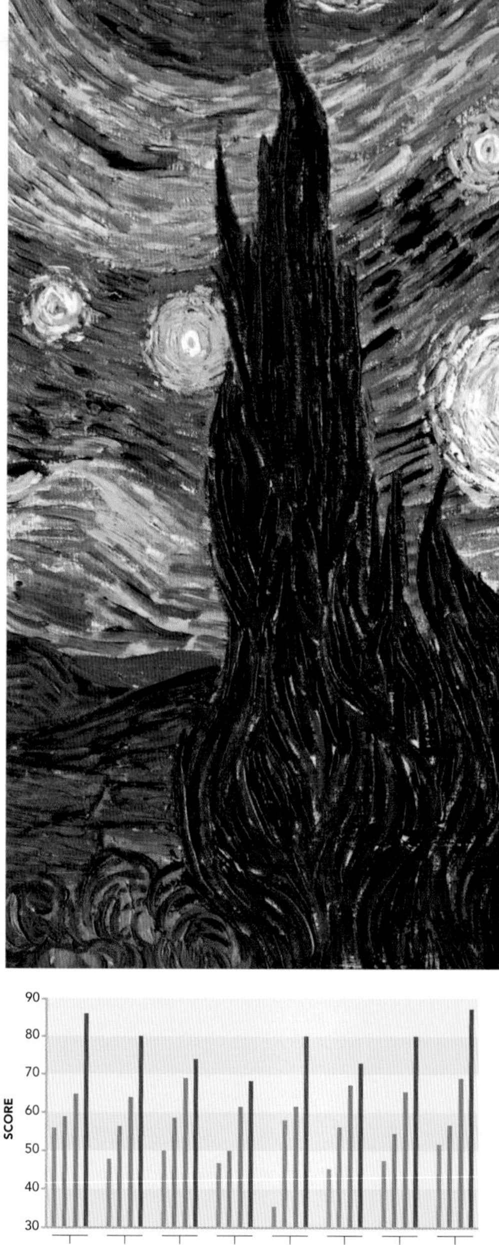

STARRY NIGHT
The artist Van Gogh worked on the painting *Starry Night* while in an asylum. He may have had temporal lobe epilepsy and/or bipolar disorder, both of which are associated with high levels of creativity.

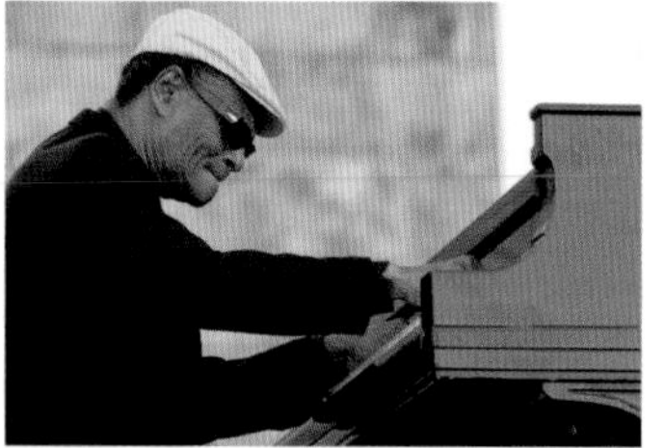

MUSICIANS
Brain-imaging studies of musicians at work show that frontal areas keep attention targeted when they play by rote, but turn off in improvization so ideas can "float".

CREATIVITY AND MADNESS

Creativity and some types of insanity share certain features, such as intense imagination, a tendency to link things that may seem unconnected to others, and openness to ideas that others may swiftly discount. The difference between highly creative people and those who tip into madness is that creative people maintain insight. They recognize that their imaginings are not real and remain able to control any bizarre symptoms and channel them into their work.

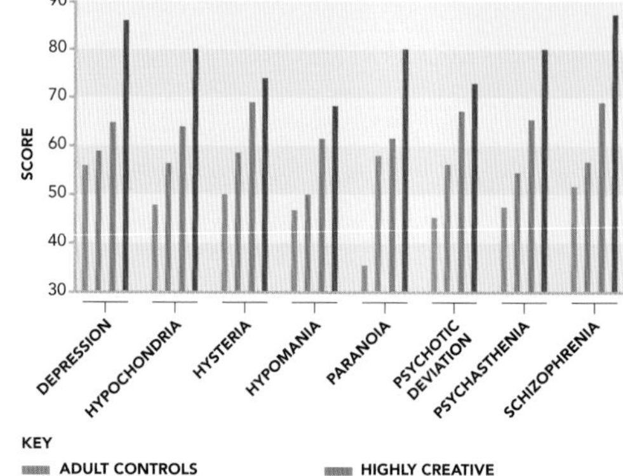

MENTAL-DISORDER TESTING
Very creative people score highly on tests for mental disorders but rarely fulfill the diagnostic criteria for these conditions, so their mental states can be seen as being somewhere between normal and insane.

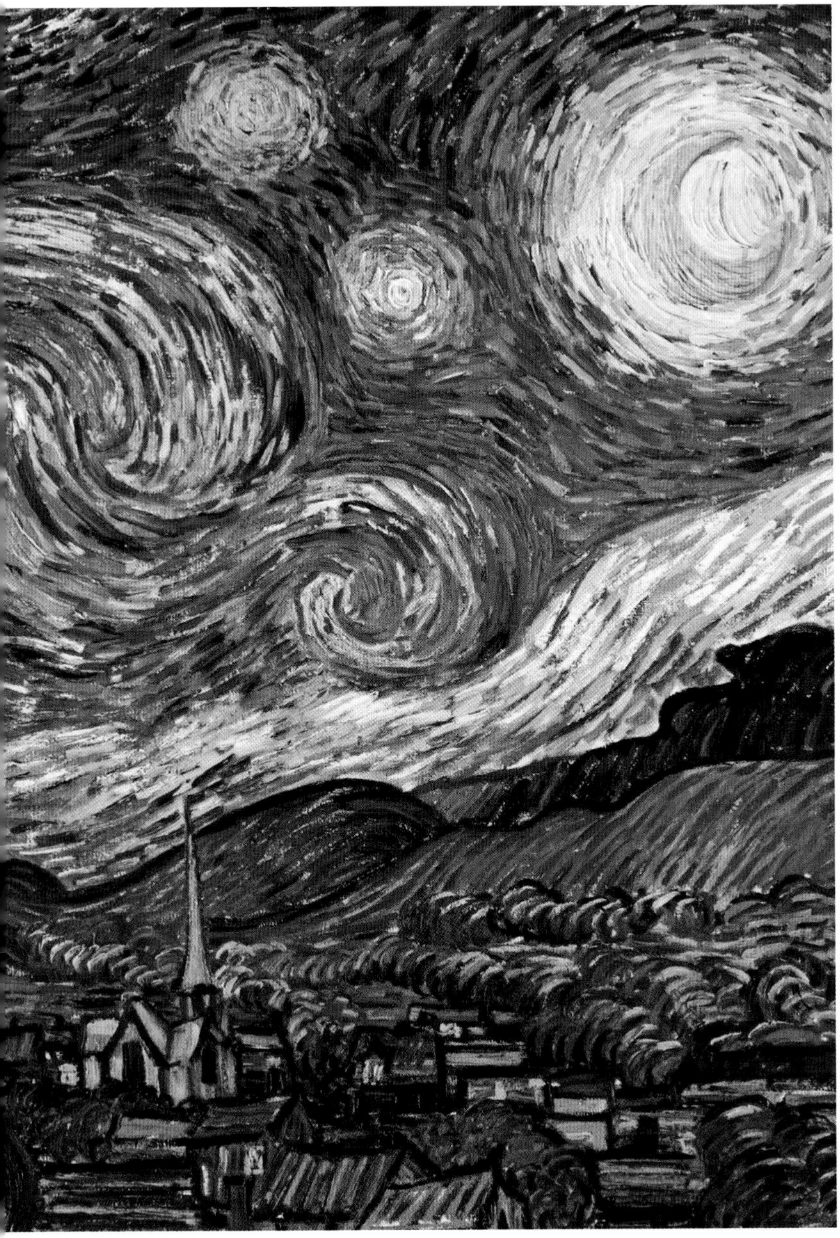

HUMOUR

A lot of humour arises from the juxtaposition of apparently unconnected ideas, which is similar to the process underlying creativity. Studies looking at how humourous interplay between co-workers affects workplace innovation suggest that keeping workers laughing may "jump-start" their creative faculties, perhaps because humour forces people to attend to "distractions", making them more open to new information. Brain-imaging studies have shown that humour stimulates the brain's "reward" circuit and elevates circulating levels of dopamine, which is linked to motivation and pleasurable anticipation.

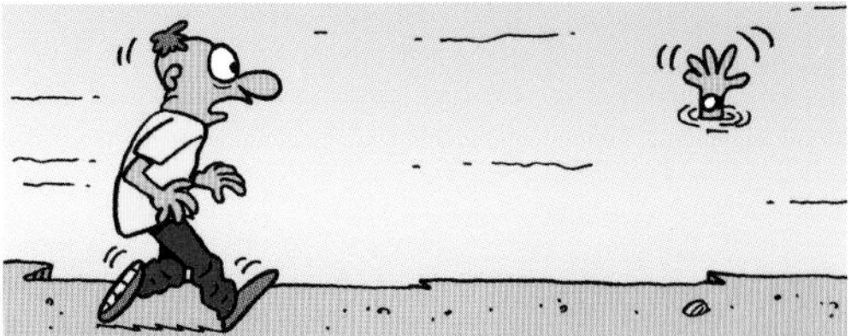

EXPECTATION OF INTENTION

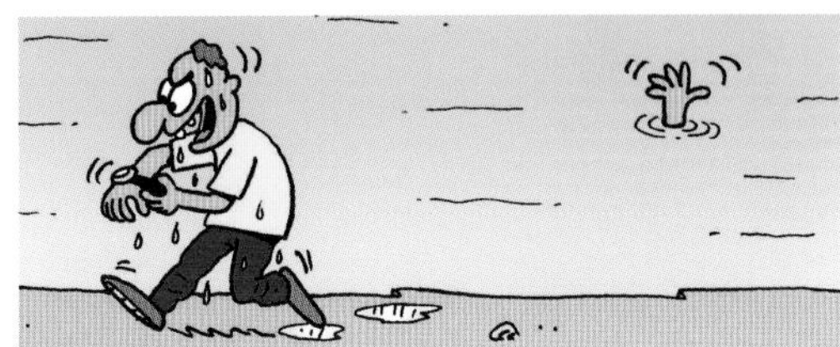

INCONGRUITY

BRAIN AREAS LINKED TO HUMOUR
The first frame above sparks activity in brain areas linked to predicting intention – here, the cartoon character's. The next frame activates areas linked to surprise and emotion, suggesting that such incongruity is central to humour.

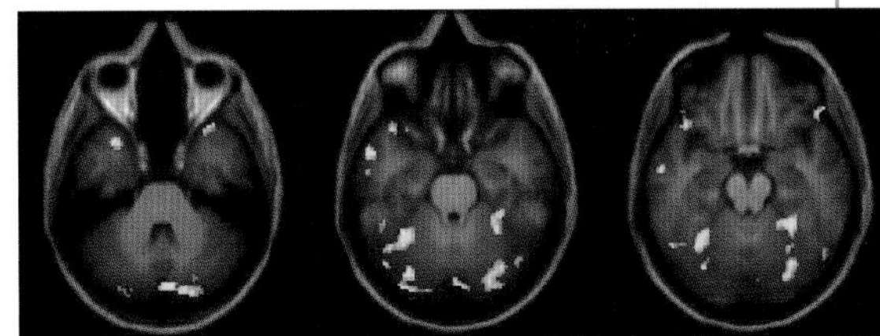

EXPECTATION OF INTENTION

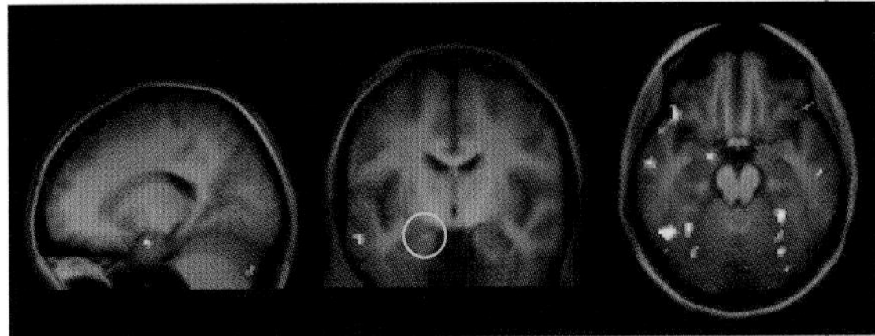

APPRECIATION

BRAIN IMAGING DURING CARTOON READING
The top row of fMRI scans show brain areas activated by the first frame of the cartoon above, including the temporal and parietal areas and the cerebellum. These become active when, by observing a person's actions, we "know" what their intentions are. When the expectation is subverted, as in the second frame, it creates activity in the left amygdala (bottom row, circled). The amygdala is active in emotion, and the left side is particularly linked to pleasant feelings.

TURNING ON CREATIVITY

As soon as we can categorize a stimulus we tend not to scrutinize it further, but immediately edit it out. So, when we see a dog, we mentally label it as "dog" and do not stop to take in every detail. The frontal lobes manage this editing process, and there is some evidence to suggest that if activity in this area is inhibited, people "take in" more. Tests using transcranial magnetic stimulation (TMS) to "turn off" the frontal lobes show that creative skills can emerge as frontal-lobe activity decreases.

TMS TEST
Volunteers subjected to TMS displayed new creative drawing skills when frontal-lobe activity was turned off.

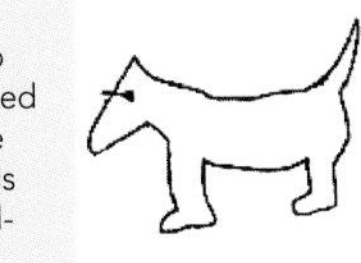

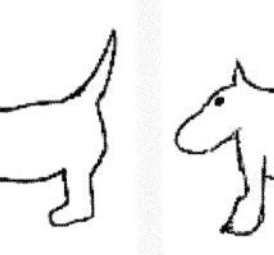

PRACTICE

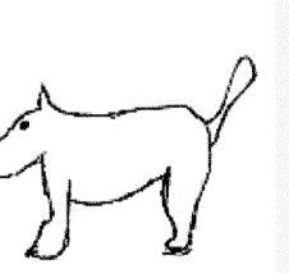

BEFORE

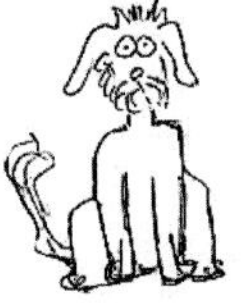

DURING

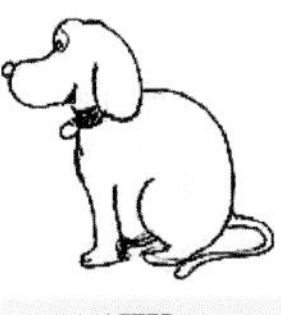

AFTER

BELIEF AND SUPERSTITION

OUR BRAINS ARE CONSTANTLY TRYING TO MAKE SENSE OF THE WORLD IN ORDER TO GUIDE OUR ACTIONS. ONE WAY OF DOING THIS IS BY CREATING EXPLANATORY STORIES OR IDEAS INTO WHICH WE FIT OUR EXPERIENCES. SUCH FRAMEWORKS ARE OFTEN USEFUL, BUT MAY NOT ALWAYS BE CORRECT.

BELIEVING IS SEEING

Most people have some kind of belief system, which forms a framework for their experience. Some were taught their beliefs, while others arrived at them by examining their experience and working out their own interpretation. Once a belief system has been formed, it acts both as an explanation for what has happened in the past and also a "working hypothesis" that is projected onto the world. For example, if a person believes that the world is governed by a benign supernatural being, they will "see" events such as coincidences or strokes of good fortune as evidence of this, while a person with a materialist belief system would interpret them merely as chance happenings. People who are quick to see meaningful connections between, for example, random events are more inclined than others to have a magical or superstitious belief system.

HOLY TOAST
People with a tendency towards magical thinking are quicker to see patterns like the "face" in this piece of toast. They are also more likely to see such things as "meaningful" – perhaps even as signs from God.

PATTERN-MAKING
The ability to "see" patterns helps us to make sense of the world and respond appropriately. But we can be both too good and too poor at it.

AUTISM
Autistic people do not see patterns that are obvious to most of us, so get swamped by information, all of which seems equally important.

LITERAL-MINDEDNESS
Failure to recognize subtle patterns leads to concrete-mindedness, such as failure to understand metaphors (as seen in Asperger's syndrome).

SUPERSTITION
Too much pattern-making may lead people to "see" things that are not there, or make links between events that are not actually connected.

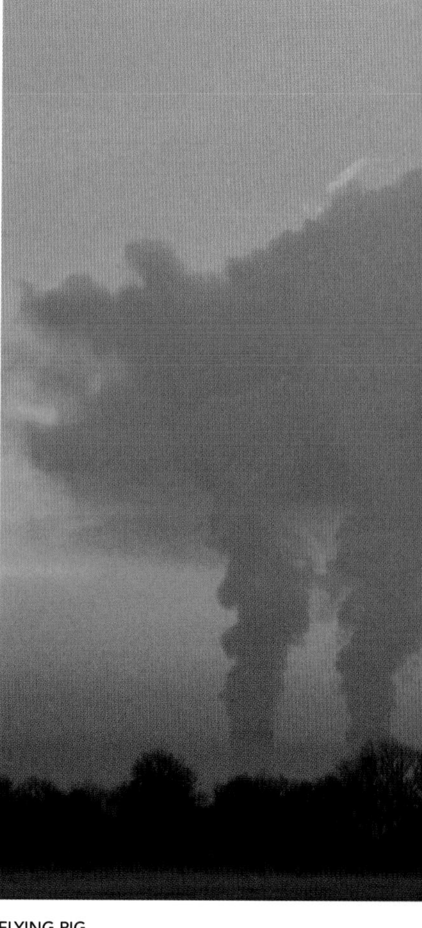

FLYING PIG
The human brain has evolved to pick up very quickly on visual stimuli that might signal danger or opportunity. Hence faces, human bodies, and animal forms are among the most likely things to be "seen" in clouds.

RELIGION IN THE BRAIN

Religious practice is largely determined by cultural factors. However, studies of identical twins who have been brought up separately suggest that the likelihood of a person experiencing a religious conversion or spiritual transcendence may be due more to genes than to upbringing. Spiritual transcendence shares some features with other "weird" experiences, such as out-of-body experiences, auras, and "the sensed presence" (see opposite page). These are associated with flurries of unusually high activity in the temporal lobes. The areas involved in intense religious experiences seem to be more widespread, however. For example, a study of nuns from a meditative order showed that, as they recalled an intense religious experience, many different areas were activated. So there does not seem to be a single "God-spot".

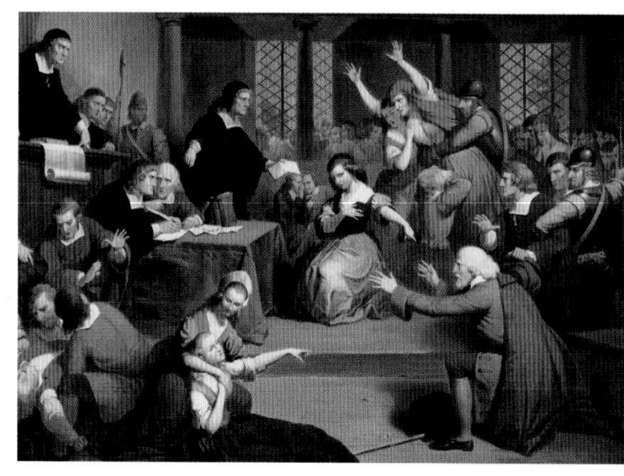

SALEM WITCH TRIALS
Rigid belief systems can lead people to "see" things that do not exist. During the Salem witch trials of 1692, for example, religious bigots "saw" evidence of the devil in the behaviour of entirely ordinary people.

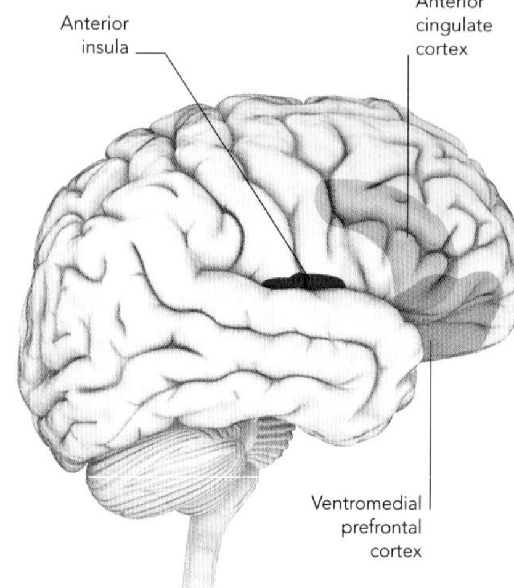

THE BASIS OF BELIEF
Belief and disbelief are driven by parts of the brain to do with emotions, not reasoning. Belief activates the ventromedial prefrontal cortex, which processes reward, emotion, and taste, while disbelief is registered by the insula, which generates feelings of disgust.

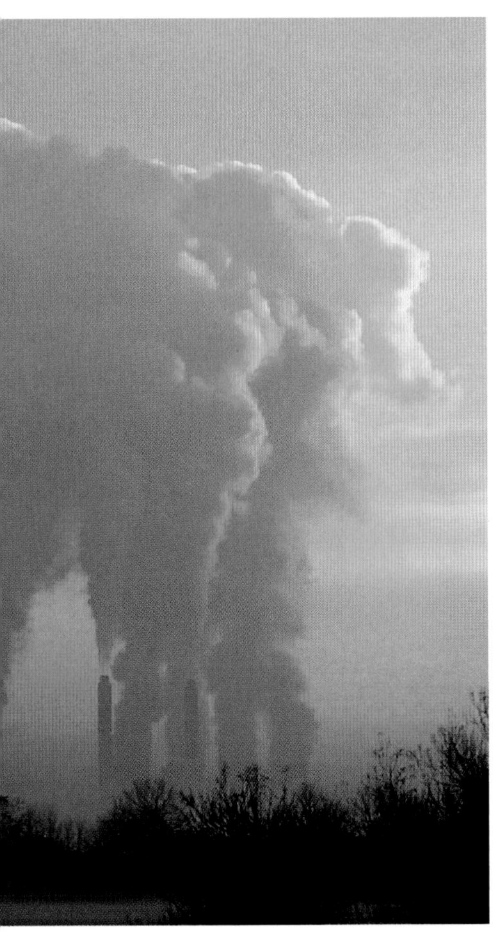

BRAIN CHEMISTRY

High natural levels of the neurotransmitter dopamine may explain why some people are unusually quick to pick out patterns. Believers are known to be more likely than sceptics to see a word or face in nonsense images, and sceptics more likely to miss real faces or words that are partly hidden by visual "noise". One study found that sceptics' tendency to see hidden patterns increased when they were given L-dopa, a drug that increases dopamine levels.

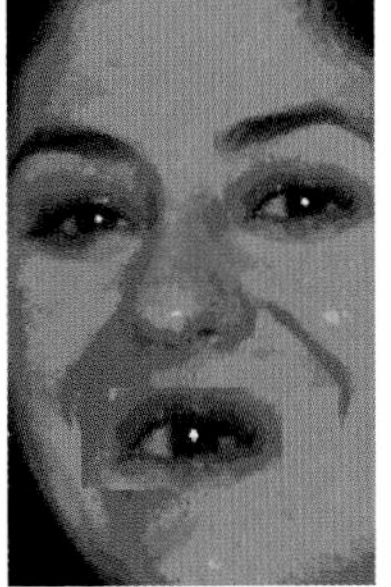

SCRAMBLED FACE

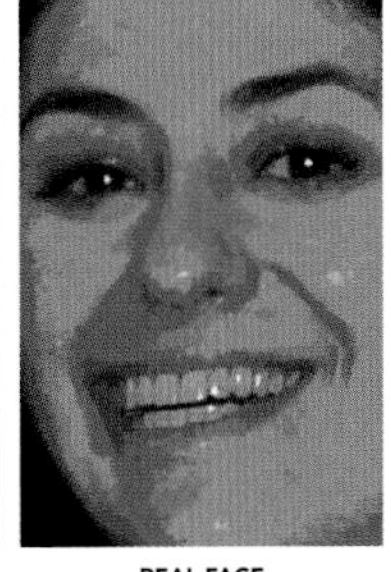

REAL FACE

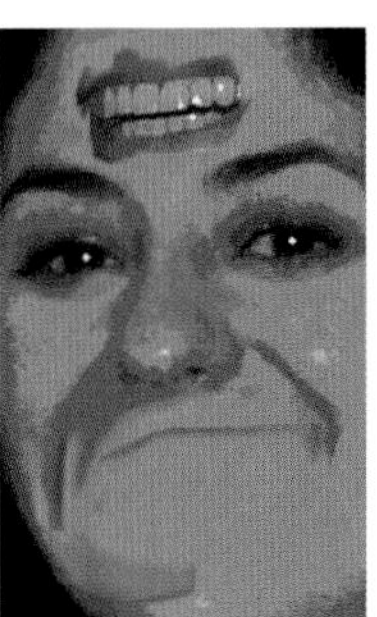

SCRAMBLED FACE

SCRAMBLED FACES STUDY
Believers are more likely than sceptics to see "real" faces when presented with a rapid sequence of "scrambled" faces. Sceptics, by contrast, are more likely to fail to spot "real" faces mixed in with the scrambled ones.

SEEING LITTLE PEOPLE

The content of supernatural "sightings" varies according to culture. Fairies were once commonly seen, while today it is more usual for people to report seeing alien beings. Claims of being abducted by aliens seem to be more common at times when the magnetic effects of solar radiation are high. One theory is that the radiation causes tiny temporal-lobe seizures in susceptible people, creating hallucinations.

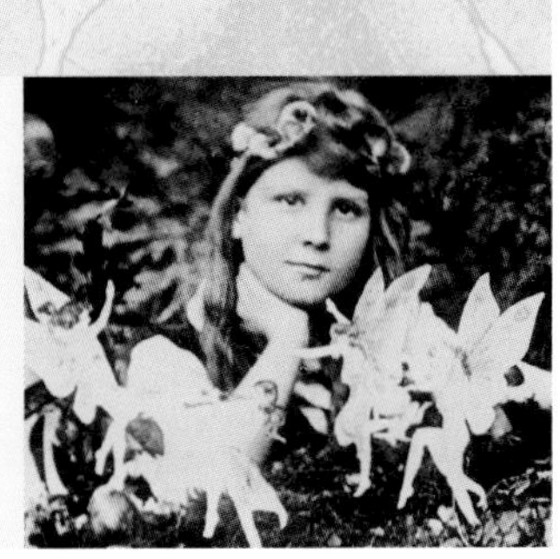

THE COTTINGLEY FAIRIES
This faked photograph (part of a series) was made by two mischievous children in 1917. Many adults believed that the fairies were real.

THE HAUNTED BRAIN

Apparently "supernatural" experiences may be due to disturbances in various parts of the brain. Tiny seizures in the temporal lobes are thought to be responsible for many of the emotional effects reported in such events, such as feelings of ecstasy or intense fear. Temporal-lobe disturbance is also associated with the sense of an invisible presence that often accompanies perceiving ghosts. Distortions of space and embodiment, such as the illusion of looking down at oneself, known as an "out-of-body" experience, are linked to a change in activity in the parietal lobes, which normally maintain a relatively stable sense of space and time. Hallucinations may result from faulty visual or auditory processing or failure to interpret sights and sounds normally.

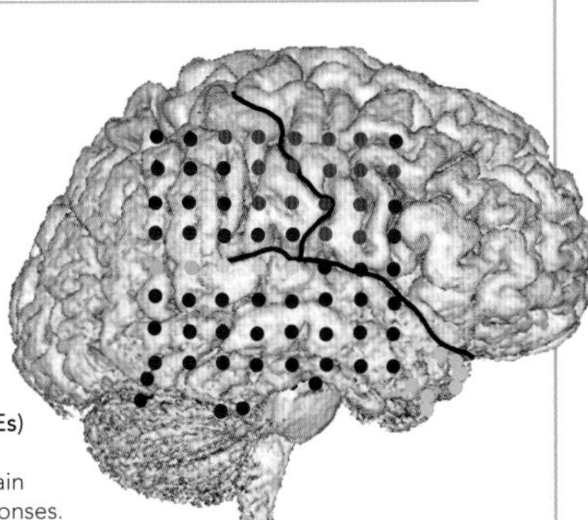

KEY
- TEMPORO-PARIETAL JUNCTION (TPJ)
- MOTOR CORTEX
- SOMATOSENSORY CORTEX
- AUDITORY CORTEX
- FOCUS OF EPILEPTIC ACTIVITY IN TEMPORAL LOBE

OUT-OF-BODY EXPERIENCES (OBEs)
This diagram shows areas where electrodes were implanted in the brain of an epileptic person to evoke responses. Stimulation of the TPJ (blue dots) was found to induce OBEs.

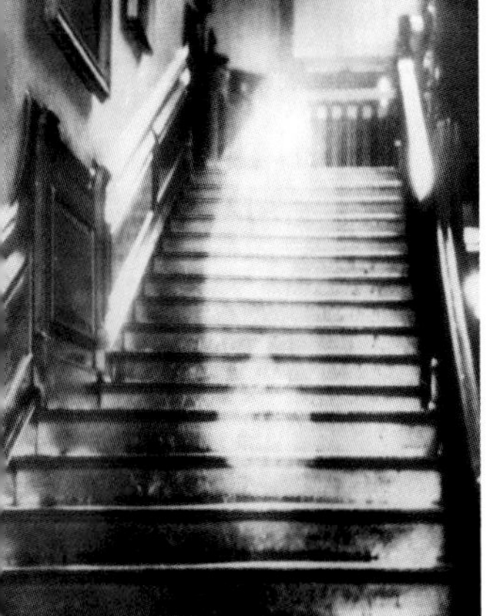

WHITE LADY
Expectation has a strong effect on what a person sees. Many "hauntings" arise because people have been led to expect to see a ghost in a certain place. Any unusual sensory effect is then interpreted as a spectre.

SO YOU THINK YOU'RE CLAIRVOYANT?

Our brains are continually making predictions about the near future, using knowledge of past and present to guess what will happen next. Sometimes things happen that the brain can't predict because they are random. Usually we are alerted to such events by snapping to attention, but if the change is very fast we may become aware of it unconsciously before we know consciously that it has happened, giving the impression that we have perceived the event in the future. This "out-of-synch" brain glitch occurs more often in people who hold superstitious beliefs.

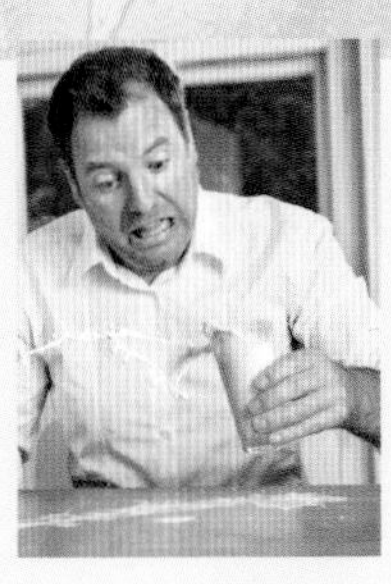

FORESIGHT
Sometimes it feels as though we foresaw an event, because our emotional reaction to it occurs before we consciously see it happen.

ILLUSIONS

ILLUSIONS OCCUR WHEN SENSORY DATA CLASHES WITH OUR ASSUMPTIONS ABOUT THE WAY THINGS ARE. THE BRAIN ATTEMPTS TO MAKE THE INFORMATION "FIT". THE RESULTING CONFUSION GIVES US A GLIMPSE OF HOW THE BRAIN WORKS.

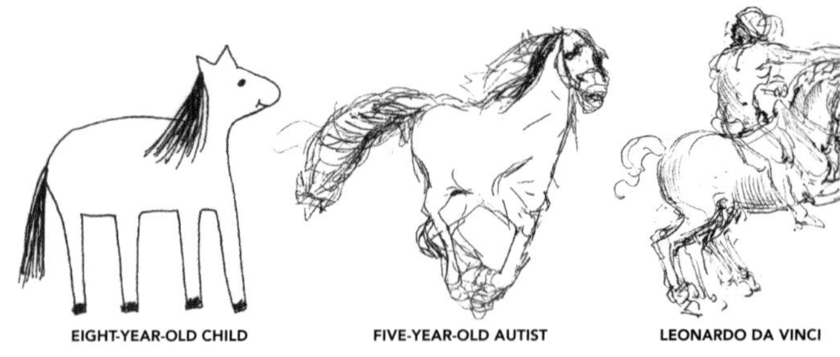

EIGHT-YEAR-OLD CHILD | FIVE-YEAR-OLD AUTIST | LEONARDO DA VINCI

TYPES OF ILLUSION

The brain has certain rules that it applies to incoming information in order to make sense of it quickly. If we hear a voice and at the same time see a mouth moving, for example, we assume the voice comes from the mouth. Like all such rules, though, this is only a best guess and can be wrong. Hence it leaves us open to the illusion of ventriloquy. Low-level illusions – those created in the early stages of perception – are unavoidable, but those that arise due to higher-level cognition are less robust. It is impossible not to see the after-image that occurs when you have been looking at a bright light, for example, because this is created by low-level nerve activity, which cannot be affected by conscious thought. However, once you know the voice comes from the ventriloquist rather than the dummy, a result of higher-level cognition, the illusion is less convincing. Illusions may be generated by both conscious and unconscious assumptions. A child's concept of how a horse looks, for example, includes four distinct legs (top left), which governs how the horse is visualized. An "expert" viewer of horses – such as the artist Leonardo Da Vinci (top right) - has a more realistic concept.

ARTIST'S EYE
The middle drawing is by a five-year-old autistic savant, who probably had no concept of a horse at all. Unlike the normal child, her concepts do not mislead her.

CANALS ON MARS

Until the early 20th century, some astronomers believed that Mars was crossed by canals. Maps were made, and for nearly a decade the canals seemed to be visible to people with fairly strong telescopes. The canals did not "vanish" until analysis of the Martian atmosphere proved that life there was not possible. Acceptance that the canals could not exist stopped people seeing them.

MARTIAN MAP

DISTORTING MIRRORS

Information from the outside world, including sensations from the rest of the body, is constantly compared to a "virtual" world within the brain, which includes a conceptual map of the body. When the two fail to match up, the brain assumes that something outside has changed. It can even be fooled that the body has shrunk. The shrinking-body illusion involves stimulating the arm muscles with vibrators, to create the feeling that the limbs are moving in, beyond the sides of the body. The brain decides that the body has shrunk.

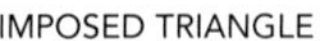

IMPOSED TRIANGLE
The brain imposes things that are not there, like this white triangle, when it is the most likely explanation for what we see.

Impulse travels through thalamus to parietal cortex

Impulse travels up to spinal cord

Vibrators strapped to wrists cause sensation of arms moving inwards

SHRINKING BODY
The brain's body map is encoded in the parietal cortex, the part of the brain dealing with space. This illusion activates the area as though it is registering an actual change in body shape.

AMBIGUOUS ILLUSIONS

Something strange happens when we look at ambiguous figures. The input to the brain stays the same, but what we see flips from one thing to another. This demonstrates that perception is an active process, driven by information that is already in our brains as well as information from the outside world. The switching occurs because the brain is searching for the most meaningful interpretation of the image. Normally, the brain settles quickly on a solution by using basic rules such as, "if one thing surrounds another, the surrounded shape is the object and the other thing is the ground". Ambiguous figures confound such rules. For instance, in the vase illusion (left) it is impossible to see which shape is on top, so the brain tries one way of seeing it, then another. You see both images, but you can never see both of them simultaneously.

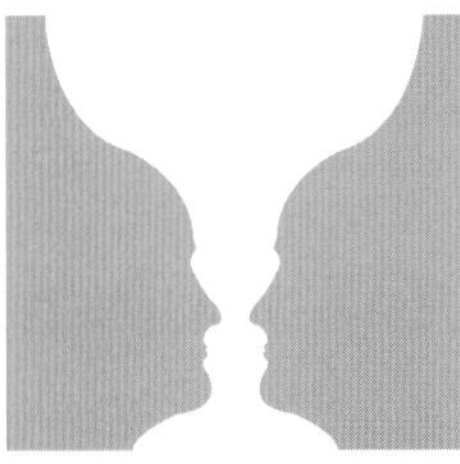

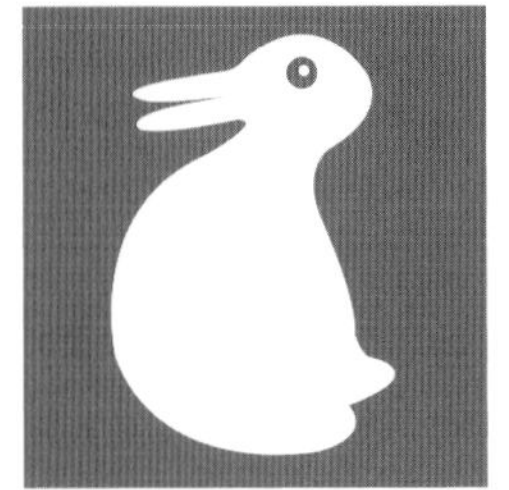

SHAPE SHIFTERS
In the vase–face illusion (top), the figures switch between two facing profiles and the outline of a vase. The bottom figure can be seen as either a rabbit or a duck.

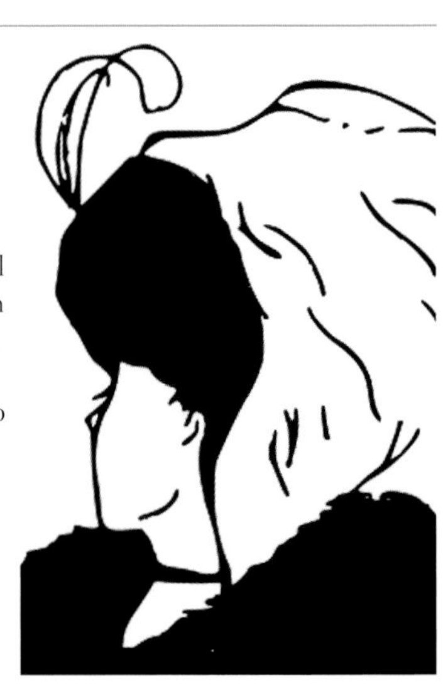

MY WIFE AND MY MOTHER-IN-LAW
In this illusion, the figure of either a young woman or an old hag may dominate at first, but once you have "seen" the alternative, the brain finds it again easily.

DISTORTING ILLUSIONS

Distorting illusions are characterized by visual images that generate a false impression of an object's size, length, or curvature. They generally exploit the "allowances" the brain normally makes in order to make sense of what it sees. For example, the brain "allows" that objects of the same size will look smaller if they are farther away, and that larger objects in an array should command greater attention than small ones. Like other illusions, distortions may occur at low or high levels of perception (see opposite page). Those that happen in the earliest stages, before the brain "recognizes" what it is looking at, are the most robust because they cannot be influenced by conscious thought.

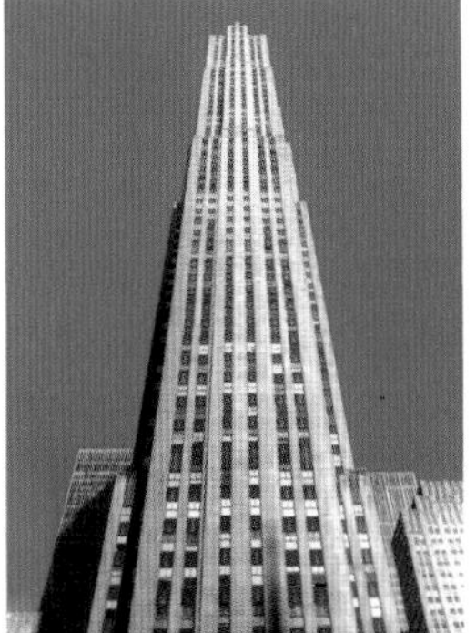

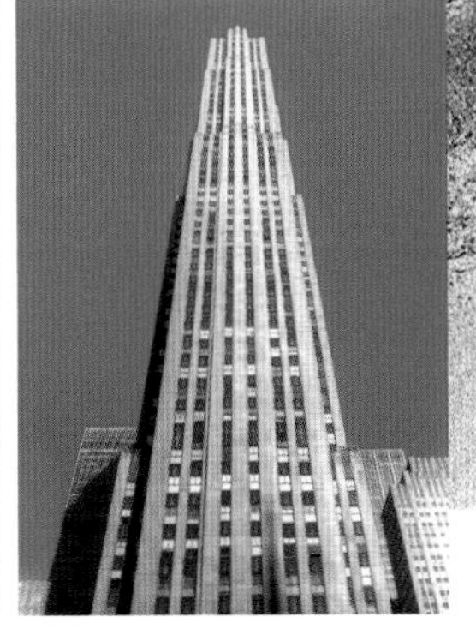

TOWER ILLUSION
These images of the Rockefeller Plaza in New York are identical but the one on the right seems to lean to the right. This is because the brain treats them as a single scene. Usually, if two adjacent towers rise in parallel their outlines converge due to perspective. When seeing two towers with parallel outlines, the brain assumes the towers are diverging.

PERSPECTIVE ILLUSION
Even though the figures walking along the road are the same height, the brain insists that the one farthest away looks taller. This is because the rule of perspective – things shrink with distance – is applied at an early stage of perception.

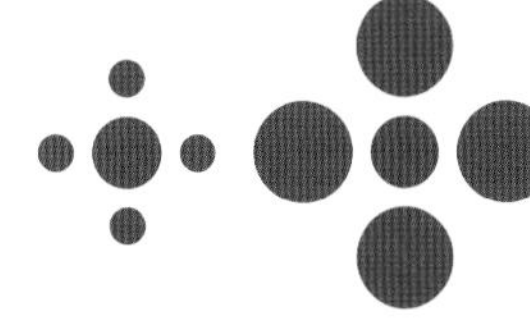

EBBINGHAUS ILLUSION
The central circle is the same size in both images, but we see it as bigger when compared to smaller circles, rather than larger ones.

PARADOX ILLUSIONS

It is possible to represent objects in two dimensions that cannot actually exist in the real, three-dimensional world. Paradox illusions are generated by such images, which are often dependent on the brain's erroneous assumption that adjacent edges must join. Although impossible, the best examples are oddly convincing, and the conscious brain is teased and intrigued by them. As with ambiguous illusions, the brain tries first one interpretation and then another, but is unable to settle because none of the available views make sense. Brain-imaging scans show that impossible images are recognized by the brain very early in the process of perception, well before conscious recognition. Unlike the conscious brain, the unconscious part is not very concerned with such images, and spends less time trying to process them than it spends on "real" objects.

THE TRIBAR
The Penrose triangle, also known as the tribar, is a perspective drawing that comprises three three-dimensional bars that appear to be connected, but in reality could not be.

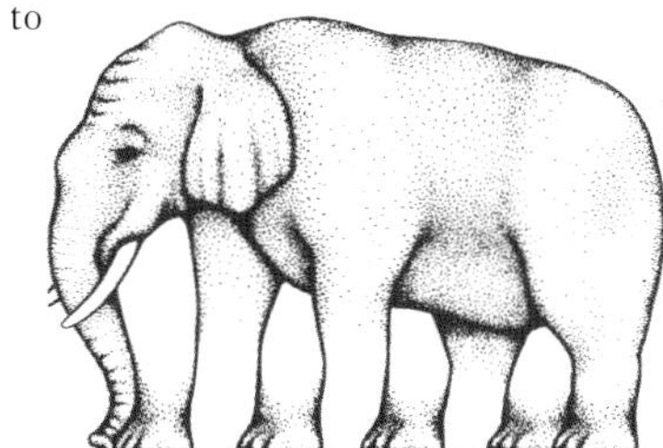

THE IMPOSSIBLE ELEPHANT
Although it is impossible to determine how many legs this elephant has, the brain keeps trying to match up the shaded areas of "legs" with the apparently detached feet.

M.C. ESCHER

"Mauk" Escher, a Dutch graphic artist, started drawing elaborate impossible realities in the 1930s and produced a huge quantity of now famous illusions. He created the images from imagination rather than by reference to observation, and incorporated many sophisticated mathematical concepts into his artworks. His images are both tantalizing and emotionally charged – some of his landscapes are witty, while others have a dark, surreal quality. Several of his works show buildings that could never actually be constructed.

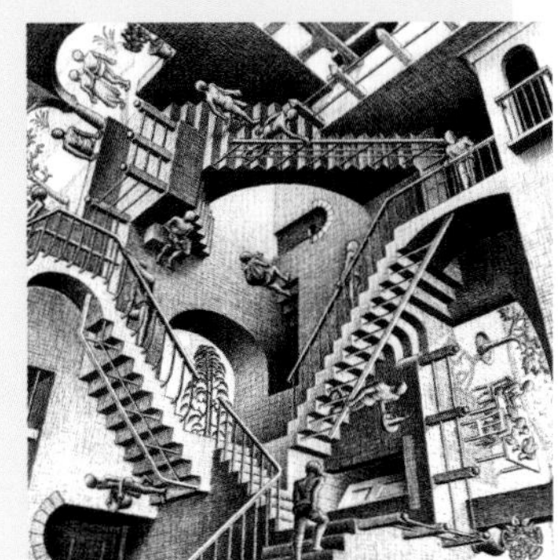

RELATIVITY
The scene shown here is impossible in that it could exist only in a world in which gravity worked in three directions rather than one.

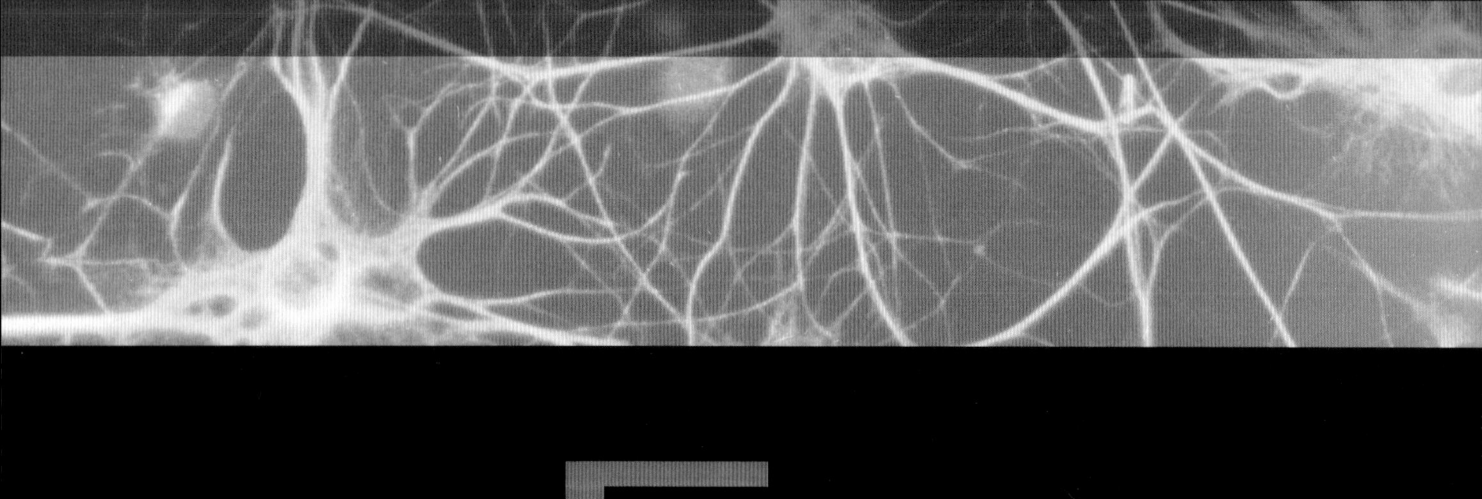

HOW DOES THE ELECTRICAL FIRING OF CELLS IN OUR BRAIN PRODUCE OUR CONSCIOUS EXPERIENCE OF THE WORLD, AND WITH IT SUCH THINGS AS OUR SENSE OF A PRIVATE SELF AND OUR ABILITY FOR ABSTRACT THOUGHT AND REFLECTION? THIS IS A FAMOUSLY DIFFICULT QUESTION. ANSWERING IT INVOLVES BUILDING A BRIDGE BETWEEN THE PHYSICAL AND MENTAL WORLDS. AS NEUROSCIENCE ADVANCES, WE ARE GETTING CLOSER TO UNDERSTANDING WHAT CONSCIOUSNESS IS AND HOW IT COMES ABOUT. FOR EXAMPLE, DIFFERENT CONSCIOUS STATES CAN NOW

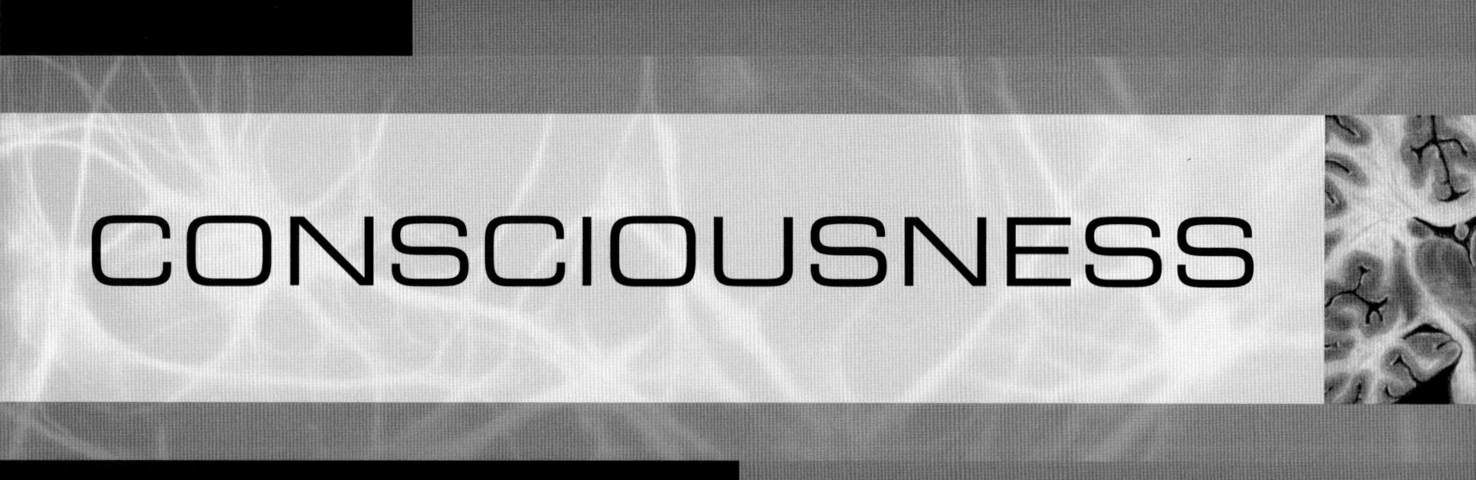
CONSCIOUSNESS

WHAT IS CONSCIOUSNESS?

CONSCIOUSNESS IS ESSENTIAL – WITHOUT IT, LIFE WOULD HAVE NO MEANING. WE CAN IDENTIFY THE SORT OF BRAIN ACTIVITY THAT GENERATES CONSCIOUS AWARENESS, BUT HOW THIS APPARENTLY INTANGIBLE PHENOMENON ARISES FROM A PHYSICAL ORGAN REMAINS A MYSTERY.

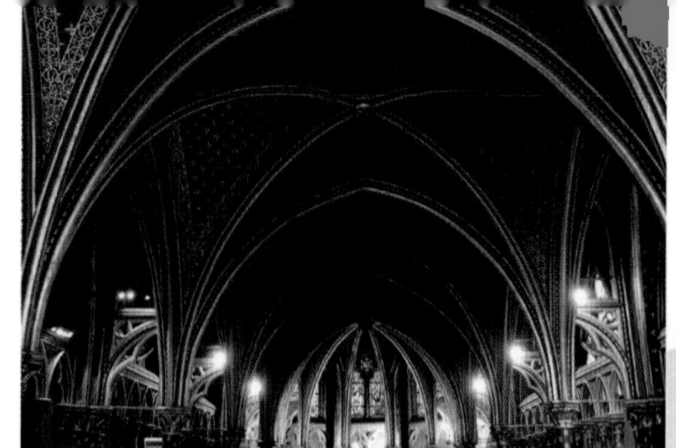

SPANDRELS
This is the name given to the spaces between arches. Although we talk of them as objects, without the arch they cease to exist. Consciousness may have appeared in the same way, as a result of other evolved features.

THE NATURE OF CONSCIOUSNESS

Consciousness is like nothing else. A thought, feeling, or idea seems to be a different kind of thing from the physical objects that make up the rest of the universe. The contents of our minds cannot be located in space or time. Although they appear to be produced by particular types of physical activity in the brain, it is not known if this activity itself forms consciousness (the Monist/materialist view) or if brain activity correlates with a different thing altogether that we call "the mind" or consciousness (the dualist view). If consciousness is not simply brain activity, this suggests the material universe is just one aspect of reality and that consciousness is part of a parallel reality in which entirely different rules apply.

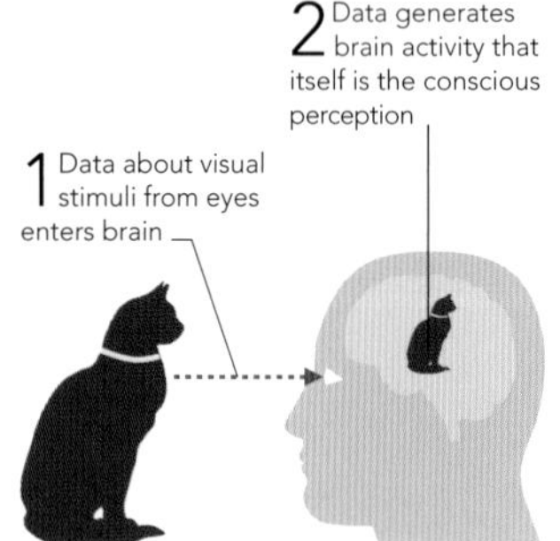

MONISM
According to this theory, consciousness is part of the material universe. It is identical to the brain activity that correlates with it. It developed when cognitive mechanisms evolved, but only as a result of them, rather than for any purpose of its own.

2 Data generates brain activity

3 Brain activity allows mind to make conscious perception

1 Data about visual stimuli from eyes enters brain

DUALISM
Consciousness is non-physical and exists in another dimension to the material universe. Certain brain processes are associated with it, but are not identical to it. Some dualists believe consciousness may exist without the brain processes associated with it.

DESCARTES AND THE MIND/BODY PROBLEM

The French philosopher René Descartes (1596–1650) is generally held to have founded modern dualism when he proposed that matter is separate and distinct from the mind (things like emotions, thoughts, and perceptions). This presented a problem: how can the two "kinds" of things interact? Descartes' solution was that "mind-stuff" affected the body via the pineal gland – a small nucleus in the centre of the brain. His solution to what has become known as the mind/body problem is now generally discounted, especially as the function of the pineal gland – hormone modulation – becomes clearer.

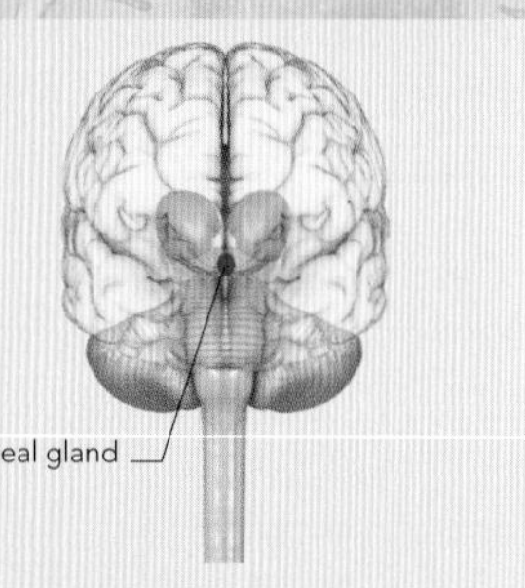

THE THIRD EYE
The pineal gland produces melatonin, a hormone that modulates sleep cycles. It is sometimes called the third eye – a reference to the mystical role attributed to it.

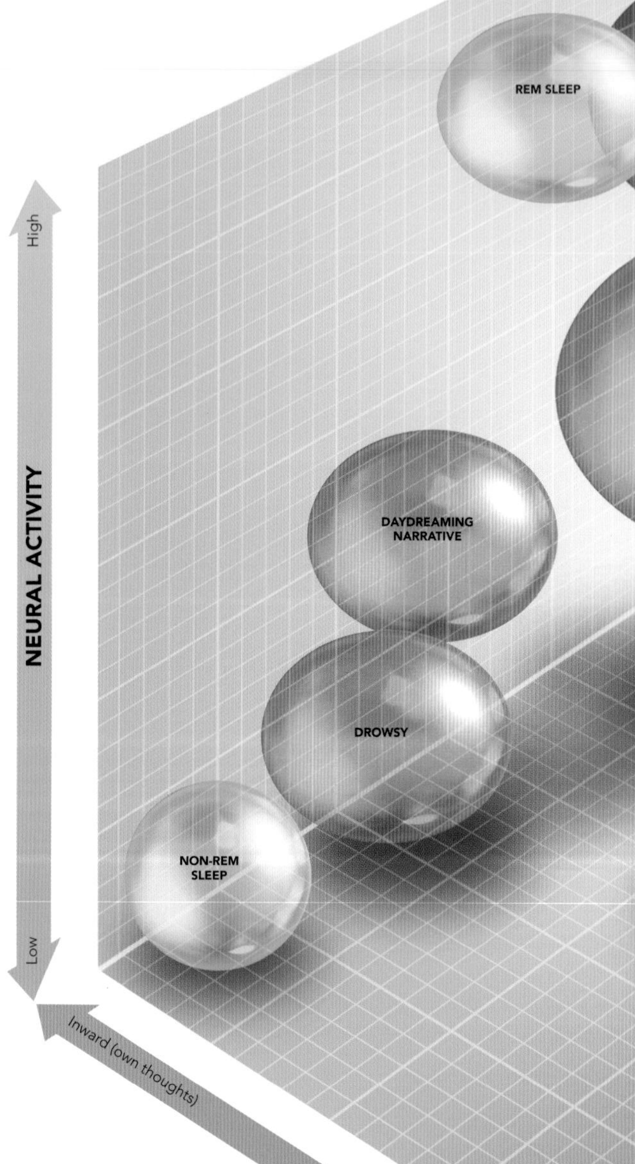

VISUALIZING THE MIND
This diagram is a representation of different states of mind, or modes of consciousness, framed within a box that represents the mind itself. The states of mind are positioned within the box according to the degree of neural activity that correlates with each, the direction of the focus of its attention (towards the outer world or inwards towards thoughts themselves), and the level of concentration each state of mind commands.

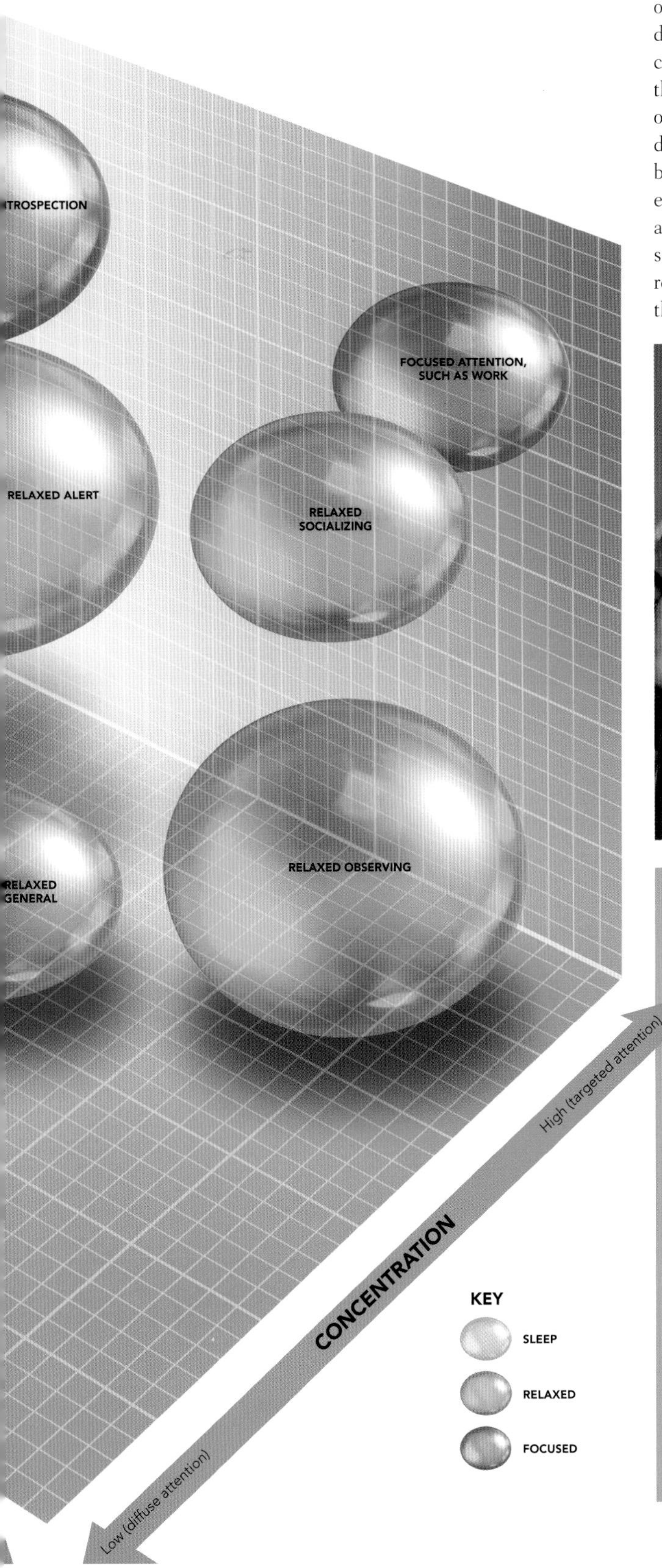

INTROSPECTION

FOCUSED ATTENTION, SUCH AS WORK

RELAXED ALERT

RELAXED SOCIALIZING

RELAXED OBSERVING

RELAXED GENERAL

High (targeted attention)

CONCENTRATION

Low (diffuse attention)

KEY

SLEEP

RELAXED

FOCUSED

TYPES AND LEVELS OF CONSCIOUSNESS

Consciousness has different modes, such as emotions, sensations, thoughts, and perceptions, which are all experienced at different levels of neural activity, focus, and concentration. The level of neural activity determines the intensity of consciousness. The direction of focus can be towards the outside world or the inner world (thinking about thoughts). Concentration can be loosely targeted, involving a range of objects or fixed, involving just one particular aspect. Consciousness also divides into three types of awareness: awareness in the moment – the brain registers and reacts to moment-by-moment events but does not encode them in memory; conscious awareness – events are registered and encoded in memory; and self-consciousness – events are registered and remembered, and the person is conscious of doing this.

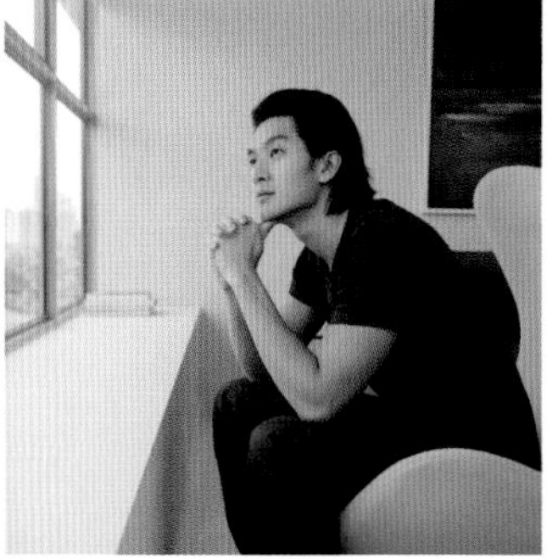

THE THINKER
Most conscious thinking is couched in language. Words function as symbolic "handles", used to grasp the objects they represent. However, about 25 per cent of thoughts are experienced as sensations or perceptions.

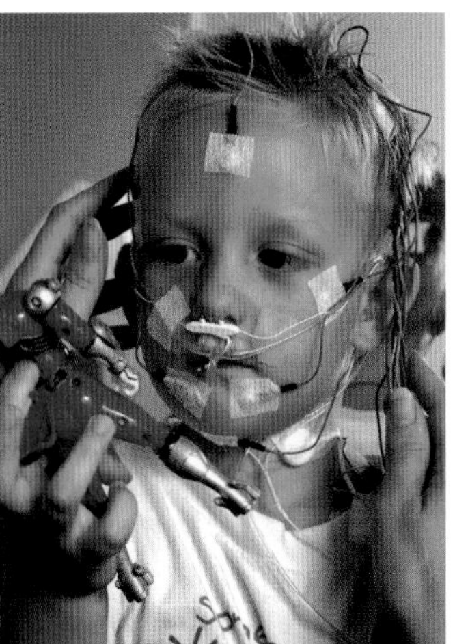

FIXED CONCENTRATION
When focusing on an object, attention narrows. Other potential focal points are neglected. This can be useful – this child notices less of a potentially traumatizing medical procedure when focused on a toy.

THE CHINESE ROOM

Is consciousness needed for "understanding"? Philosopher John Searle invented the idea of a room in which every dictionary and rule relating to the Chinese language was stored. Inside is a man who is able to translate and respond to questions written in Chinese by manipulating these resources, despite not being able to speak a word of Chinese. Hence, someone posting the words "How does your dog smell?" in Chinese may receive the reply, in Chinese, "Awful!". From outside it looks as though the man inside must have "understood" the question, but Searle argues that merely behaving this way is not the same as understanding. In the same way, a computer could never be described as "having a mind" or "understanding". Other philosophers argue that understanding – and perhaps every other type of consciousness – is merely the process of behaving as though one understands.

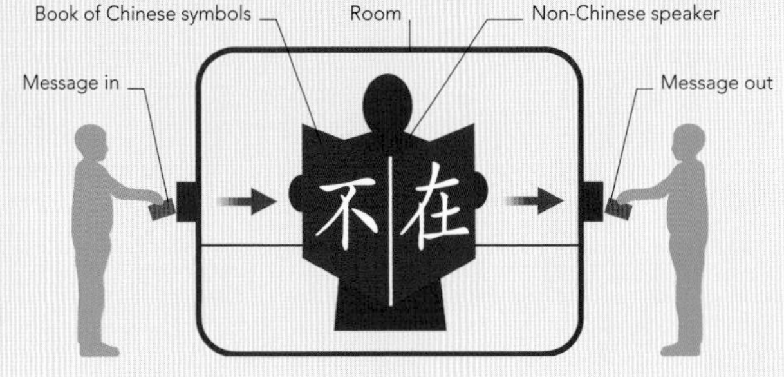

LOCATING CONSCIOUSNESS

HUMAN CONSCIOUSNESS ARISES FROM THE INTERACTION OF EVERY PART OF A PERSON WITH THEIR ENVIRONMENT. WE KNOW THAT THE BRAIN PLAYS THE MAJOR ROLE IN PRODUCING CONSCIOUS AWARENESS, BUT WE DO NOT KNOW HOW. CERTAIN PROCESSES WITHIN THE BRAIN, AND NEURONAL ACTIVITY IN PARTICULAR AREAS, CORRELATE RELIABLY WITH CONSCIOUS STATES, WHILE OTHERS DO NOT. THESE PROCESSES AND AREAS SEEM TO BE NECESSARY FOR CONSCIOUSNESS, ALTHOUGH THEY MAY NOT BE SUFFICIENT FOR IT.

SIGNIFICANT BRAIN ANATOMY

Different types of neuronal activity in the brain are associated with the emergence of conscious awareness. Neuronal activity in the cortex, and particularly in the frontal lobes, is associated with the arousal of conscious experience. It takes up to half a second for a stimulus to become conscious after it has first been registered in the brain. Initially, the neuronal activity triggered by the stimulus occurs in the "lower" areas of the brain, such as the amygdala and thalamus, and then in the "higher" brain, in the parts of the cortex that process sensations. The frontal cortex is activated usually only when an experience becomes conscious, suggesting that the involvement of this part of the brain may be an essential component of consciousness.

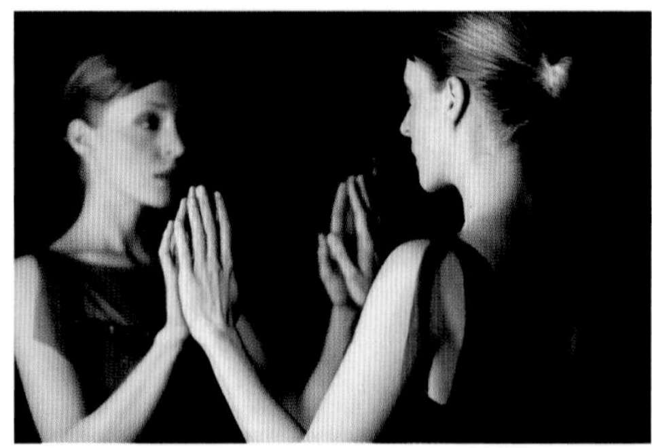

SELF AWARENESS
In order to be conscious, the brain needs to "own" its perceptions – that is, to recognize that those perceptions are occurring within itself. To do this it has to generate a sense of self (as opposed to unconscious awareness). Without this, consciousness may not be possible.

THE "BRAIN-IN-A-VAT"

The idea of a conscious but disembodied brain is central to many science fiction and horror films, and is often used as a thought experiment in philosophical debates about the nature of reality. In recent years, the notion has ceased to be entirely theoretical as modern technology edges towards the possibility of inducing in the brain a virtual reality, indistinguishable from the reality experienced through the body. It is even possible that such a thing has been achieved already, and the external world, as we experience it, is not "real" at all.

VIRTUAL REALITY
The idea that we are simply disembodied brains hooked up to a supercomputer that simulates conscious experience is a famous thought experiment.

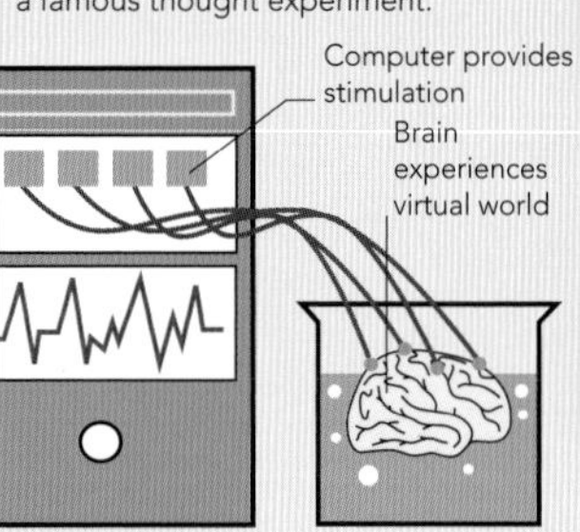

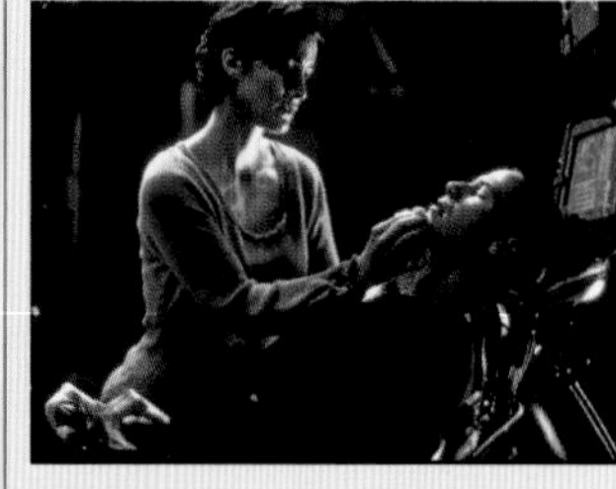

THE MATRIX
This 1999 film explores the idea of virtual reality being the only "reality" humans experience. People's brains are "plugged" into the Matrix, a huge computer program simulating physical experience.

CRUCIAL PARTS OF THE BRAIN
Various areas of the brain are involved in generating conscious experience, even though none of them alone is sufficient to sustain it. If any of these are severely damaged, consciousness is compromised, altered, or lost.

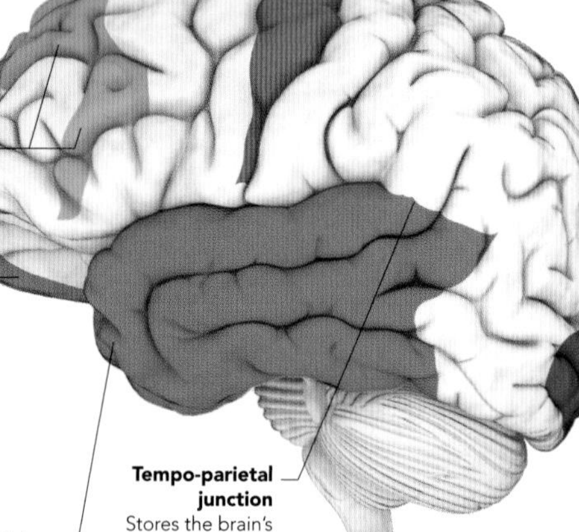

Motor cortex
Body awareness (involving motor cortex) may be crucial to sense of self, which seems necessary for consciousness

Supplementary motor area
Deliberate actions are "rehearsed" here, distinguishing them from unconscious reactions

Primary visual cortex
Without this there is no conscious vision, even if other parts of visual cortex are functioning

Dorsolateral prefrontal cortex
Different ideas and perceptions are "bound" together here – a process thought to be necessary for conscious experience

Orbitofrontal cortex
Conscious emotion arises here; if inactive, reactions to stimuli are merely reflexive body actions with no emotion

Tempo-parietal junction
Stores the brain's "map" of self in relation to world and pulls information together from many areas

Temporal lobe
Personal memories and language depend on these; without these faculties consciousness is severely curtailed

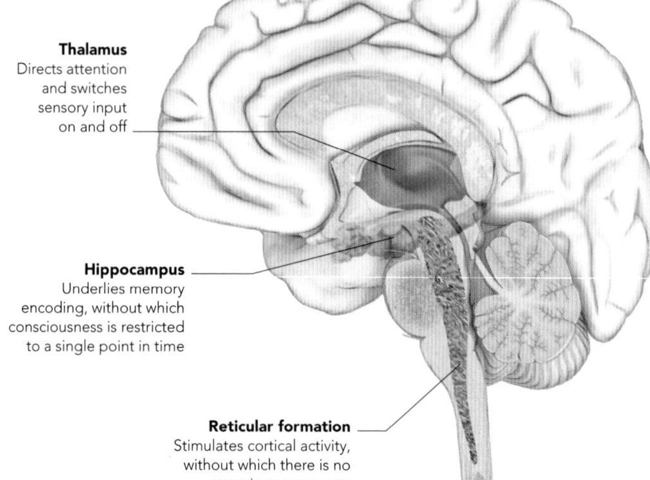

Thalamus
Directs attention and switches sensory input on and off

Hippocampus
Underlies memory encoding, without which consciousness is restricted to a single point in time

Reticular formation
Stimulates cortical activity, without which there is no conscious awareness

REQUIREMENTS OF CONSCIOUSNESS

Every state of conscious awareness has a specific pattern of brain activity associated with it. For example, seeing a patch of yellow produces one pattern of brain activity, hearing speech another. These patterns of activity are commonly referred to as the neural correlates of consciousness. If the brain state changes from one pattern to another, so does the experience of consciousness. The processes relevant to consciousness are generally assumed to be found at the level of brain cells rather than at the level of individual molecules or atoms. It is likely that, for consciousness to arise, the four factors listed below need to be present. Yet it is also possible that consciousness does arise at the far smaller atomic (quantum) level, and if so may be subject to very different laws.

VISUAL PHANTOMS

Conscious perception does not rely solely on external stimuli – it can also arise internally. Our brains constantly "fill in" missing information to make sense of the world. For example, you may see phantom-like vertical lines connecting the two blocks in the first column. This "imaginary" perception depends on similar neural-activity patterns as conscious perceptions of "real" stimuli.

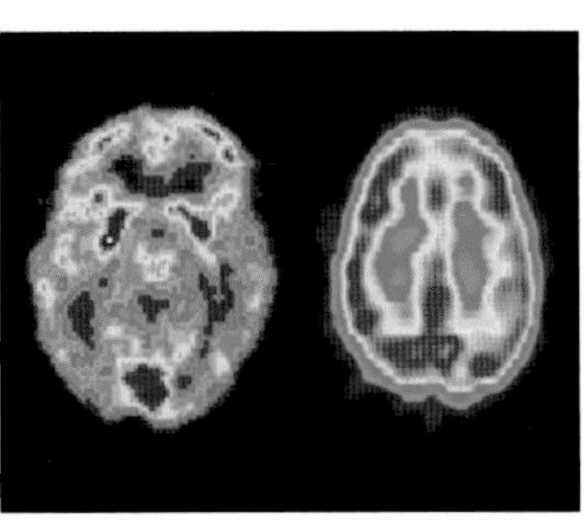

LEVEL OF COMPLEXITY

Neural activity must be complex for consciousness to occur, but not too complex. If all the neurons are firing, such as in an epileptic seizure, consciousness is lost.

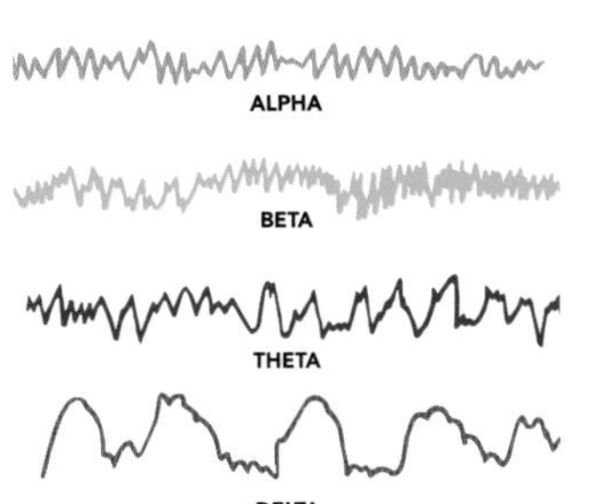

FIRING THRESHOLDS

Consciousness arises only when brain cells fire at fairly high rates. The high firing rate of Beta waves indicates alertness, while the low rate of Delta waves indicates deep sleep.

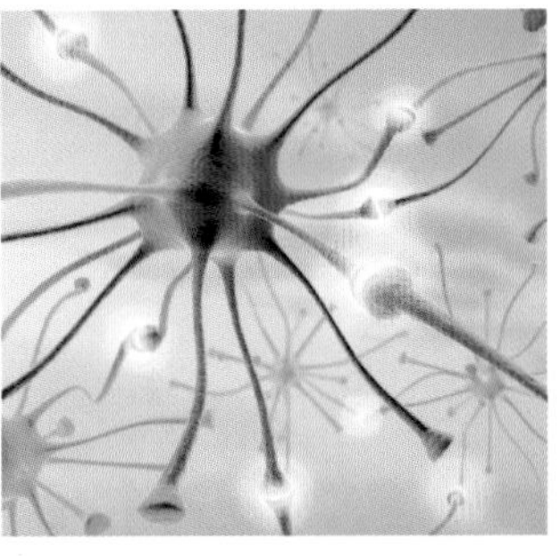

SYNCHRONOUS FIRING

Clusters of cells across the brain fire in unison. This seems to "bind" independent perceptions (say, the left and right visual fields) into one conscious perception.

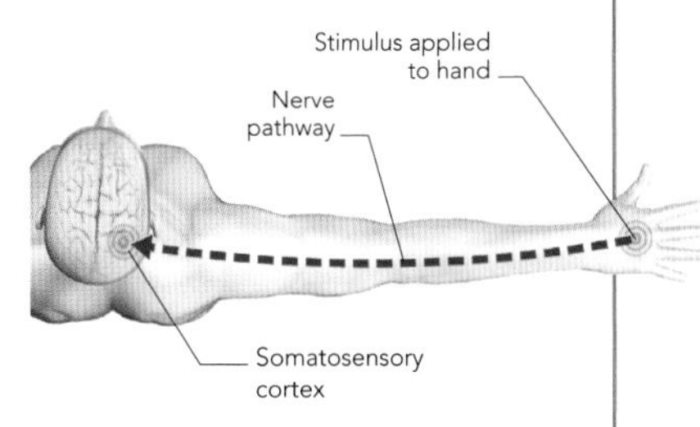

TIMING

It takes $\frac{1}{2}$ a second for the unconscious brain to process stimuli into conscious perceptions, but the brain fools us into thinking we experience things immediately.

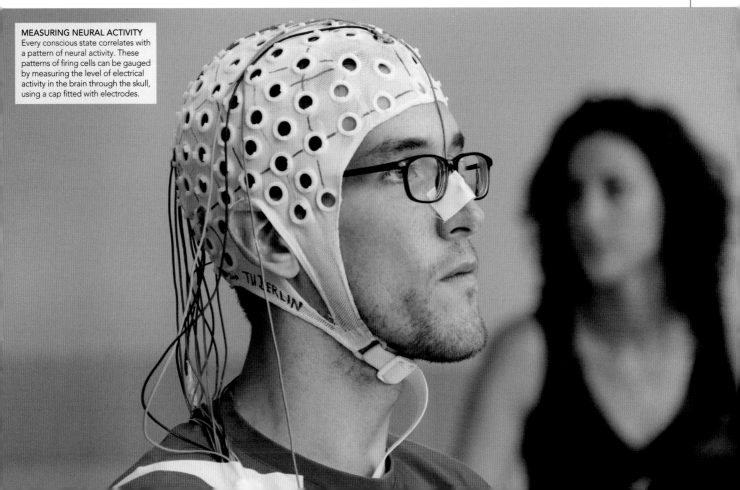

MEASURING NEURAL ACTIVITY

Every conscious state correlates with a pattern of neural activity. These patterns of firing cells can be gauged by measuring the level of electrical activity in the brain through the skull, using a cap fitted with electrodes.

ATTENTION AND CONSCIOUSNESS

ATTENTION CONTROLS AND DIRECTS CONSCIOUSNESS. IT ACTS LIKE A HIGHLIGHTER THAT MAKES CERTAIN PARTS OF THE WORLD "JUMP OUT" AND CAUSES THE REST TO RECEDE. IT SELECTS THE FEATURE THAT IS CURRENTLY MOST IMPORTANT IN THE ENVIRONMENT AND AMPLIFIES THE BRAIN'S RESPONSE TO IT.

WHAT IS ATTENTION?

Attention causes you to select one item from the sensory inputs you are receiving and allows you to become more fully or sharply conscious of it. Consciousness and attention are so closely linked that it is almost impossible to attend to something and not be conscious of it. Overt attention involves consciously directing the eyes, ears, or other sense organs towards a stimulus and processing information from it. Covert attention involves switching attention to a stimulus without directing the sense organs towards it. Attention may seem continuous, but maintaining focused attention is actually rare and difficult. It is also hard to switch attention from one object to another: the more attentive you are to one stimulus, the slower you are to turn your attention away from it. Hence an event that captures your attention will "blot out" anything else for a fraction of a second.

ATTENTION TYPES

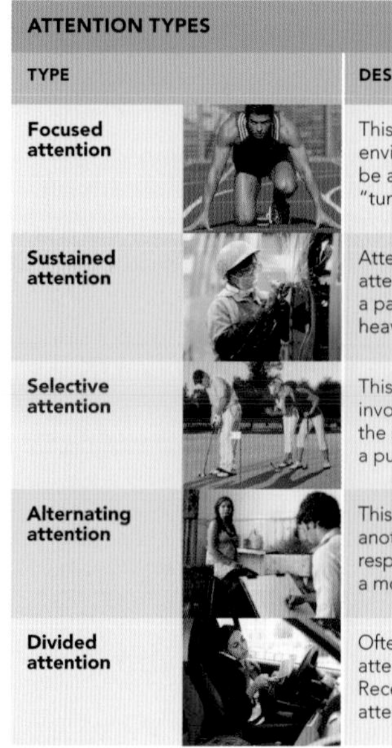

TYPE	DESCRIPTION
Focused attention	This is the ability to single out one object in one's environment and respond to it. An example might be an athlete focusing on the starter's gun, while "tuning out" the noise from the crowd.
Sustained attention	Attention naturally tends to wander. Sustained attention is the ability to maintain concentration on a particular object or activity, such as operating heavy machinery for a continuous period of time.
Selective attention	This form is similar to sustained attention, but involves the ability to resist shifting attention from the selected target, for example when focusing on a putt despite other competing stimuli.
Alternating attention	This involves shifting quickly from one stimulus to another, which requires a different sort of cognitive response – for example, when shifting attention from a model you are painting to the actual painting.
Divided attention	Often known as "multi-tasking", this involves dividing attention between two or more competing tasks. Recent research suggests that apparently divided attention is actually very quick alternating attention.

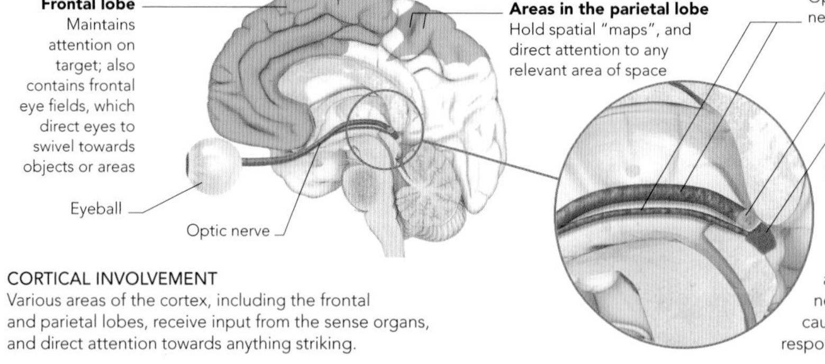
Frontal lobe
Maintains attention on target; also contains frontal eye fields, which direct eyes to swivel towards objects or areas
Eyeball
Optic nerve
Areas in the parietal lobe
Hold spatial "maps", and direct attention to any relevant area of space
Optic nerve
Lateral geniculate nucleus
Superior colliculus
SUPERIOR COLLICULUS
This is part of a network of brain areas that direct eye movements. Signals from the retina arrive here via the optic nerve; activity in this area causes attention to shift in response to notable stimuli.

CORTICAL INVOLVEMENT
Various areas of the cortex, including the frontal and parietal lobes, receive input from the sense organs, and direct attention towards anything striking.

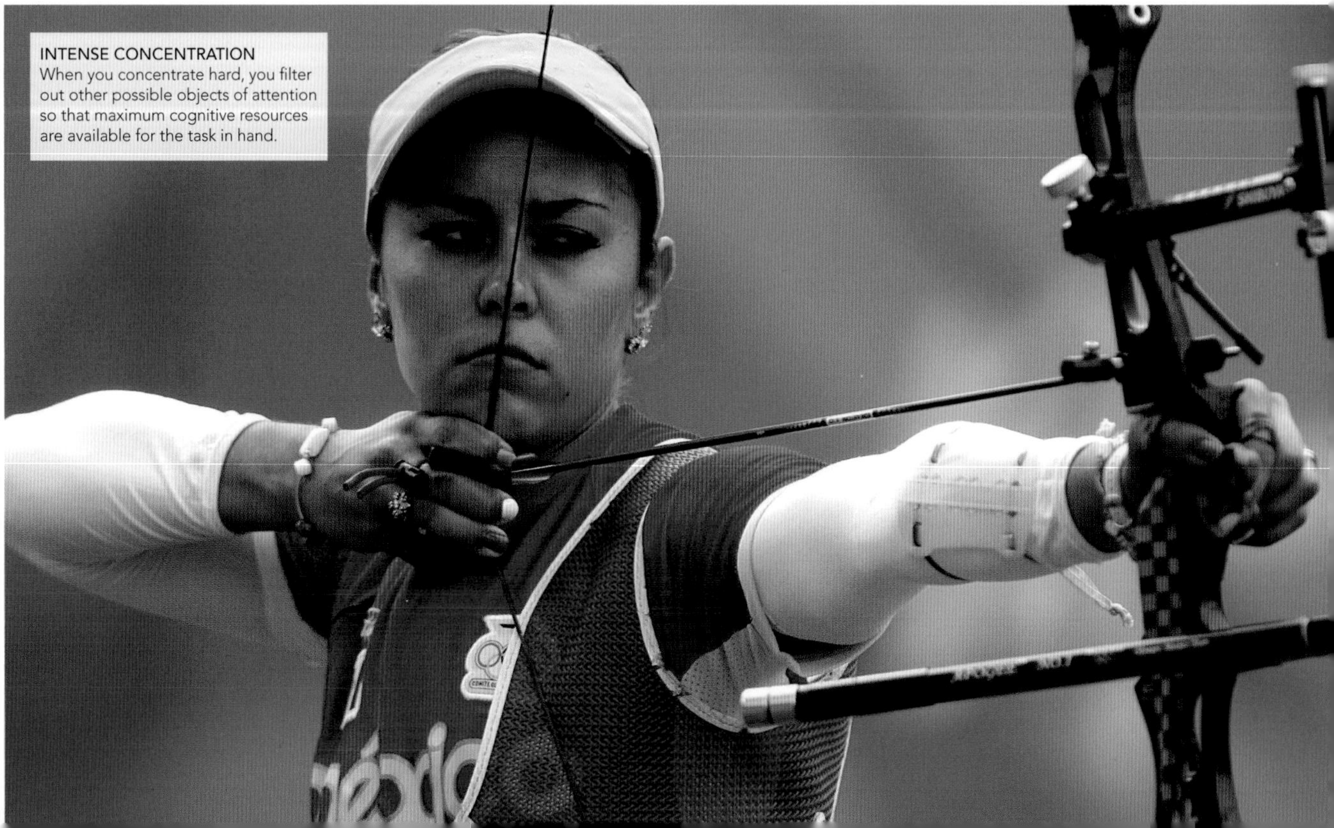

INTENSE CONCENTRATION
When you concentrate hard, you filter out other possible objects of attention so that maximum cognitive resources are available for the task in hand.

NEURAL MECHANISMS

If the brain registers an unexpected movement, a loud sound, or some other potentially significant stimulus, it directs the sense organs towards it – for example, by swivelling the eyes in the direction of a sudden movement. This happens automatically, in the lower regions of the brain, and it does not in itself create consciousness of the stimulus. However, attention also increases activity in the neurons that are concerned with the stimulus. If the stimulus is a person, for example, neural activity increases in the visual areas that monitor the place in space where the person is located; the face-recognition area; the amygdala; the temporal-parietal areas, which work out their intentions; and the supplementary motor area, which works out what to do about them. If the neurons are excited beyond a certain point, consciousness "kicks in".

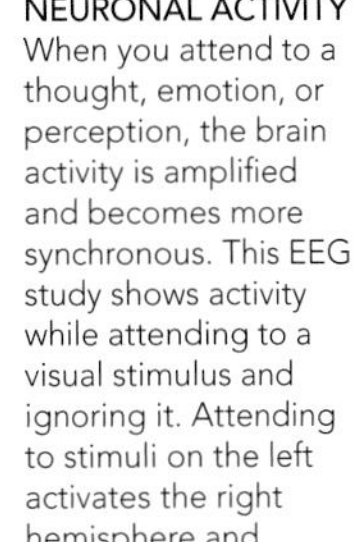

NEURONAL ACTIVITY
When you attend to a thought, emotion, or perception, the brain activity is amplified and becomes more synchronous. This EEG study shows activity while attending to a visual stimulus and ignoring it. Attending to stimuli on the left activates the right hemisphere and vice versa.

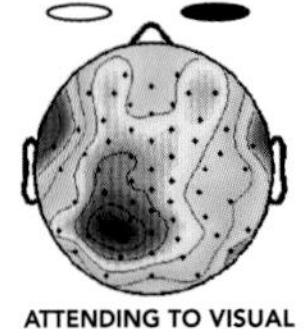

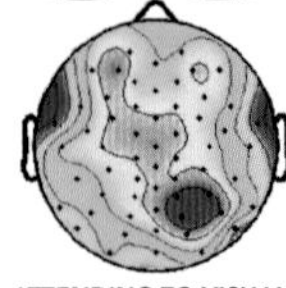

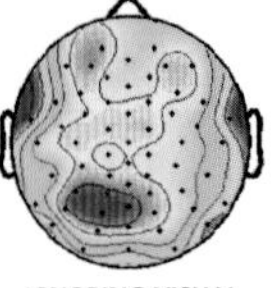

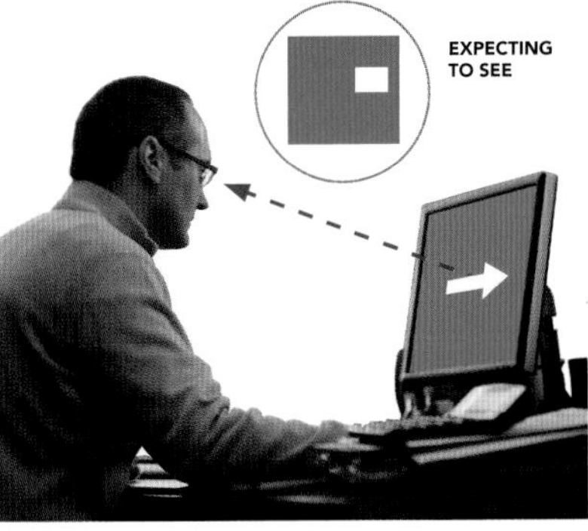

ATTENTION TO LOCATION
In this experiment, an arrow directs the subject's attention to a location where he expects a subsequent target stimulus to appear. While focusing on the location, waiting for something to appear, fMRI scans (below) show sustained activity in the frontal eye fields and parietal cortex – areas concerned with focusing on a particular area in space. Activity in the temporal lobe suggests readiness to identify the target when it appears.

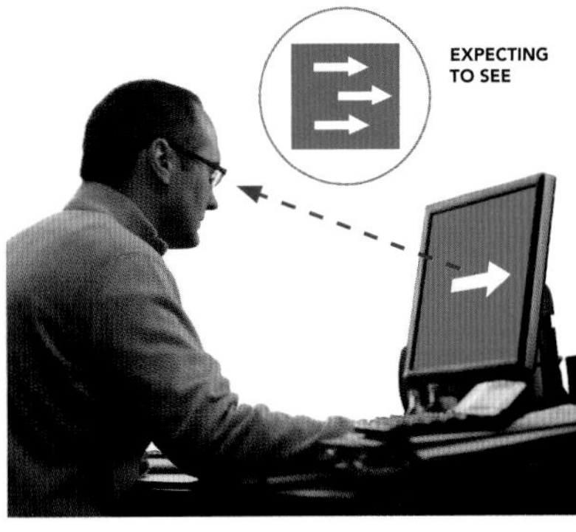

ATTENTION TO DIRECTION
In this experiment, the arrow tells the subject to look out for a moving target that will be travelling from left to right. This directional cue produces sustained signals in the frontal eye fields, as in the location task, but greater activity in the parietal lobes, where calculations are made about spatial direction as well as location. These calculations prime the brain to react to the target when it appears.

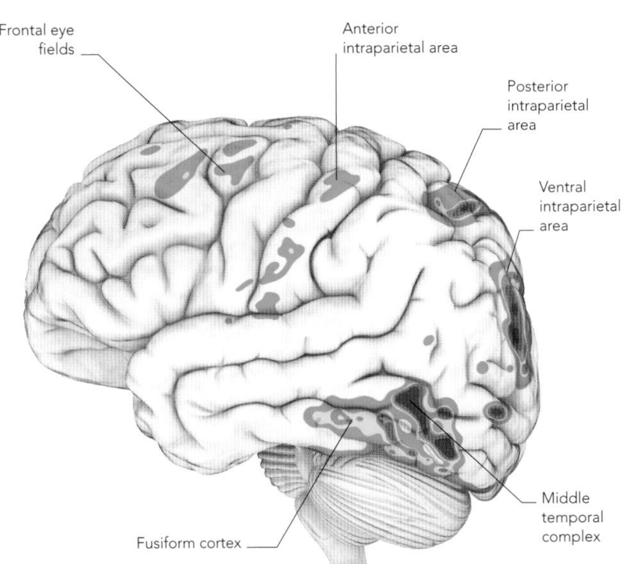

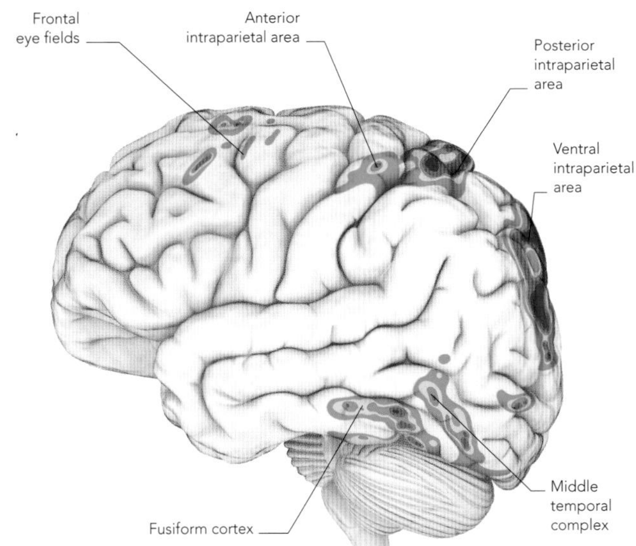

ABILITY TO FOCUS

The best-known attention disorder is ADHD (see p.246) but there are many others, affecting adults as well as children. Any variation from a normal ability to focus or shift attention might be considered a disorder if it disrupts a person's ability to function in their environment. Someone who gets absorbed in things that interest them and fails to notice other people talking to them might do very well in a job that calls for intense focus (scrutinizing medical images for abnormalities, say) but could be considered strange, or even ill, in a highly sociable environment. One type of attention failure – so-called "inattention blindness" – occurs when a person is so intent on focusing on one aspect of a scenario that they completely miss some other, major, component. It is so common that it is considered normal.

CARD TRICK
If the ace = 14, what number do the cards add up to? Focusing on this mathematical task might cause you to miss an unusual detail.

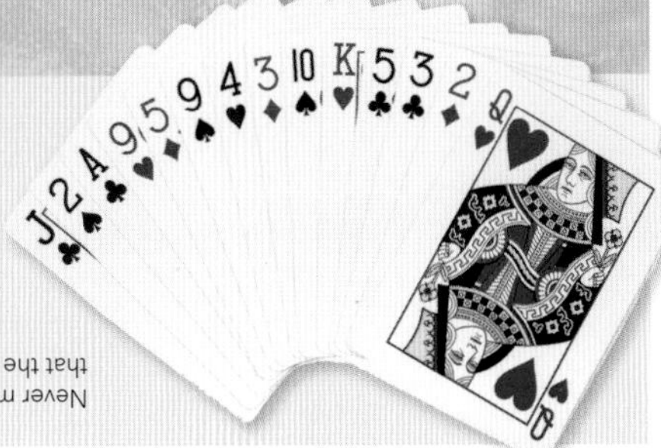

Never mind the total – did you spot that the four of hearts is black?

THE IDLING BRAIN

THE BRAIN HAS DISTINCT MODES, EACH OF WHICH USES A DIFFERENT NETWORK OF NEURONS. "RESTING-STATE NETWORKS" BECOME ACTIVATED WHEN WE CEASE TO BE FULLY ENGAGED WITH THE OUTSIDE WORLD.

THE RESTING STATE NETWORK

When the brain is not actively engaged in a task it falls into one of a number of resting states. The most common of these involves the default-mode network (DMN). When the brain is in task mode it responds to sensation by creating action plans, which are then turned into actual actions. In contrast, while in a resting state, the brain creates action plans but does not act them out – they are imagined scenarios. The medial frontal cortex is active in the resting state, indicating social rumination, while the lateral frontal cortex is active in task mode, indicating sequential thought patterns suited to handling objects.

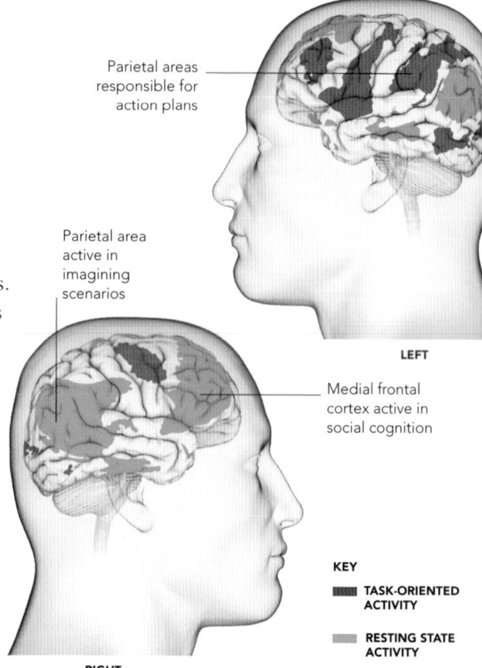

TASK AND RESTING STATES

These scans show the brain in two different states – at rest and while performing a task. The green areas show the areas of high activity in the resting state. When a person is actively engaged in a task, the purple areas become active and the green ones calm down.

READING THE DEFAULT-MODE NETWORK

Although default mode network activity is recognizably similar in everyone, there are small individual differences, which seem to tally with differences in personality. Researchers at several centres are charting individuals' DMN activity by EEG and correlating the information with those people's personalities. Drawing on this information, it may be possible to produce a brain-activity-related personality test.

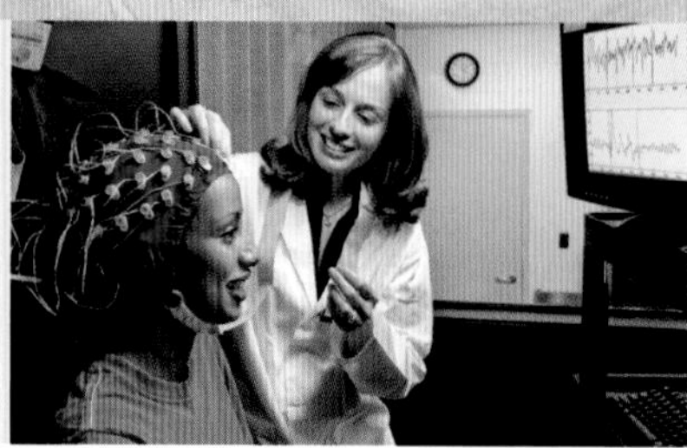

THE DMN AND SOCIAL AWARENESS

The areas of brain activated in the default-mode network are very similar to those activated when a person is asked to interpret a social situation and, in particular, their own situation with regard to other people. This suggests that whenever we are free of immediate mental tasks we fall back into a state of rumination about our relationships with others, and our place in the social world.

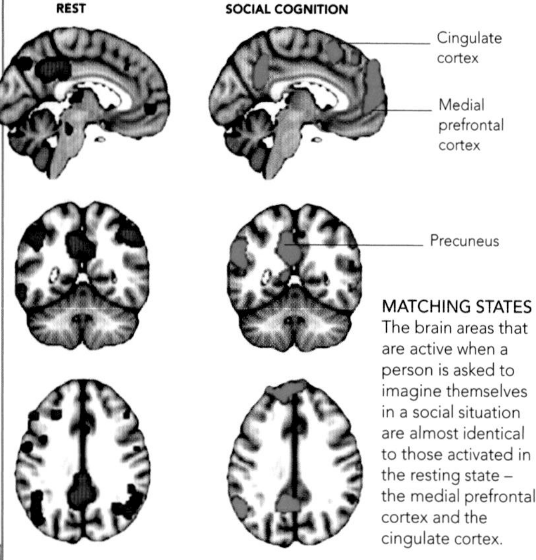

MATCHING STATES

The brain areas that are active when a person is asked to imagine themselves in a social situation are almost identical to those activated in the resting state – the medial prefrontal cortex and the cingulate cortex.

THE BRAIN'S EGO

The thoughts associated with the default-mode network are mainly self-centred and driven by one's own autobiography and place in the social hierarchy. They often draw on half-forgotten memories and are coloured by emotion. These are the concerns that Sigmund Freud identified with the half-submerged mind-state that he called the ego. Some researchers have suggested the DMN is functionally the same as the Freudian ego.

FREUD'S THEORY OF MIND

Freud thought that most brain processes were unconscious. The ego, part of the mind involved in self, was partly conscious. The rest of the conscious mind controlled thoughts and actions, and roughly matches the "task-oriented" mind state.

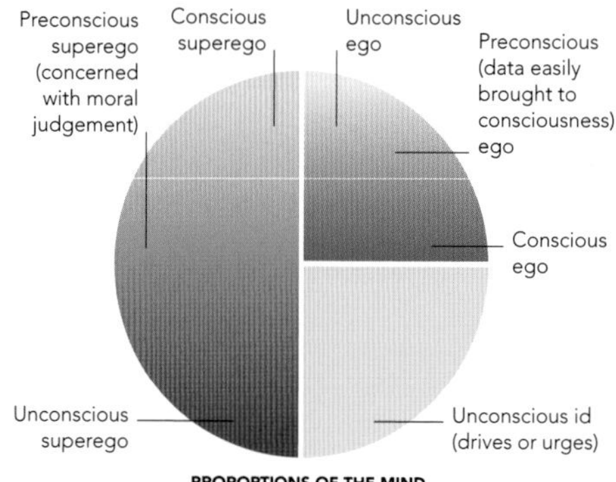

THE WANDERING MIND

People seem to spend about one-third of their waking hours in a resting state mode, and if they are doing something untaxing, such as driving down a straight, empty road, the proportion is even higher. In one experiment, people were invited to sit in a laboratory and do nothing except read a novel and report whenever their mind wandered. Over the course of half an hour, they typically reported one to three episodes of mind-wandering.

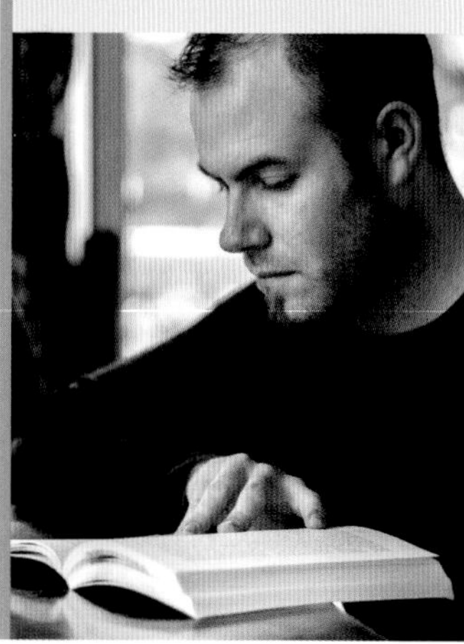

RESTING STATE AND CREATIVITY

Most people switch very cleanly from default mode to task mode if they are suddenly called upon to engage with the outside world. In some people, though, the two modes run concurrently. This may make them more creative, because the free-floating, discursive nature of thinking in the default mode may drift towards a solution to a problem that would escape the more targeted, constrained thinking associated with task-oriented cognition. However, overlap between the two modes is also associated with schizophrenia and depression. This may account for some of the unconventional thinking associated with schizophrenia and the lack of concentration displayed by many depressed people.

FIRING THE DMN
The connections between areas involved in the DMN are tighter in schizophrenics and their relatives. This means that if one of the areas is triggered, it is more likely to fire up the whole network.

CONTROL

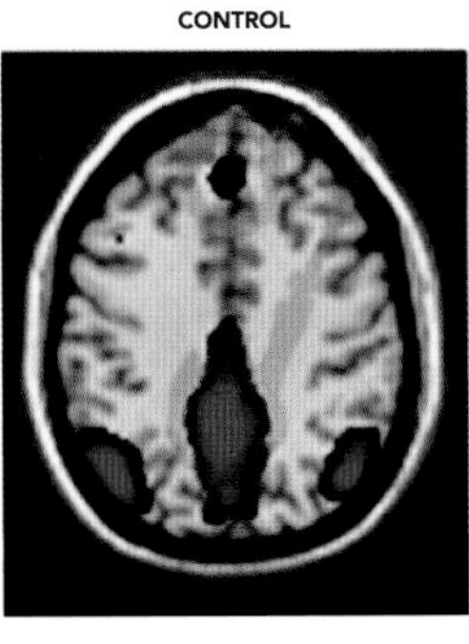

RELATIVE OF SCHIZOPHRENIC

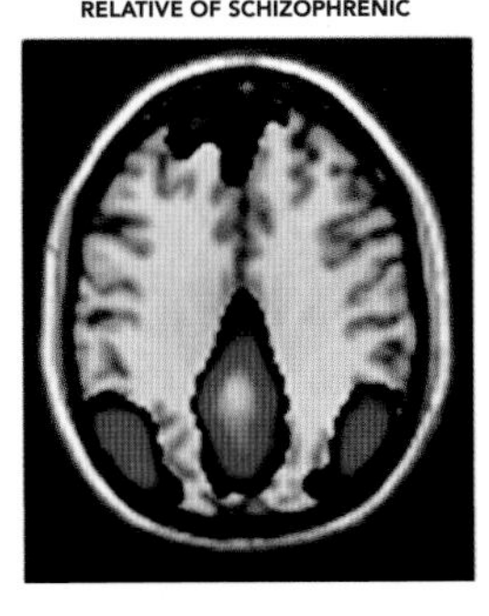

SCHIZOPHRENIC

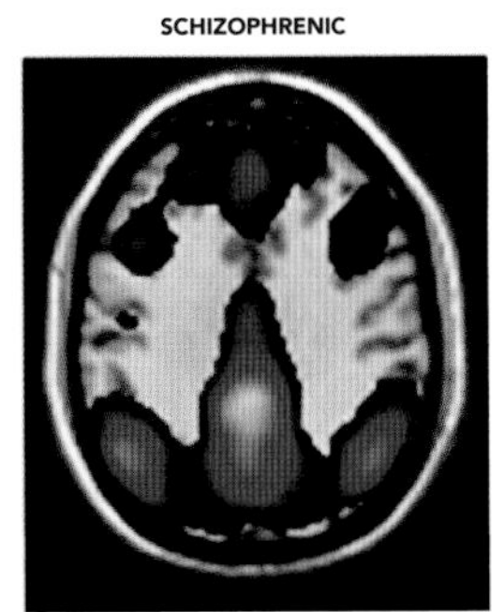

DMN IN ANIMALS

The default-mode network has been observed in animals other than humans. In fact, researchers have found it in all animal species tested so far, including dogs and rats. The regions of the brain most active in the DMN appear to be more highly developed the more social the animal species is – with humans forming the largest social groups of any animal and having correspondingly large "social brain" areas. One theory is that the DMN may allow all social animals to keep themselves secure and "up to speed" in their societies.

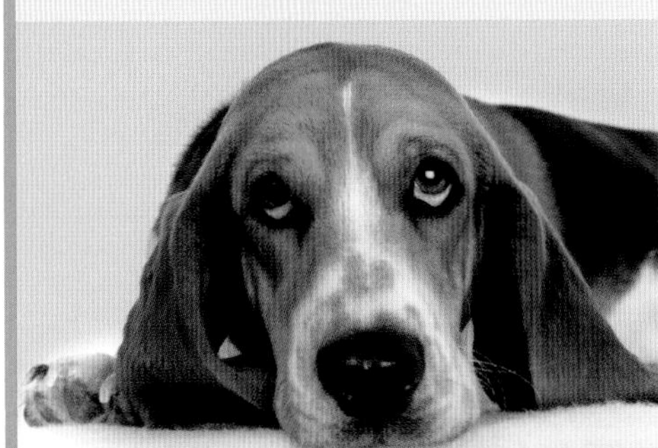

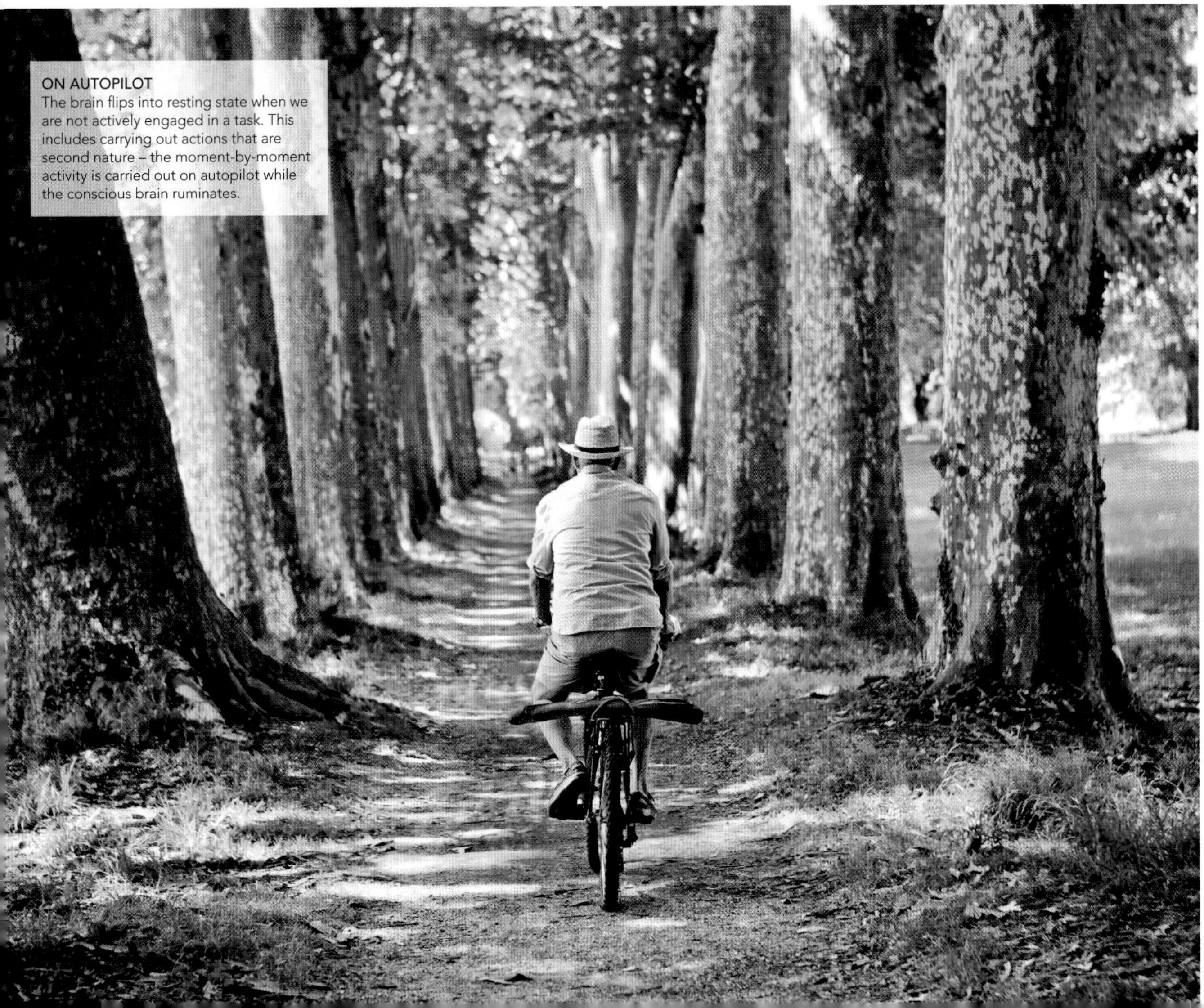

ON AUTOPILOT
The brain flips into resting state when we are not actively engaged in a task. This includes carrying out actions that are second nature – the moment-by-moment activity is carried out on autopilot while the conscious brain ruminates.

ALTERING CONSCIOUSNESS

THE BRAIN IS CAPABLE OF GENERATING A WIDE RANGE OF CONSCIOUS EXPERIENCES, INCLUDING SOME STATES THAT ALTER OUR PERCEPTIONS AND EMOTIONS TO SUCH AN EXTENT THAT THE ENTIRE WORLD SEEMS DRAMATICALLY DIFFERENT. SUCH "ALTERED STATES" ARE NOW THE SUBJECT OF INTENSE NEUROSCIENTIFIC RESEARCH.

ALTERED BRAIN STATES

Our normal waking state varies from daydreaming, through relaxed awareness, to sharply focused. The brain is capable of generating a much wider range of conscious experiences than this, though. Sometimes we slip outside the normal range spontaneously, when feverish or exhausted, for instance, or during or after an emotionally overwhelming event. We may also deliberately seek to get out of our normal state by engaging in rituals such as prolonged dancing, or through meditation, or by taking drugs.

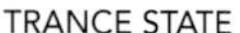

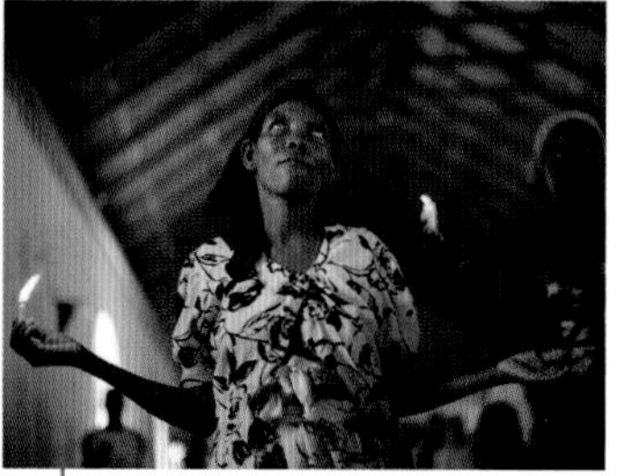

TRANCE STATE
A trance is an altered state of consciousness that may be induced by hypnosis, drugs, or ritual. It can be pleasurable or frightening.

Frontal lobe
May go "offline" in altered states, reducing critical thinking; can be hyperactive during meditation, indicating increased attention

Parietal lobe
Altered activity here may create out-of-body feeling or distorted experience of space and time

Corpus callosum
Allows the two hemispheres to communicate; blissful states are linked with greater synchrony between hemispheres and sudden switches of activity from one hemisphere to another

Temporal lobe
Flurries of activity here are associated with unexplainable experiences including hallucinations and sensing auras or an invisible presence

Thalamus
May shut off incoming information, sending a person into "a world of their own"

Reticular formation
Alerting signals from reticular formation to cerebral cortex may be reduced, causing increased relaxation and sense of wellbeing

BRAIN AREAS INVOLVED IN ALTERED STATES
Altered states may range from blissful to terrible, and they are generated by correspondingly varied changes in neural activity in the brain, particularly involving the areas shown here.

DISSOCIATION

Dissociation refers to instances when elements of consciousness (the sensations, thoughts, and emotions of the moment) that are sometimes bound together as a whole are, instead, experienced separately or are cut out of conscious awareness. Many altered states fall into this category. Usually, dissociation is referred to as a mental or behavioural disorder, but some "normal" conscious states, such as daydreaming or concentrating, are dissociative. It is more accurate to look at these conscious states as a spectrum (see below), with highly unified or "bound" experience at one end and "fractured" consciousness at the other.

HYPNOSIS

Hypnosis is a form of dissociation in which a person's field of attention is narrowed to a single thought, feeling, or idea. When experiencing this state of mind, normal distractions and preoccupations may be kept out of mind. People undergoing hypnosis voluntarily may become very suggestible to the hypnotist's ideas, so it is often used therapeutically, for instance, to break a habit such as smoking.

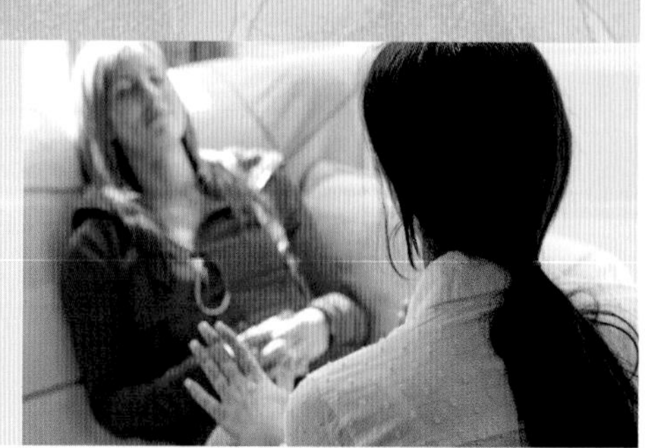

BOUND TOGETHER — **NORMAL** — **FRACTURED**

FEELING OF ONENESS OR "MEANINGFULNESS"

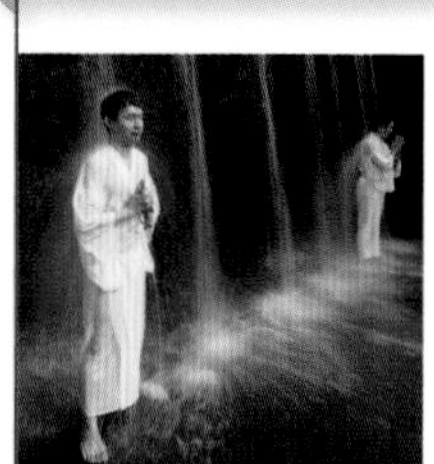

STATE OF EXTREME RELAXATION WITH FEWER INTROSPECTIVE THOUGHTS

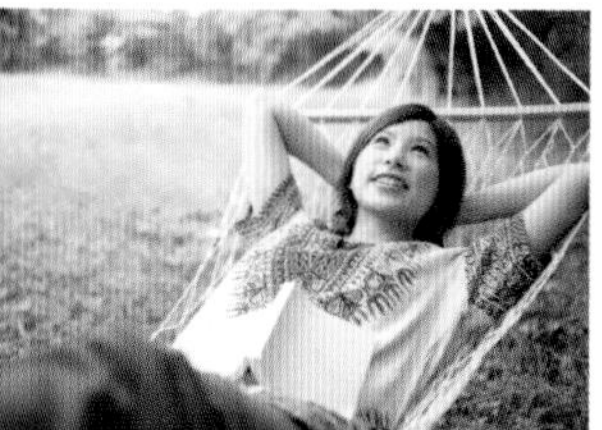

DAYDREAMING; CAN SPRING BACK TO ALERT IMMEDIATELY

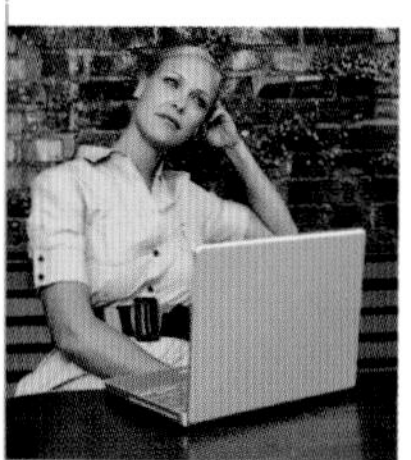

HIGH LEVEL OF ALERTNESS AND AWARENESS

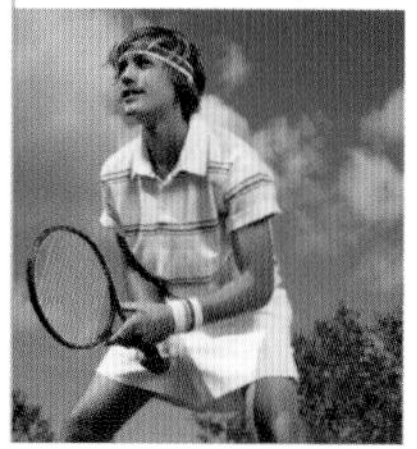

SEPARATION FROM SELF OR SENSE OF BEING DISTANCED FROM REALITY

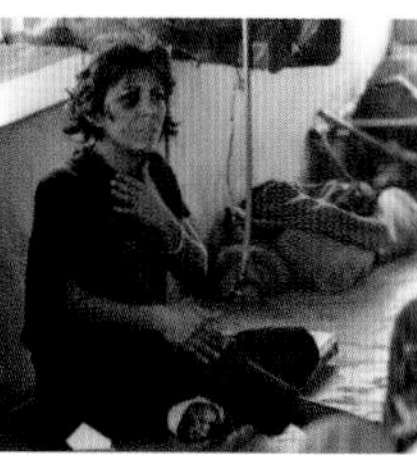

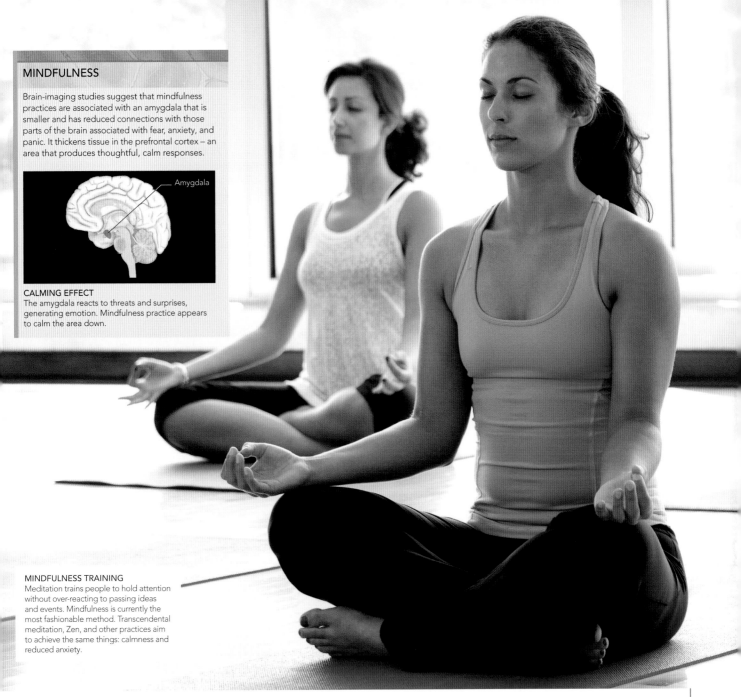

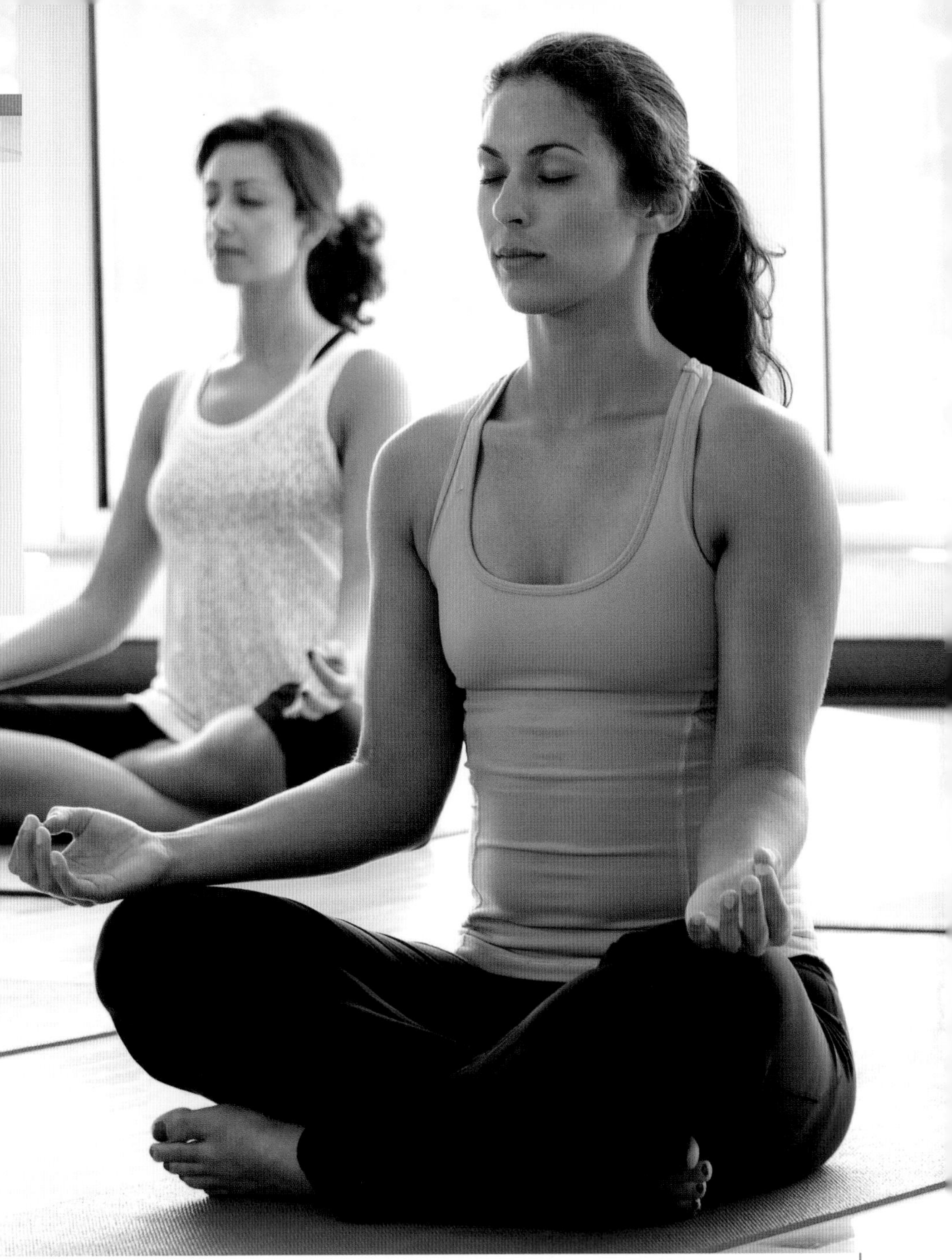

MINDFULNESS

Brain-imaging studies suggest that mindfulness practices are associated with an amygdala that is smaller and has reduced connections with those parts of the brain associated with fear, anxiety, and panic. It thickens tissue in the prefrontal cortex – an area that produces thoughtful, calm responses.

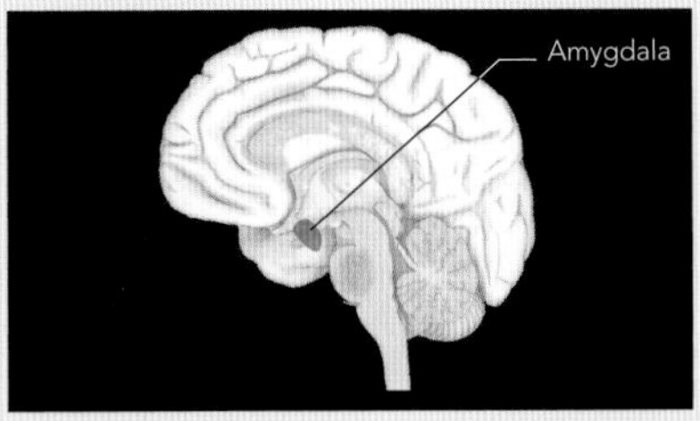

Amygdala

CALMING EFFECT
The amygdala reacts to threats and surprises, generating emotion. Mindfulness practice appears to calm the area down.

MINDFULNESS TRAINING
Meditation trains people to hold attention without over-reacting to passing ideas and events. Mindfulness is currently the most fashionable method. Transcendental meditation, Zen, and other practices aim to achieve the same things: calmness and reduced anxiety.

OUT-OF-BODY EXPERIENCES

Out-of-body experiences (OBEs) occur when the internal representation of the body is out of kilter with the real body. This often happens in dreams, but when you are awake it may be interpreted as a supernatural event. OBEs typically occur as you wake up, before the brain has properly reconnected with the external world (see p.173) and are associated with activity in the temporo-parietal junction.

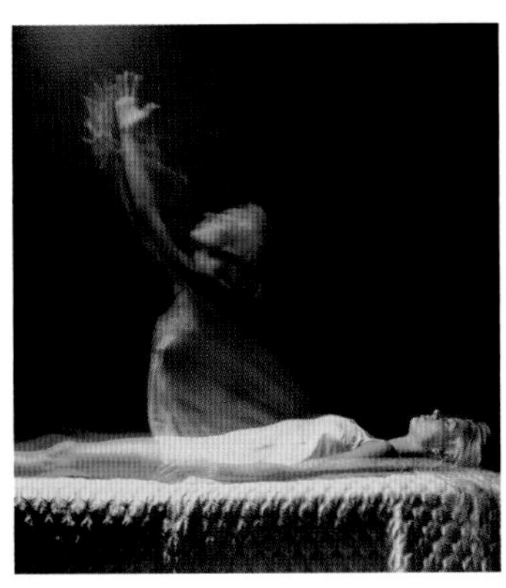

NEAR-DEATH EXPERIENCES
OBEs are often accompanied by feelings of ecstasy, and they are a central feature of many so-called "near-death experiences".

THE COLLECTIVE UNCONSCIOUS

Carl Jung (1875–1961) was a Swiss psychiatrist who developed the idea of the collective unconscious – a part of the unconscious mind shared by everyone as a product of ancestry, which can be accessed in certain states of mind. He thought it included "archetypes" (innate, universal concepts) such as the mother, God, hero and so on, and that we detect their influences in the form of myths, symbols, and instinct. Presumably he saw the collective unconscious as a sort of "folk memory", embodied in the structure of the brain.

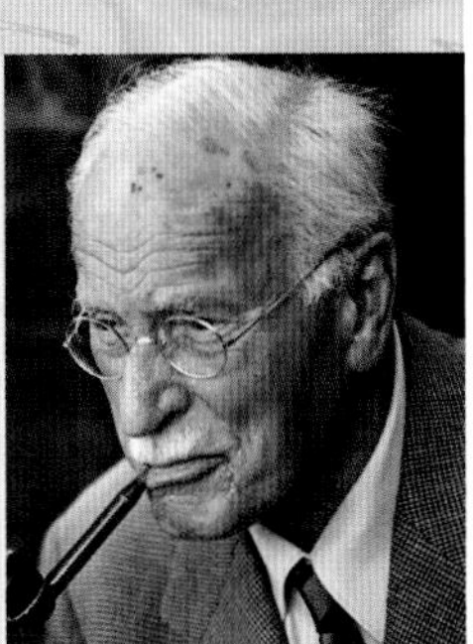

SLEEP AND DREAMS

ABOUT A THIRD OF LIFE IS SPENT ASLEEP, DURING WHICH TIME THE BRAIN REMAINS ACTIVE, FULFILLING A RANGE OF IMPORTANT FUNCTIONS. DURING SLEEP, THE BRAIN GENERATES DREAMS, WHICH PROVIDE US WITH SOME OF THE MOST INTENSE AND STRANGE EXPERIENCES THAT WE HAVE.

THE SLEEPING BRAIN

No one is quite sure what it is about sleep that makes it so important. One theory is that it allows "downtime" for the body to repair itself. One way it may do this is by draining away detritus – the broken-down molecules that accumulate in cerebrospinal fluid during cell activation. Another is that it simply keeps the person out of danger for a period of time during each day, by keeping them still. A third is that the brain needs to switch off from the outside world in order to sort, process, and memorize information. Certainly, important memory functions do occur during sleep, but whether or not this is the primary purpose of sleep remains unclear. Sleep–wake cycles are controlled by neurotransmitters that act on different parts of the brain to induce sleep or waking up. Research also suggests that a chemical called adenosine builds up in the blood while we are awake and causes drowsiness; while we sleep, the chemical is gradually broken down.

SLEEP PROBLEMS

About one in five people suffer problems with sleep. The most common complaint is insomnia – the inability to fall or stay asleep. Insomnia is treated with drugs that bind to receptors for GABA (the brain's inhibitory neurotransmitter). Narcolepsy is a sleep disorder that causes people to fall asleep suddenly and inappropriately, or to feel exhausted through the day. Narcoleptics cannot experience the amount of restorative deep sleep that healthy people have and live in a state of sleep deprivation. When they fall asleep – which may occur with little warning – they enter REM sleep almost immediately and have vivid dreams. Sleepwalking occurs in deep sleep when a block that stops motor impulses is lifted but other sleep mechanisms remain. Sleepwalkers do complex things, such as driving cars, but they perform actions robotically, as they are following automatic action plans stored in the unconscious brain.

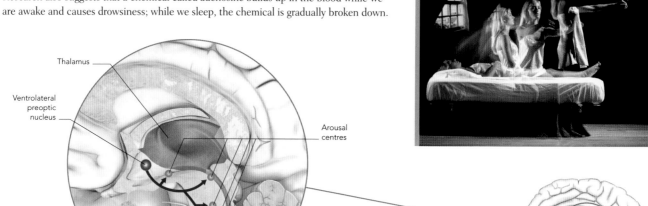

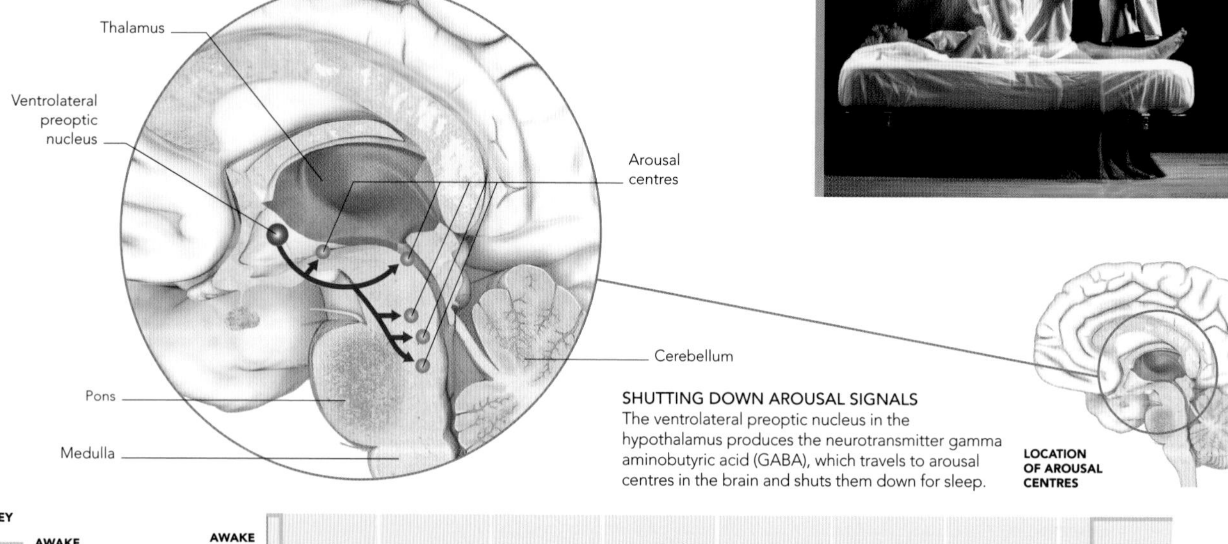

SHUTTING DOWN AROUSAL SIGNALS
The ventrolateral preoptic nucleus in the hypothalamus produces the neurotransmitter gamma aminobutyric acid (GABA), which travels to arousal centres in the brain and shuts them down for sleep.

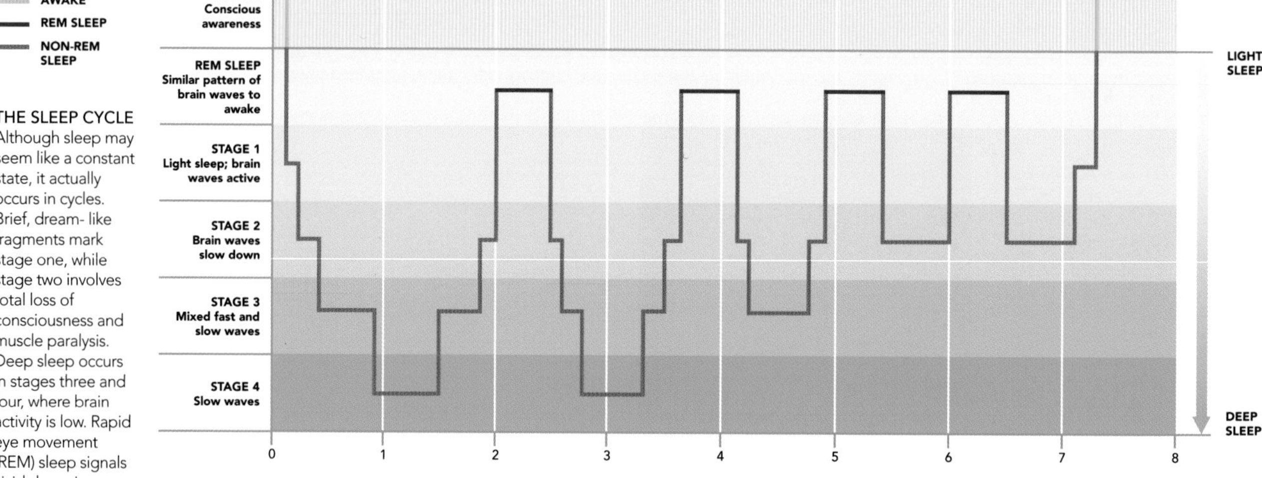

THE SLEEP CYCLE
Although sleep may seem like a constant state, it actually occurs in cycles. Brief, dream- like fragments mark stage one, while stage two involves total loss of consciousness and muscle paralysis. Deep sleep occurs in stages three and four, where brain activity is low. Rapid eye movement (REM) sleep signals vivid dreaming.

THE DREAMING BRAIN

There are two types of dreaming. During deep sleep we have vague, often emotionally charged and nonsensical dreams that are often forgotten immediately. The brain is not very active, but seems to be gently processing information in order to lay it down in memory. In REM sleep the brain becomes very active and produces vivid, intense "virtual realities", typically with a narrative. The part of the brain that processes sensations is very active during REM dreaming. The frontal lobes, which include areas that apply critical analysis to our experience, are effectively turned off, so when crazy events happen in our dreams, we just accept them.

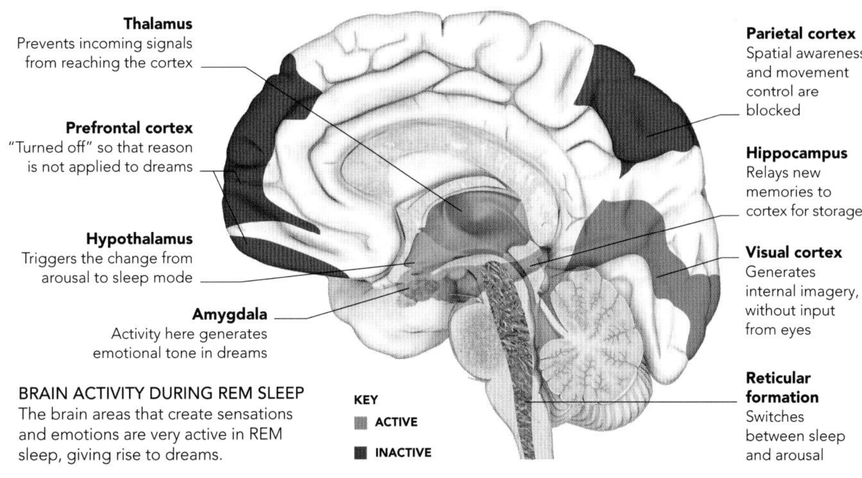
Thalamus
Prevents incoming signals from reaching the cortex
Prefrontal cortex
"Turned off" so that reason is not applied to dreams
Hypothalamus
Triggers the change from arousal to sleep mode
Amygdala
Activity here generates emotional tone in dreams
Parietal cortex
Spatial awareness and movement control are blocked
Hippocampus
Relays new memories to cortex for storage
Visual cortex
Generates internal imagery, without input from eyes
Reticular formation
Switches between sleep and arousal
KEY
ACTIVE
INACTIVE

BRAIN ACTIVITY DURING REM SLEEP
The brain areas that create sensations and emotions are very active in REM sleep, giving rise to dreams.

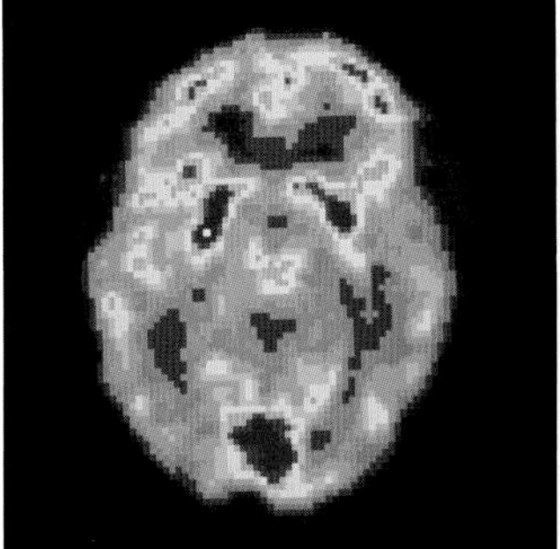

AWAKE
This PET scan shows the areas that are active when a person is awake (shown in red and yellow). The green and blue areas are less active.

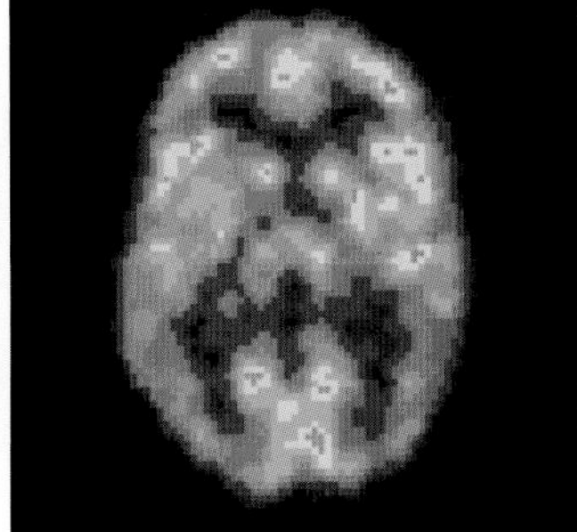

DEEP SLEEP
This PET scan shows that activity quietens down in many areas of the brain during deep sleep. The purple areas are the least active.

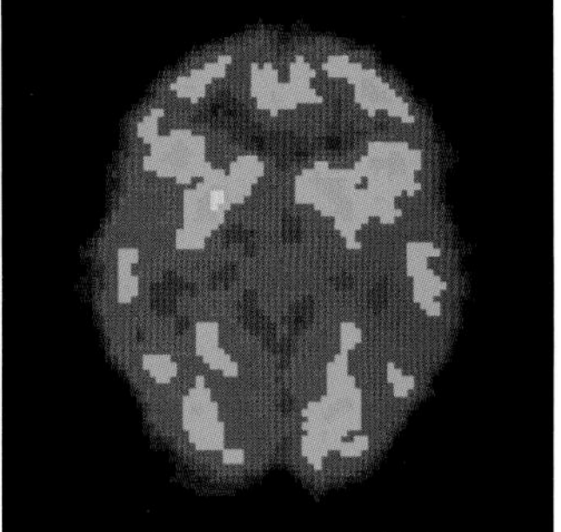

DRUGGED SLEEP
Most sleeping drugs induce a deeper sleep than normal. The purple areas on this PET scan show that much of the brain is inactive.

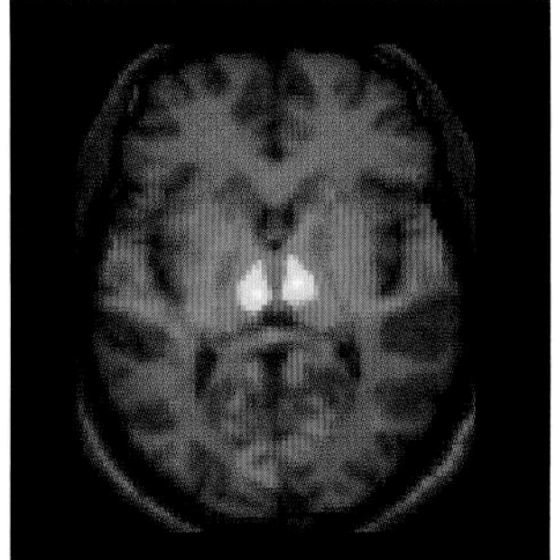

REM SLEEP
This fMRI scan shows activity during REM sleep (yellow most active, then red), it spans areas involved with generating sensations.

WAKING AND LUCID DREAMS

Usually, when shifting from dreaming to waking, several changes occur together in the brain. The block on incoming stimuli is lifted, so external sensory inputs enter the brain again, which overrides and turns off the internally generated sensations that comprise dreams. The block on outgoing signals from the motor cortex is also lifted, so that it becomes possible to move again. Additionally, the frontal lobes are reactivated, shifting us back into a normal state of consciousness in which we know who and where we are, and can tell the difference between fantasy and reality. Lucid dreams occur when the frontal lobes "wake up" during sleep, but the block on incoming and outgoing signals continues. As the frontal lobes are active, the dreamer is able to deduce that they are actually dreaming and experience events in a normal state of mind.

ANYTHING IS POSSIBLE
In lucid dreams you can control the action just as in a waking daydream, but the experience is more intense and seems real.

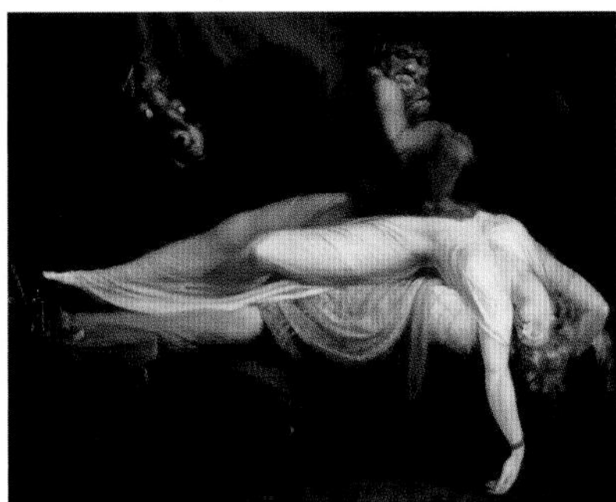

SLEEP PARALYSIS
Waking up while the motor-impulse blockade is still operating is known as sleep paralysis. This frightening sensation feels like being weighed down, which may be the origin of the myth of the incubi and succubi, evil spirits that were thought to squat on sleepers.

FREUD AND PSYCHOANALYSIS

Sigmund Freud was an Austrian psychiatrist, who founded the study of psychoanalysis. He called dreaming the "royal route to the unconscious", because he thought that dreams revealed the emotions and desires that we suppress when we are awake. He postulated that these suppressed desires are often too shocking to be consciously admitted, and even in dreams they have to be disguised in symbols. Freudian dream analysis aimed to decode the symbols to reveal the true nature of the desires of the dreamer.

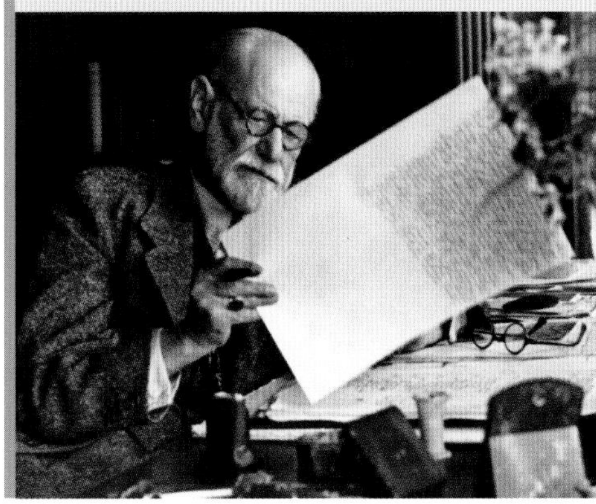

TIME

TIME IS NOT A CONSTANT IN THE BRAIN – IT SPEEDS UP AND SLOWS DOWN ACCORDING TO WHAT IS BEING EXPERIENCED. THE BRAIN HAS MANY DIFFERENT WAYS OF MEASURING TIME. LONGER DURATIONS, SUCH AS DAY LENGTH, ARE MEASURED BY THE EBB AND FLOW OF HORMONES, WHILE THE MILLISECOND INTERVALS INVOLVED IN MANY BRAIN PROCESSES ARE MARKED BY THE OSCILLATION OF NEURONS.

SUBJECTIVE TIME

The passage of time as we experience it (known as subjective time) is not the same as the regular passage of time as measured out by our clocks (objective time). The crucial difference is that subjective time can speed up and slow down, according to what we are experiencing. On a moment-by-moment scale, the rate at which time seems to pass is dictated by the rate of firing, or oscillation, of clusters of neurons. The faster they fire, the more events we register in any given second, giving us the impression that time lasts longer. Neuronal firing is controlled by neurotransmitters - excitatory ones speed it up, and inhibitory ones slow it down. Young people have more excitatory neurotransmitters and, therefore, are able to cope with faster external events.

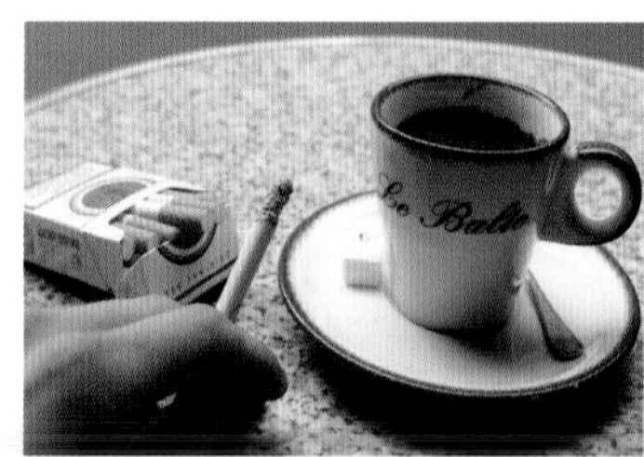

TIME PASSING SLOWLY
Stimulants like caffeine speed up the brain, allowing more external events to be registered. This produces a sense of time stretching out.

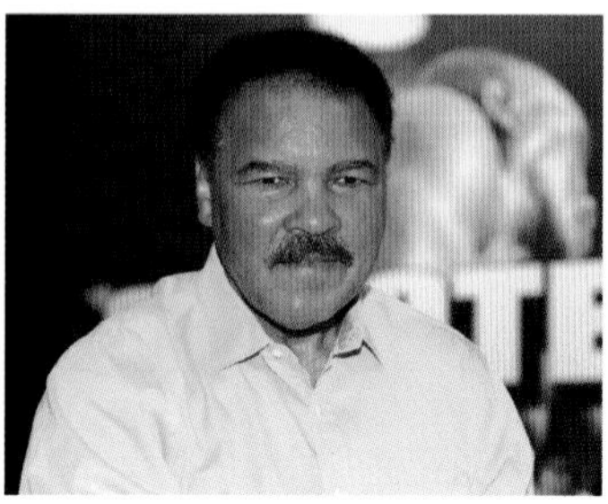

TIME RUSHING BY
Severe depletion of dopamine, as in Parkinson's disease, may slow the brain down so much that the external world seems to be rushing by.

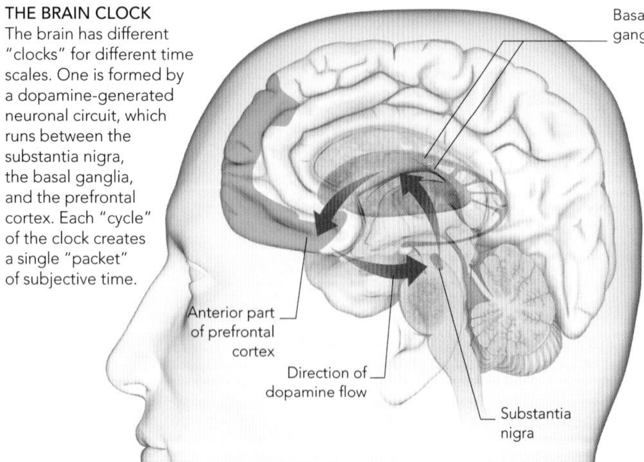
Basal ganglia
Anterior part of prefrontal cortex
Direction of dopamine flow
Substantia nigra

THE BRAIN CLOCK
The brain has different "clocks" for different time scales. One is formed by a dopamine-generated neuronal circuit, which runs between the substantia nigra, the basal ganglia, and the prefrontal cortex. Each "cycle" of the clock creates a single "packet" of subjective time.

CATATONIA

Catatonia is a state most commonly observed in people with certain types of schizophrenia. The sufferer becomes motionless and stops reacting to external stimuli. They may remain mute, or rigid, for days on end, sometimes striking bizarre poses, which would normally be impossible to maintain. The state seems to come about when the flow of dopamine slows right down, and people who have experienced this condition report that they lose all sense of time.

PACKETS OF TIME
The brain divides time into "packets" (a cycle of neural activity), each of which registers a single event. The size of the packet depends on how fast the relevant neurons are firing, but regardless of the size of the packet, the brain will only be able to take in one event from that packet. If two events happen, the brain will miss the second one. Some events will always appear blurred to us, such as the beating of a dragonfly's wings, as several flaps occur in each packet.

EXPERIENCING EVENTS
If the "clock" neurons fire only once in 1/10 of a second, only one event will be registered in that time, although many more may actually occur. If the neural clock doubles its speed, both events will be registered because the neural clock will have created two "packets" of subjective time.

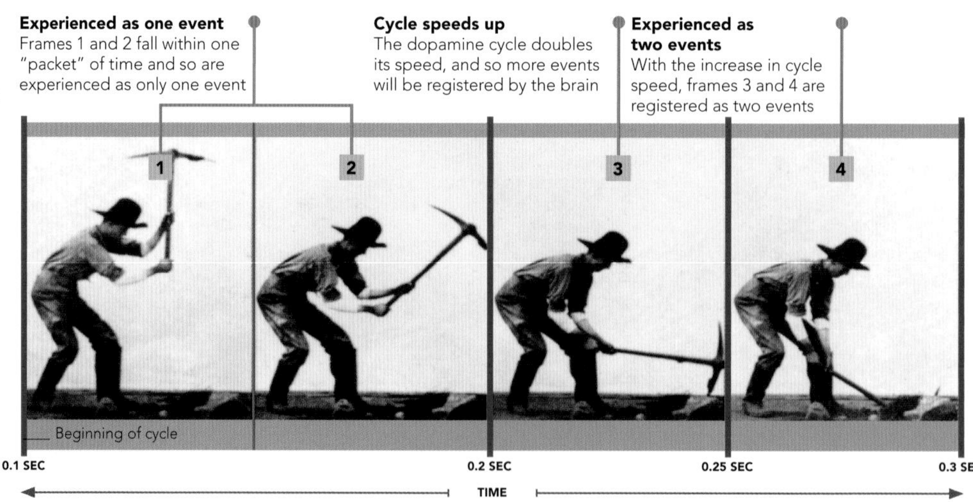
Experienced as one event
Frames 1 and 2 fall within one "packet" of time and so are experienced as only one event
Cycle speeds up
The dopamine cycle doubles its speed, and so more events will be registered by the brain
Experienced as two events
With the increase in cycle speed, frames 3 and 4 are registered as two events
1
2
3
4
Beginning of cycle
0.1 SEC
0.2 SEC
0.25 SEC
0.3 SEC
TIME

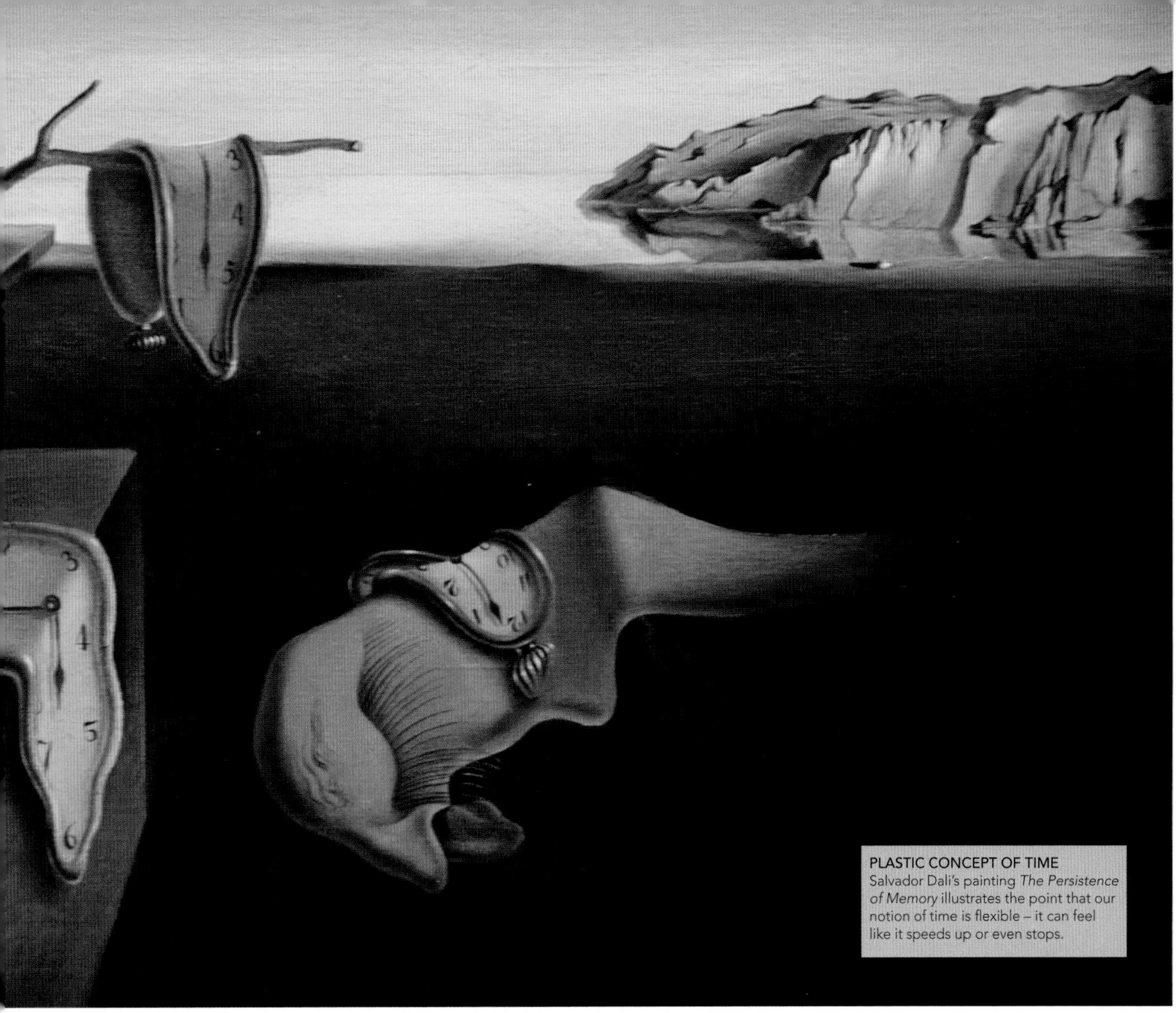

PLASTIC CONCEPT OF TIME
Salvador Dali's painting *The Persistence of Memory* illustrates the point that our notion of time is flexible – it can feel like it speeds up or even stops.

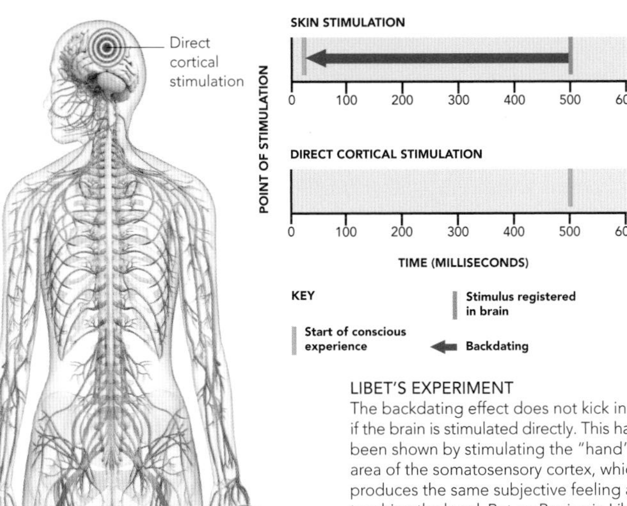

LIBET'S EXPERIMENT
The backdating effect does not kick in if the brain is stimulated directly. This has been shown by stimulating the "hand" area of the somatosensory cortex, which produces the same subjective feeling as touching the hand. But, as Benjamin Libet discovered, if you stimulate the brain and the hand at the same time, the feeling brought on by touching the hand is reported before the one produced by stimulating the brain.

BACKDATING TIME

It takes on average half a second for the unconscious mind to process incoming sensory stimuli into conscious perceptions. Yet we are not aware of this time lag – you think you see things move as they move, and when you stub your toe you get the impression of knowing about it straight away. This illusion of immediacy is created by an ingenious mechanism, which backdates conscious perceptions to the time when the stimulus first entered the brain. On the face of it, this seems impossible because cortical signals take the same "real" time to process to consciousness, but somehow we are tricked into thinking we feel things earlier. One way it might be explained is that consciousness consists of many parallel streams and that the brain jumps from one to another, revising them and redrafting them.

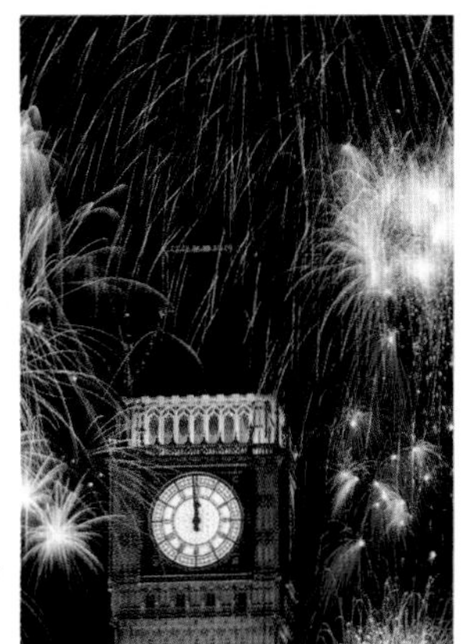

HALF A SECOND LATE
We become conscious of events around us nearly half a second after they occur, but we do not notice this time lag.

THE SELF AND CONSCIOUSNESS

THE HUMAN BRAIN GENERATES AN IDEA OF "SELF" THAT ALLOWS US TO "OWN" OUR EXPERIENCES AND FORGES A CONNECTION BETWEEN OUR THOUGHTS AND INTENTIONS, OUR BODIES, AND OUR ACTIONS. OUR SENSE OF SELF ALSO ALLOWS US TO EXAMINE OUR OWN MINDS AND TO USE WHAT WE SEE TO GUIDE OUR BEHAVIOUR.

WHAT IS THE SELF?

We divide the world into that which is subjective and internal and that which is objective and external. The boundary between the two acts like a container, which holds the former and places the latter outside. This container is what we know as the "self". Among other things, it includes our thoughts, intentions, and habits, as well as our actual bodies. Except in altered states (see p.186), all experiences we report include a sense of self, but most of the time the sense is unconscious. This "consciousness-with-self" is what we generally call "consciousness". When the sense of self becomes conscious, we talk of being "self-conscious".

LEVELS OF CONSCIOUSNESS	
The sense of self lies at the heart of our experiences. It takes various forms and operates at different levels of our consciousness.	
Introspection	You think about your own thoughts or action; one form is being "self-conscious" about your performance of an act.
Normal consciousness	You feel that your thoughts are your own, and your actions are the result of your decisions; you can report experiences.
Knowledge	You react to the environment, perhaps by doing complex actions (such as driving), but if asked you can't recall doing it.
Unconsciousness	In deepest sleep, your brain does not perceive the outside world or generate a sense of self to experience anything.

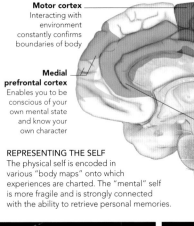

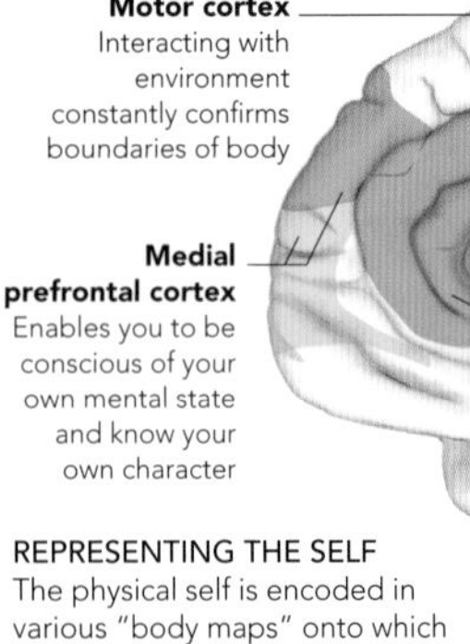
Motor cortex
Interacting with environment constantly confirms boundaries of body
Medial prefrontal cortex
Enables you to be conscious of your own mental state and know your own character
Somatosensory cortex
Sensations from body give repeated reminders of physical embodiment
Parietal cortex
This "maps" the body and its relationship to outside world
Posterior cingulate cortex
Active in personal memory retrieval, awareness of social interactions, and a crucial player in default-mode network (see p.184)
Anterior cingulate cortex
This monitors our own actions

REPRESENTING THE SELF
The physical self is encoded in various "body maps" onto which experiences are charted. The "mental" self is more fragile and is strongly connected with the ability to retrieve personal memories.

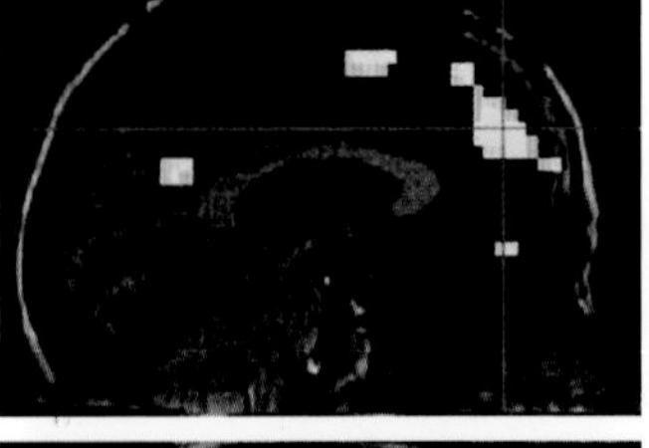
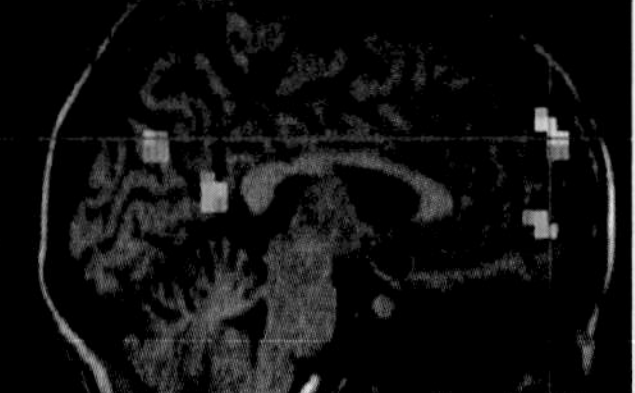
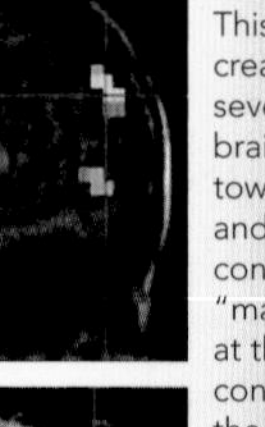
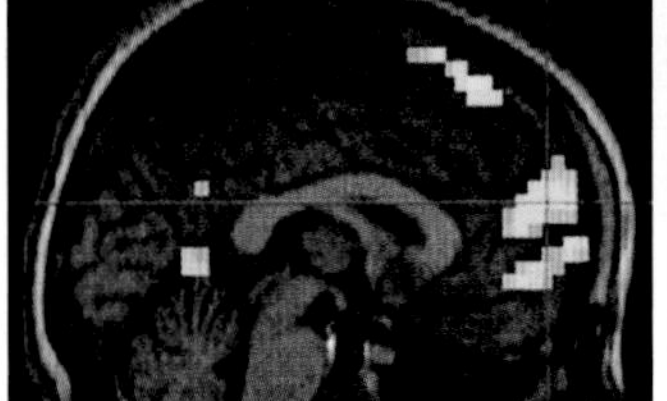
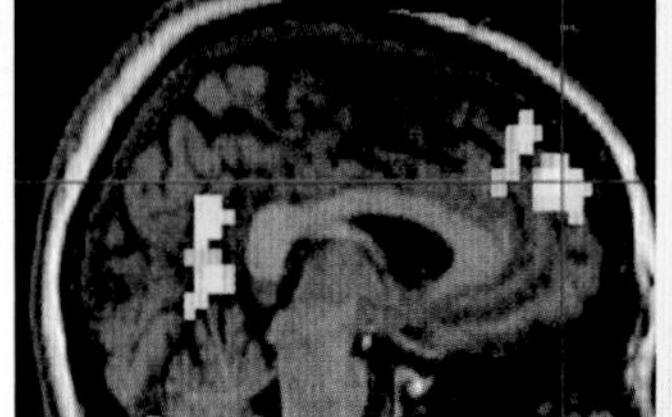

SELF-REFLECTIVE THOUGHT
This kind of thought creates activity in several areas of the brain. The areas towards the top and back are mainly concerned with body "maps", while those at the front are concerned with the mental self.

EXAMINING THE "I"
Trying to examine the "I" is like trying to look at your own eye – it is impossible because you are trying to see the thing you are using to see with. In effect, a shadow self arises, observing the "I".

AGENCY AND INTENTION

Agency is our sense of control over our actions. We feel that our conscious thoughts dictate what we do, but this appears to be incorrect. A famous experiment by Benjamin Libet (see below) revealed that a person's brain starts to plan and execute a movement unconsciously, before the person has consciously decided to do it. This is often interpreted to show that our sense of agency and of making "decisions" is illusory. The sense of agency we experience may actually have evolved primarily to give us early warning not of our own actions but of the actions of others. Because we feel ourselves to be agents, we also intuit agency in others and thus think we know their intentions and can predict what they will do.

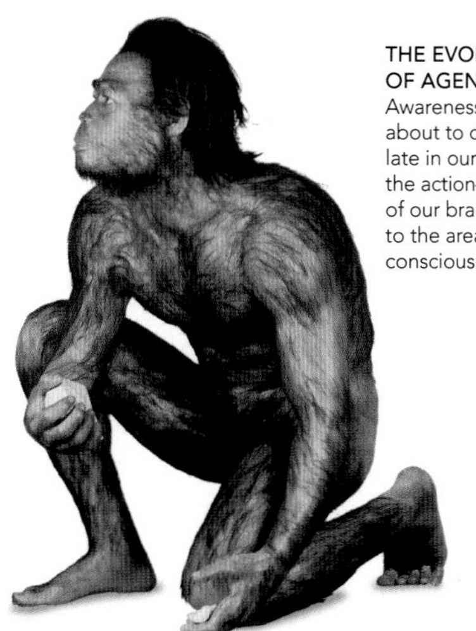

THE EVOLUTION OF AGENCY
Awareness of what we are about to do may have arisen late in our evolution, once the action–planning part of our brain had connected to the areas that support consciousness.

SCHIZOPHRENIA AND AGENCY

People with schizophrenia may have a disturbed sense of agency. Some attribute their own actions to the intentions of others, claiming they are being "controlled" by outside forces; others, that they "cause" events unconnected with their own actions, such as moving the Sun. Studies have suggested that these disturbances of the sense of agency are the result of failure to predict the consequences of an action.

FREE WILL EXPERIMENT
Libet asked volunteers to make a finger movement when they wanted to and to report the exact moment they "decided" to move by noting the time on a huge clock face with a sweep hand. Meanwhile, their brain activity was monitored, and EEGs showed the unconscious activity that planned the movement and sent the message to move to the relevant muscles. The timing of this activity was also noted, along with the time that the movement became visible. The experiment revealed that the conscious decision to make the movement occurred about one-fifth of a second after the brain had instructed the muscles to move.

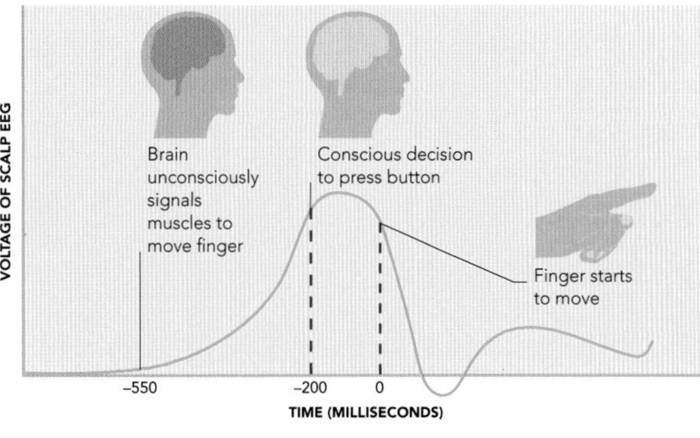

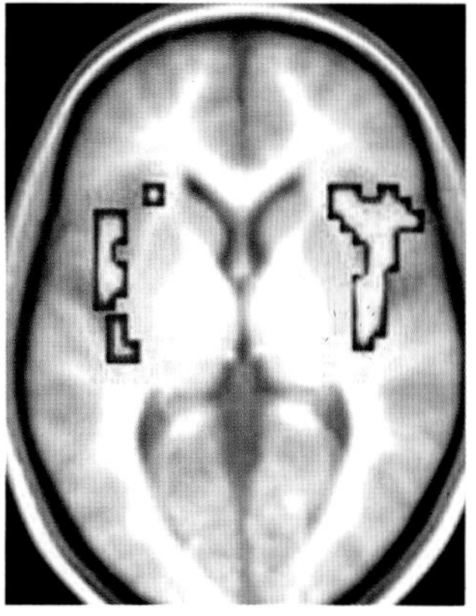

AUDITORY HALLUCINATION
This fMRI shows activity in a hallucinating schizophrenic. The speech areas in the right hemisphere may produce subvocal speech that could be interpreted as an external voice, distorting a sense of agency.

DISLOCATED SELF

The brain holds various "body maps" – internal representations of the physical self. The earliest, most basic map to emerge tells us where our body ends and the rest of the world begins. A more developed body "atlas" enables us to know our spatial location in the world. Normally, the internal maps and the body itself are closely matched, but it is possible for them to be askew. If a person loses a limb, for example, they may develop what is known as a phantom limb – a feeling that they have a limb that, in fact, no longer exists (see p.104). People can also be tricked into "owning" a limb or even a body that is not actually theirs.

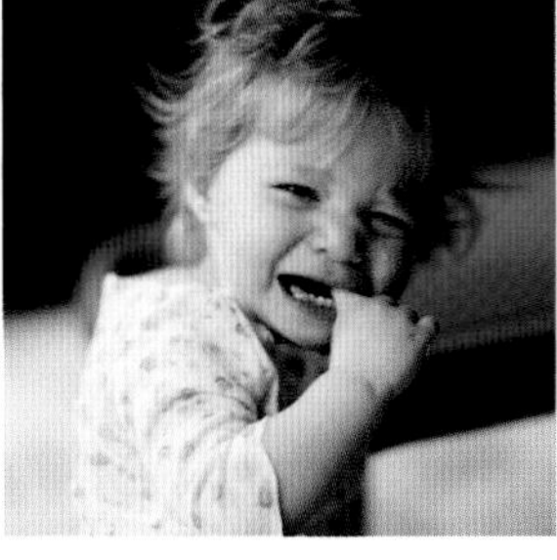

INFANT BODY MAPS
Babies probably do not distinguish between their body and external objects until their body maps start to take in information from the world.

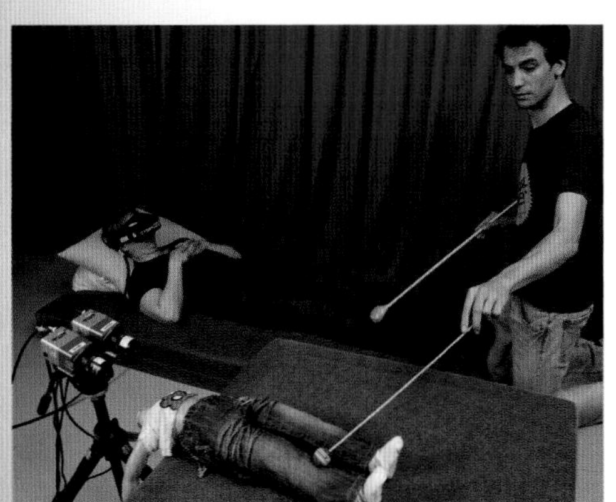

VIRTUAL BODY
People can be fooled into "losing" their real body and adopting another. In one experiment, volunteers wore virtual-reality headsets that substituted their view of their legs for those of an adjacent doll-sized mannequin. When the model was touched, the person reported feeling that the model's limbs were theirs. They also felt as though they had shrunk in relation to their surroundings.

LOSING THE SELF

Normal conscious activity involves keeping our "self" in mind, at least unconsciously. This means we see the world from our own, embodied perspective, and colour our perceptions and behaviour with the background notion of ourselves as agents. Sometimes, though, the self temporarily disappears – for example, when we enter mental states such as "flow" or "loss of control" (see below). These states can be both joyous and potentially perilous experiences.

Flow	In this pleasant state, we become so absorbed in something outside ourselves that self-consciousness vanishes, and with it the self's tendency to inhibit and interfere with whatever else the brain is doing. This allows us to perceive things more intensely and may help us perform better.
Loss of control	Failing to exercise control of our emotions is another instance of self-diminishment, but, unlike flow, it can be seriously disadvantageous. Brain imaging studies suggest that people "lose it" when the prefrontal area of the brain fails to respond adequately to alerts sent by the anterior cingulate cortex (ACC), which monitors one's own actions. Under provocation, the ACC registers that the emotional brain is tending to produce impulsive behaviour, and this usually triggers activity in the prefrontal cortex that inhibits the response. When someone is unusually stressed or tired, however, the prefrontal cortex may not respond, so the emotions are acted out. People in this state often report a sense of being "taken over", as though their agency has been hijacked.

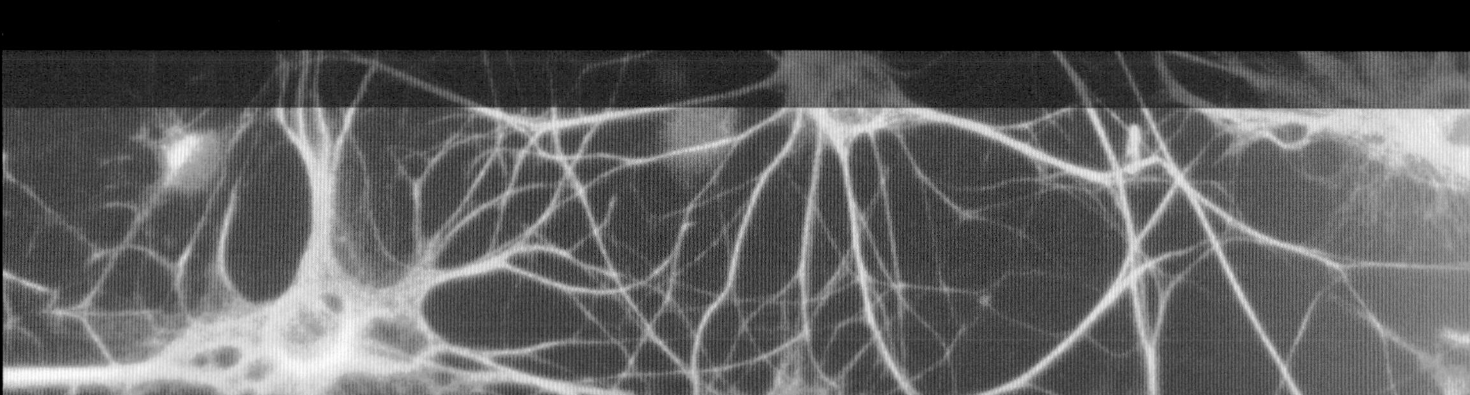

NO TWO BRAINS ARE EXACTLY ALIKE. ALTHOUGH THEY ARE BUILT ACCORDING TO THE SAME BASIC PLAN, EACH ONE IS PRODUCED FROM INSTRUCTIONS ENCODED IN A UNIQUE SET OF GENES, WHICH ARE ENGAGED IN COMPLEX INTERACTION WITH THE ENVIRONMENT. WE OFTEN THINK THAT OUR INDIVIDUALITY IS EXPRESSED THROUGH OUR PERSONALITY, BUT RECENT STUDIES SUGGEST THAT PERSONALITY IS A MUTABLE PHENOMENON. WE HAVE A NUMBER OF SUBTLY DIFFERENT PERSONALITIES THAT WE EXHIBIT IN DIFFERENT SITUATIONS.

THE INDIVIDUAL BRAIN

of it regulates gene expression, while other parts of it have no known function and are sometimes referred to as "junk" DNA. Genes are like dimmer switches – they can turn their activity (expression) on, off, up, or down. In the brain, gene expression affects the levels of neurotransmitters, which, in turn, influences complex functions like personality, memory, and intelligence. However, neurotransmitters also affect gene expression. Environmental influences affect patterns of gene expression, so that brain function also depends upon factors such as diet, geographical surroundings, social networks, and even stress levels. Chemical tags attach to DNA and alter gene expression – a process known as epigenetic alteration (see opposite).

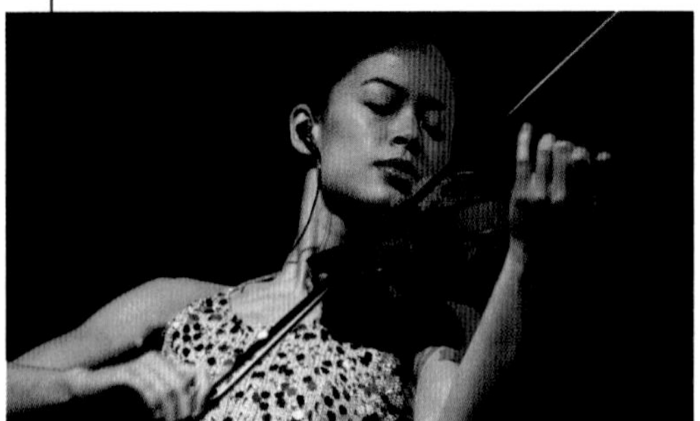

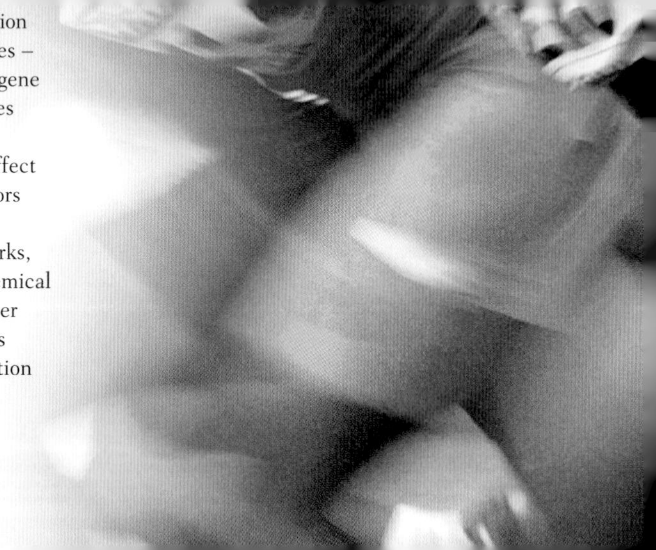

GENETICS AND THE BRAIN

Genes make proteins, which have many roles in the body. Some form structures, such as hair, while others, such as enzymes, regulate processes. For example, several genes in the genome may code for the protein molecules that make serotonin, one of the neurotransmitters involved in mood. Each variant of this gene makes a slightly different protein molecule, which may carry out its job more, or maybe less, efficiently. Thus, gene variants may result in one person having more serotonin and another person less serotonin. Less serotonin may mean a predisposition to depression or a tendency to overeat. This is also true of other neurotransmitters, such as dopamine – a lack of dopamine has been linked to increased risk-taking behaviour. Therefore, your genotype can affect the structure and functioning of your brain which, in turn, will influence behaviour. Another way that behaviour may be altered by genes is through epigenetic changes. These occur when the pattern of gene activation – rather than the genes themselves – is altered by molecular changes in DNA near to the genes. The changes may be passed on through several generations. Trauma provokes epigenetic changes in brain cells, probably due to raised stress hormones. People who commit suicide following childhood abuse have been found to have more epigenetic changes affecting genes, which act in the brain. Their offspring also show such changes and are also more likely than others to commit suicide. Research is underway to find a method of reversing epigenetic alterations.

Long, thin backbone of DNA molecule

New DNA strand made during cell copying

Base pair

Mutations occur when base pairs are changed during copying

MUTATION
Genes are a series of base pairs, linked molecules that form rungs in a DNA ladder (see opposite). Molecules of guanine (G), cytosine (C), adenine (A), and thymine (T) join in G-C and A-T pairs. The pair sequence in a particular gene is similar in all of us, but variations in the sequence help to make us unique. These may be introduced as a result of errors, or mutations, during the process of cell copying.

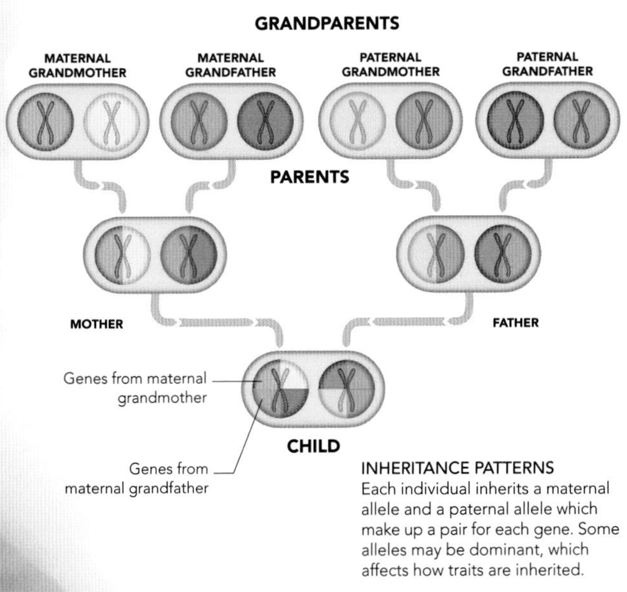

INHERITANCE PATTERNS
Each individual inherits a maternal allele and a paternal allele which make up a pair for each gene. Some alleles may be dominant, which affects how traits are inherited.

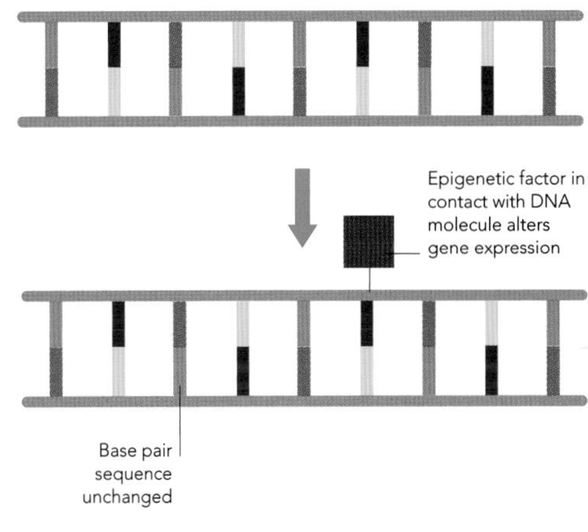

EPIGENETIC CHANGES
Epigenetic changes alter how the gene works, without actually changing the base pairs. Molecules from outside the gene, known as epigenetic factors, attach to the DNA and make it difficult for one or more genes to act in the normal way in the body. Epigenetic factors can be passed through a number of generations but, unlike mutations, they will finally disappear.

THE PLASTIC BRAIN

The brain was once believed to be immutable from birth, with a certain number of brain cells and fixed neuronal circuits. The only changes thought to occur were the loss of brain cells and a reduction in brain volume. But researchers have shown that experience and learning remodel brain circuits. Examples of such neuronal plasticity include long-term potentiation, where memory and learning generate new circuits (see p.158); the remodelling of the brain after a stroke or in drug addiction to strengthen pathways or create new ones; and the formation of new brain cells (neurogenesis). The brain, it seems, has a certain ability to repair itself and continue to grow and develop throughout life.

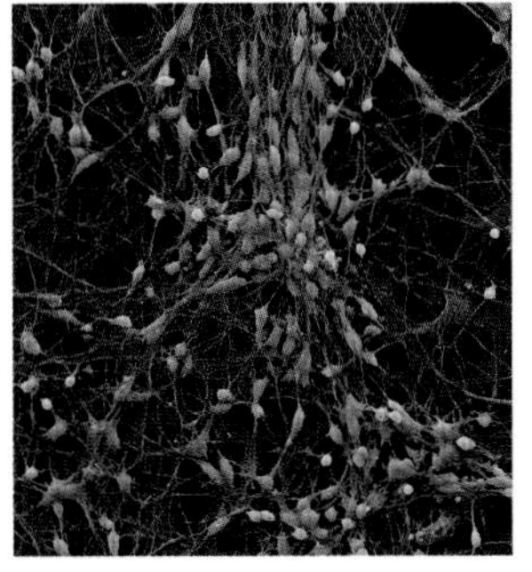

BIRTH OF NEURONS
This coloured electron micrograph shows neural progenitor cells. These cells lie between stem cells and fully differentiated cells. They are capable of developing into neurons and other neural cells.

INFLUENCING THE BRAIN

EVERYONE'S BRAIN IS DIFFERENT AND SOME STUDIES SUGGEST THAT GENDER AND SEXUAL ORIENTATION ARE REFLECTED IN DIFFERENCES IN THE BRAIN'S ANATOMY AND FUNCTIONING. THE BRAINS OF RIGHT- AND LEFT-HANDED PEOPLE ARE ORGANIZED DIFFERENTLY, AND EVEN SOCIAL AND CULTURAL INFLUENCES CAN SHAPE THE WAY THE BRAIN CARRIES OUT CERTAIN TASKS.

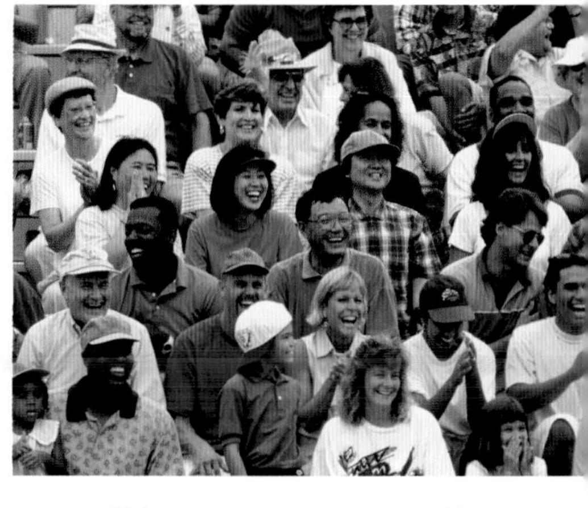

ONE OF THE CROWD
Just as each individual's face in this crowd is different, and unique to them, so too are their brains. Genetic differences at birth are just one factor – cultural and environmental influences during life can also have a profound effect.

MALE AND FEMALE BRAINS

Research into brain differences between the sexes is controversial. Some are convinced that differences are culturally, not biologically, determined. However, many studies have found anatomical differences between female and male brains. The corpus callosum and anterior commissure (linking the hemispheres) are larger in women. This may be why women are more emotionally aware – the emotional right is better connected to the analytical left. It may allow emotion to be built more readily into thought and speech. Imaging studies may reflect stereotypical differences between the sexes, showing different areas connected in each – though this could be culturally influenced.

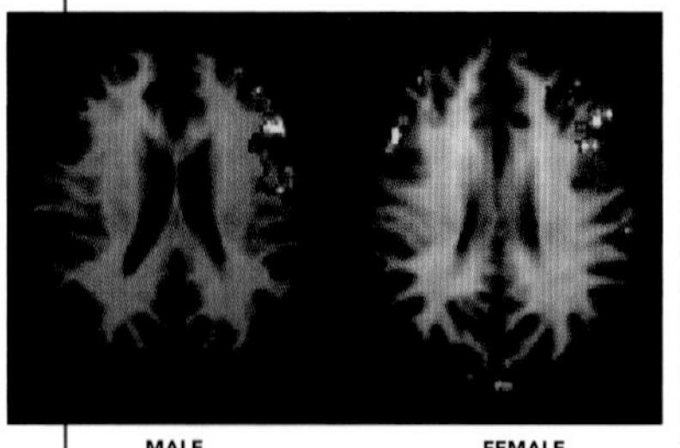

RESPONDING TO LANGUAGE
These fMRI scans reveal that women show activity on both sides of the brain when responding to language. In men, however, the activity is restricted more to the left hemisphere (shown on the right side of the scan).

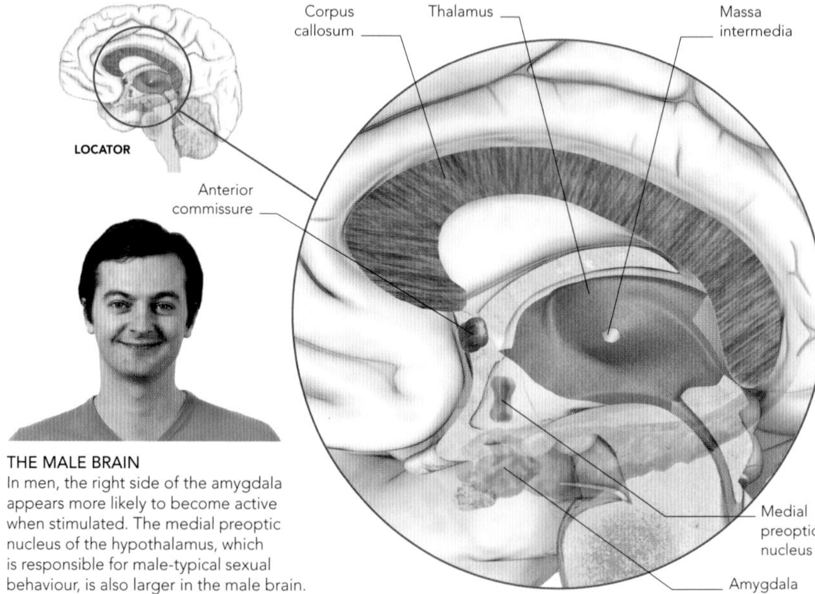

THE MALE BRAIN
In men, the right side of the amygdala appears more likely to become active when stimulated. The medial preoptic nucleus of the hypothalamus, which is responsible for male-typical sexual behaviour, is also larger in the male brain.

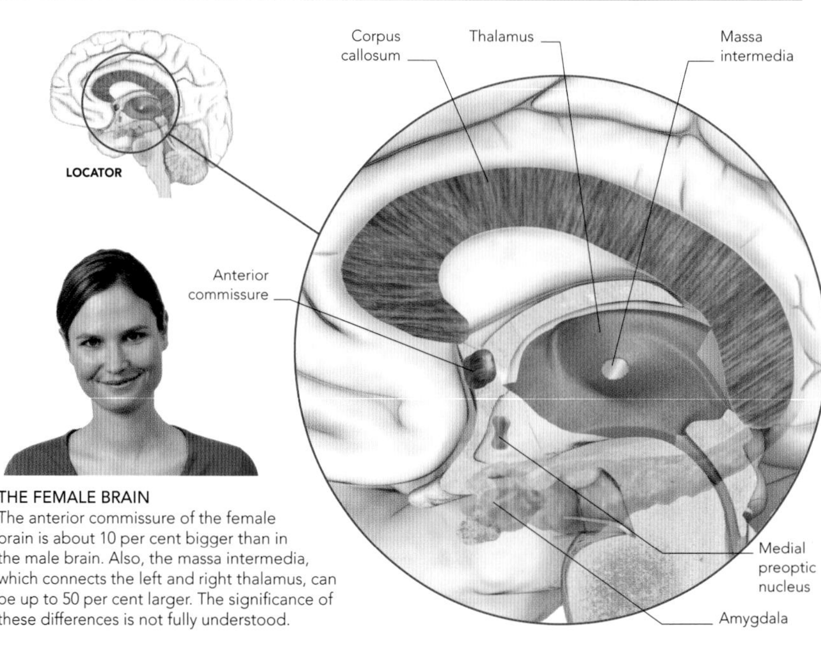

THE FEMALE BRAIN
The anterior commissure of the female brain is about 10 per cent bigger than in the male brain. Also, the massa intermedia, which connects the left and right thalamus, can be up to 50 per cent larger. The significance of these differences is not fully understood.

THE GAY BRAIN

Brain imaging studies suggest that in homosexual people, important brain structures involved in mood, emotion, anxiety, and aggression, tend to resemble those of heterosexuals of the opposite sex. Heterosexual men tend to have asymmetric brains (the right hemisphere is slightly larger), a characteristic shared by gay women. Patterns of brain connectivity are similar between heterosexual women and gay men, particularly in areas involved with anxiety.

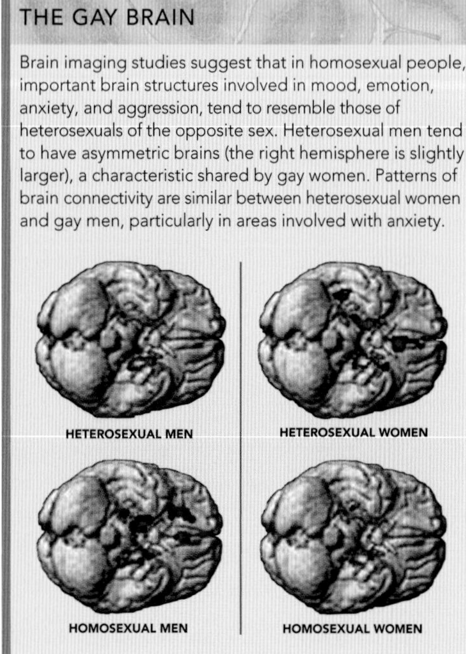

LEFT OR RIGHT HAND?

About 88 per cent of people are right-handed – that is, they use their right hands rather than left for tasks requiring fine motor skills, such as signing their name. Archaeological evidence, such as tools, suggests this has been the case for several million years. About 70 per cent of left-handers have language dominance in the left hemisphere, like right-handers, but 30 per cent show language distributed between the hemispheres. This unusual arrangement may help those who have it to integrate ideas more easily than others, but there is little evidence to support this.

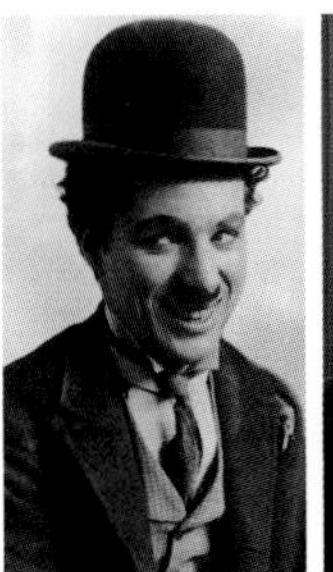

CHARLIE CHAPLIN

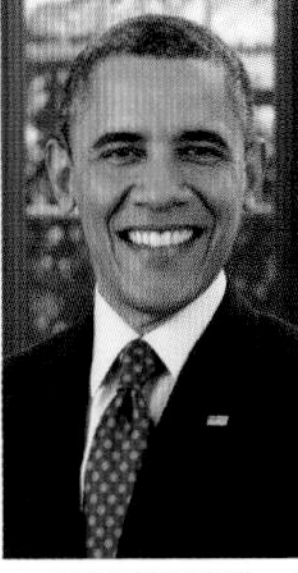

BARACK OBAMA

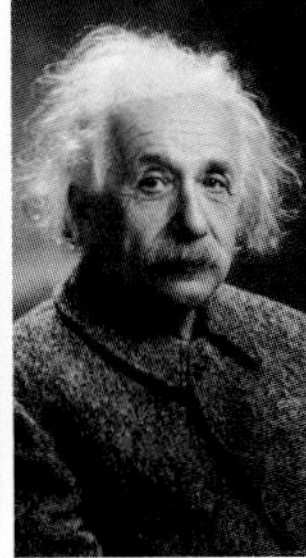

ALBERT EINSTEIN

LEFT-HANDED LUMINARIES
Many talented and brilliant people are or have been left-handed, including five of the last eight US presidents. This has led to a widespread notion that left-handed people are particularly gifted. Statistical analysis, however, suggests there are little or no consistent differences between left- and right-handers in IQ or other cognitive skills.

FAMILY EFFECTS

The way a person reacts to stress throughout their life is set, at least in part, by their very earliest experiences. In one study, fMRI scans were taken of sleeping babies' brains, which revealed activity stimulated by the sound of angry voices in two areas that react to emotional stimuli. Babies who came from homes where parents argued frequently showed greater activity than those from peaceful homes. The study suggests that the strength of a person's response to angry voices is primed in the cradle.

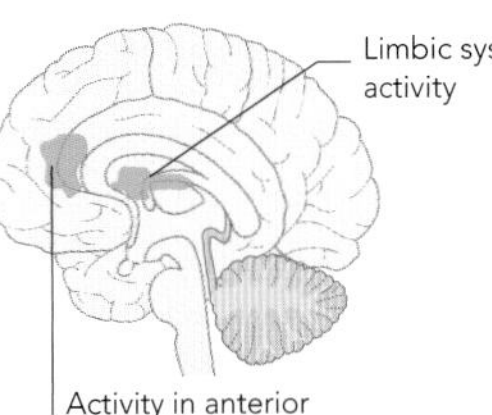

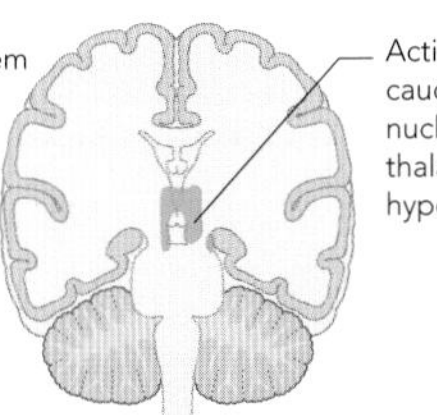

STRESSED BABY
Studies in which sleeping babies' brains were imaged as they were read to in an angry voice show activity in areas regulating emotion and stress.

TWINS

Studies of identical twins who were separated at birth and brought up in different families show that, even as adults, they are very similar in terms of interests and personality, as well as looks. This demonstrates how genes continue to exert their effects throughout life and often override environmental influences. Twin fetuses, including fraternal twins, effectively compete for resources, and a baby's position in the womb can affect the hormones they receive. In the case of boy twins, for example, one may partially block the other's uptake of testosterone, reducing the degree of brain masculinization that happens to the other. Girls with a boy twin may receive a higher-than-normal dose of testosterone because the mother's release of the hormone is elevated if she is carrying a male fetus. Studies have shown such girls are more likely than those with girl twins to display "tomboyish" behaviour.

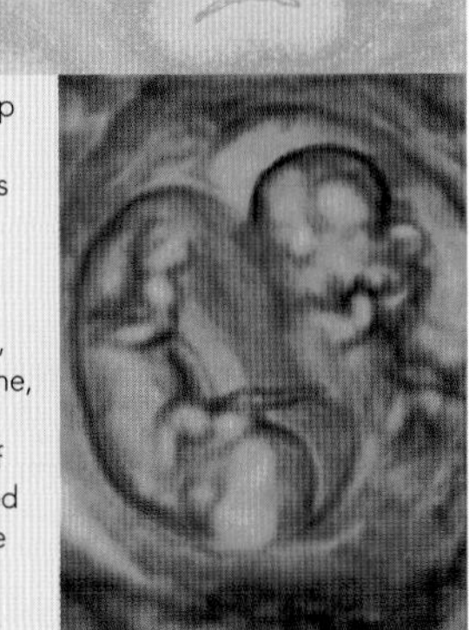

CULTURAL INFLUENCES

Researchers have shown that culture influences the way the brain works. They carried out tests during fMRI scans on people raised in the US and people raised in East Asia, in which participants did puzzles involving lines in a square (see below). US culture is perceived to be focused upon the individual, while East Asian culture tends to be more focused on family and community. The brains of the US participants had to work harder when they were doing tasks involving context, while those of the East Asians worked harder when they had to judge individual lines. Brain activity lessened when participants undertook tasks related to their culture's comfort zone. Participants were also asked how closely they identified with their culture, and the brains of those who identified most strongly had to work the hardest when doing tasks related to the "opposite" culture.

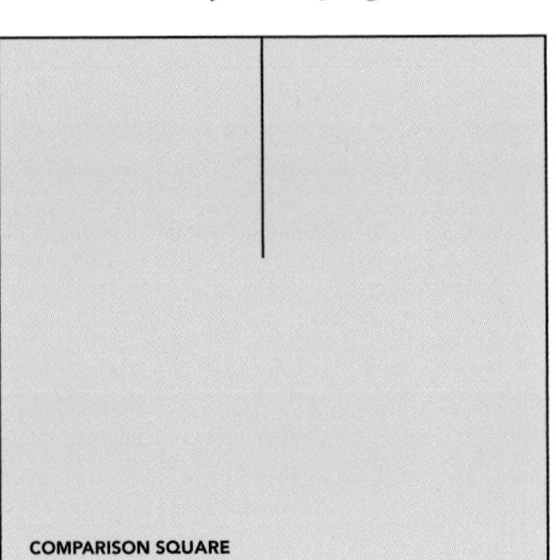

PERCEPTUAL TEST
The length of the line in this square may be perceived differently if it is compared to another line. Whether the brain is comfortable judging its length depends on the context of the test and cultural background.

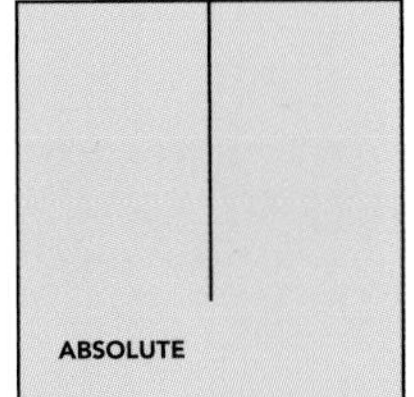

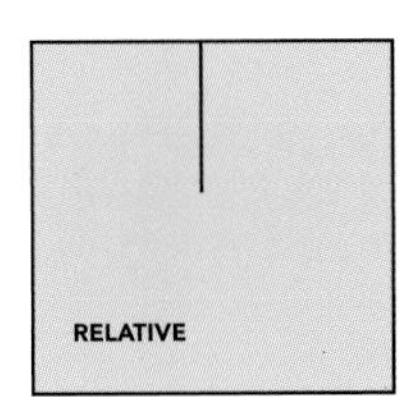

ABSOLUTE AND RELATIVE TASKS
In an absolute task, the line's length is compared to that of the line in the comparison square. In the relative task, the length of the line and its relation to the size of the square is compared to the same relationship in the first square.

RELATIVE TASK
ABSOLUTE TASK
EAST ASIANS
AMERICANS

BRAIN ACTIVATION PATTERNS
East Asian brains have to work less at the relative line perception task, whereas Americans are the opposite, with the absolute task being less demanding of their brains. This is because these tests are "easier" when the tasks are more in line with cultural norms.

PERSONALITY

PERSONALITY IS GENERALLY AGREED TO BE A GROUP OF BEHAVIOURAL CHARACTERISTICS TYPICALLY EXHIBITED BY AN INDIVIDUAL. SOME PEOPLE DISPLAY THE SAME BEHAVIOUR IN DIFFERENT SITUATIONS AND AT DIFFERENT TIMES, WHILE OTHERS ARE MUCH MORE CHANGEABLE.

LEARNING TO BE YOU

Each one of us has a genetic blueprint that predisposes us to characteristics such as aggression or extroversion. Although genes contribute greatly to personality development, the way we turn out to be also depends on how we learn to behave. Personality can be seen as a bundle of habitual responses. These may be learned by copying behaviour from caregivers or even from television. If a response is repeated frequently, it is encoded as a memory. Thereafter it is as much a "part" of the person as a genetic inclination.

MIMICKING BEHAVIOUR
Many of the mind habits that make up personality are initially learned by mimicking the adults that care for us as infants.

PERSONALITY AND THE BRAIN

Many different personality traits have been linked to specific patterns of activity in the brain, some of which are linked to the expression of certain genes or particular genetic mutations. For example, a person who produces more excitatory neurotransmitters is less likely to feel the need to seek thrills than someone who needs a lot of stimulation to experience the same level of excitement.

PERSONALITY MARKERS IN THE BRAIN		
Extroversion	Extroverts have reduced activity, in response to stimuli, in the neural circuit that keeps the brain aroused (shown here). As a result they need more environmental stimuli to keep them feeling energized.	Dorsolateral prefrontal cortex; Anterior cingulate cortex; Thalamus
Aggression	People with a version of a gene previously linked to impulsive violence show abnormally reduced volume and unusually low activity in the cingulate cortex – an area concerned with monitoring and guiding behaviour.	Cingulate cortex
Social behaviour	Socially secure people have a stronger response to friendly-looking people in the striatum – an area concerned with reward – than shy people. Avoidant types show a stronger reaction in the amygdala to unfriendly-looking people.	Striatum; Amygdala
Novelty seeking	People who like novelty may have better connections between areas shown here. The hippocampus sends signals to the striatum – which registers pleasure – when it identifies an experience as new.	Striatum; Hippocampus
Co-operation	Co-operative people show increased activity in the insula if they think their treatment is unfair. Unco-operative people do not register unfairness to the same extent, suggesting an under-developed sense of trust.	Insula
Optimism	Optimism is linked to enhanced activation in the amygdala and in the anterior cingulate cortex when imagining positive future events relative to negative ones.	Cingulate cortex; Amygdala

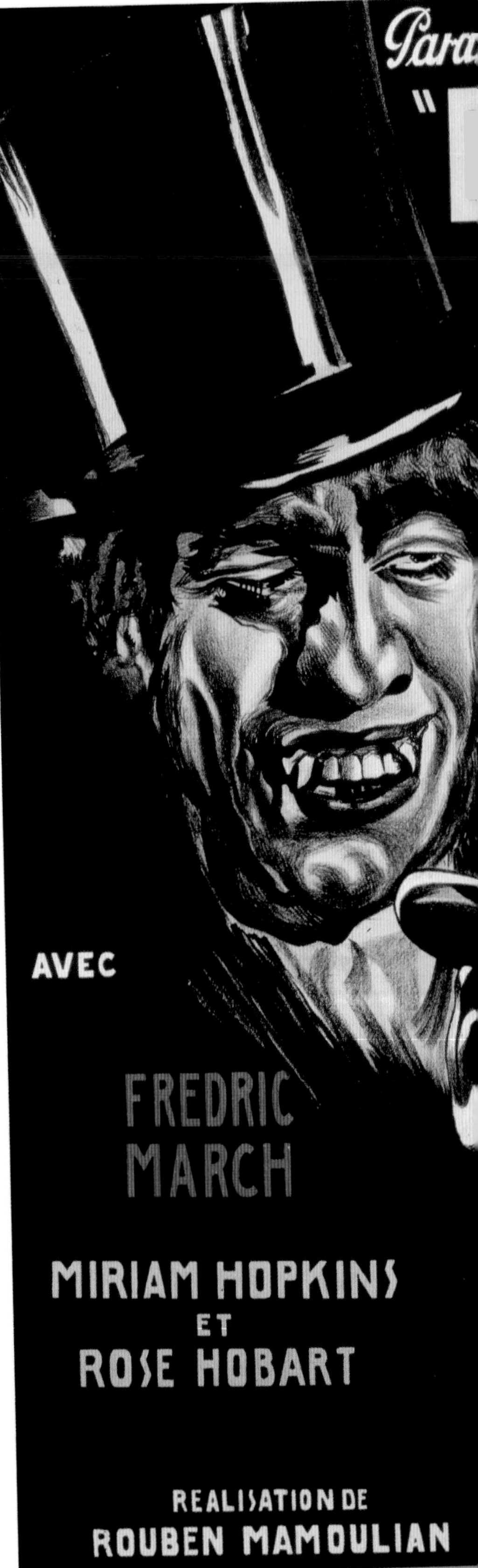

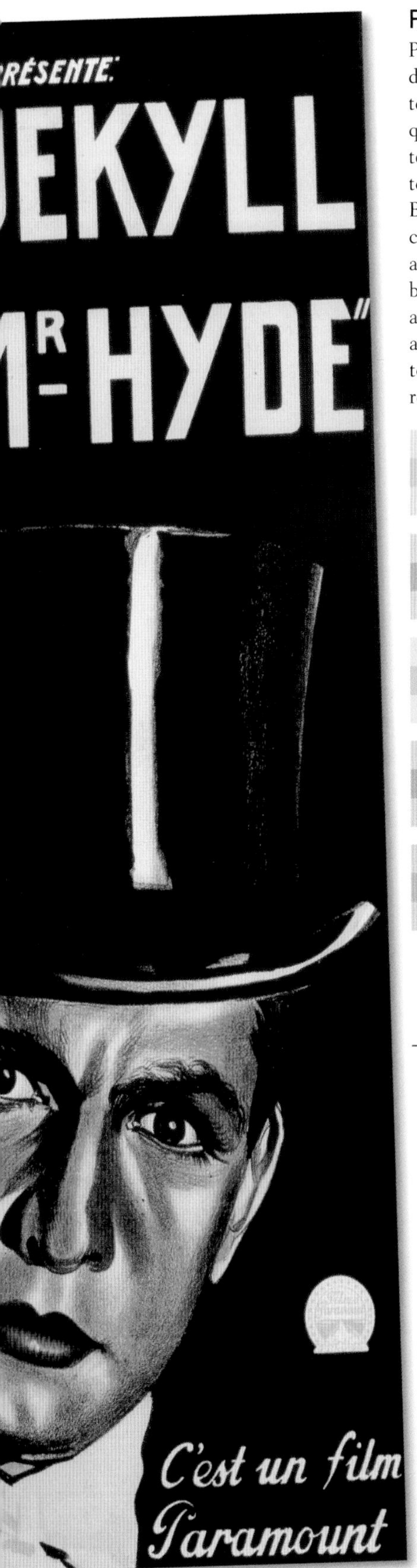

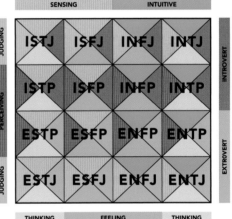

PERSONALITY ASSESSMENT

Personality testing is used for many reasons, such as for determining a person's suitability for a job or promotion. Some tests are standardized assessments that require people to answer questions about their typical behaviour. The results are used to determine the individual's personality profile. Type tests place people in a particular category. Myers–Briggs, for example (below, right) sorts people into categories based on the predominance of certain attributes. Trait tests do not fit people into types, but draw up a profile based on where they lie along a number of dimensions. Projective tests, such as the Rorschach inkblot test, invite people to "reveal" aspects of their personality when responding to ambiguous stimuli.

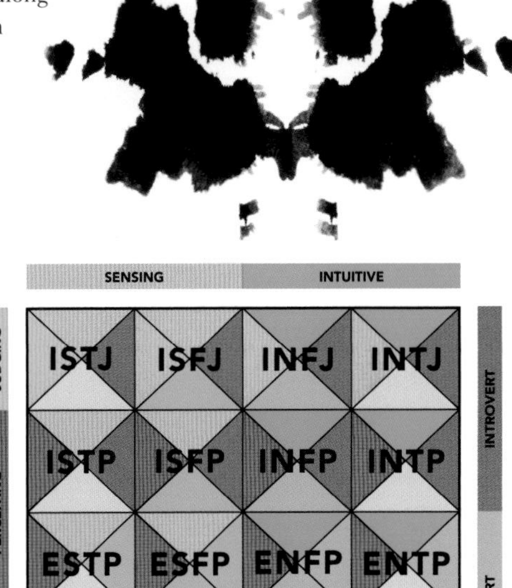

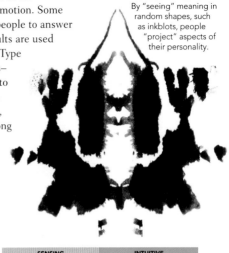

PROJECTIVE TESTS
By "seeing" meaning in random shapes, such as inkblots, people "project" aspects of their personality.

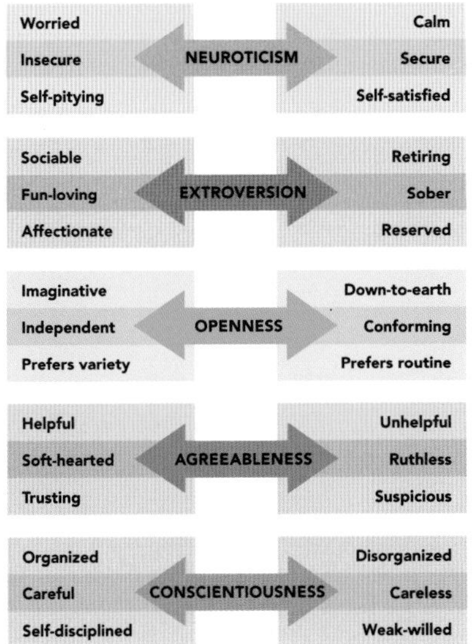

THE BIG FIVE
According to this trait test model, basic differences in personality can be "boiled down" to five dimensions. People may fall anywhere on each dimension.

	SENSING	SENSING	INTUITIVE	INTUITIVE	
JUDGING	ISTJ	ISFJ	INFJ	INTJ	INTROVERT
PERCEIVING	ISTP	ISFP	INFP	INTP	INTROVERT
PERCEIVING	ESTP	ESFP	ENFP	ENTP	EXTROVERT
JUDGING	ESTJ	ESFJ	ENFJ	ENTJ	EXTROVERT
	THINKING	FEELING	FEELING	THINKING	

MYERS–BRIGGS INDICATORS
The Myers–Briggs test asks people a very wide range of questions and places the person in one of 16 types. Despite criticisms of its lack of validity, it is the most widely used personality test in use in business.

MANY PERSONALITIES?

Type tests like the Myers–Briggs (above) have been found to give different results according to the situation in which the person is tested. Trait tests allow for people to be different at different times, but still assume they have a "major" personality that is more real than others. Some evidence suggests, however, that practically everyone has more than one personality, and that many people have a large number of them. Memories that are available to a person in one situation may not be accessible in another. In extreme cases, this results in dissociative identity disorder (DID), but in normal people it merely shows up as mood changes, memory "glitches", and the coming and going of different skills, behaviours, and ways of seeing the world.

DR JEKYLL AND MR HYDE
Dramatic personality changes, such as a "split personality", are a staple of horror films and ghost stories. They reflect a distrust of people who appear not to have stable personalities.

DISSOCIATIVE IDENTITY DISORDER

Extreme multiplicity, in which personalities are completely compartmentalized, results in a person switching from one personality to another without retaining any memory of their previous state. They may behave differently according to which personality they are, and may even adopt a different name and history for each one. Because they have no memory of the others, each of them is likely to have memory gaps. Some people with DID find, for example, that they do things of which, in another personality, they disapprove.

BRAIN MONITORING AND STIMULATION

IT IS NOW POSSIBLE TO WATCH THE BRAIN'S ACTIVITY TAKING PLACE ON AN EXTERNAL DISPLAY AND DELIBERATELY CHANGE IT. THIS IS KNOWN AS NEUROFEEDBACK. MORE DIRECTLY, ACTIVITY CAN BE STIMULATED BY ELECTRICAL INPUT SENT THROUGH THE SKULL OR FROM ELECTRODES IMPLANTED INTO THE BRAIN ITSELF.

NEUROFEEDBACK

Brain activity is constantly altered by what an individual feels, thinks, or senses. The neurofeedback process works by turning the brain's activity itself into an external stimulus, which the person then responds to. For instance, EEG sensors may be used to pick up a person's brainwaves. Different mind-states, such as relaxation or anxiety, have characteristic wave-forms that are translated into a dynamic visual display. The activity registered by the EEG is then sent to a device that turns them into a form that the person can easily understand and manipulate. This may be as simple as a line that moves up or down, or a more complex game. The person tries to change the on-screen information just by using their brain. The result of their effort is then displayed, so the person learns what to do in order to achieve the effect they want. Repeatedly doing this makes it increasingly easy for them to gain a desired state of mind, such as relaxation or focused attention.

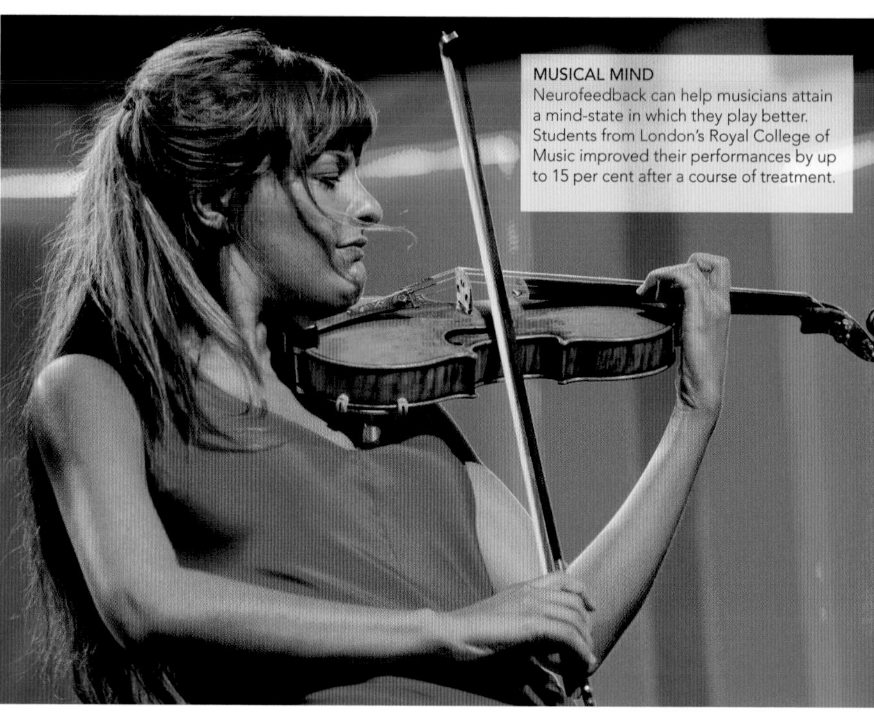

MUSICAL MIND
Neurofeedback can help musicians attain a mind-state in which they play better. Students from London's Royal College of Music improved their performances by up to 15 per cent after a course of treatment.

Step 1 EEG (or a similar brain "reading" device) charts the neural activity in the person's brain. The information is then transferred to a computer.

Step 2 The computer turns the neural patterns into a dynamic visual display, such as an interactive game with a clear goal like making an on-screen object move.

Step 3 The person plays the game just by altering their brain-state. The machine registers neural changes, such as those marking relaxation, and "rewards" them with wins.

Step 4 The player associates the "wins" in the game with certain brain states. The process then begins again, and through repetition the player learns to achieve them more easily.

FEEDBACK LOOP
The neurofeedback process teaches people to change their brain-state. Once people have learned to do this with the equipment, they find it easier to do so at will.

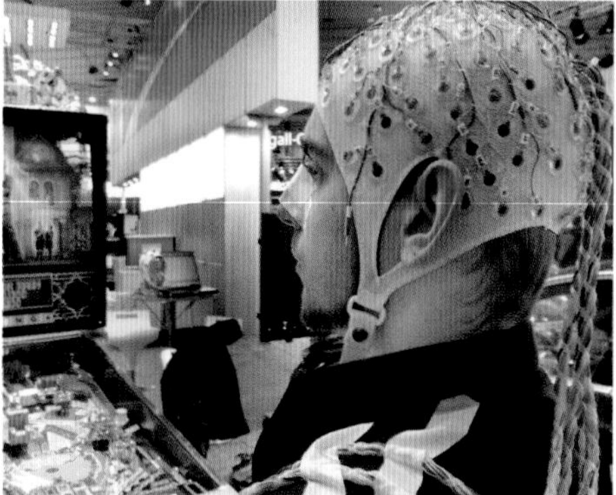

MIND CONTROL
EEG is the usual brain "reading" process used for neurofeedback. Dozens of scalp-mounted electrodes pick up oscillations of underlying neurons and convert them into waves.

ECT

Electroconvulsive therapy (ECT) involves sending an electric current through the brain until the neurons are so stimulated that they produce a seizure (see p.226). It is used as a treatment of last resort for chronic depression, and it often works when drugs and psychotherapy have no effect. The way that it works is not fully understood, but it is thought that the seizure resets certain neurons' potential to fire, making them more or less sensitive. The seizure induced by ECT is short-lasting and harmless, and muscle relaxants are used to prevent convulsions. However, patients often complain of memory problems following the treatment.

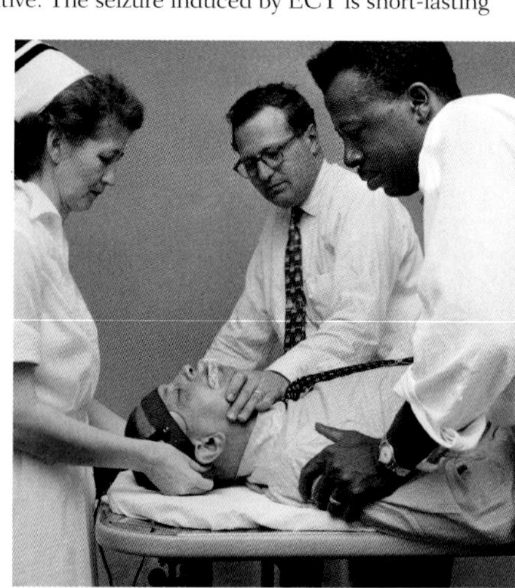

HISTORIC ECT
ECT was widely used in the 1950s in mental institutions. At that time it was a crude technique, which involved creating a whole-brain seizure that caused the patient to thrash about.

TMS

Transcranial magnetic stimulation (TMS) sends a magnetic pulse through the skull and into the brain. The pulse temporarily disrupts normal activity in the part of the brain beneath it. Repeated stimulation of a particular area causes long-term changes in the way it functions. For example, it can increase activity in parts of the brain that are known to be underactive in people with depression, or decrease it in areas known to be overactive in those with obsessive compulsive disorder. Repeated sessions of TMS are increasingly used as treatment for these and other conditions.

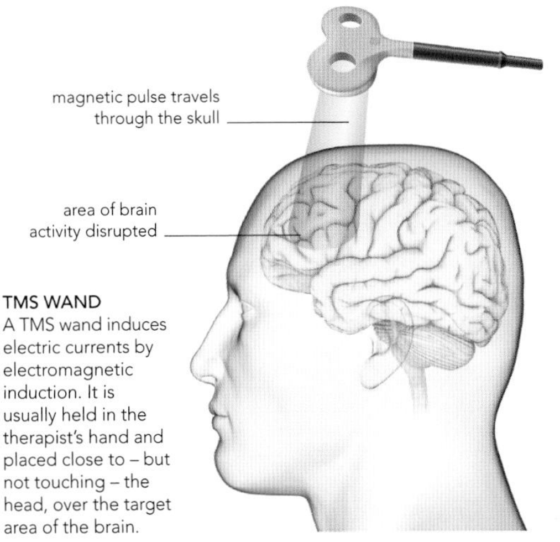

TMS WAND
A TMS wand induces electric currents by electromagnetic induction. It is usually held in the therapist's hand and placed close to – but not touching – the head, over the target area of the brain.

DEEP BRAIN STIMULATION

In deep brain stimulation, tiny electrodes are placed surgically in the brain. They radiate current to nearby target areas, activating otherwise sluggish neurons, which in turn create local changes in brain chemistry. The electrodes are attached to very fine wires, which are inserted deep into the brain through small holes in the skull. They are situated in different brain areas according to the condition being treated and may be sited quite differently in each patient. In some cases, the wires are connected to an external switch that allows the patient to turn the current on and off as required.

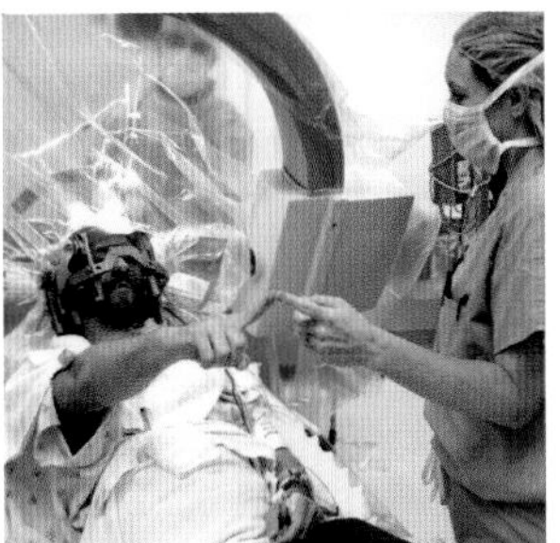

BRAIN SURGERY
Patients are operated on while conscious so that they are able to communicate. Their reactions guide the surgical team to implant the electrodes in the right spot.

TREATING STROKE

Neurostimulation may be used to help people recover from the effects of stroke. The damaged area of the brain is stimulated in order to help neighbouring neurons grow and take over the work of the cells that have been killed off. Conversely, inhibitory stimulation may be applied to the brain cells corresponding to the damaged area on the opposite side of the brain. This prevents the opposite side of the brain compensating for the damaged area and interfering with its recovery.

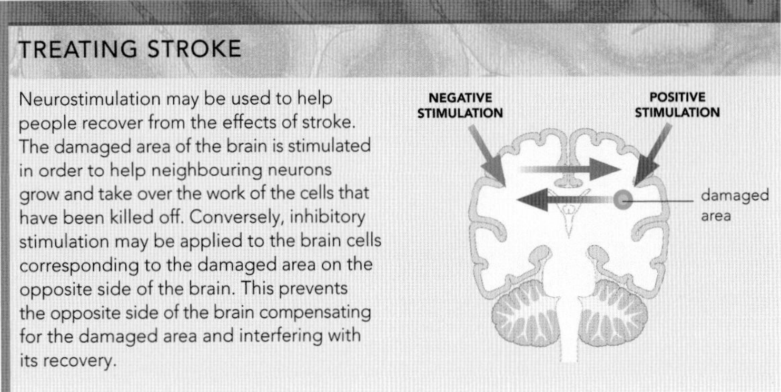

TDCS

Transcranial direct current stimulation (tDCS) is a way of stimulating – or inhibiting – selected neurons by sending a minute charge of electricity through the cortex via scalp-mounted electrodes. The current used is less than 2 milliAmps – so small that most people can barely feel it. Thousands of studies show that it is safe and that it may reduce symptoms of mood disorders, chronic pain, tinnitus, motor and speech disorders – especially after stroke – and possibly schizophrenia and dementia. It also enhances brain function in healthy people – using it can improve maths skills and creativity, and lead to swifter learning.

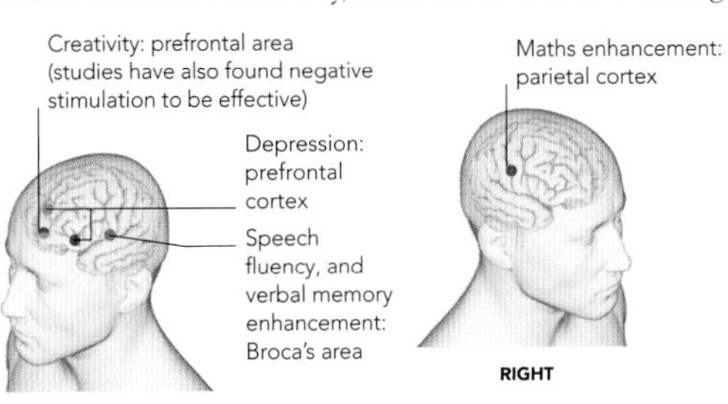

BRAIN AREAS
Stimulating (or inhibiting) different brain areas with tDCS has different effects. These are some of the areas where anode stimulation (red) or cathode inhibition (blue) has been shown to alter experience or enhance a particular skill.

OPTOGENETICS

Optogenetics allows specific neural pathways in the brain to be turned on and off by light. At the moment it is used only in research animals to map brain circuits, but eventually it is expected to have a number of medical uses. The first application is likely to be to repair retinal cells in the eye that have ceased to be sensitive to light. The technique involves taking light-sensitive molecules from algae, then inserting them into specific brain cells. A fibre-optic light is then inserted into the brain, and, when the light is switched on, the cells containing the inserted molecules become active. Depending on where the neurons are, the stimulation can alter behaviour and create new memories and habits.

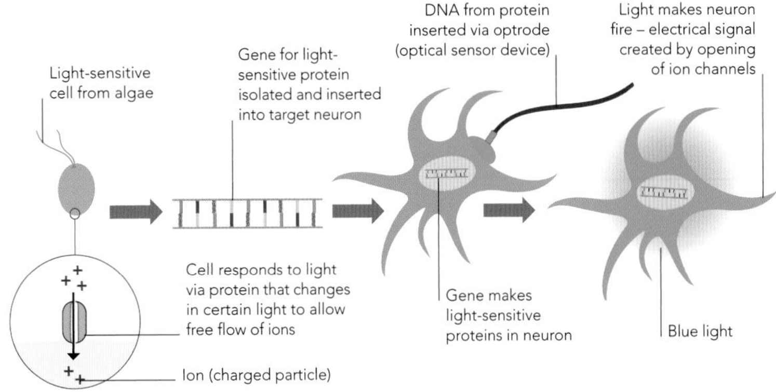

INSERTING MOLECULES
There are various methods of inserting light-sensitive molecules into brain cells. The most common involves using a virus that targets particular neurons as a carrier.

STRANGE BRAINS

ON THE WHOLE ONE BRAIN LOOKS VERY MUCH LIKE ANOTHER, GIVE OR TAKE A SMALL VARIATION IN SIZE. SOME BRAINS, HOWEVER, ARE DRAMATICALLY DIFFERENT FROM NORMAL, AND IN MANY CASES PHYSICAL ECCENTRICITY PRODUCES UNUSUAL WAYS OF BEHAVING AND SEEING THE WORLD.

THE SPLIT BRAIN

The corpus callosum carries signals between the two hemispheres. Rarely, this tissue is surgically severed in people with epilepsy, in order to prevent the spread of seizures. Researchers projected images separately to each hemisphere (see split-brain experiment, below) of split-brain patients. Normally the two sides would share the information via the corpus callosum, but without it each side only recognized its own image. The patients could identify the picture known by the language dominant left brain, but denied seeing anything else. Yet they were able to select the object seen by the right brain, using the left hand (which is controlled by the right hemisphere). Asked why they selected that object, however, they were unable to say. This suggests that the right hemisphere (in right–handers) is unconscious – even though the information it holds affects behaviour.

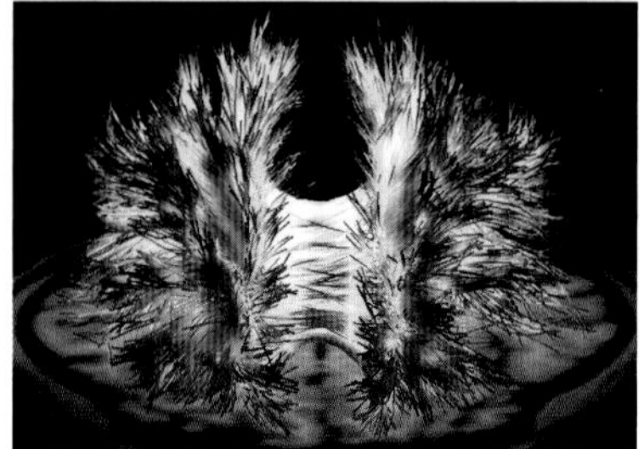

CONNECTING THE HEMISPHERES
This diffusion tensor image clearly shows the wide band of fibres that forms the corpus callosum, which connects the left and right hemispheres of the brain.

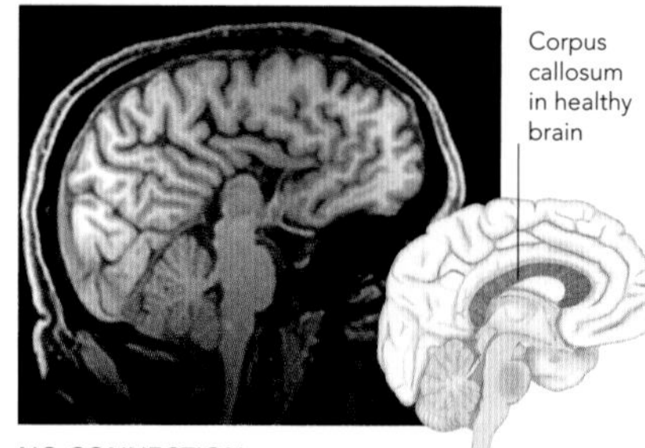

NO CONNECTION
Occasionally the corpus callosum fails to develop, in a condition known as agenesis of the corpus callosum (shown here in an MRI scan). This leaves the two hemispheres of the brain unconnected.

TESTING YOUR CORPUS CALLOSUM

Close your eyes and spread out your hands, palms facing upwards. Get someone to touch one of your fingertips, and with your opposite hand try to touch the corresponding finger with thumb of the same hand (see below). If information is flowing properly between the hemispheres, you should be able to do this without opening your eyes.

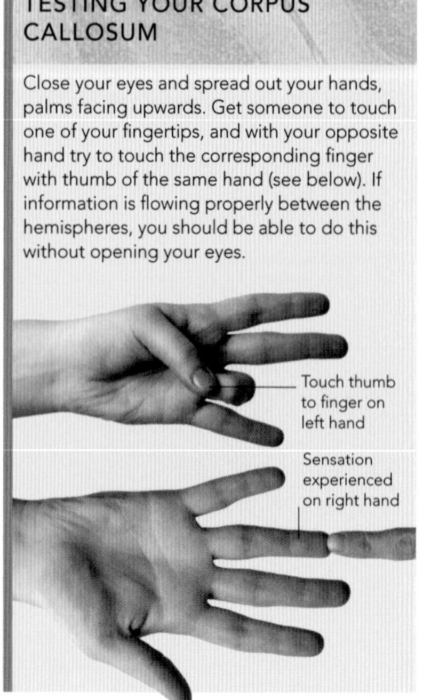

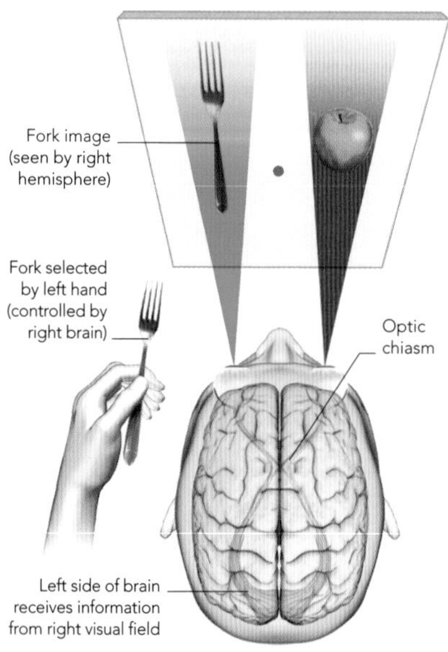

SPLIT-BRAIN EXPERIMENT
In a split-brain experiment, the image shown to the right side of the brain can guide the actions of the left hand to select an object, even though the person is not conscious of seeing the image and is only aware of seeing the apple.

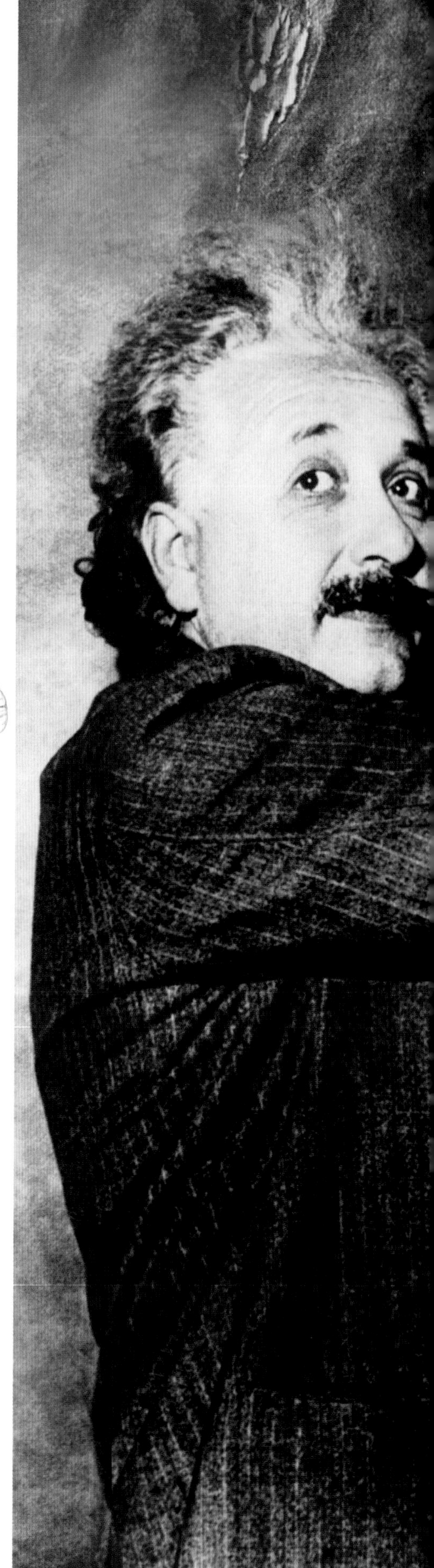

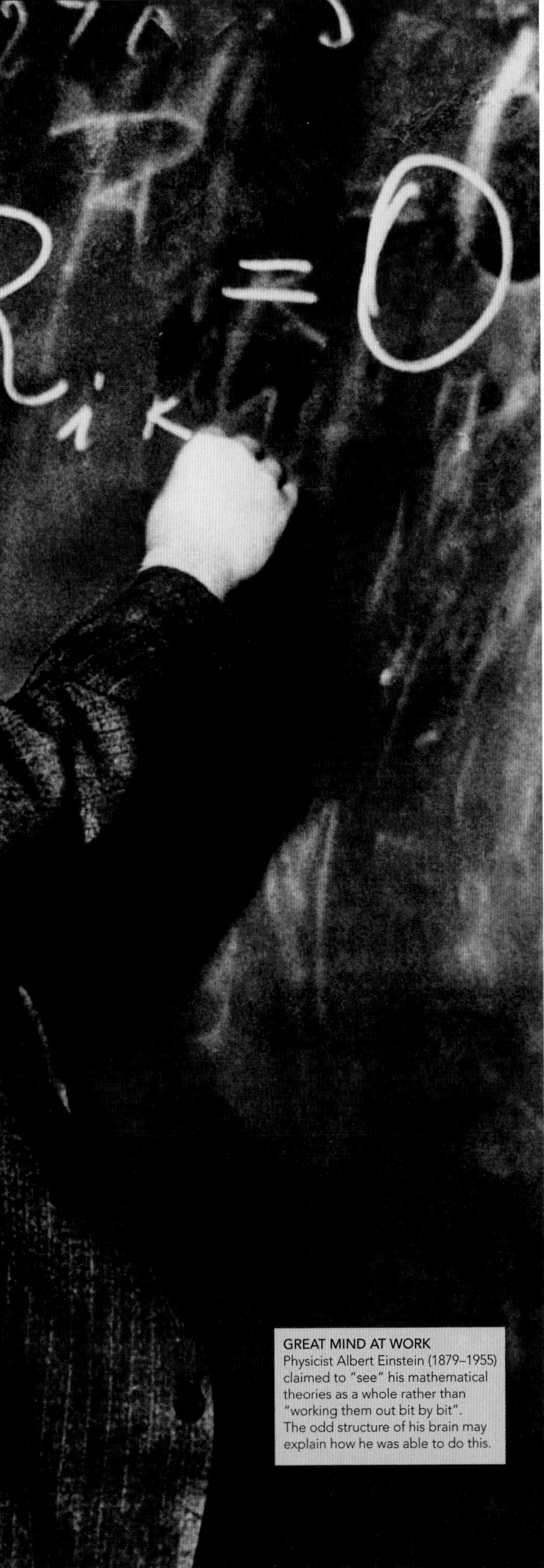

WEIRD BRAINS

Brain scans have revealed some astonishing physical abnormalities, such as brains that are missing an entire hemisphere. The effect of losing half a brain would be catastrophic if it happened in later life. However, several cases have come to light in which brain growth has been severely restricted in infancy and yet the person has gone on to live a near normal life with few, if any, adverse symptoms.

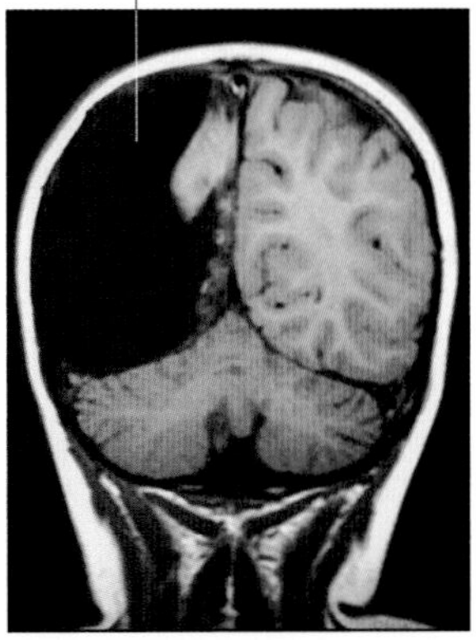

Left hemisphere missing

HALF A BRAIN
Despite having one side of her brain removed, this girl learned to be fluent in two languages.

SIZE DOESN'T MATTER

Brains do not, generally, vary greatly in size, and there is little evidence to suggest that bigger brains produce greater intelligence. At one extreme, Irish writer Jonathan Swift (1667–1754) had a brain that, at the time of his death, weighed a relatively enormous 2,000g (70½oz). In 1928, the Moscow Brain Research Institute started collecting and mapping the brains of famous Russians, including that of the physiologist Ivan Pavlov (1849–1936). His brain was at the other end of the size scale, weighing a mere 1,517g (53½oz).

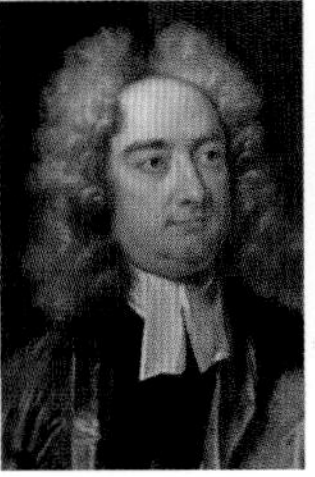

JONATHAN SWIFT

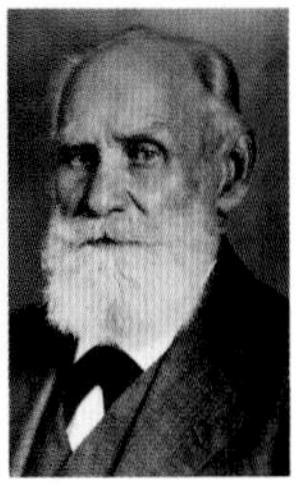

IVAN PAVLOV

VARYING SIZES
The brains of famous intellectuals vary greatly in size, so the connection between IQ and size is unclear.

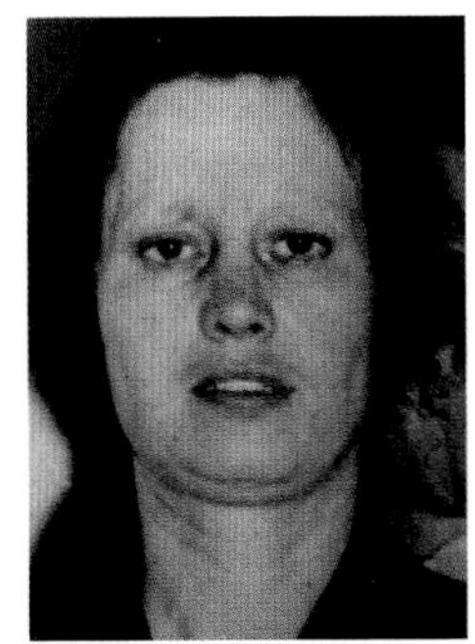

THE TERRORIST'S BRAIN

Ulrike Meinhof (1934–76) was a member of the infamous Baader–Meinhof Gang, which was responsible for a number of killings, bombings, and kidnappings in Germany during the 1970s. She was captured and committed suicide in prison. After her death, studies suggest that brain damage resulting from an operation on a swollen blood vessel might have accounted for her violent behaviour.

FACE OF A KILLER
This rare image of Meinhof was taken when she was arrested in 1972. In 1962, she had a metal clip inserted in her brain during surgery, which helped police identify her.

EINSTEIN'S BRAIN

Albert Einstein's brain was removed after his death. Many years later, it was examined by Dr. Sandra Witelson and compared with other brains in a brain bank. It was found to be wider than normal, and part of a groove that normally runs through the parietal lobe was missing. The area affected is concerned with mathematics and spatial reasoning, and it is possible the missing groove allowed neurons there to communicate more easily, giving him his extraordinary talent for describing the universe mathematically.

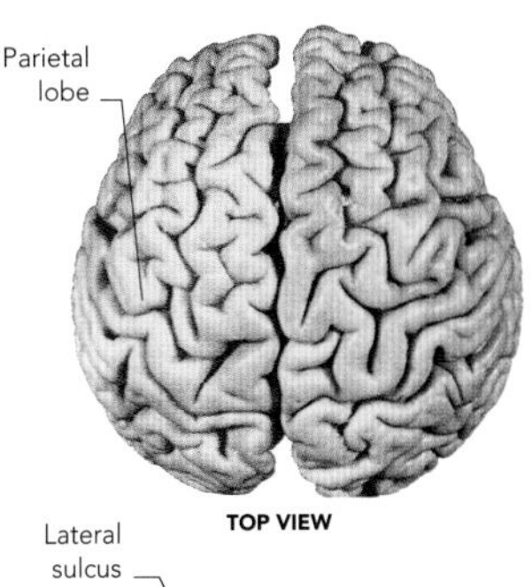

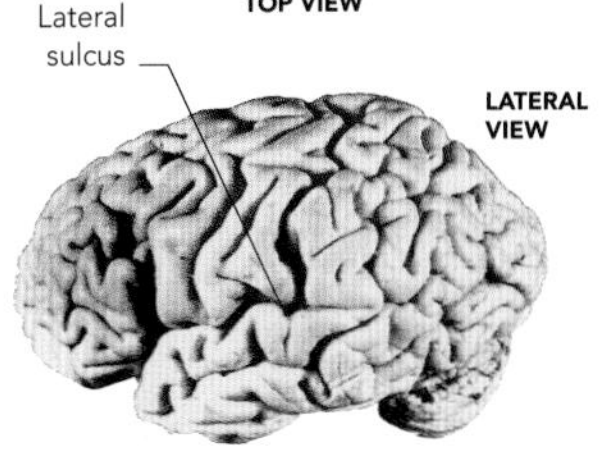

A MATHEMATICAL BRAIN?
Einstein's brain was wider than normal (top) and the part of the lateral sulcus normally found in the parietal cortex, was apparently missing.

GREAT MIND AT WORK
Physicist Albert Einstein (1879–1955) claimed to "see" his mathematical theories as a whole rather than "working them out bit by bit". The odd structure of his brain may explain how he was able to do this.

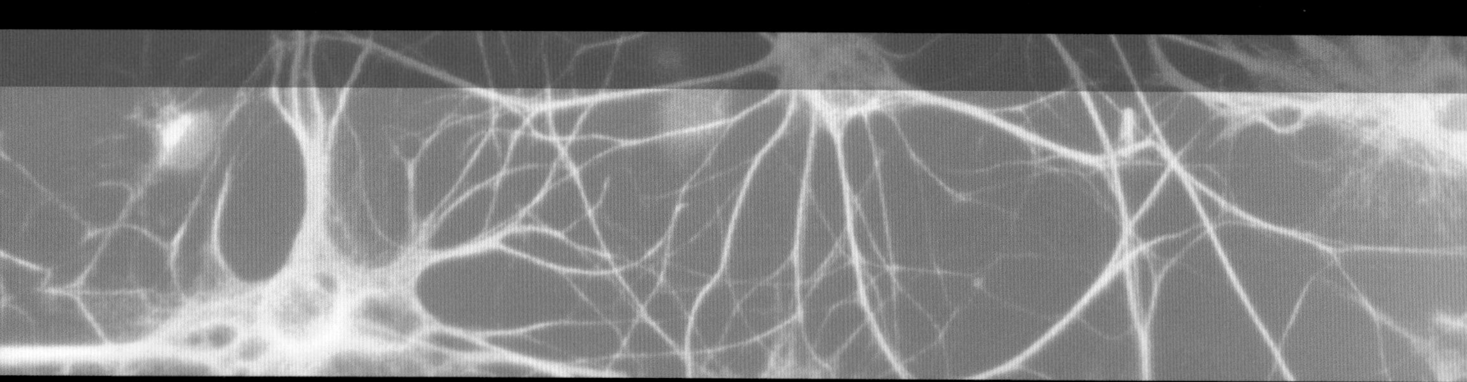

OUR BRAIN CHANGES OVER THE COURSE OF OUR LIFE, AND THIS HAS FAR-REACHING EFFECTS ON WHAT WE CAN DO AND HOW WE BEHAVE. DEVELOPMENT STARTS A FEW WEEKS AFTER CONCEPTION, AND TO BEGIN WITH IS INCREDIBLY RAPID, WITH HUNDREDS OF THOUSANDS OF NEURONS BEING ADDED EVERY MINUTE. THE PACE GRADUALLY SLOWS, AND WE ARE WELL INTO OUR 20S BEFORE OUR BRAINS ARE FULLY DEVELOPED. AS WE AGE FURTHER, NATURAL AND IRREVERSIBLE DEGENERATION SETS IN, BUT THE BRAIN HAS VARIOUS MECHANISMS TO COMPENSATE FOR THIS.

DEVELOPMENT AND AGEING

THE INFANT BRAIN

THE HUMAN BRAIN FORMS FROM THE OUTERMOST LAYER OF TISSUE IN A DEVELOPING EMBRYO, AND IT UNDERGOES SEVERAL TRANSFORMATIONS BEFORE EMERGING AS THE RECOGNIZABLE ORGAN. AFTER A PERIOD OF RAPID CELL GROWTH, NEWLY GENERATED NEURONS MOVE AROUND TO FORM THE VARIOUS PARTS OF THE BRAIN. IT TAKES MORE THAN 20 YEARS FOR THE BRAIN TO BECOME FULLY MATURE.

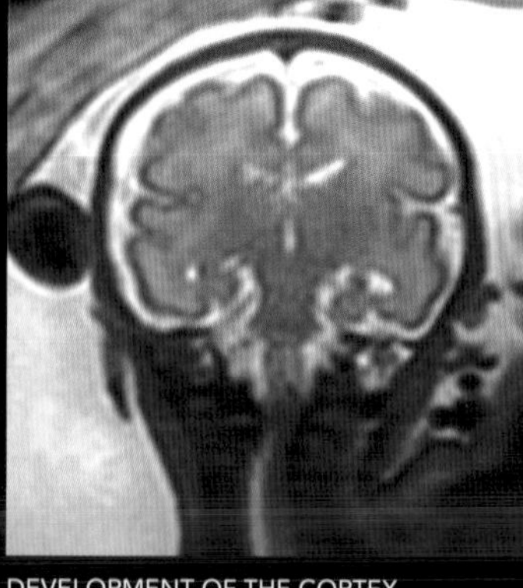

DEVELOPMENT OF THE CORTEX
The cerebral cortex develops from the forebrain, one of three vesicles formed from the neural tube. The frontal lobes form first, followed by the parietal, then temporal and occipital lobes.

CONCEPTION TO BIRTH

In the days after conception, the embryo is just a minute ball of cells. Development of the brain and nervous system starts at about three weeks as the cells differentiate into layers, the outermost of which thickens and flattens to form a feature called the neural plate (see below) along the back of the embryo. This broadens and folds to form the liquid-filled neural tube, which will become the brain and spinal cord. The brain starts to develop at about four weeks as a bulb at the upper end of the neural tube, while the lower part begins to form the spinal cord. The main sections of the brain, including the cerebral cortex, are visible within seven weeks. Over the next weeks, the brain grows, develops, and becomes more complex.

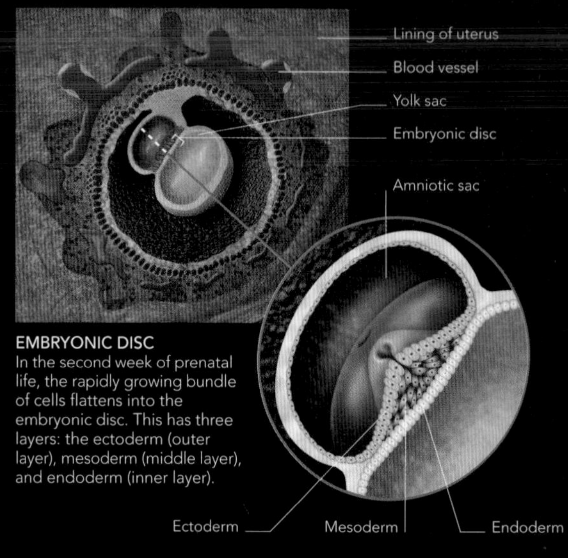

EMBRYONIC DISC
In the second week of prenatal life, the rapidly growing bundle of cells flattens into the embryonic disc. This has three layers: the ectoderm (outer layer), mesoderm (middle layer), and endoderm (inner layer).

KEY FOR EMBRYO DEVELOPMENT

- FOREBRAIN (PROSENCEPHALON)
- MIDBRAIN (MESENCEPHALON)
- HINDBRAIN (RHOMBENCEPHALON)
- SPINAL CORD

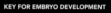

Neural tube forms

Forebrain prominence

3 WEEKS
Within three weeks of conception, the neural tube is well developed along the back of the embryo and the prominence that will develop into the forebrain is clearly defined.

Ear bud

Eye bud

Neural tube

5 WEEKS
The future forebrain, midbrain, and hindbrain can be seen clearly by five weeks, and rudimentary eye and ear buds emerge. The optic nerve, retina, and iris start to form.

Cranial nerves

Ear bud

Eye bud

7 WEEKS
The embryo is around 2cm (3/4in) long, and the bulges that will become the brainstem, cerebellum, and cerebrum are now clearly visible. The cranial and sensory nerves also start to develop.

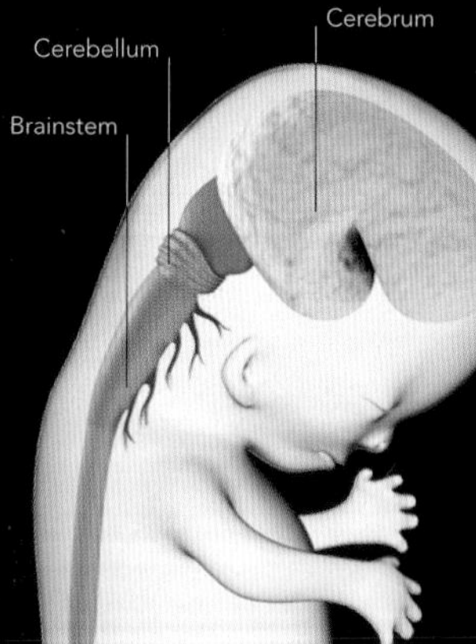

11 WEEKS
The cerebrum enlarges, and the eyes and ears mature, moving into position. The fetus's head is still large relative to the body. The hindbrain divides into the cerebellum and the brainstem.

FORMATION OF THE NEURAL TUBE

The key event in the development of the nervous system is the formation of the neural tube. This process is known as neurulation, and begins when the primitive spinal cord (notochord) sends a signal to the tissue above it to thicken, forming the neural plate. The neural plate turns inwards and forms a depression, known as the neural groove. Folds within the groove fuse together and then close in on themselves to form the neural tube. Some neural-fold tissue is pinched off to form the neural crest, which will become the peripheral nervous system.

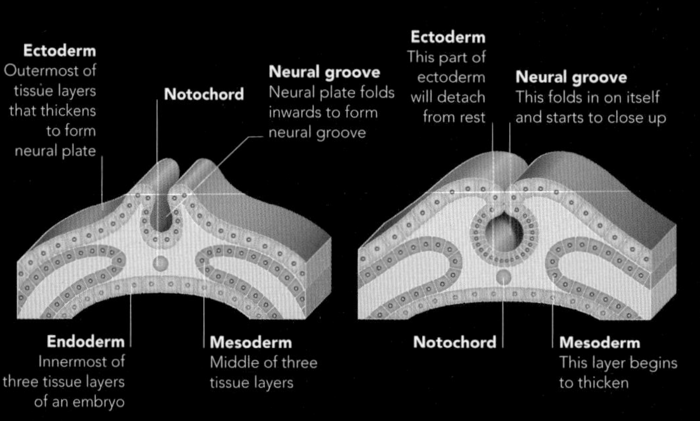

NERVE GROWTH AND PRUNING

nly one-sixth of the brain develops before birth, and the growth ate in the first three years of life is phenomenal. Most of the growth, owever, is connective tissue, as pathways are forged between eurons. By the age of three, this dense network of fibres requires pruning" back, a process known as apoptosis. The pruning allows he preserved connections to work more efficiently. It is similar to he way in which "noise" can be extracted from a radio signal to leave nly the intended content without the interference.

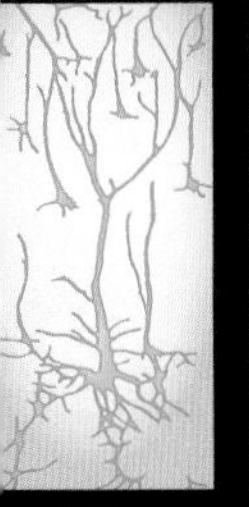
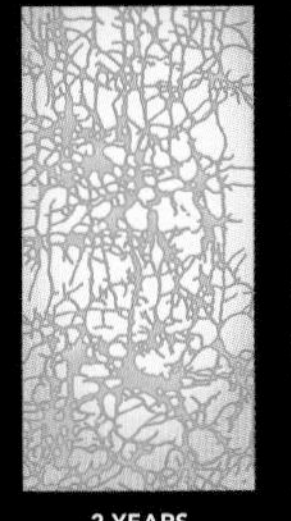
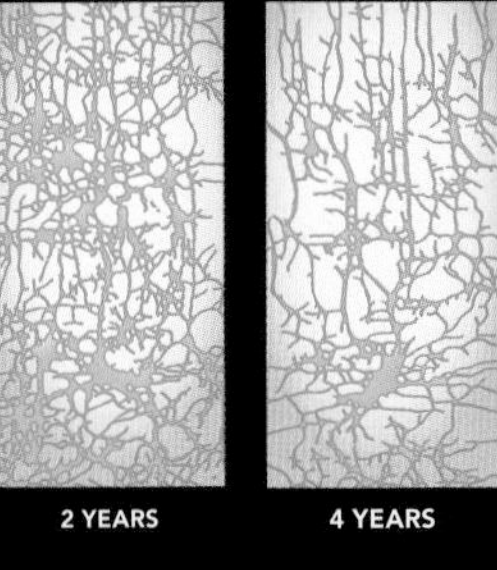
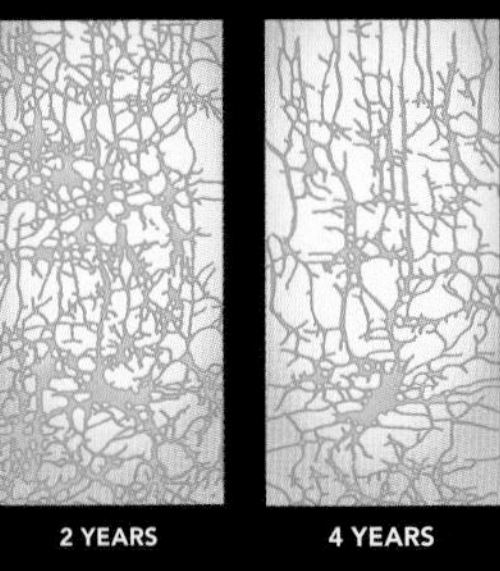
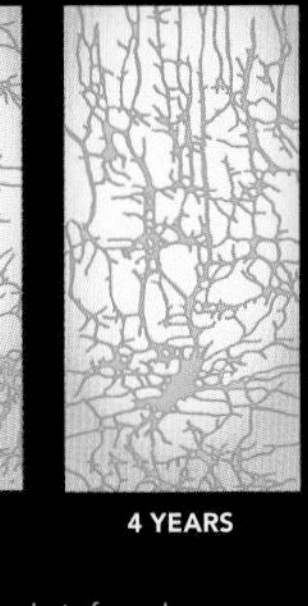

NEURAL NETWORKS
A dense network of connecting fibres forms between the brain's neurons during the first few years of life. By the age of four, these connections have been pruned back.

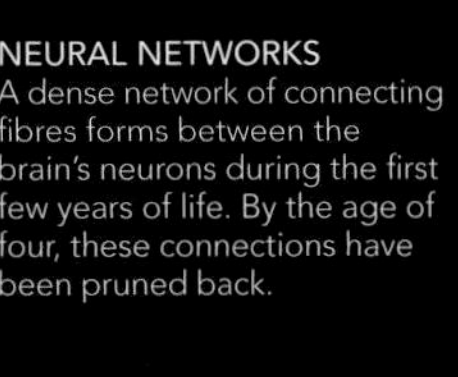

LANGUAGE DEVELOPMENT

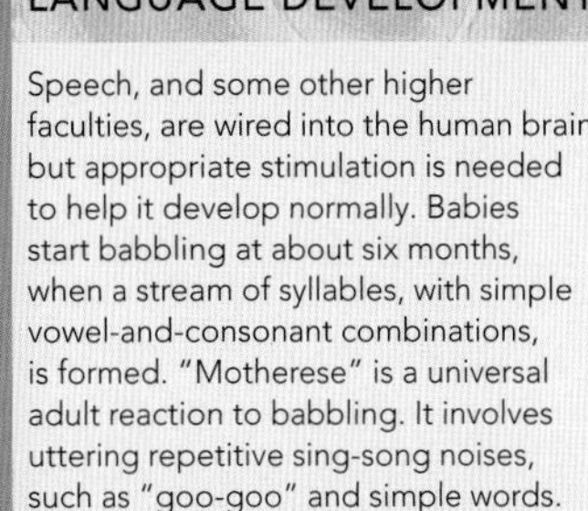

Speech, and some other higher faculties, are wired into the human brain but appropriate stimulation is needed to help it develop normally. Babies start babbling at about six months, when a stream of syllables, with simple vowel-and-consonant combinations, is formed. "Motherese" is a universal adult reaction to babbling. It involves uttering repetitive sing-song noises, such as "goo-goo" and simple words. It aids speech development in the child and promotes bonding.

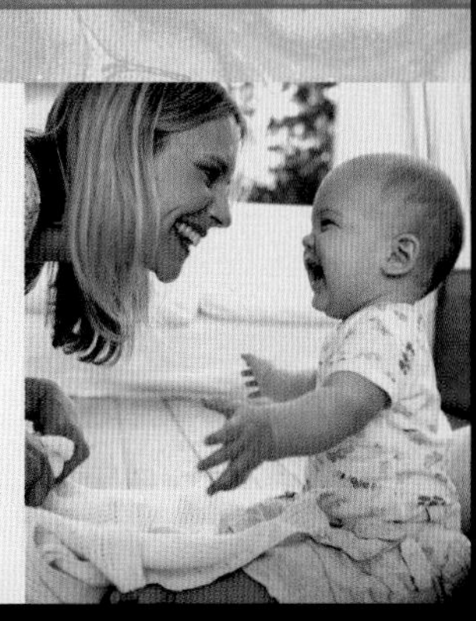

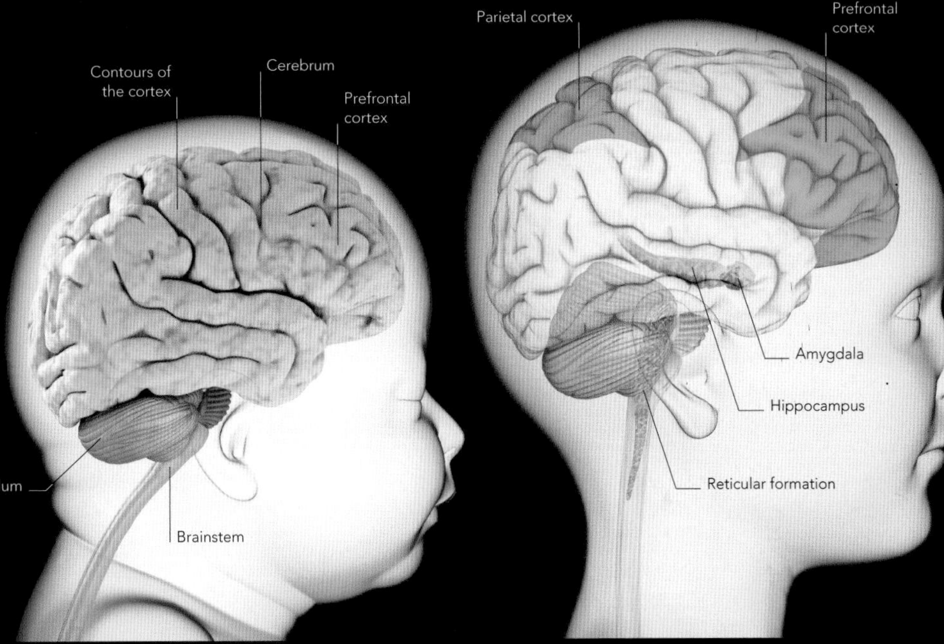

5 WEEKS
he hemispheres are now clearly dissected, nd some of the deeper grooves that form ne bulges and valleys – gyri and sulci – are ecoming visible. The cerebellum is tucked nder the cerebrum.

BIRTH
The cerebrum develops, and the ridges (gyri) and fissures (sulci) increase in complexity. At birth, a baby has as many neurons as an adult – 100 billion. Most are formed in the first six months of gestation but are not yet mature.

3 YEARS
Parts of the brain, like the prefrontal cortex, develop but large areas are offline as the connections between areas are yet to form or are yet to be coated in myelin, so signals can't travel along them reliably. This limits the ability of the frontal brain to think and judge. Growth of the amygdala and hippocampus allows memories to be retained.

PLACES AND FACES

'he basic functional blueprint f the brain is in place even t birth. The back of the brain s already wired to receive nformation from the eyes, or example, which it will tart to turn into visual images, nd the limbic areas, which egister "good" and "bad" vents, are already working. ...

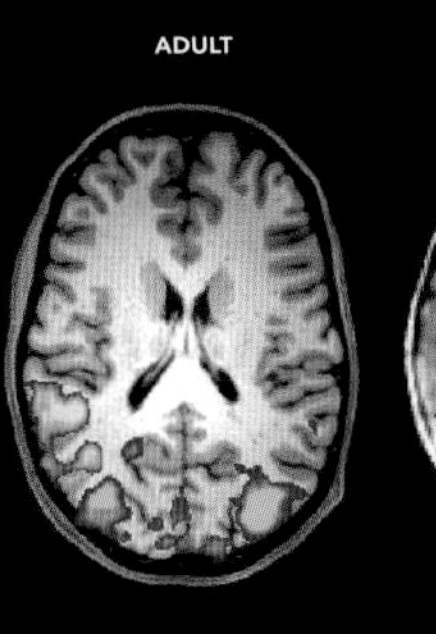
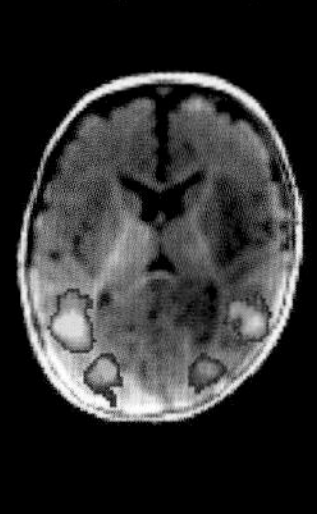
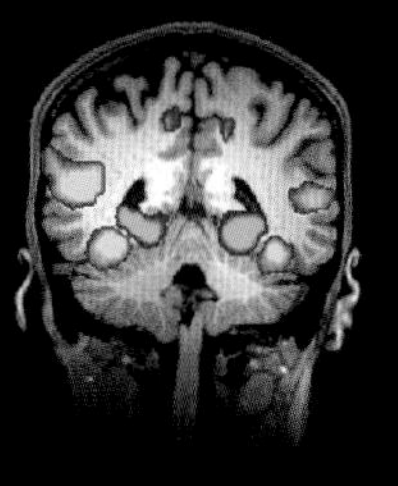
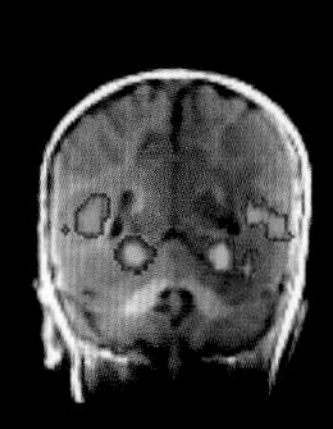

PRIMED TO SEE
Brain scans of six-month-old infants show they already process faces in a different area from

CHILDHOOD AND ADOLESCENCE

THE BRAIN DEVELOPS BY CREATING MORE AND MORE NEURAL PATHWAYS, WHICH CONNECT UP THE VARIOUS FUNCTIONAL AREAS. THE EARLIEST PARTS TO BECOME FULLY INTEGRATED ARE CONCERNED WITH PERCEPTION, CLOSELY FOLLOWED BY MOTOR AREAS.

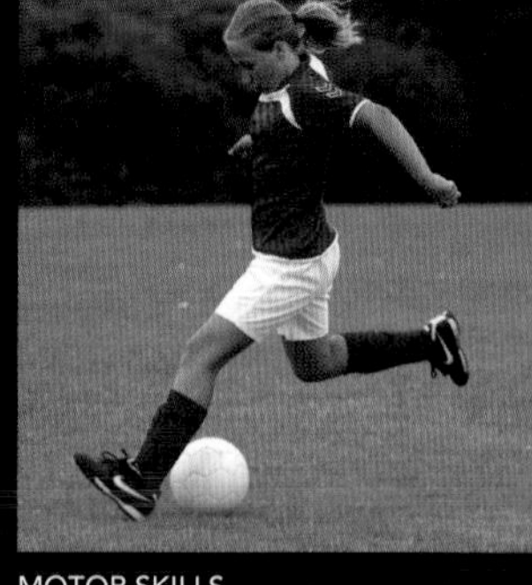

MOTOR SKILLS
Physical dexterity develops fairly early as perception and motor areas of the brain become connected.

THE BRAIN IN CHILDHOOD

The brain matures throughout childhood and young adulthood – the process is not complete until a person is in their late twenties. During that time different areas of the brain connect, producing increasingly complex and controlled behaviour. Connection occurs as the neurons grow axons – threads that reach out to other neurons – and the axons become covered in fatty sheaths (myelin), which allow electrical signals to move faster and more reliably along them.

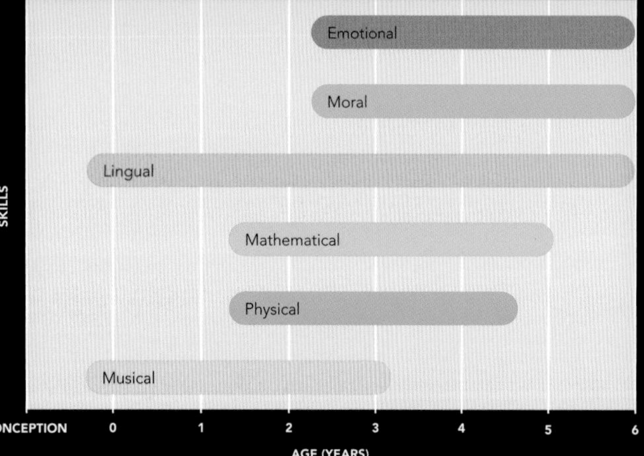

WINDOWS OF LEARNING

Human skills and faculties develop as the associated parts of the brain mature. The timetable is under genetic control, and no amount of teaching can instil in a child an ability that their brain is not ready to acquire. Until they are about three, for instance, an infant cannot make moral judgements because their prefrontal cortex, where such decisions are made, is not fully "online". When the area is maturing, however, a child will learn the skill associated with it easily and rapidly, given the right stimuli. If a window of learning is missed, the child will have difficulty acquiring the skill later.

CHANGING CONNECTIONS

Scientists have devised a typical growth chart of the human brain, formed by taking more than 200 fMRI scans of individuals with an age range of 7–10 years. They found that fibres connecting peripheral brain areas decreased, while increases occurred in those connecting the limbic areas with the frontal cortex as the brain matured.

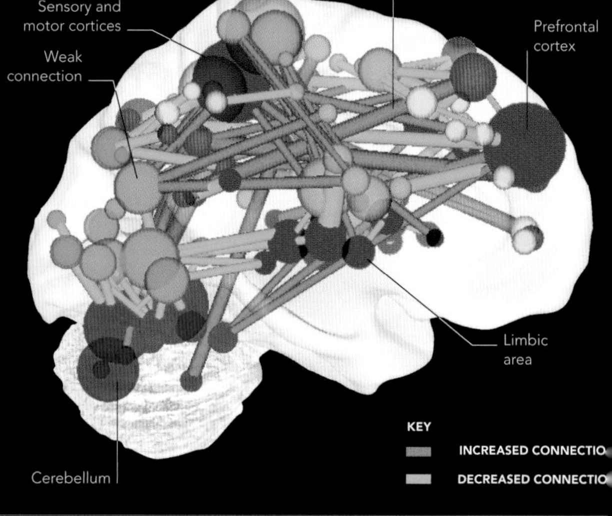

JOINING UP

In order to think and behave as an adult a person's brain needs to be "joined up". This allows perceptions to be fully understood and actions to be considered. Connection depends on a process called myelination, during which neuronal pathways between areas are coated with fat to allow the transmission of electrical signals.

MYELINATION
These scans show, on average, the degree of connection that exists at various ages. Yellow shows full myelination, green is partial, and blue is none.

KEY
FULL MYELINATION
PARTIAL MYELINATION
NO MYELINATION

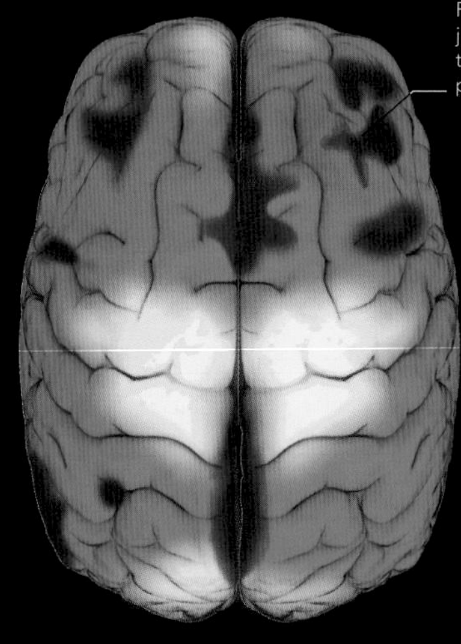

5 YEARS

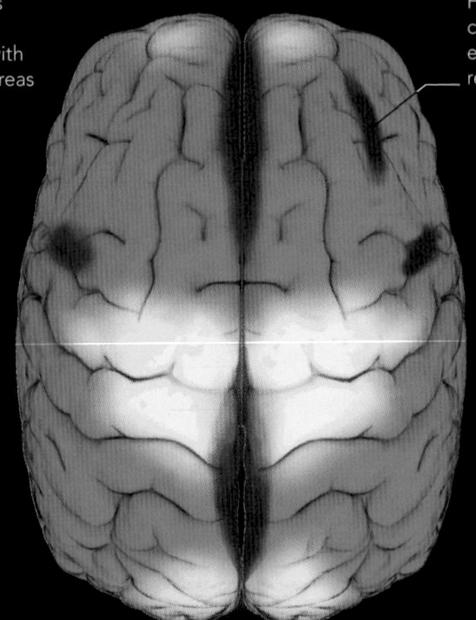

8 YEARS

Between puberty and early adulthood the human brain undergoes a dramatic restructuring. This process is often reflected in impulsive and rebellious behaviour, and sudden personality changes. While all these changes take place, the teenage brain is particularly vulnerable. Personality traits such as risk-taking or pessimism may be amplified to the extent that they cause dysfunction such as heavy drug-taking, reckless or criminal behaviour, intense anxiety, or depression. In many cases, the issue passes as the brain becomes more mature, but sometimes it signals the start of a serious, long-term mental health problem.

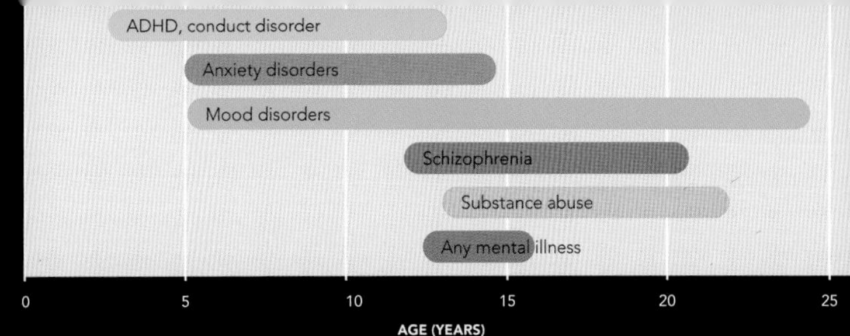

ADHD, conduct disorder
Anxiety disorders
Mood disorders
Schizophrenia
Substance abuse
Any mental illness
0
5
10
15
20
25
AGE (YEARS)

MENTAL HEALTH RISKS

The dramatic brain changes that occur during adolescence make teenagers particularly susceptible to mental ill-health. One in five adolescents has a mental illness that will persist into adulthood.

BRAIN CHANGES

Teenage brain changes, in both sexes, are driven by testosterone release. The hormone makes neural pathways exceptionally plastic for a while, so connections make and break easily. This allows teenagers to learn new things quickly, and to adopt new habits and personality traits, which in turn will be changed again if they are not advantageous. The instability of the teenage brain results in baffling changeability, and a tendency towards risk-taking and rebellious behaviour. The prefrontal cortex is still developing, which is thought to be one reason for impulsiveness and rash decision-making. It is closely connected to the basal ganglia, which play an important role in motor skills. The fibre tract that links the two hemispheres – the corpus callosum – thickens, allowing for increased information-processing skills.

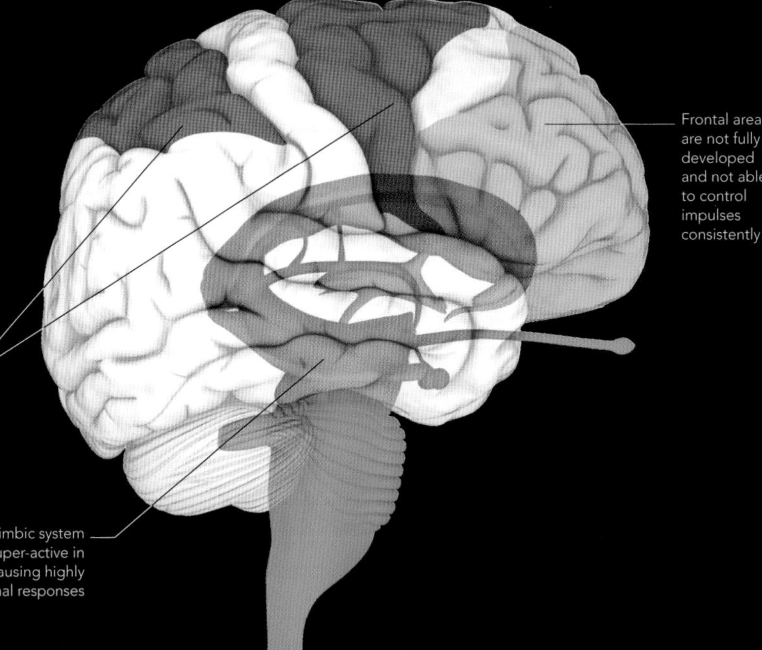

Frontal areas are not fully developed and not able to control impulses consistently
Motor areas and body maps in brain may get out of synch, causing physical gaucheness and clumsy actions
Limbic system is super-active in teenagers, causing highly emotional responses

WORK IN PROGRESS

Many different areas of the brain undergo changes, each causing a particular, temporary characteristic of teenagers.

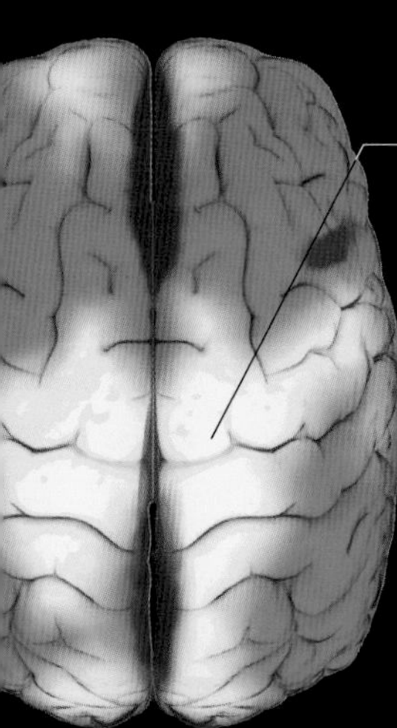

Connection is well-forged in back of brain but remains weak in frontal areas

12 YEARS

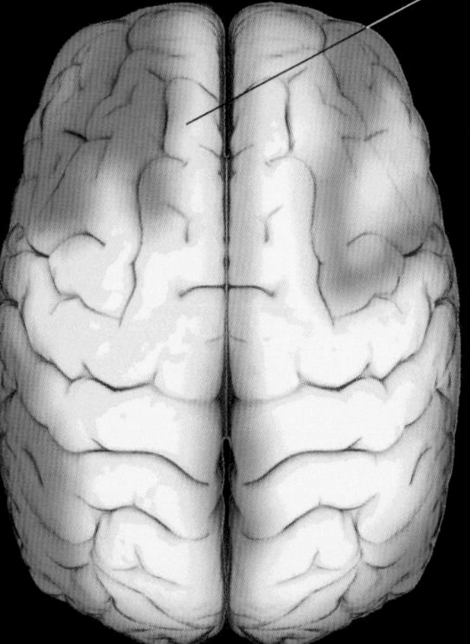

Connectivity is established, but teen brain is undergoing seismic changes, which make links unreliable

18 YEARS

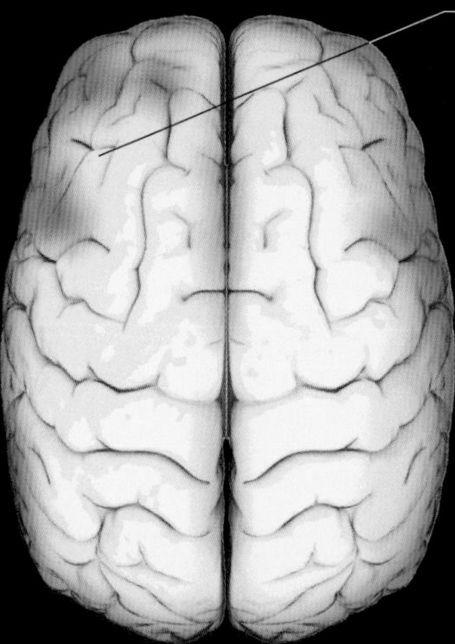

Whole brain is now connected but new links continue to be forged for another ten years or so

20 YEARS

THE BRAIN DOES NOT STOP GROWING WHEN IT REACHES MATURITY. MORE THAN ANY OTHER ORGAN, IT CONTINUES TO REFORM ITSELF LONG INTO ADULTHOOD. NEW BRAIN CELLS CONTINUE TO BE CREATED, AND THE ARCHITECTURE OF THE BRAIN IS CHANGED CONSTANTLY IN RESPONSE TO LIFE EXPERIENCES.

REACHING MATURITY

Human brains are slow to reach full maturity. The prefrontal cortex is the last part to become fully active, and full myelination – the sheathing of neuronal connections, which allows information to flow freely along them – does not occur until a person is in their late twenties or early thirties. Once the prefrontal cortex is fully online, it becomes more active in situations that have emotional content. Whereas a teenager or child might be overwhelmed by emotion, the prefrontal cortex inhibits emotion when necessary, and so allows for a more thoughtful, deliberated response.

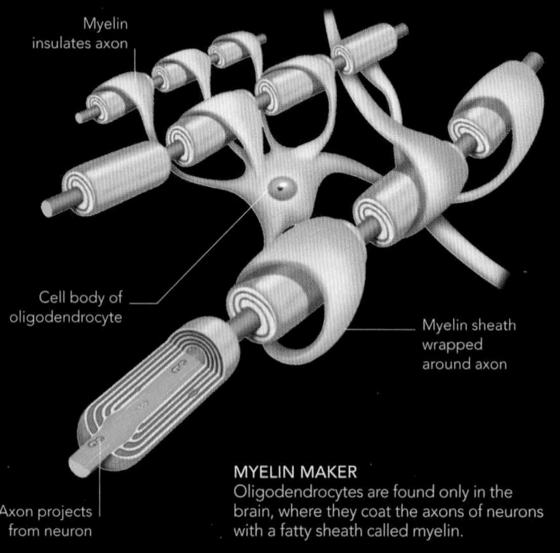

MYELIN MAKER
Oligodendrocytes are found only in the brain, where they coat the axons of neurons with a fatty sheath called myelin.

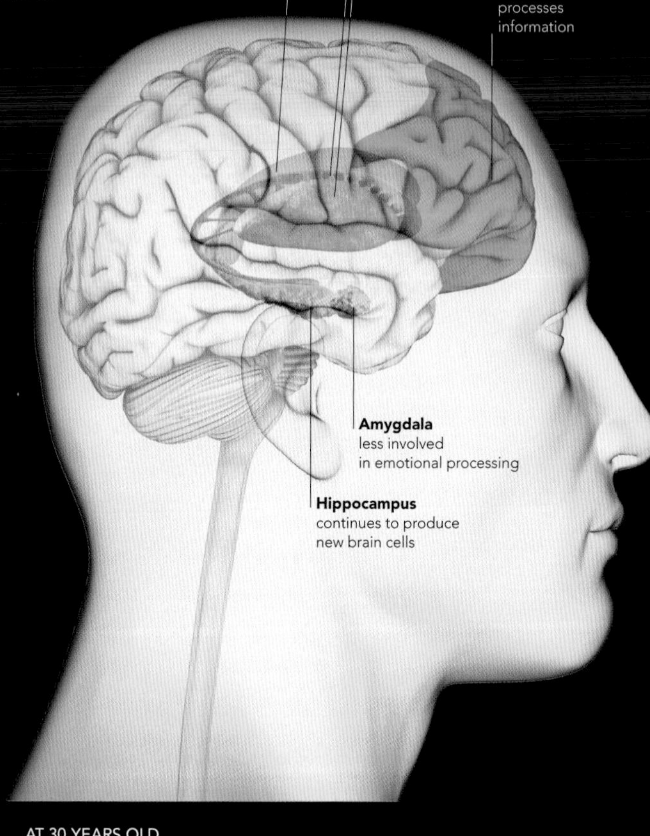

AT 30 YEARS OLD
The prefrontal cortex is now fully developed, allowing for improved executive functions. This also means that the brain is less reliant on the amygdala to process emotional information. The other areas of the brain that were still developing in adolescence have now reached maturity.

NEUROGENESIS

It used to be thought that the number of brain cells in the adult brain was fixed early in life and that laying down new memories and learning new things was achieved entirely by changes to existing neurons and their connections with one another. While this sort of rewiring is important for learning, it is now known that adults also benefit from the creation of new brain cells. Neurogenesis occurs mainly in the dentate gyrus of the hippocampus, the brain region that is centrally important for learning and memory. About one-third of the neurons in the adult hippocampus are replaced in a person's lifetime.

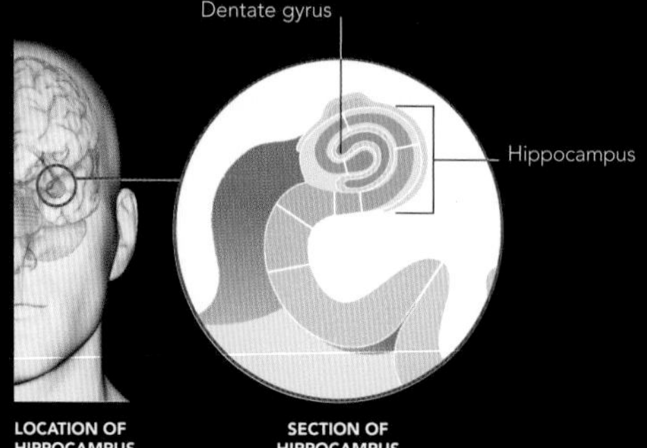

MEMORY MAKER
The hippocampus is a vital part of the brain, which is essential for laying down and recalling memories. Neurogenesis, which occurs in the dentate gyrus (see opposite), helps it to encode new information. Neurogenesis is measured in animals by injecting their brains with radioactive marker that attaches to dividing cells. Counting the marked cells when the aimals die shows how many cells have multiplied.

HIGHER FUNCTION

A person's brain continues to mature right up until their late twenties. The main changes take place inside the "higher" functional areas of the brain, such as the frontal cortex, which gradually becomes more active – pulling together information from the rest of the brain and forming a complex and holistic view of the world. Until then the emotional parts of the brain are not fully connected with these areas concerned with thought, judgement, and behavioural inhibition. As the connections between the areas become more stable, people tend to react less emotionally and impulsively – instead becoming more cautious, considered, and exercising better judgement.

NEW MEMORIES FOR OLD

The creation of new brain cells allows new information to be stored, but their arrival disrupts existing memories because they change the wiring pattern. Most memories form in the hippocampus and are transferred to long-term storage in other brain areas. For a while, the memory resides both in the hippocampus and elsewhere. After a few years, the memory is cleared from the hippocampus. Until the memory is fully transferred, the arrival of new cells in the hippocampus may weaken the connections encoding memories stored there. This may be why we rarely retain memories from when we were very young.

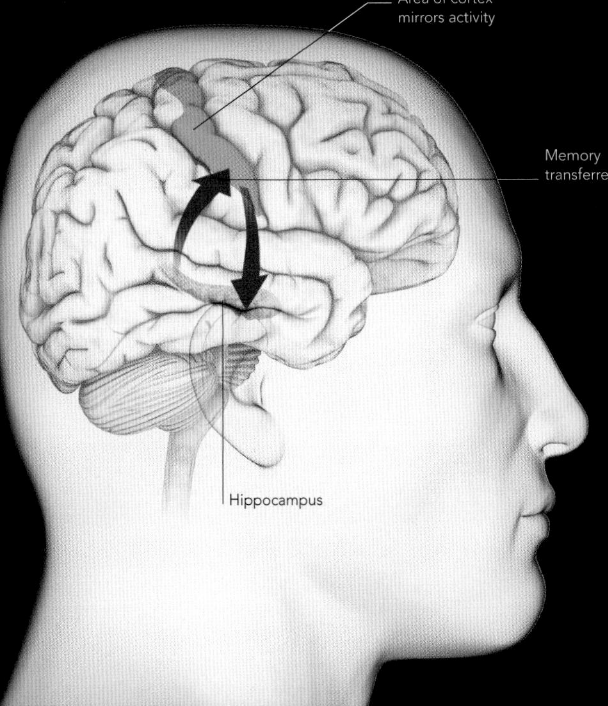

MEMORY TRANSFER
Memories are first formed as patterns of neural activity in the hippocampus, which are then echoed in areas of the cortex (see pp.160–61).

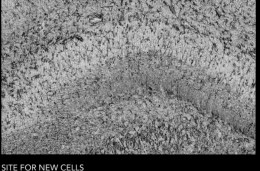

SITE FOR NEW CELLS
This light micrograph shows a section through the hippocampus, which has been magnified and stained to show nerve cells in the dentate gyrus, where new neurons are made.

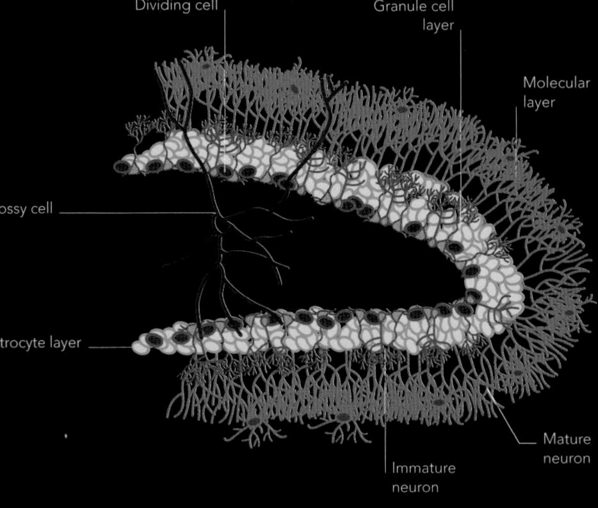

DENTATE GYRUS CELLS
In adults new neurons are made in just two areas of the brain – the olfactory cortex (the part of the frontal cortex that registers smells) and, more commonly, in part of the hippocampus called the dentate gyrus. Astrocyte cells in this area produce a protein that triggers the process. Cells divide and mature, moving up through the granular to the molecular layer of the dentate gyrus.

PARENTHOOD

Having a child is a major event in most adult lives and usually brings about profound changes in behaviour. These are accompanied by changes in the brains of both mothers and fathers. In both parents, raised levels of hormones, particularly prolactin and oxytocin, sensitize areas of the brain concerned with alarm (such as the amygdala) and action, making them more sensitive to their babies' cues, such as cries and expressions. Men's testosterone level falls, and prolactin rises, making their brains temporarily more like that of a female.

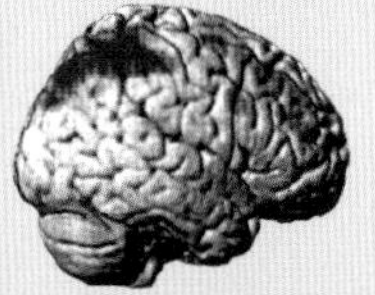

BRAIN CHANGE
Research shows that becoming a parent produces a flurry of neurogenesis. MRI studies reveal an increase in cortical thickness in new mothers' brains, shown red in the scans, left.

SEEING BABIES
Parents' brains react more strongly to the sight of their own child's face than to that of others. In mothers, the strength of response, especially in the amygdala, is correlated with the extent to which the mother is bonded with the child. Mothers suffering postnatal depression show a reduced amygdala response compared to those strongly attached to their child.

Imaging studies reveal that all adults show a particular response to the sight of a baby's face. A spot in the orbitofrontal cortex – a brain area associated with emotion – becomes active when they see an infant, but not when they see an adult face. This "signature" response is the same in men and women, and in both parents and non-parents. It suggests that we are primed by evolution to feel an emotional bond with infants of our own species.

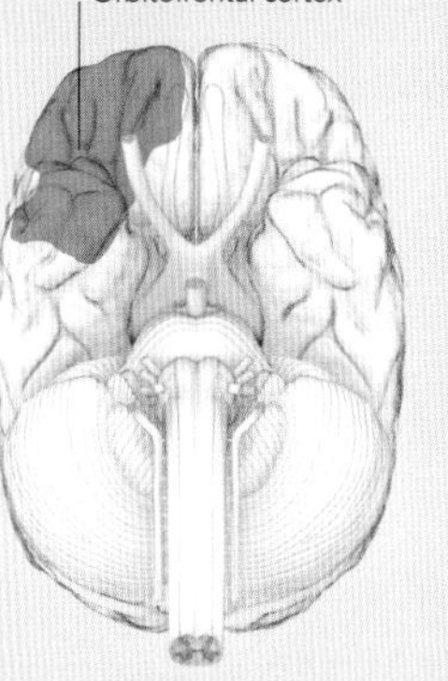

THE AGEING BRAIN

THE TRADITIONAL VIEW OF AGEING IS THAT THE BRAIN AND THE BODY START TO DEGENERATE. THIS IS TRUE IN THAT NEURONS ARE LOST AND, FOR THOSE THAT REMAIN, IMPULSES ARE TRANSMITTED MORE SLOWLY. THIS CAN LEAD TO SLOWING THOUGHT PROCESSES, MEMORY PROBLEMS, AND DETERIORATING REFLEXES, WHICH CAN CAUSE PROBLEMS WITH BALANCE AND MOVEMENT.

NATURAL DEGENERATION

In the past, it was rare for people to live to the age of 50 and beyond, so we have not evolved to use the brain in such advanced years. This makes the ageing brain a relatively new phenomenon in human history and evolution. The natural degeneration of the brain and nervous system is not caused by disease, and so should not be confused with the pathology of dementia, which is associated with a pattern of specific brain changes. Recent research shows that most neurons actually remain healthy until you die, but brain volume and size decrease 5–10 per cent from the age of 20–90. There are also changes in topography, with the grooves widening and tangles and plaques (small, disc-shaped growths) forming. However, the role of these deficits is not absolutely clear. They can occur in the brains of both healthy people and sufferers of Alzheimer's disease.

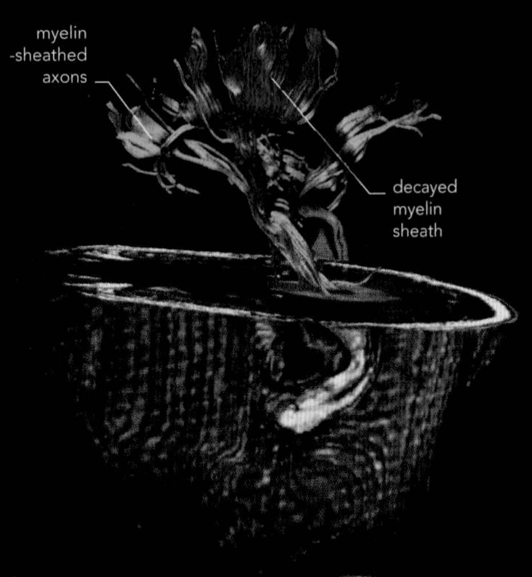

MYELIN DECAY
The myelin sheath that insulates the axons of neurons is vital for effective cell-to-cell communication. This protein-based structure decays with age, leaving brain circuits less efficient, leading to balance and memory problems. The decayed myelin sheaths travelling from the cortex to spine are shown as blue and purple on this image, while the healthy ones are shown in green.

AGE AND EXCITEMENT LEVELS

Dopamine is a neurotransmitter that triggers excitement and rapid decision-making. Brain-imaging studies suggest that, as people age, activity in their dopamine circuits decreases. This might be reflected in behavioural changes, because dopamine is linked with thrill-seeking and risk-taking. Perhaps older people prefer a quieter life than younger people because dopamine is less abundant.

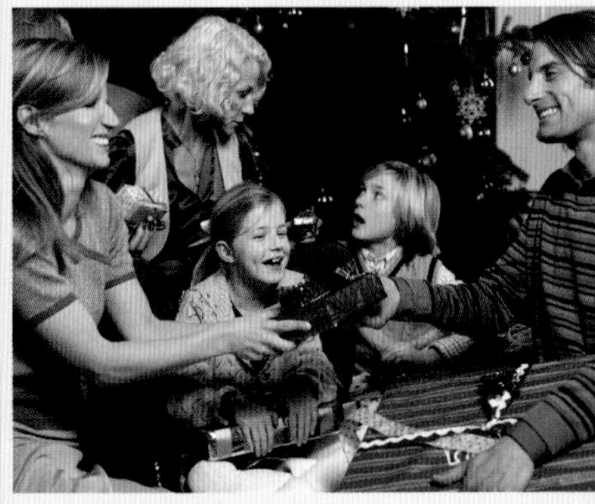

THE THRILL OF CHRISTMAS
Opening presents is highly exciting for children, but much less so for older people because dopamine, which is triggered by "rewards" (in this case, gifts), has less impact as you age.

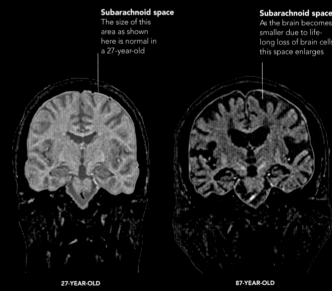

Basal ganglia
These clusters of nerve cells appear normal in the young brain

Basal ganglia
The brighter areas are the product of iron accumulation

27-YEAR-OLD

87-YEAR-OLD

BASAL GANGLIA
This series of MRI scans shows the differences between crucial areas of the brain of a young adult compared to an elderly adult. The scans above show the basal ganglia, which plays a vital role in co-ordinating movement.

Subarachnoid space
The size of this area as shown here is normal in a 27-year-old

Subarachnoid space
As the brain becomes smaller due to life-long loss of brain cells this space enlarges

27-YEAR-OLD

87-YEAR-OLD

SUBARACHNOID SPACE
The subarachnoid space is the area around the outside edge of the brain, and is known as a potential site for brain haemorrhage (see p.229). It becomes notably larger as the brain ages, reflecting a general reduction in brain volume.

POSITIVE AGEING

The brain can compensate for the effects of ageing, and mental function can even improve with age. Myelin increases in the temporal and frontal lobes in the 45–50 age group may enable people to manage their knowledge better. Also, comprehension studies have shown that high-functioning older adults use either both hemispheres together, or a different hemisphere to either young adults or lower-functioning older adults. This may be the brain's way of making up for declining functions, to keep thought and memory processes stronger.

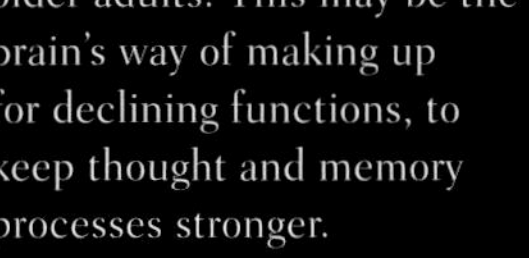

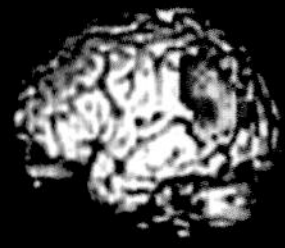

YOUNG ADULT (LEFT HEMISPHERE)

YOUNG ADULT (RIGHT HEMISPHERE)

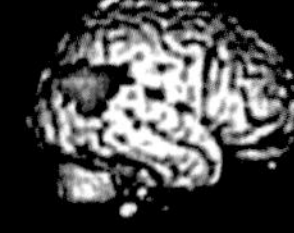

ELDERLY ADULT (LEFT HEMISPHERE)

ELDERLY ADULT (RIGHT HEMISPHERE)

BRAIN ACTIVATION CONTRASTS
One study compared fMRI scans of brain activity in young adults (top row) and older adults (bottom row) during sentence comprehension. The results suggest that older people with good comprehension compensate for the deficits in language areas of the brain by recruiting other areas.

PROTEIN ACCUMULATION

A recent study examined the brains of five people in their eighties, who had performed very well in memory tests and compared them to the brains of "normal", non-demented elderly people of a similar age. The ones who performed well in the memory tests had fewer tangles consisting of a protein called tau in their brains than the other group. These tangles grow inside brain cells and are thought to eventually kill them.

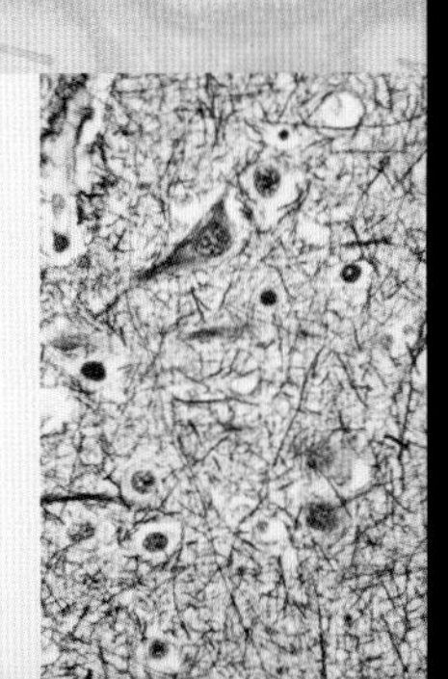

FIBRE-LIKE TANGLES
Microscopic tangles (shown as dark masses) are often found in large numbers in the brains of Alzheimer's patients.

KEEPING THE BRAIN YOUNG

New research into brain ageing indicates that the rate of decline may be slowed by lifestyle factors, such as regular exercise. Research has also found that reducing food intake, resulting in lower blood glucose levels, may slow the pace of change, because blood glucose can cause damage to proteins. Certainly, people with elevated blood glucose levels, such as those with type 1 diabetes show more signs of brain ageing than non-diabetic individuals.

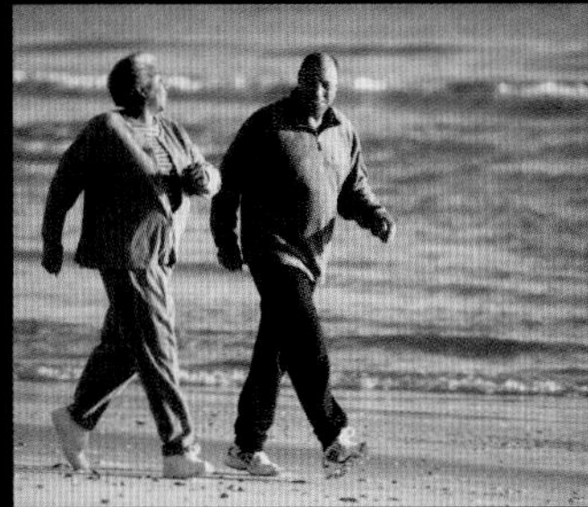

EXERCISE

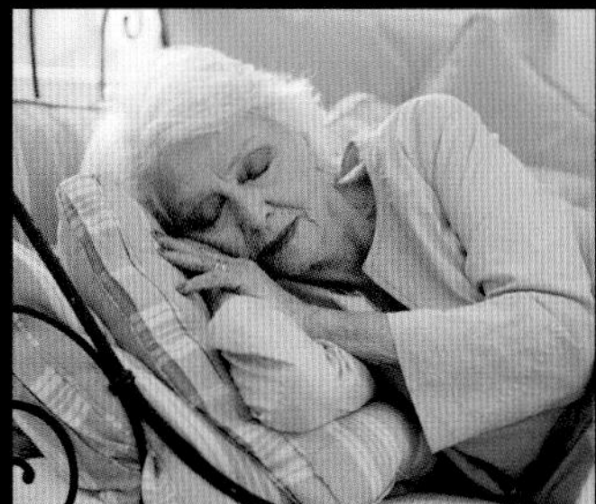

REST

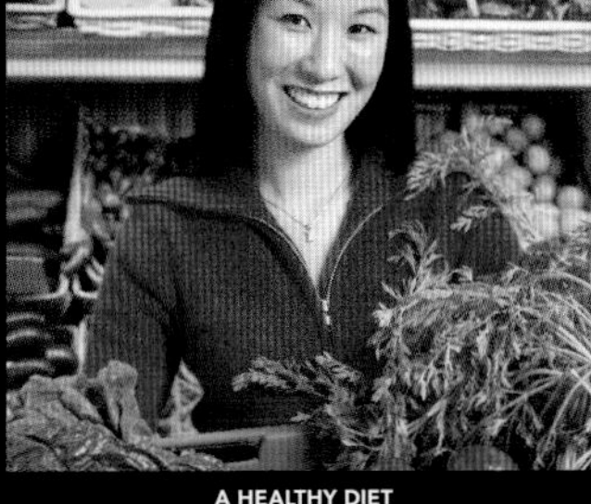

A HEALTHY DIET

MENTAL FITNESS

BENEFITS OF A HEALTHY LIFESTYLE
A number of lifestyle factors may help to stimulate the growth of neural tissue. Gentle aerobic exercise, such as rapid walking, regular sleep, a good diet, and mental exercises help to delay age-related mental decline and protect against age-related problems, such as memory loss.

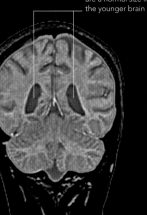

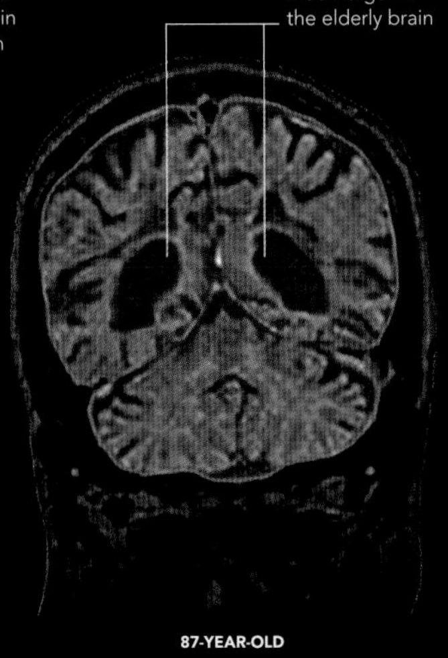
Ventricles
These hollow spaces filled with cerebrospinal fluid are a normal size in the younger brain
Ventricles
These hollow spaces are much larger in the elderly brain

27-YEAR-OLD

87-YEAR-OLD

VENTRICLES
The ventricles contain cerebrospinal fluid, which performs several functions, including protecting the brain from injury and transporting hormones. These areas become larger as the brain ages, as a result of the general loss of grey matter.

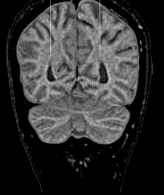

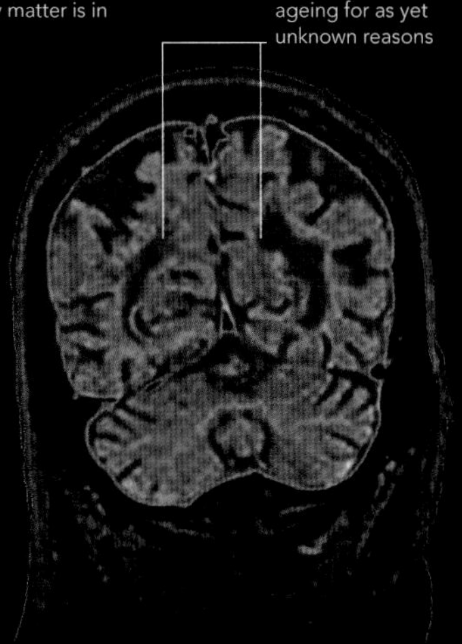
White-matter tract
This communication channel for the brain's information-processing grey matter is in good condition
White-matter tract
This changes in appearance during ageing for as yet unknown reasons

27-YEAR-OLD

87-YEAR-OLD

WHITE-MATTER TRACTS
The white matter contains mainly supporting (glial) cells, which are needed to support neurons. Because there are less supporting cells as the brain gets older, neurons function less efficiently.

AS WE DISCOVER HOW THE BRAIN WORKS, THE PROSPECT OF CHANGING IT, ENHANCING IT, AND DEVELOPING ARTIFICIAL BRAINS IS FAST BECOMING FACT RATHER THAN FICTION. TECHNOLOGIES FOR MIND READING, THOUGHT CONTROL, AND ARTIFICIAL INTELLIGENCE ARE ALREADY WITH US, AND ARE BECOMING MORE SOPHISTICATED EVERY DAY.

BRAIN–MACHINE INTERFACES

When a person is thinking, their brain produces electrical signals. Scientists have discovered ways in which the electrical signals can be picked up by sensors and sent wirelessly to other electrical devices, making it possible for a person to move or alter objects by thought alone. Most research in this field is directed towards developing devices to help people with nervous-system injuries regain the use of paralysed limbs. The technology has also been picked up by some computer-game manufacturers, who have produced games that can be played using thought power.

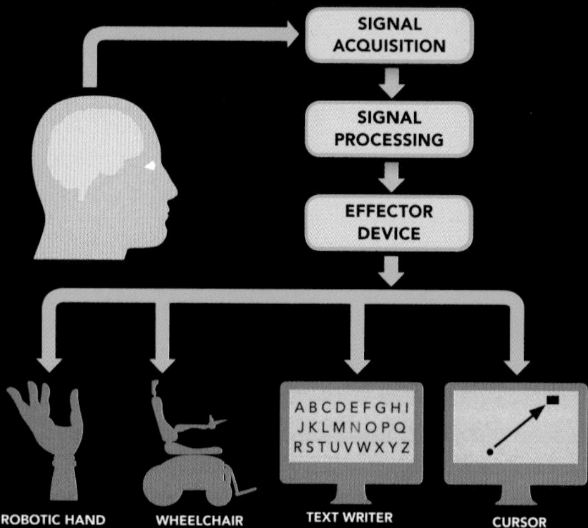

REGAINING CONTROL
Mind-control technology allows people to use devices such as artificial limbs, wheelchairs, and computers simply by directing their thoughts. Signals from the brain are received, then analysed and recoded, before being transmitted to a device as instructions.

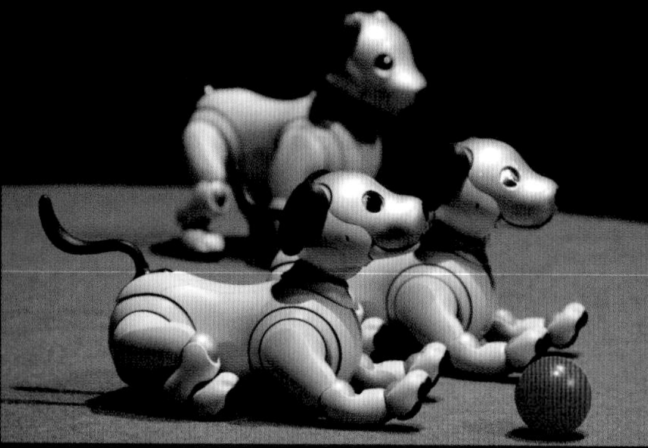

HELPFUL ROBOTS
Modern robots are designed to help people and fulfil a wide range of functions. The latest robots can serve food, do housework, help in hospitals, take risks on the battlefield, and even function as cute, playful pets.

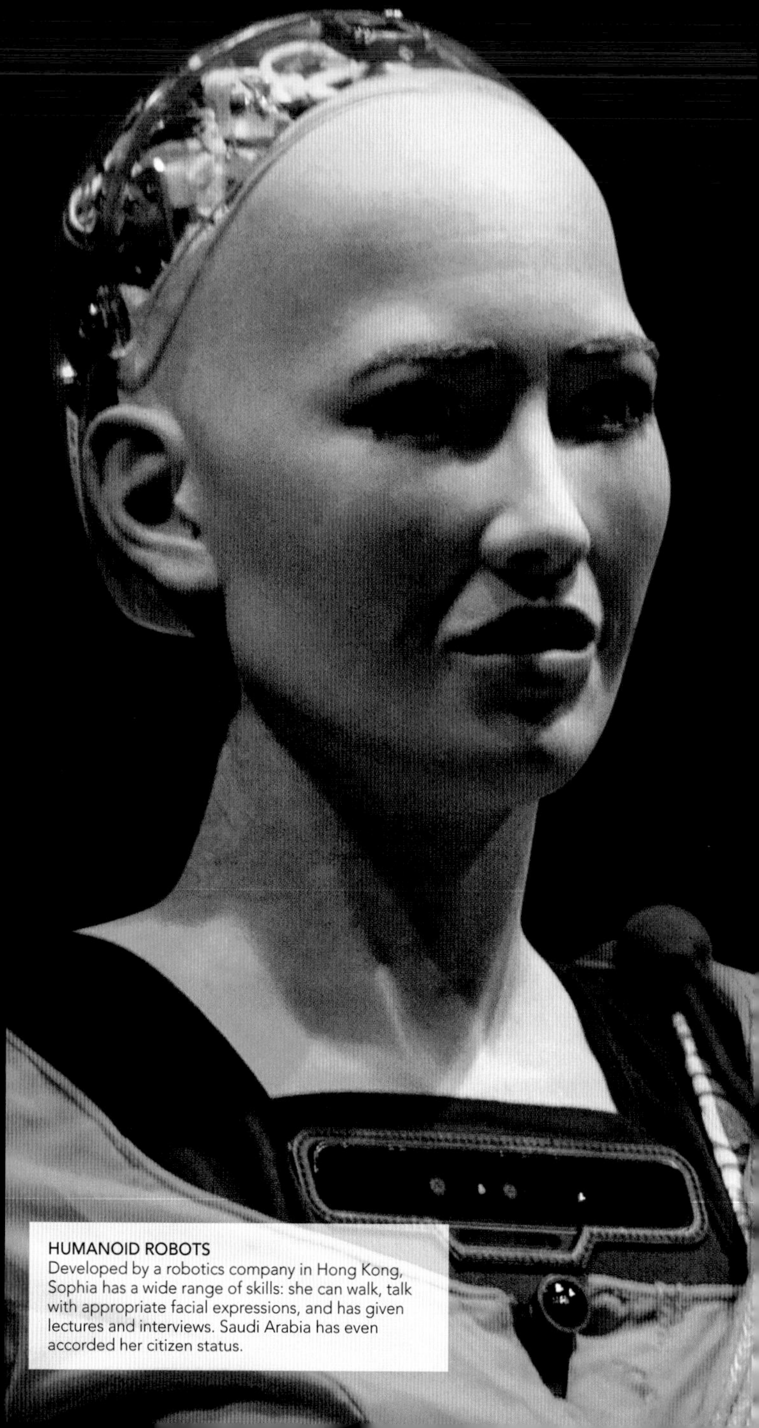

HUMANOID ROBOTS
Developed by a robotics company in Hong Kong, Sophia has a wide range of skills: she can walk, talk with appropriate facial expressions, and has given lectures and interviews. Saudi Arabia has even accorded her citizen status.

ne "picture" of neural activity created by MRI scanning can be translated into a recise description of what a person is eeing and, to some extent, what they are inking. To achieve this, the output of a erson's fMRI scan, captured while they are oking at a particular image, is processed y sophisticated computer software that anslates the pattern of activity into a visual ead out". Such "mind reading" is made ossible because neurons in the visual ortex are specialized for specific stimuli – orizontal or vertical lines, for example, so eir firing patterns are indicative of the type visual stimuli the neurons are registering.

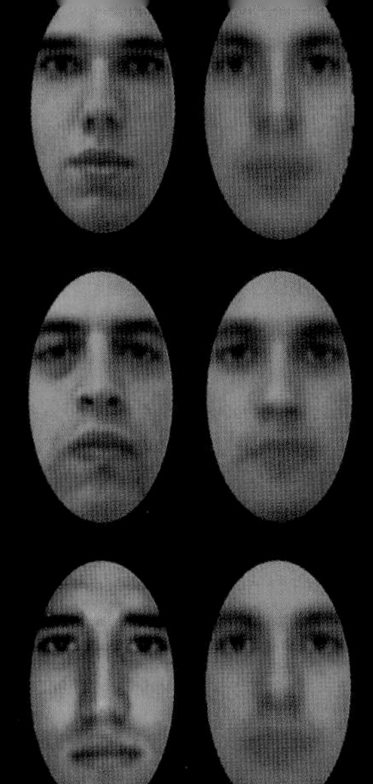

AKING FACES
EG brain scans of people looking faces have been decoded by cientists in Canada and then fed to a computer, which reproduces hat that person is seeing.

Mind reading is not limited to revealing what it is that a person is looking at. Brain-scanning studies have shown that, when a person is lying, their brain generates a different pattern of neural activity to when they are telling the truth. This has been used to develop a "lie detector" that analyses brain activity captured by fMRI. Although still in development, the technology is claimed to have an accuracy rate of over 90 per cent – significantly greater than the accuracy rate of polygraph tests.

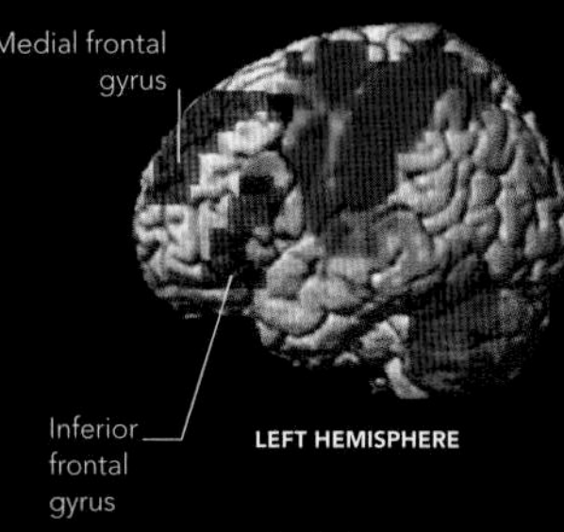

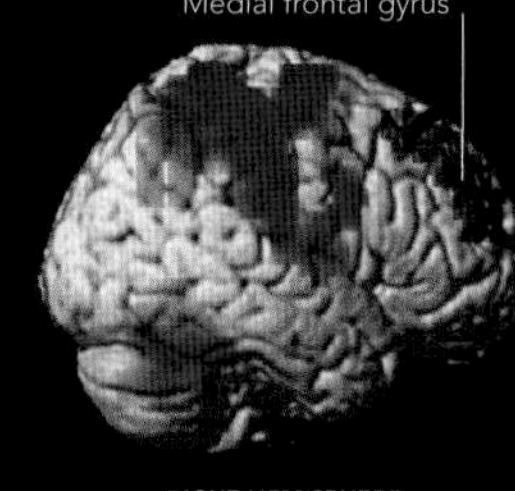

REVEALING THE TRUTH
Different areas of the brain are activated according to when someone is telling the truth and when they are lying. Here, the red areas show the telltale activity of a lie, while the blue areas are associated with telling the truth.

ARTIFICIAL INTELLIGENCE

cientists have been working for decades on producing ntelligent non-biological systems, and have been very uccessful in developing computer programs that can qual, or sometimes outperform, the human brain. Chess programs, for instance, can now compete n even terms with the best players in the world. However, it has proved difficult to develop systems hat are as flexible as the human brain, and thus able o operate in the constantly changing environments hat constitute "real" life. To overcome this, the mphasis of artificial intelligence research has recently hifted from developing more advanced computers to reating "emotional" machines that are able to make rude but quick "holistic" or "intuitive" judgements hat do not depend on enormous calculating capacity.

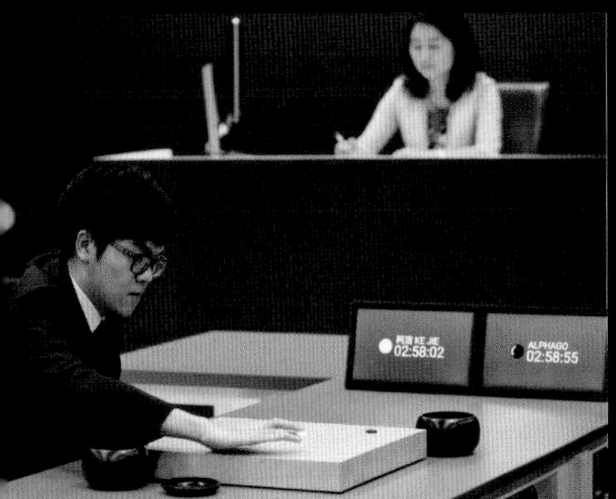

O WINNER
lphaGo – a programme developed by Google Deep Mind – eat Ke Jie, the world number-one player, at the 2017 Future of Go ummit. Go is an ancient game, even more complex than chess.

THE UNCANNY VALLEY

As robots are made to look more like humans, people find them increasingly uncomfortable. Robots such as Sophia (see opposite), fall into what is known as the "uncanny valley". This is a dip in a graph relating to a machine, which has a vertical axis measuring how comfortable people feel with it and a horizontal axis measuring how closely the machine resembles a real person. While mechanical robots do not worry people, once a device looks human yet "not quite right", a sense of uneasiness occurs.

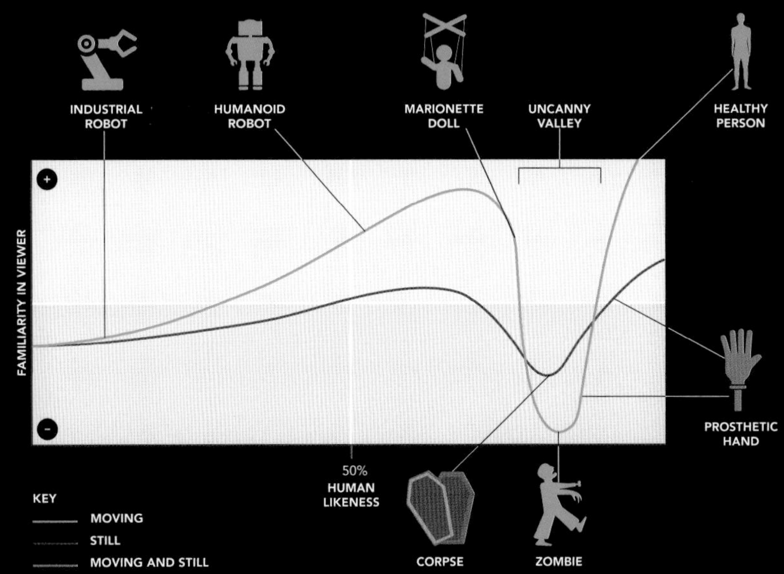

MONSTER OR MACHINE?
This graph illustrates that although humanoid robots are more familiar to people than more functional-looking industrial robots, there is a tipping point at which increased likeness to humans results in less familiarity. This is the "uncanny valley".

THE STATE OF TECHNOLOGY

Recent advances in biotechnology have made it possible to replace damaged limbs with artificial ones that can be controlled by thought, operating in much the same way as the original. Another advance involves altering brain function by inserting electrical pacemakers. Artificial sense organs, such as the bionic eye, are already on trial, and artificial brain parts such as memory add-ons and hippocampus replacements are not far behind.

Electrode

BRAIN PROBE
This X-ray shows an electrode inserted into the brain during a technique called deep brain stimulation.

THE BIONIC EYE

People who have become blind as a consequence of eye conditions (as opposed to damage to areas of the brain associated with vision) may soon be able to see again thanks to the development of artificial eyes. A "bionic" eye prototype has been created, comprising a computer chip that sits in the back of the individual's own eye socket, which is linked up to a tiny video camera built into a pair of spectacles. Images captured by the camera are beamed to the chip, which translates them into electrical impulses and sends them on to the visual cortex via the optic nerve.

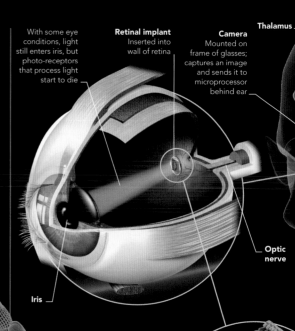

With some eye conditions, light still enters iris, but photo-receptors that process light start to die

Retinal implant Inserted into wall of retina

Camera Mounted on frame of glasses; captures an image and sends it to microprocessor behind ear

Thalamus

Optic nerve

Iris

Retina cross-section

Retinal implant Receives signals from microprocessor and emits pulses, which travel via optic nerve to visual cortex in brain

Photo-receptors destroyed by disease

ETHICS AND TECHNOLOGY

As biotechnology advances, it generates ethical and moral dilemmas. Brain technologies are particularly sensitive because most of us consider the products of our brain – thoughts, feeling, desires – as the central part of our "selves". Stem cells – immature body cells that have the potential to turn into many different types of cell – might one day be used to restore damaged neurons. Their use in other areas of medicine has already generated huge debate, because initially they had to be harvested from human fetuses, but they can now be obtained another way.

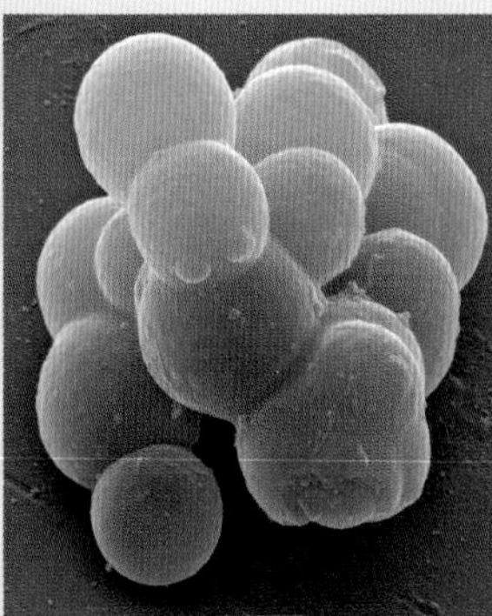

STEM CELLS
Stem cells like these can now be taken from blood flowing through the umbilical cord. Initially they came from fetuses, which caused much ethical debate.

NANOROBOTS
Microscopic robots could one day re-engineer our bodies to be stronger, more intelligent, and resistant to disease, presenting complicated life choices.

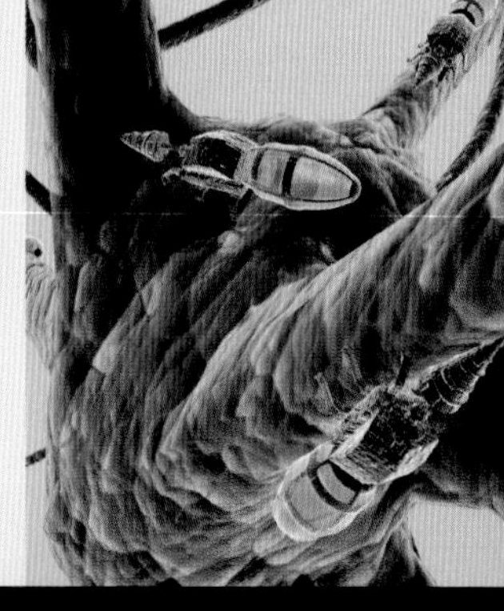

BRAIN AND BODY ENHANCEMENTS
Practically every part of the body, including the sense organs, may soon have artificial counterparts. Some of these are already in development, although of those shown above only the vagus nerve stimulator is in widespread clinical use.

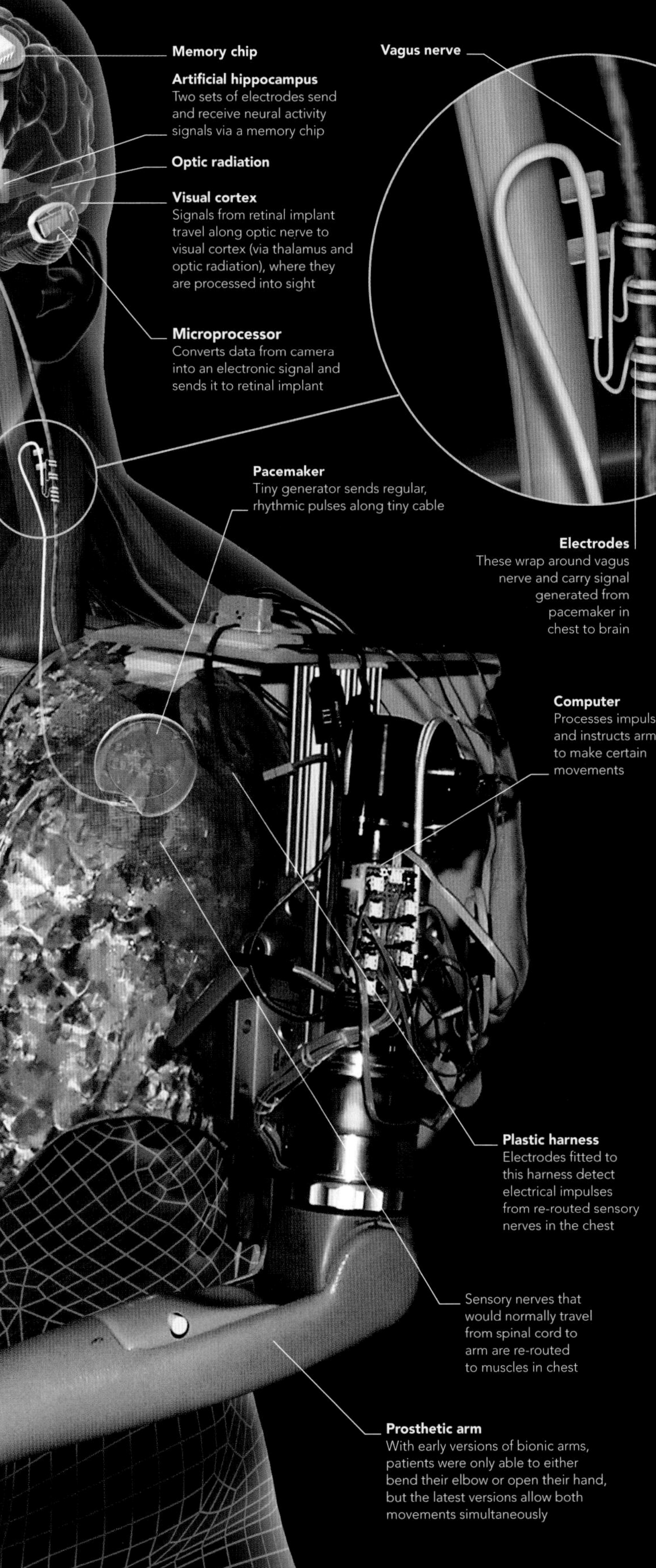
Memory chip
Artificial hippocampus
Two sets of electrodes send and receive neural activity signals via a memory chip
Optic radiation
Visual cortex
Signals from retinal implant travel along optic nerve to visual cortex (via thalamus and optic radiation), where they are processed into sight
Microprocessor
Converts data from camera into an electronic signal and sends it to retinal implant
Vagus nerve
Pacemaker
Tiny generator sends regular, rhythmic pulses along tiny cable
Electrodes
These wrap around vagus nerve and carry signal generated from pacemaker in chest to brain
Computer
Processes impulses and instructs arm to make certain movements
Plastic harness
Electrodes fitted to this harness detect electrical impulses from re-routed sensory nerves in the chest
Sensory nerves that would normally travel from spinal cord to arm are re-routed to muscles in chest
Prosthetic arm
With early versions of bionic arms, patients were only able to either bend their elbow or open their hand, but the latest versions allow both movements simultaneously

VAGUS-NERVE STIMULATION

The vagus nerve is a cranial nerve travelling from the brainstem to various internal organs, which has an important role in mediating brain arousal. A number of different types of brain disorder, such as chronic epilepsy and severe depression, benefit from the effects of stimulating this nerve. A small disc with a tiny generator fuelled by a lithium battery is surgically implanted in the chest, which sends regular, rhythmic pulses along a wire that is tethered to the left vagus nerve (the right vagus nerve runs directly to the heart). The frequency and intensity of the electrical pulses can be altered according to the severity of the condition.

THE BIONIC ARM

A bionic arm that is operated by the power of thought alone is already in use, and future models, which are currently being developed, are likely to be more lifelike and increasingly dextrous. The current versions work by re-routing motor nerves from the brain that originally ran to the hand, and terminating them instead in electrodes, which communicate with computer-driven motors in the arm itself. Sensors feed a limited degree of sensory information back to the brain, so the user can determine both temperature and pressure.

THE FUTURE

The rampant progress of biotechnology raises profound questions about what it is to be human. This is particularly true with technology that affects the human brain, because of all organs this is the one we identify with the most closely. Some of the most common questions raised include:

QUESTION	ANSWER
What changes in the way our brains function might we see if technology advances at its present rate?	"Thought" devices enabling us to control the world by mind power alone; synthetic brain "modules" to replace failing ones; conscious mood control by direct stimulation of the relevant brain areas.
Won't these things change what it means to be human? Will they even be acceptable?	Many of them, in crude form, are with us already and proving to be quite acceptable. We have "bionic" limbs, brain pacemakers, and even a prototype replacement hippocampus (see p.161).
What are the main technical problems still to be overcome?	The main problem is to do with mapping – despite the advances of the last ten years, the complex interconnections between different brain areas are still largely unknown.
Will machines ever be conscious?	There seems no reason why not. The ultimate challenge may not be technical at all, but rather the ethical implications of human consciousness being embodied in a non-human form.

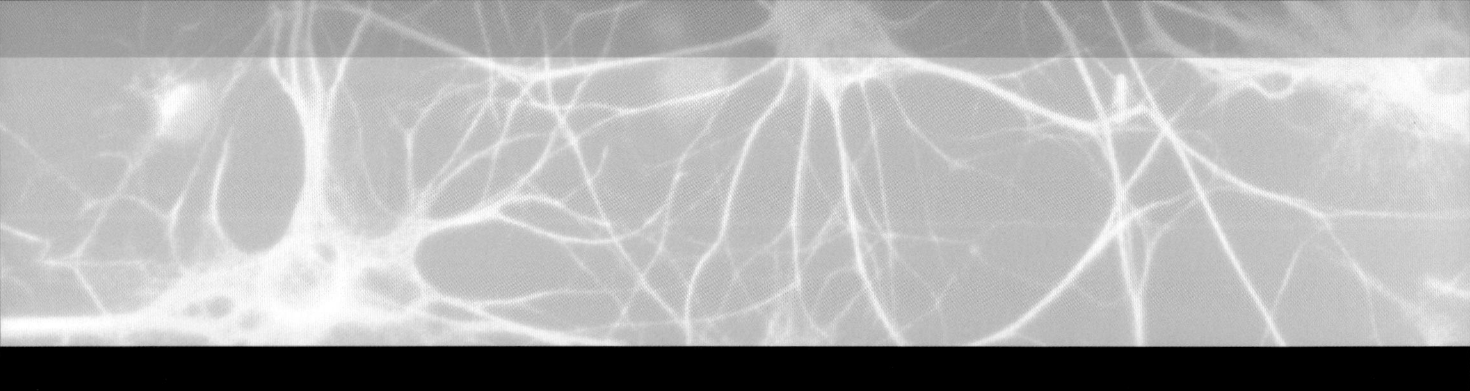

THE PERCEPTION OF BRAIN DISORDERS AND THEIR CAUSES HAS CHANGED PROFOUNDLY OVER THE COURSE OF HUMAN HISTORY. EVEN TODAY, DIFFERENT CULTURES HOLD MARKEDLY DIFFERENT VIEWS ABOUT THE DIVIDING LINE BETWEEN NORMAL AND DISORDERED STATES OF MIND. BUT, JUST AS OUR KNOWLEDGE OF HOW THE BRAIN WORKS IS CURRENTLY UNDERGOING A REVOLUTION, SO TOO IS OUR UNDERSTANDING OF WHAT CAN GO WRONG. NEVERTHELESS, THERE ARE MANY DISORDERS WITH CAUSES THAT REMAIN MYSTERIOUS.

DISEASES AND DISORDERS

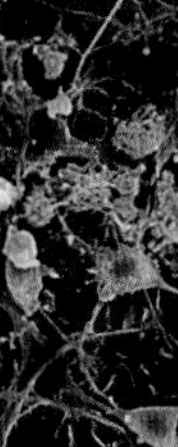

THE DISORDERED BRAIN

EVERY MENTAL STATE HAS A CORRESPONDING BRAIN STATE, CONSISTING OF A PARTICULAR PATTERN AND SEQUENCE OF NEURAL PROCESSES. UNTIL RECENTLY, MOST OF THESE PROCESSES WERE UNDETECTABLE, BUT THE ADVENT OF HIGH-TECH IMAGING HAS MADE THEM VISIBLE, WITH THE RESULT THAT MENTAL DISORDERS ARE INCREASINGLY BEING RECOGNIZED AS NEUROLOGICAL BRAIN DISORDERS.

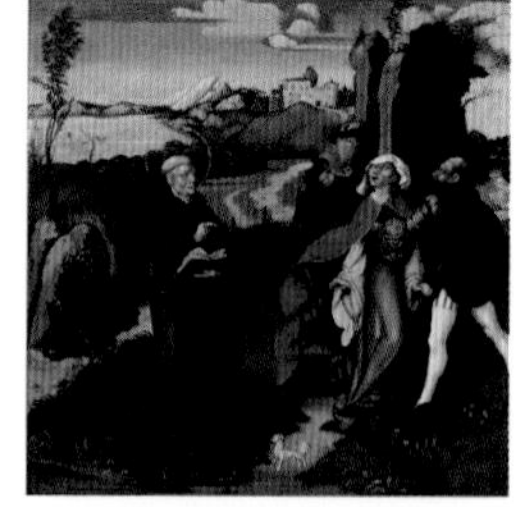

EXORCISM
Exorcism is a ritual designed to expel bad spirits from the living. It was very widespread in the Middle Ages, when demonic possession was often thought to be the cause of mental illness.

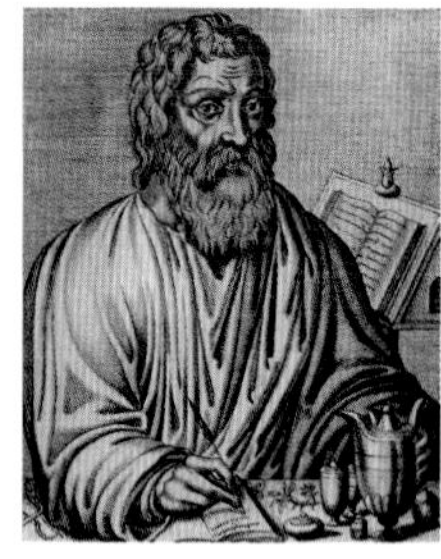

FOUR HUMOURS
Hippocrates developed the idea that illness was the result of a lack of balance among four humours – blood, phlegm, and black and yellow bile.

HISTORICAL THEORIES OF MENTAL ILLNESS

Mental illness has commonly been regarded as disease of the spirit. In the Middle Ages it was assumed that devils (foul spirits) entered people and made them depressed (poor-spirited) or insane. Physical theories of mental illness include an imbalance of the "four humours", which were thought to determine a person's general mood and health, and fluctuations or blockages of various types of "forces". The 19th-century physician Franz Mesmer, for example, thought he had discovered "animal magnetism", which could cause ill health, including madness, if it was blocked. His treatment to control the magnetic flow was, effectively, hypnotism. Sigmund Freud (see p.189) popularized the concept of the unconscious, and believed that suppressed desires caused neurosis. He developed psychoanalysis, based on the idea of bringing hidden conflicts to consciousness.

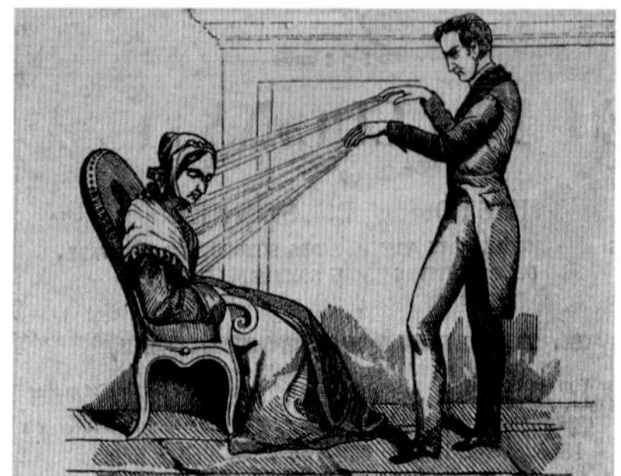

HEALING ENERGY
"Mesmerists" healed anxious minds by hypnotism, though at the time they thought they were using animal magnetism (energy flow).

WHAT IS MENTAL DISORDER?

Mental illness is generally diagnosed when a person reports that they are experiencing the world in a way that is radically different from others or when their behaviour makes it difficult for them to function in society. The shifting nature of mental illness makes diagnosis notoriously difficult. Yet standard diagnosis is important because the presence or absence of mental illness may decide whether a person is criminally responsible, suitable for particular types of employment, or eligible for state aid. Medical practice also makes diagnosis essential before treatment can be given. The most commonly consulted guide to mental disorders is the US Diagnostic and Statistical Manual (DSM) published by the American Psychiatric Association (see panel below).

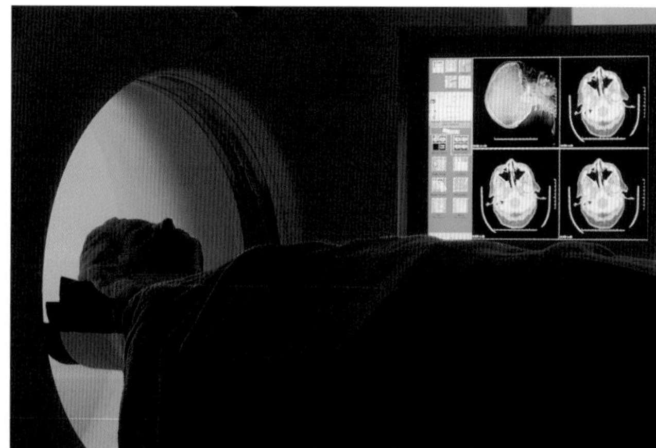

MODERN DIAGNOSTIC TOOLS
Some mental illnesses may be diagnosed by brain imaging – CT and MRI scans are good at showing up tumours and areas of damage. Functional brain imaging may be used to explore abnormal brain patterns, such as those found in epilepsy.

DIAGNOSING MENTAL DISORDERS

The first edition of the DSM was published in 1952 following research by the US military during the Second World War. The current edition, DSM-5, was published in 2013 after 14 years of research. DSM-5 includes new diagnostic and classification criteria for some conditions – for example, Asperger's is now part of the autistic spectrum rather than a condition in its own right. But controversy has arisen over whether the manual has changed sufficiently to reflect advances in brain research. Diagnosis is still based firmly on behavioural tests not brain imaging or biological markers. The failure of DSM-5 to take a neuroscientific approach to mental illness has led the largest US centre for psychiatric research, the National Institute of Mental Health, to reject the manual.

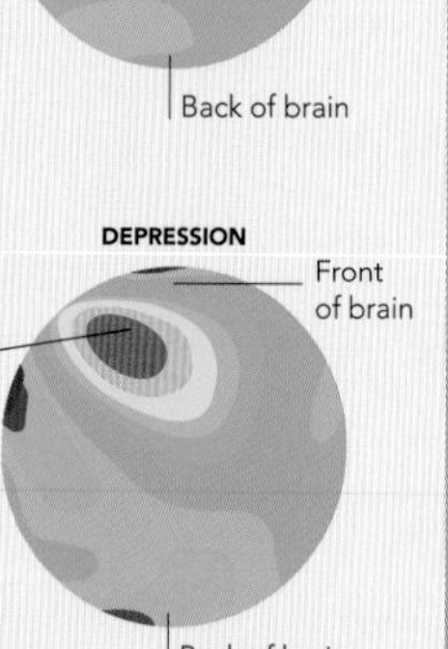

IMAGING DEPRESSION
Brain imaging can help diagnose disorders such as anxiety and depression. One method is to use EEGs to reveal abnormal electrical activity. The map below right, for example, shows an area of orange, which represents an excess amount of slow brainwave activity. This pattern is associated with depression.

PHYSICAL DISORDERS

All mental illness is physiological in that the behaviour and experience associated with it is created by a pattern of neuronal activity, but only conditions that are clearly linked to damage are considered to be physical.

DEVELOPMENTAL Growing brains are very sensitive to environmental assault, such as oxygen deprivation. A problem before or during birth may cause permanent damage.

TRAUMATIC Brain trauma may arise from external events such as accidents that cause head injuries, and also from "cerebral" accidents, such as strokes and aneurysms.

DEGENERATIVE Brains, like all the organs, degenerate, and this can result in mental conditions such as memory loss, cognitive impairment, and, in severe cases, dementia.

ROOTS OF DISORDER

Some disorders are caused by physical damage, such as a head injury, or degeneration that disrupts normal brain function. Others are caused by "faulty" genes, or developmental problems – things that go wrong during gestation or infancy. In many cases, the root causes of mental illness cannot be traced and simply manifest as "functional" problems. Functional disorders may be marked by abnormalities in brain function, but it is often unclear if these are the cause or effect of the condition.

MANY CAUSES

Most mental illness is due to a combination of causes, as shown in this Venn diagram. The placements of the conditions are open to revision because in very few cases is the precise contribution of any one factor certain. As more is learned about the brain, the apparent causes may change.

DEGENERATION

- ALZHEIMER'S DISEASE
- PARKINSON'S DISEASE
- MOTOR NEURONE DISEASE

INJURY, TRAUMA, INFECTION

- EPILEPSY
- MENINGITIS
- ENCEPHALITIS
- HAEMORRHAGE
- HYDROCEPHALUS
- CREUTZFELD–JACOB DISEASE
- ABSCESS
- COMA
- PARALYSIS
- CEREBRAL PALSY

DEVELOPMENTAL/ GENETIC

- NARCOLEPSY
- DOWN'S SYNDROME
- HUNTINGTON'S DISEASE
- NEURAL-TUBE DEFECTS

FUNCTIONAL

- ATTENTION-DEFICIT HYPERACTIVITY DISORDER
- MUNCHAUSEN'S SYNDROME
- PHOBIAS
- CONDUCT DISORDER
- BODY DYSMORPHIC DISORDER
- HYPOCHONDRIA

- MULTI-INFARCT DEMENTIA
- STROKE
- TUMOURS
- MULTIPLE SCLEROSIS
- DELUSIONAL DISORDERS
- DEPRESSION
- AUTISTIC SPECTRUM
- DEVELOPMENTAL DELAY
- ADDICTIONS
- CHRONIC FATIGUE SYNDROME
- BIPOLAR DISORDER
- POST-TRAUMATIC STRESS DISORDER
- TOURETTE'S SYNDROME
- PERSONALITY DISORDERS
- ANXIETY DISORDERS
- EATING DISORDERS
- SEASONAL AFFECTIVE DISORDER
- OBSESSIVE–COMPULSIVE DISORDER
- SCHIZOPHRENIA
- SOMATIZATION DISORDER

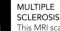

MULTIPLE SCLEROSIS
This MRI scan shows a demyelinated lesion (pink) in a person with MS (see p.235) It is the result of degeneration, which in turn may be due to genetic vulnerability or injury.

CONSTELLATIONS AND SPECTRUMS

Many disorders that have conventionally been seen as discrete conditions are now being recognized as related. People with autism, for example, have a core problem with understanding other people's mental processes. Around this core lies a constellation of symptoms grouped into three overlapping "suites" of behaviour. These suites are conventionally seen as different types of problem, but their common relationship to the core deficit suggests that they share a genetic underpinning. Psychosis has a core that is characterized by over-interpretation of other minds. It too can be seen as the core of symptoms from overlapping suites.

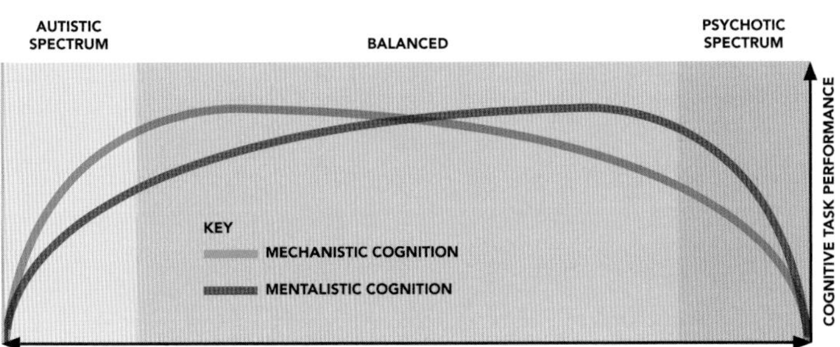

OPPOSITE PROBLEMS?

Although they appear entirely different, autistic constellation disorders and psychotic spectrum conditions may actually be related. The two clusters of symptoms may be envisaged as existing on a single spectrum (above) with normal behaviour in the middle.

BIPOLAR DEPRESSION
UNIPOLAR DEPRESSION
SCHIZOPHRENIA
PSYCHOTIC SPECTRUM

Psychotic spectrum core
Hypermentalistic cognition and behaviour; overly sensitive (to the point of delusion) about other minds

RESTRICTED INTERESTS, REPETITIVE BEHAVIOUR
PROBLEMS WITH SOCIAL RECIPROCITY
LANGUAGE, COMMUNICATION DIFFICULTIES
AUTISTIC SPECTRUM

Autistic spectrum core
Hypomentalistic – problems with understanding other people's mental processes or reflecting on their own

SUITES OF BEHAVIOUR

Psychotic and autistic spectrum disorders are shown here as separate suites of behaviour, with the common symptoms forming the core of each spectrum.

HEADACHE AND MIGRAINE

Headache is a common symptom, but the mechanism underlying it is not known for certain. The brain itself has no pain-sensitive nerve receptors. In many cases, it is thought that tension in the meninges or in blood vessels or muscles of the head and/or neck stimulates pain receptors, which send impulses to the sensory cortex of the brain, resulting in a headache. However, in some types of headache, such as migraine, the pain is thought to be due to overactivity of neurons that affects the brain's sensory cortex.

TENSION HEADACHE

ALSO KNOWN AS STRESS HEADACHES, TENSION HEADACHES ARE PROBABLY THE MOST COMMON TYPE OF HEADACHE.

The pain tends to be constant, although it may throb, and it may occur in the forehead or more generally over the head. The pain may be accompanied by tightening of the neck muscles and a feeling of pressure behind the eyes and/or tightness around the head. Tension headaches are typically brought on by stress, which causes tension in the muscles of the neck and scalp. This, in turn, is thought to stimulate pain receptors in these areas, which send "pain impulses" to the sensory cortex.

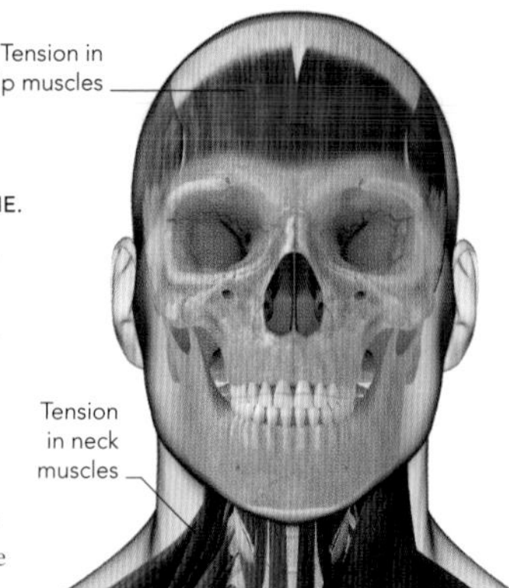

MUSCULAR TENSION
Pain receptors in the muscles of the scalp and neck are stimulated by muscular tension, leading to the pain of a tension headache.

CLUSTER HEADACHE

THESE HEADACHES OCCUR IN CLUSTERS OF RELATIVELY SHORT ATTACKS OF SEVERE, OFTEN EXCRUCIATING, PAIN.

During cluster headaches there are several attacks (typically one to four) a day, followed by an attack-free remission period. The cluster period usually lasts for a few weeks to about a couple of months. A remission period may last for months or even years, although some people experience no significant remissions. The cause of cluster headaches is not known, although there is some evidence that abnormal nerve-cell activity in the hypothalamus may be involved.

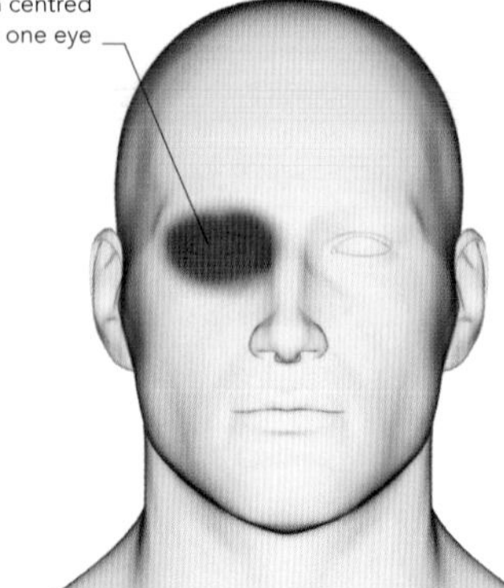

AREA OF PAIN
A cluster headache typically affects one side of the head and is centred around the eye, which may also water and become inflamed.

MIGRAINE

A MIGRAINE IS AN INTENSE, OFTEN THROBBING HEADACHE, MADE WORSE BY MOVEMENT AND OFTEN ACCOMPANIED BY SENSORY DISTURBANCES AND NAUSEA.

A migraine headache usually occurs at the front or one side of the head, although the area of pain can move during an attack.

Migraine is classified into two types: classical migraine and common migraine. In classical migraine, the headache is preceded by aura, a group of warning symptoms that includes: visual disturbances, such as flashing lights and other distortions; stiffness, tingling, or numbness; difficulty speaking; and poor co-ordination. In common migraine there is no aura. In both types there may be an early stage, known as the prodrome, with features such as difficulty concentrating, mood changes, and tiredness or excessive energy. In common migraine, the prodrome is followed by the headache; in classical migraine, it is followed by aura, which is then succeeded by the headache. The headache gets worse with movement, and it is accompanied by symptoms including nausea and/or vomiting, and increased sensitivity to sound, light, and sometimes smells. It is often followed by a postdrome stage, in which there may be tiredness, difficulty focusing, poor concentration, and persistence of increased sensitivity.

Causes and triggers

The underlying cause of migraine is not known, but recent research suggests that it may be due to a surge of neuronal activity that sweeps through parts of the brain, eventually stimulating the sensory cortex, which results in the sensation of pain. However, many external factors that trigger migraine attacks have been identified: dietary factors, such as irregular meals, specific foods, and dehydration; physical factors, such as tiredness and hormonal changes; emotional factors, such as stress or shock; and environmental conditions, including changes in the weather or a stuffy atmosphere.

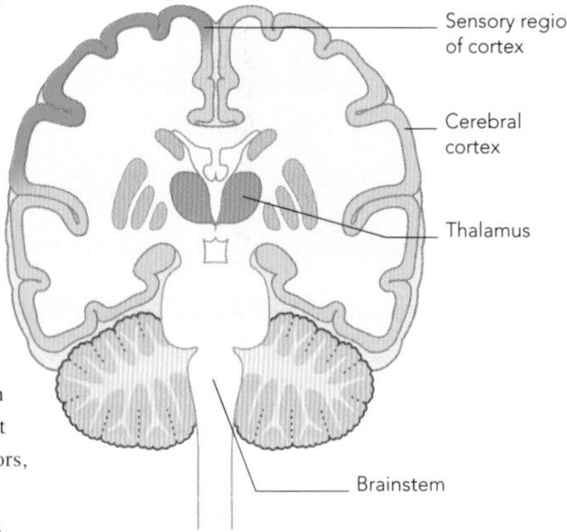

MECHANISM OF MIGRAINE
The neurological pathways that cause migraine are unknown, but may involve intense neuronal activity in the brainstem, thalamus, and sensory cortex.

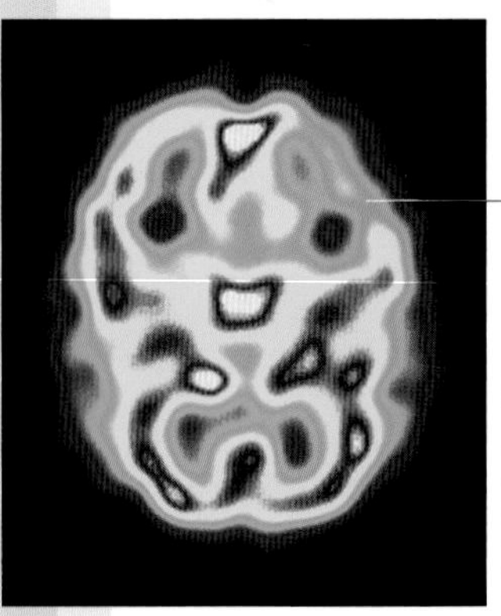

DURING AN ATTACK
This SPECT scan shows different levels of brain activity during a migraine: red and yellow indicate high activity; areas of low activity are shown in green and blue.

Aura
Typically lasts about an hour

Headache
May last for hours or days

Prodrome
May last for hours or days

Postdrome
May last for hours or days

INTENSITY

TIME

COURSE OF MIGRAINE ATTACK
A classical migraine attack typically comprises four stages, which can vary in intensity and duration. Prodrome is followed by aura, during which there are warning signs such as visual disturbances, abnormal sensations, poor co-ordination, and difficulty speaking. After the aura stage comes the headache, which is in turn followed by the postdrome stage.

CHRONIC FATIGUE SYNDROME

ALSO KNOWN AS MYALGIC ENCEPHALOMYELITIS (ME), CHRONIC FATIGUE SYNDROME IS A COMPLEX CONDITION THAT CAUSES EXTREME TIREDNESS THAT LASTS FOR A PROLONGED PERIOD OF TIME.

The cause of chronic fatigue syndrome is not known. It can develop after a viral infection or a period of emotional stress, but in many cases there is no specific preceding factor. The principle symptom is persistent, overwhelming tiredness that lasts for at least several months.

Other symptoms vary, but commonly include poor concentration, impaired short-term memory, muscle and joint pain, and feeling ill and/or extremely tired after even mild exertion. The disorder is also often associated with depression or anxiety, but it is unclear whether these are a cause or a result of the condition.

Chronic fatigue syndrome is usually diagnosed from the symptoms, although various tests and psychological assessments can be carried out to exclude other possible conditions. It is a long-term disorder, although there may be periods of remission and sometimes the disorder clears up spontaneously.

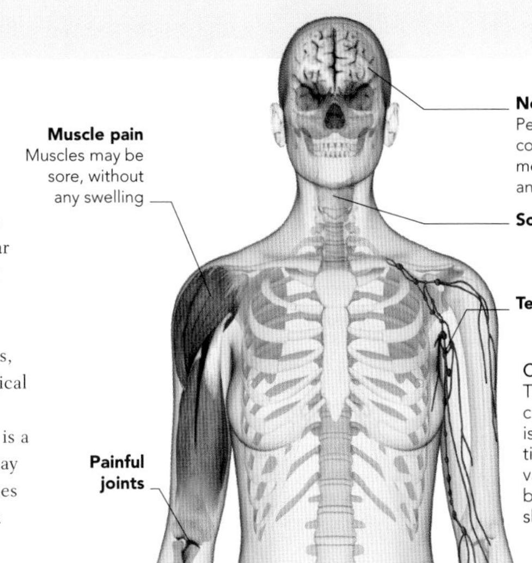

COMMON SYMPTOMS
The main indication of chronic fatigue syndrome is persistent, overwhelming tiredness. Other symptoms vary from person to person, but common symptoms are shown here.

HEAD INJURIES

HEAD INJURIES RANGE FROM MINOR BUMPS WITH NO LONG-TERM EFFECTS TO BRAIN DAMAGE THAT CAN BE FATAL.

Injuries to the head are often classified as closed, in which the skull is not broken, or open, in which the skull is fractured, leaving the brain exposed. Closed head injuries may cause indirect damage to the brain. For example, a hard blow to the head that does not fracture the skull may cause brain injury at the site of impact as the inside of the skull hits the brain. Such a trauma may also cause brain injury at the opposite side of the head (a contrecoup injury). Open head injuries are caused by a strong impact from a sharp object that fractures the skull and may penetrate the brain, for example, a stab wound.

Effects

Head injuries can rupture blood vessels, causing a brain haemorrhage (see p.229). Minor head injuries typically produce only mild, short-lived symptoms, such as a bruise on the head. In some cases, a temporary disturbance of brain function (concussion) may follow even relatively minor injuries, particularly if the injury has caused unconsciousness, and this may cause confusion, dizziness, and blurred vision, which may last for several days. Postconcussive amnesia can also occur. Repeated concussions eventually cause detectable brain damage, which may result in punchdrunk syndrome, symptoms of which may include impaired cognitive abilities, progressive dementia, parkinsonism (see p.234), tremors, and epilepsy.

Severe head injury may produce unconsciousness or coma, and usually brain damage, which in very severe cases may be fatal. In nonfatal cases, the effects of brain damage vary widely according to the severity and location of damage. The effects may include weakness, paralysis, problems with memory and/or concentration, intellectual impairment, and even personality changes. Such effects can be long-term or permanent.

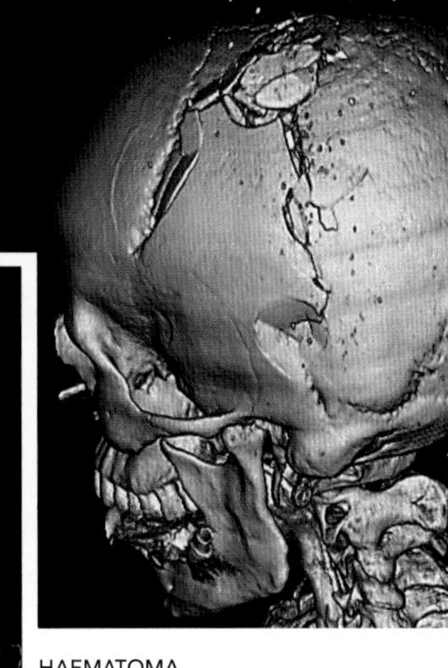

FRACTURED SKULL
This three-dimensional CT scan of the skull reveals multiple fractures, including two large depressed fractures in which the skull has been pushed inwards and fragmented. Such injuries are usually the result of a powerful blow from a blunt object and, in severe cases, may cause brain damage or even death.

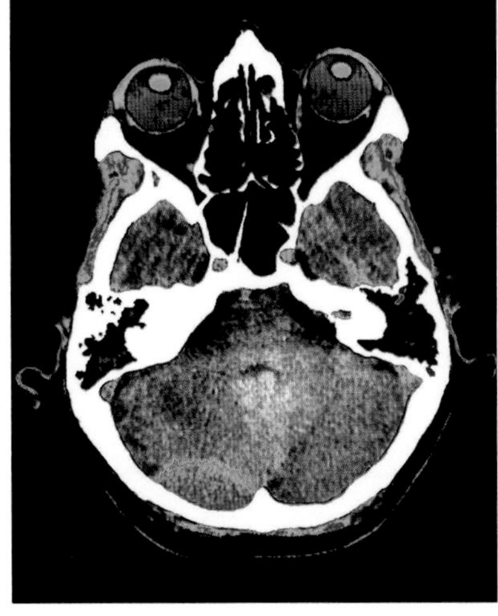

HAEMATOMA
This colour-enhanced CT scan shows a large extradural haematoma (orange) – a mass of clotted blood caused by a haemorrhage that occurred due to a head injury. Without treatment, it may press on the brain, causing brain damage or death.

MOVING PERSON

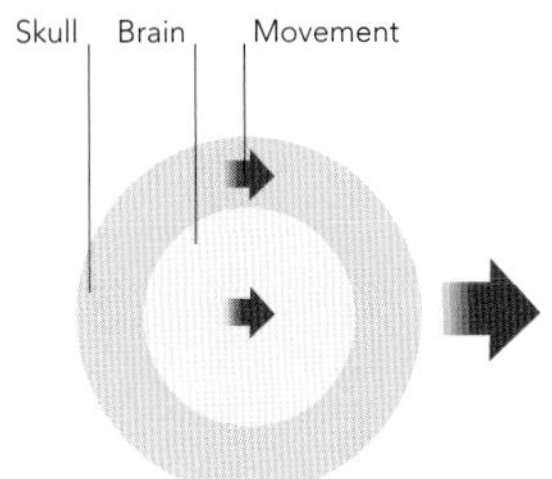

1 In a person who is moving rapidly – for example, when travelling in a car – the skull and brain enclosed within it are moving at the same speed.

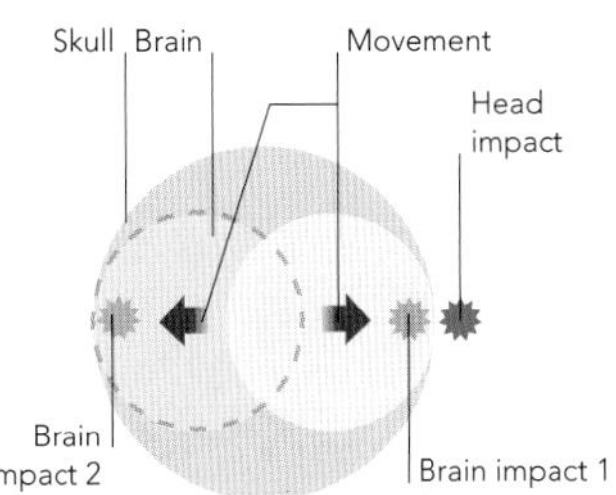

2 If movement is suddenly stopped due to an impact, the brain hits the front of the skull, and a coutrecoup injury occurs when it rebounds and hits the back of the skull.

STATIONARY PERSON

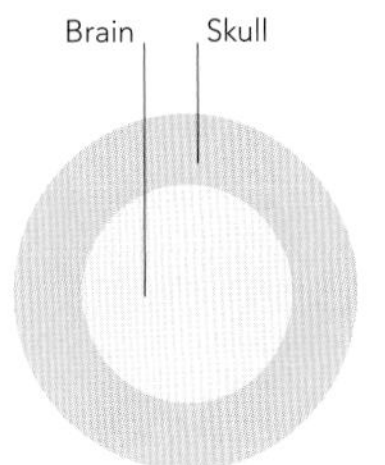

1 In the situation where a person is stationary, both the skull and the brain within it are motionless.

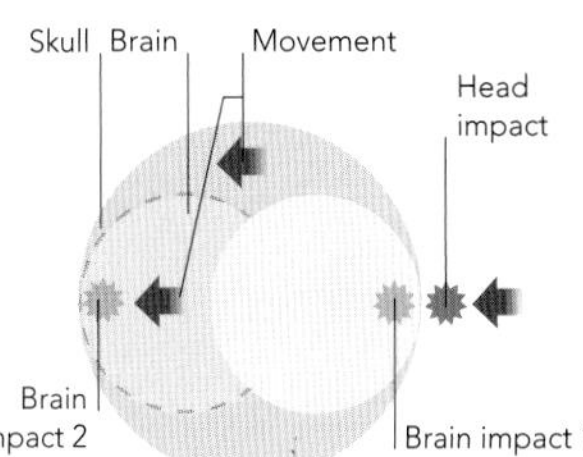

2 If the head is struck suddenly, the front of the skull is pushed against the brain, and the brain then rebounds and hits the back of the skull, causing a coutrecoup injury.

EPILEPSY

EPILEPSY IS A BRAIN FUNCTION DISORDER IN WHICH THERE ARE RECURRENT SEIZURES OR PERIODS OF ALTERED CONSCIOUSNESS.

Normally, neuronal activity in the brain occurs in a regulated way. However, during an epileptic seizure, neurons start firing in an abnormal way, disrupting normal brain function. Although seizures are a defining feature of epilepsy, they can occur without epilepsy being the cause.

The mechanism underlying epileptic seizures is not known for certain, but it is thought to involve a chemical imbalance in the brain. Normally, the neurotransmitter gamma-aminobutyric acid (GABA) helps regulate brain activity by inhibiting neurons in the brain. When the level of GABA falls too low – which itself may be due to abnormal amounts of enzymes that regulate GABA levels – neurons are not inhibited and they send a flood of impulses through the brain, resulting in a seizure. Epilepsy can have a number of causes, although often the cause is unclear. A genetic factor may be involved in some cases. Other causes include head injury; birth trauma; an infection such as meningitis or encephalitis; a stroke; a brain tumour; and abuse of drugs or alcohol.

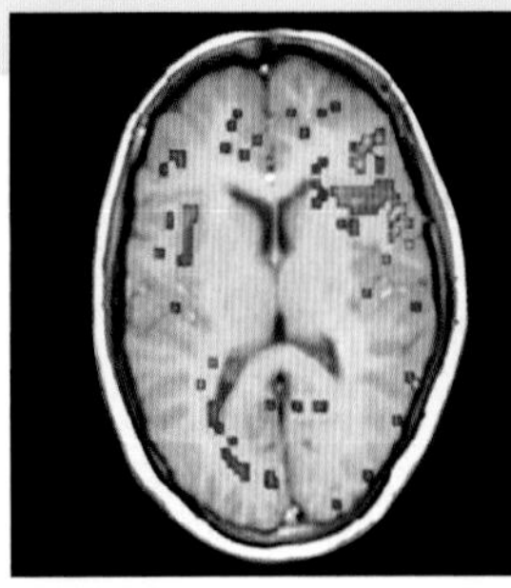

SEIZURE This colour-enhanced brain scan of a person with epilepsy reveals that the focus of seizure activity is in the right frontal lobe, as shown by the large orange cluster at the top right of the image.

Many people find that specific factors can trigger a seizure. These triggers include stress; lack of sleep; fever; flashing lights; and drugs such as cocaine, amphetamines, Ecstasy, and opiates. Some women who suffer from epilepsy are more likely to have a seizure before the start of a menstrual period.

Broadly, epileptic seizures fall into two main types: generalized seizures and partial seizures (see table below). Seizures often start in one area of the brain, which might contain scar tissue or some structural abnormality, and then spread throughout the rest of the brain.

Some people experience warning signs (called an aura) before an epileptic seizure. Warning signs may include a strange smell or taste; a feeling of foreboding; déjà vu; and a sense of unreality. In most cases, seizures stop by themselves. Sometimes a seizure can persist or seizures follow on from each other without the person recovering in between. This is known as status epilepticus and is a medical emergency.

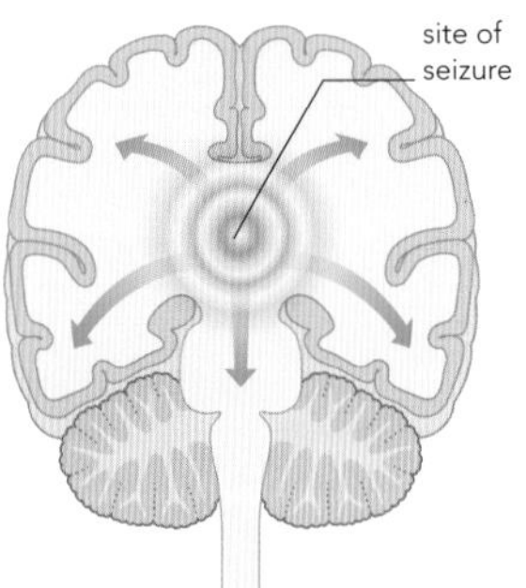

PARTIAL EPILEPTIC SEIZURES
In a partial seizure, the seizure starts in and affects only part of the brain (above left). Sometimes, a seizure may start as a partial seizure and then become generalized and spread (above right).

GENERALIZED EPILEPTIC SEIZURE
In generalized seizures, most or all of the brain is affected by abnormal neuron activity.

STATUS EPILEPTICUS

Status epilepticus is the term used to refer to a potentially life-threatening condition in which there is a prolonged epileptic seizure or a series of repeated seizures that occur one after the other without recovery of consciousness between attacks. Precise definitions of status epilepticus vary, but generally it is defined as a single seizure that lasts for longer than 30 minutes, or a series of repeated seizures that lasts for longer than this time. In people who are known epileptics, the most common cause of status epilepticus is failure to take anti-epileptic medication. In other cases, the causes include a brain tumour, brain abscess, brain injury, cerebrovascular disease (such as a stroke), metabolic disorders, and drug abuse. Status epilepticus is a serious condition that may result in long-term disability or even death without prompt treatment with intravenous medications to control the seizures.

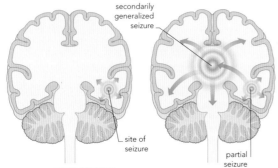

TYPES OF SEIZURES

Epileptic seizures can be categorized into two broad types, partial seizures and generalized seizures, depending on how much of the brain is affected by the abnormal neuron activity.

Partial seizures
In these types of seizures, abnormal neuron activity is restricted to a relatively small region of the brain. There are two main subtypes: simple partial seizures and complex partial seizures.

Simple partial seizures During these seizures there may be twitching on one side of the body; numbness or tingling; stiffness of the muscles in the arms, legs, and face; hallucinations of vision, taste, or smell; and sudden intense emotions. The person remains conscious throughout.

Complex partial seizures In these seizures the person is confused and unresponsive; may make peculiar, repetitive, apparently purposeless movements; and may scream or cry out, although there is no pain. The person remains conscious but usually has no memory of the seizure.

Generalized seizures
In these types of seizures, abnormal neuron activity affects most or all of the brain. There are six main subtypes, described below.

Tonic seizures In these seizures the muscles suddenly become stiff, which often causes the person to lose balance and fall over, usually backwards. Tonic seizures tend to happen without warning, are usually short-lived, and the person recovers quickly.

Clonic seizures These seizures are very similar to myoclonic ones, causing jerking or twitching of the limbs or body, although they last longer, typically up to about two minutes. In addition, a person suffering a clonic seizure may lose consciousness.

Myoclonic seizures These generally happen shortly after waking up. During such seizures the arms, legs, or body twitch or jerk. A seizure usually lasts only a fraction of a second, but sometimes several seizures may occur in quick succession. Myoclonic seizures may occur on their own, but usually happen in association with other types, such as tonic–clonic seizures.

Atonic seizures These seizures are also sometimes called drop attacks. During the seizures the muscles suddenly relax and the person becomes floppy, which often causes them to lose balance and fall over, usually forwards. Like tonic seizures, atonic seizures happen without warning, are short-lived, and the person recovers quickly after the seizure.

Tonic–clonic seizures Also sometimes known as grand mal, this type of seizure first causes the body to become rigid, this is followed by uncontrollable jerking or twitching. The person becomes unconscious and often loses bladder control. Typically, the seizure ends spontaneously after a few minutes, and afterwards the person may be drowsy and confused.

Absence seizures Sometimes also known as petit mal, this type of epileptic seizure mainly affects children. During an absence seizure, the person loses awareness of his or her surroundings and appears to be staring vacantly into space. A seizure typically lasts for less than about 30 seconds, and in some cases seizures occur several times a day.

MENINGITIS

MENINGITIS IS INFLAMMATION OF THE MENINGES, THE MEMBRANES COVERING THE BRAIN AND SPINAL CORD, OFTEN AS A RESULT OF A VIRAL OR BACTERIAL INFECTION.

Typically, the infection reaches the meninges through the bloodstream from elsewhere in the body, although it may occasionally result from direct infection of the meninges after an open head injury. It may occur as a complication of various other diseases, including Lyme disease, encephalitis, tuberculosis, and leptospirosis. Viral meningitis may be caused by viruses such as herpes simplex or chickenpox virus. It tends to be relatively mild and causes symptoms similar to those of flu. Rarely, it may cause serious symptoms, such as weakness or paralysis, speech problems, visual impairment, seizures, and coma.

Bacterial meningitis is less common than the viral form, but is more serious and can be fatal. It may be caused by various bacteria, though is usually due to infection with meningococcal or pneumococcal bacteria. Symptoms may develop rapidly, over only a few hours, and include fever, stiff neck, severe headache, nausea, vomiting, abnormal sensitivity to light, confusion, and drowsiness, and sometimes seizures and loss of consciousness. In meningococcal meningitis, the bacteria may multiply in the blood, leading to a reddish-purple rash that does not fade when pressed. If left untreated, bacterial meningitis can enter the cerebrospinal fluid, triggering an immune response that causes increased intracranial pressure, which in turn can cause brain damage.

MENINGITIS BACTERIA
The five bacterial cells in the micrograph (right) are *Neisseria meningitidis* (also known as meningococcus), which is one of the most common causes of bacterial meningitis.

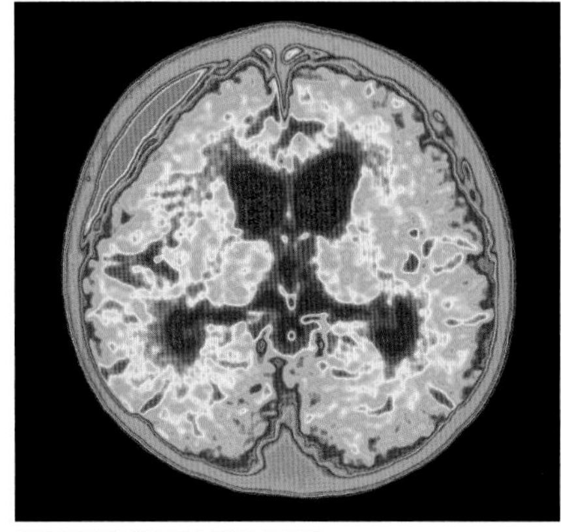

ABSCESS DUE TO MENINGITIS
This colour-enhanced MRI scan of a baby's brain shows a large abscess (pale orange at the upper left of the image) between the dura mater and arachnoid that has formed as a result of infection of the meninges.

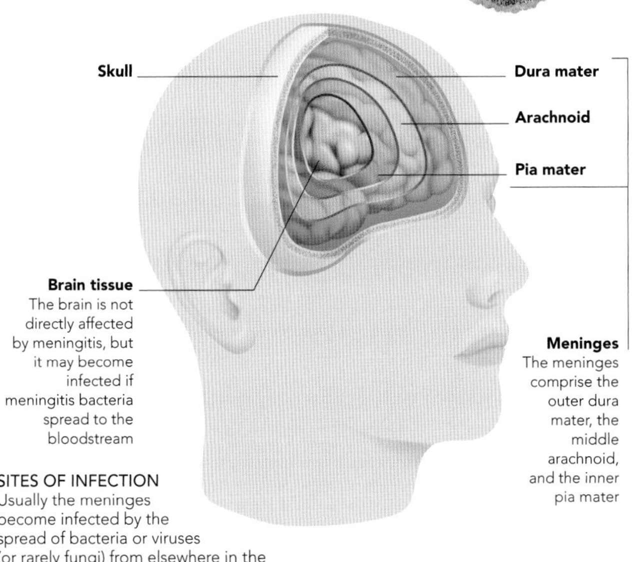
Skull
Dura mater
Arachnoid
Pia mater
Brain tissue
The brain is not directly affected by meningitis, but it may become infected if meningitis bacteria spread to the bloodstream
Meninges
The meninges comprise the outer dura mater, the middle arachnoid, and the inner pia mater

SITES OF INFECTION
Usually the meninges become infected by the spread of bacteria or viruses (or rarely fungi) from elsewhere in the body. In some cases, infective bacteria may cause septicaemia, which may affect the brain and other organs and may be fatal.

LUMBAR PUNCTURE

A lumbar puncture is a procedure in which a hollow needle is inserted into the subarachnoid space in the lower back to obtain a sample of cerebrospinal fluid or sometimes to inject drugs or other substances, such as dyes for specialized scans. The extracted fluid is examined to look for evidence of meningitis or other nervous system disorders, such as multiple sclerosis. The procedure is carried out under local anaesthesia and takes about 15 minutes. There are usually no after-effects except occasionally a headache.

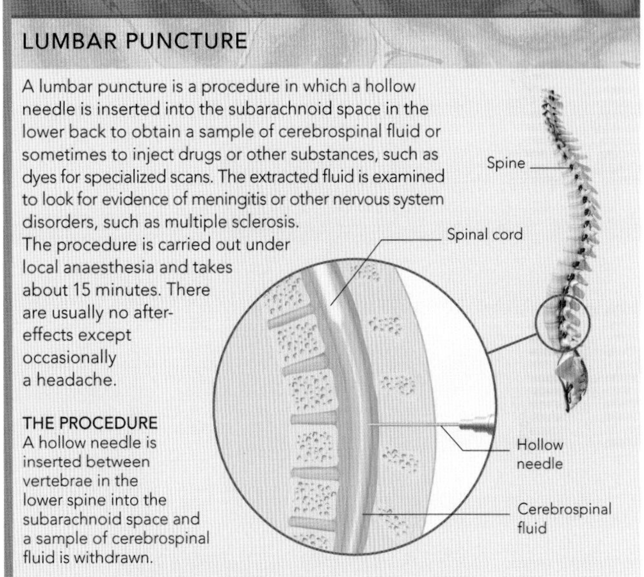
Spine
Spinal cord
Hollow needle
Cerebrospinal fluid

THE PROCEDURE
A hollow needle is inserted between vertebrae in the lower spine into the subarachnoid space and a sample of cerebrospinal fluid is withdrawn.

ENCEPHALITIS

ENCEPHALITIS IS INFLAMMATION OF THE BRAIN. IT IS USUALLY DUE TO INFECTION BY A VIRUS OR MAY OCCUR AS A RESULT OF AN AUTOIMMUNE REACTION.

A rare condition, encephalitis varies in severity from a mild, barely noticeable illness to one that can be life-threatening.

Only certain viruses are able to gain access to the central nervous system and affect nerves, and therefore potentially cause encephalitis. These viruses include the herpes simplex virus (which also causes cold sores), chickenpox virus, and measles virus. Occasionally, the infection may also affect the meninges, causing meningitis. In most cases, the immune system deals with the viral infection before it can affect the brain. However, if the immune system is compromised, there is a greater risk of developing encephalitis. When encephalitis develops, the infection causes swelling, and parts of the brain may be damaged when it compresses against the skull. Rarely, encephalitis is due to an autoimmune reaction, in which the immune system attacks the brain, leading to inflammation and brain damage.

Mild encephalitis usually causes only a slight fever and headache. In more severe cases, there may also be nausea and vomiting; weakness, loss of co-ordination, or paralysis; abnormal sensitivity to light; loss or impairment of speech; memory loss; uncharacteristic behaviour; stiff neck and back; drowsiness; confusion; seizures; and coma. In very severe cases, encephalitis can cause permanent brain damage and may even be fatal.

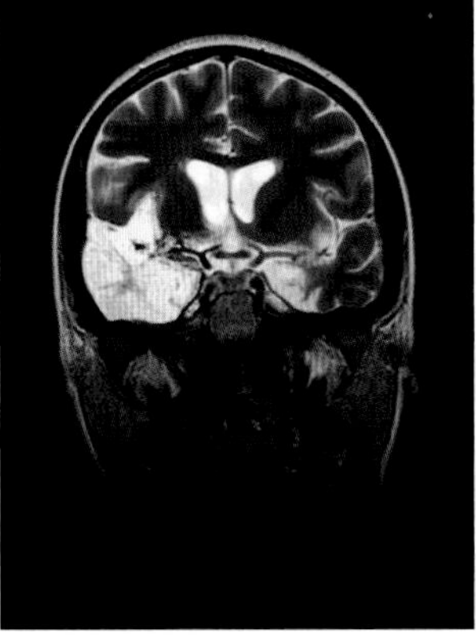

VIRAL ENCEPHALITIS
This colour-enhanced MRI scan of a brain reveals a large area of abnormal tissue in the temporal lobe (the pale orange area) that is due to infection with the herpes simplex virus, one of the most common causes of viral encephalitis.

BRAIN ABSCESS

AN ABSCESS IS A COLLECTION OF PUS, SURROUNDED BY INFLAMED TISSUE. IT CAN FORM IN THE BRAIN OR ON ITS SURFACES, AND THERE MAY BE SEVERAL AT ONCE.

A brain abscess can result from a bacterial or, more rarely, a fungal or parasitic infection. Fungal and parasitic infections are usually restricted to people whose immune systems have been impaired – for example, those with HIV/AIDS, people undergoing chemotherapy, or those taking immunosuppressants.

A brain abscess can occur as a result of a penetrating head injury or an infection spreading from elsewhere in the body, such as from a dental abscess, middle-ear infection, sinusitis, or pneumonia. It can also result from injecting drugs using a non-sterile needle.

Symptoms and effects

Once an abscess has formed, the tissue around it becomes inflamed, which may cause brain swelling and increased pressure in the skull. Symptoms may develop over a few days or weeks and depend on the area of the brain affected. Common general symptoms include: headache; fever; nausea and vomiting; stiff neck; drowsiness; confusion; and seizures. A person may also experience speech difficulties, vision problems, and weakness of the limbs.

A brain abscess can be diagnosed by a scan and tests to identify the infecting organisms. Without treatment, an abscess can cause unconsciousness, and a coma (see p.238) may develop. It may also lead to permanent damage, and in some cases can be fatal. Drug treatment can eliminate the infection and reduce the swelling in the brain, but a craniotomy (a procedure to make a small opening in the skull) may be needed to drain pus from a large abscess.

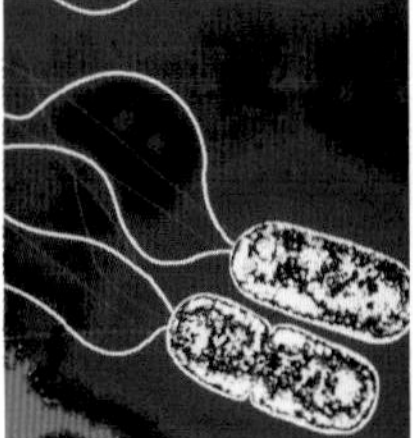

INFECTIOUS BACTERIA
A brain abscess may be caused by a wide variety of bacteria, including *Pseudomonas* (above left) and *Streptococcus* (above right), the most common cause.

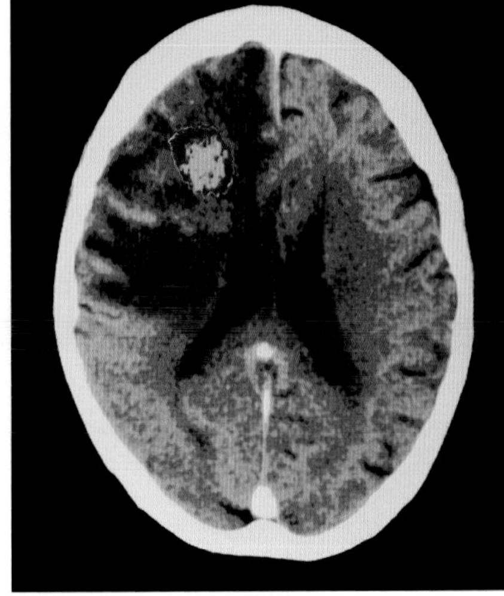

ABSCESS IN BRAIN TISSUE
This colour-enhanced CT scan shows a large abscess in the brain (orange area) of a person with AIDS. People who are immunocompromised, such as those with HIV/AIDS, are particularly vulnerable to abscesses.

TRANSIENT ISCHAEMIC ATTACK

THIS IS AN EPISODE OF TEMPORARY LOSS OF BRAIN FUNCTION DUE TO AN INTERRUPTION OF THE BLOOD SUPPLY TO PART OF THE BRAIN.

Also called a "mini-stroke", a transient ischaemic attack (TIA) is most commonly caused by a blood clot that temporarily blocks an artery supplying blood to the brain. It can also occur due to excessive narrowing of an artery as a result of atherosclerosis (build-up of fatty deposits on the artery wall). There are numerous risk factors that contribute to the likelihood of a TIA, such as diabetes mellitus, previous heart attacks, high blood-fat levels, high blood pressure, and smoking.

Symptoms usually develop suddenly and vary according to the part of the brain affected by the restricted blood flow, but they include visual disturbances or loss of vision in one eye, problems speaking or understanding speech, confusion, numbness, weakness or paralysis on one side of the body, loss of co-ordination, dizziness, and possibly brief unconsciousness. If symptoms last for more than 24 hours, the attack is classed as a stroke. Having had a TIA indicates increased risk of stroke.

Treatment for TIA is aimed at preventing a stroke and includes endarterectomy (a procedure to remove the lining of an artery affected by atherosclerosis), anticoagulant drugs, or aspirin. It is also important to treat any risk factors, and stopping smoking is essential.

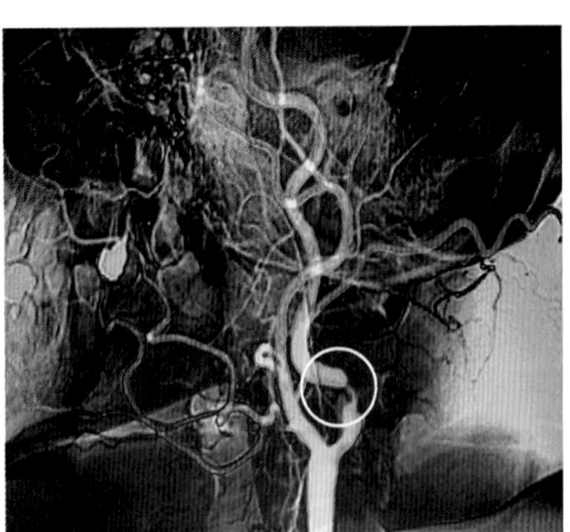

NARROWED CAROTID ARTERY
This X-ray shows an area of narrowing (circled) in the carotid artery in the neck. If an embolus temporarily lodges here, it may cause a TIA.

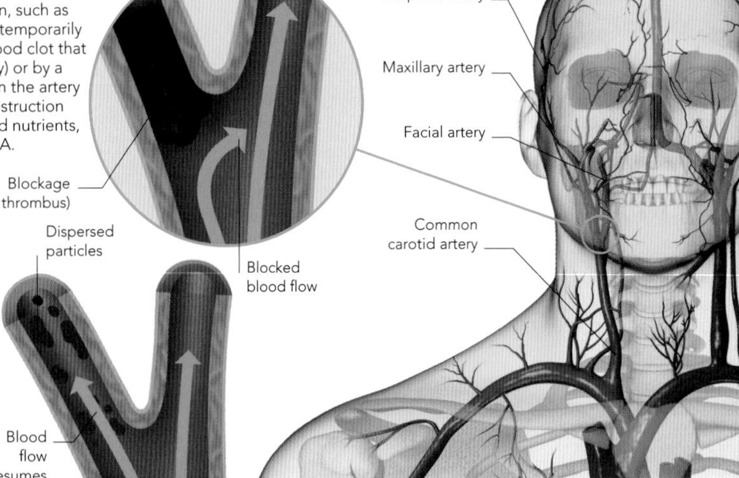

1 TEMPORARY BLOCKAGE
An artery supplying the brain, such as the carotid artery, may become temporarily obstructed by an embolus (a blood clot that originates elsewhere in the body) or by a thrombus (a clot that develops in the artery itself). The temporary arterial obstruction deprives the brain of oxygen and nutrients, producing the symptoms of a TIA.
Blockage (embolus or thrombus)
Blocked blood flow
2 DISPERSAL OF BLOCKAGE
As blood flow breaks up the obstruction, blood supply to the brain resumes and the symptoms disappear as oxygen and nutrients once again reach the brain. Transient ischaemic attacks tend to recur, and the occurrence of one or more attacks indicates an increased risk of a stroke.
Dispersed particles
Blood flow resumes
Temporal artery
Maxillary artery
Facial artery
Common carotid artery

BLOOD SUPPLY TO HEAD AND NECK
The common carotid artery is the main blood vessel supplying oxygenated blood to the head and neck. A temporary blockage of the carotid artery could result in a TIA.

STROKE

DAMAGE TO PARTS OF THE BRAIN CAN OCCUR WHEN BLOOD SUPPLY TO THE BRAIN IS INTERRUPTED.

Interruption of the blood supply to the brain can occur as a result of a blockage of an artery in the brain (ischaemic stroke), bleeding into the brain from a ruptured artery (haemorrhagic stroke), bleeding from a blood vessel in the brain (possibly from a ruptured aneurysm), or a subarachnoid haemorrhage (see below right). Risk factors include age, high blood pressure, atherosclerosis, smoking, diabetes mellitus, heart-valve damage, previous or recent heart attack, high blood-fat levels, certain heart-rhythm disorders, and sickle cell disease.

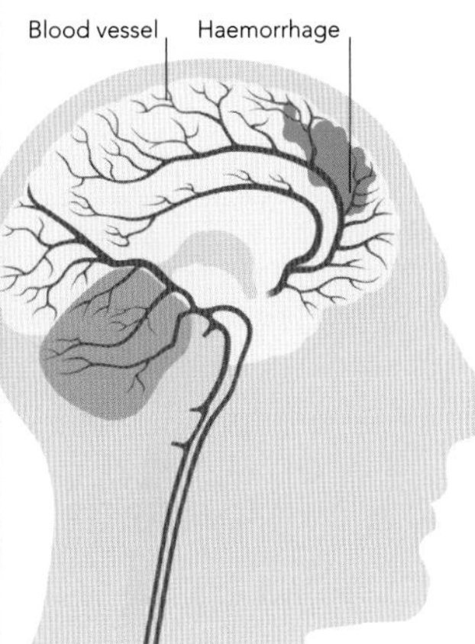
Blood vessel
Haemorrhage

Symptoms and effects

Symptoms develop suddenly and vary depending on the brain areas affected, but can include sudden headache, numbness, weakness or paralysis, visual disturbances, problems speaking or understanding speech, confusion, loss of co-ordination, and dizziness. If severe, a stroke can cause loss of consciousness, coma, and death.

Treatment depends on the cause – strokes due to a clot require drugs and haemorrhagic strokes may require surgery. Non-fatal strokes can cause long-term disability or impairment of function, for which rehabilitative therapies (such as physiotherapy and speech therapy) may be required.

HAEMORRHAGIC STROKE
A haemorrhagic stroke is caused by bleeding into the brain from a ruptured blood vessel. High blood pressure is a significant risk factor because the increased pressure makes the vessels more likely to rupture.

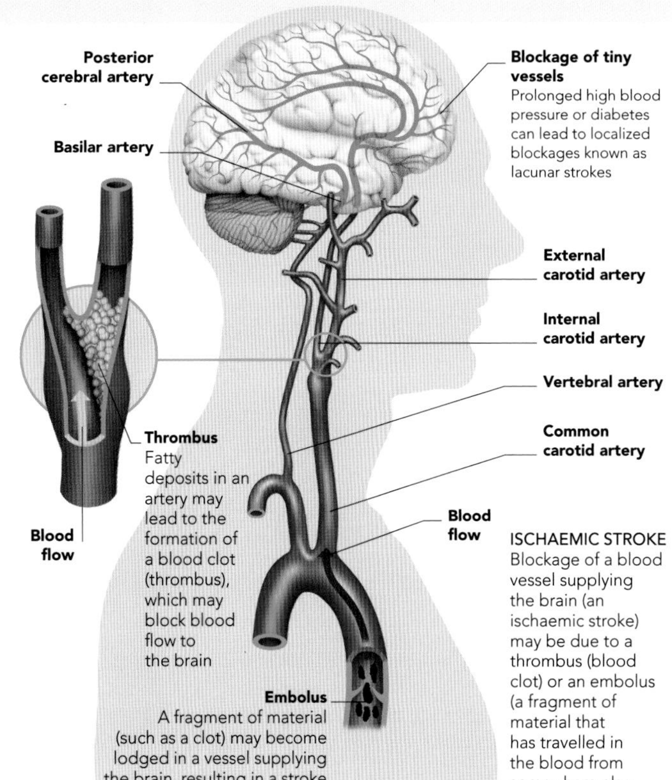
Posterior cerebral artery
Basilar artery
Blockage of tiny vessels
Prolonged high blood pressure or diabetes can lead to localized blockages known as lacunar strokes
External carotid artery
Internal carotid artery
Vertebral artery
Common carotid artery
Thrombus
Fatty deposits in an artery may lead to the formation of a blood clot (thrombus), which may block blood flow to the brain
Blood flow
Blood flow
Embolus
A fragment of material (such as a clot) may become lodged in a vessel supplying the brain, resulting in a stroke

ISCHAEMIC STROKE
Blockage of a blood vessel supplying the brain (an ischaemic stroke) may be due to a thrombus (blood clot) or an embolus (a fragment of material that has travelled in the blood from somewhere else in the body).

SUBDURAL HAEMORRHAGE

A RUPTURED BLOOD VESSEL CAN CAUSE BLEEDING BETWEEN THE TWO OUTER MENINGES THAT SURROUND THE BRAIN.

The most common cause of a subdural haemorrhage is a head injury – it can occur from minor injuries, especially in the elderly.

After the injury, bleeding may occur rapidly (within minutes) in the case of an acute subdural haemorrhage, or slowly over days or weeks for a chronic subdural haemorrhage. The trapped blood forms a clot in the skull that compresses brain tissue and causes symptoms. These are variable and may fluctuate depending on the area of the brain affected. They may include headache, one-sided paralysis, confusion, drowsiness, and seizures. In severe cases, there may be unconsciousness and coma. The long-term outcome depends on the size and location of the haemorrhage. A severe subdural haemorrhage may be fatal.

A subdural haemorrhage is usually diagnosed with a brain scan (CT or MRI). An X-ray may be taken if skull fracture is suspected. A small haemorrhage may not need treatment and can clear up on its own, but usually surgery is needed.

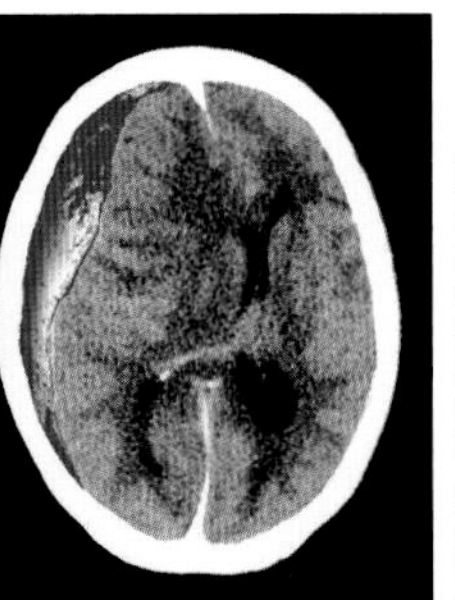

SUBDURAL HAEMATOMA
A CT scan shows a large subdural haematoma (orange), which occurs when blood from a subdural haemorrhage forms a solid mass.

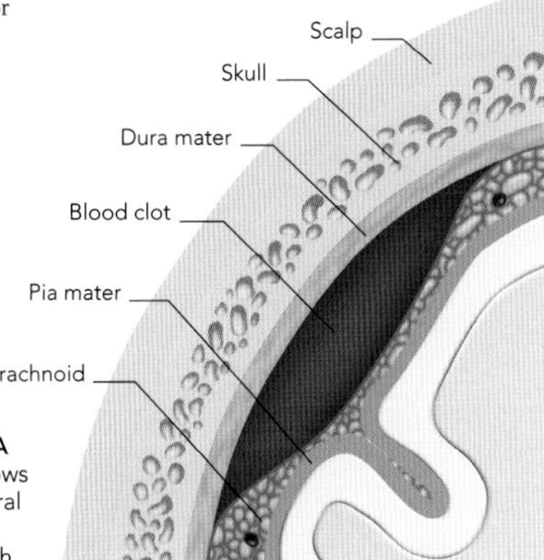
Scalp
Skull
Dura mater
Blood clot
Pia mater
Arachnoid

SITE OF SUBDURAL HAEMORRHAGE
A subdural haemorrhage is bleeding into the space between the dura mater (outermost of the three meninges) and the arachnoid (the middle meninx).

SUBARACHNOID HAEMORRHAGE

A SUBARACHNOID HAEMORRHAGE IS CAUSED BY BLEEDING INTO THE SPACE BETWEEN THE TWO INNER MEMBRANES SURROUNDING THE BRAIN.

This type of haemorrhage is most commonly caused by rupture of a berry aneurysm or, rarely, is due to the rupture of an arteriovenous malformation.

High blood pressure is a significant risk factor. Symptoms occur suddenly, without warning, and often develop rapidly (over minutes). Some people recover completely, some are left with residual disability, and some die. Arteries in the brain may constrict to reduce blood loss, which can reduce blood supply to part of the brain and cause a stroke.

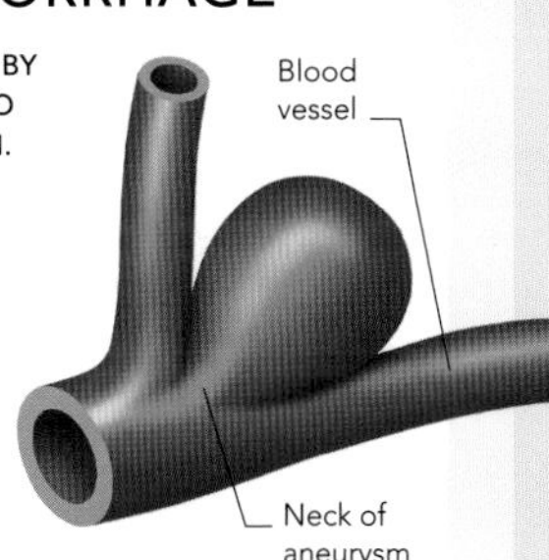
Blood vessel
Neck of aneurysm

BERRY ANEURYSM
A berry aneurysm is a swelling that develops at a weak point in a blood vessel. It is usually present from birth.

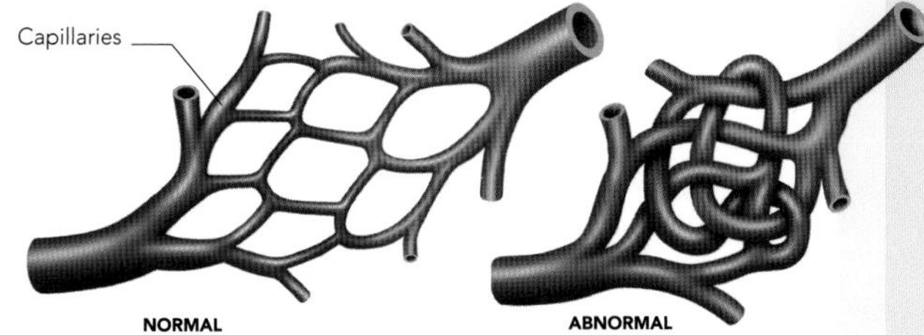
Capillaries
NORMAL
ABNORMAL

ARTERIOVENOUS MALFORMATION
An abnormal knot of blood vessels on the brain's surface that is present from birth, an arteriovenous malformation is susceptible to rupture, causing a subarachnoid haemorrhage.

BRAIN TUMOURS

BENIGN OR MALIGNANT GROWTHS CAN FORM IN THE BRAIN OR IN THE MEMBRANES AROUND THE BRAIN AND SPINAL CORD.

Primary brain tumours first develop in the brain itself and can be malignant or benign. They can arise in various types of brain cells and in any part of the brain, but primary tumours in adults are most common in the front two-thirds of the cerebral hemispheres.

Secondary tumours result from the spread of malignant cancer (metastasis) from elsewhere in the body, most commonly the lungs, skin, kidney, breast, or colon. Several secondary tumours can develop simultaneously and the cause of most tumours is not known. Rarely, some tumours may be associated with certain genetic conditions.

A tumour compresses surrounding brain tissue and raises pressure inside the skull. Symptoms therefore depend on the size and location of the tumour, but may include severe, persistent headaches, blurred vision or other sensory disturbances, speech problems, dizziness, muscle weakness, poor co-ordination, impaired mental functioning, behavioural or, personality changes, and seizures. If left untreated, a tumour may be fatal.

Brain tumours are diagnosed through brain scans and neurological tests. Treatment may involve a surgical removal (if possible), radiotherapy, and/or chemotherapy. Drugs to reduce the brain swelling may also sometimes be given.

MENINGIOMA
This micrograph shows a section through a meningioma, a type of benign tumour that develops in the meninges, the membranes that cover the brain and spinal cord.

PITUITARY TUMOURS

The pituitary gland is a pea-sized structure that hangs from the base of the brain, connected by a stalk of nerve fibres to the hypothalamus just above it. Pituitary tumours are comparatively rare and are usually benign. However, they can have a wide range of effects. A tumour may press on nearby nerves, particularly the optic nerve that passes directly above it, causing symptoms such as visual disturbances and headaches. In other cases, a tumour may cause underproduction or overproduction of hormones.

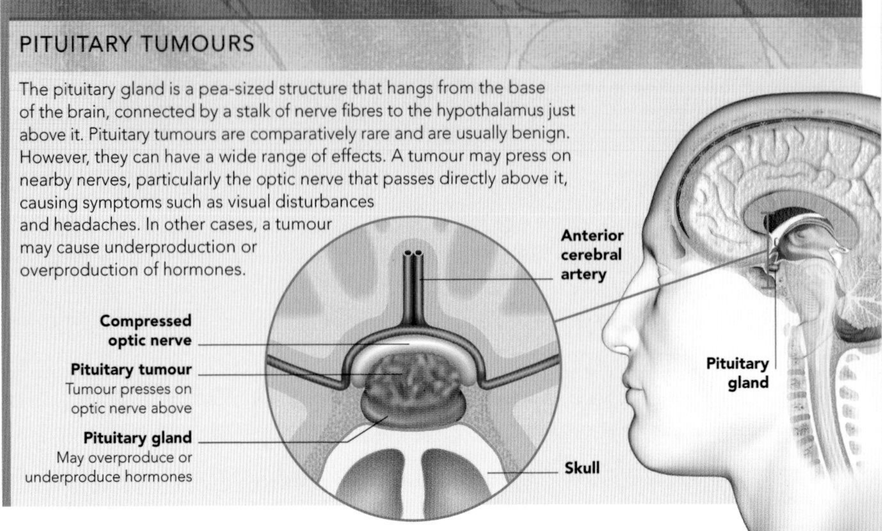

DEMENTIA

THIS DISORDER IS CHARACTERIZED BY A GENERALIZED DECLINE IN BRAIN FUNCTION, PRODUCING MEMORY PROBLEMS, CONFUSION, AND BEHAVIOURAL CHANGES.

Dementia is caused by microscopic damage to brain tissue that leads to atrophy. It can be caused by various disorders, some of which are covered on the following pages. Most commonly, it is due to Alzheimer's disease (see opposite page). Another common cause is vascular dementia, in which reduced or blocked blood supply causes death of brain cells. This can occur suddenly due to a stroke or gradually through a series of small strokes. Other causes include Lewy body dementia, in which small, round structures appear in brain cells, leading to the degeneration of affected brain tissue; and neurological deterioration associated with conditions such as AIDS, Wernicke–Korsakoff syndrome, Creutzfeldt–Jakob disease (see opposite page), Parkinson's disease (see p.234), Huntington's disease (see p.234), head injury, brain tumours (see above), and encephalitis (see p.227). It may rarely occur due to vitamin or hormone deficiency, or as a side-effect of certain medications. Rarely, dementia may be caused by inherited genetic mutations.

Symptoms and effects

Dementia is characterized by progressive memory loss, confusion, and disorientation. It can also give rise to atypical or embarrassing behaviour, personality changes, paranoia, depression, delusions, unusual irritability, and anxiety. The affected person may make up explanations to account for memory gaps or strange behaviour. As the condition progresses, a person with dementia may become indifferent towards other people and external events, and towards personal care and hygiene.

In rare cases dementia may be due to a treatable cause, such as a side-effect of medication or a vitamin deficiency, but usually there is no cure. Most forms are progressive, and a person may need total nursing care. Treatment with drugs may slow the deterioration of mental function and improve behavioural symptoms.

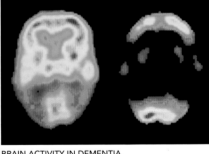

BRAIN ACTIVITY IN DEMENTIA
These two PET scans show the level of metabolic activity in a normal brain (left) and in the brain of a person with dementia (right), with yellow and red indicating areas of high activity, blue and purple areas of low activity, and black indicating minimal or no activity.

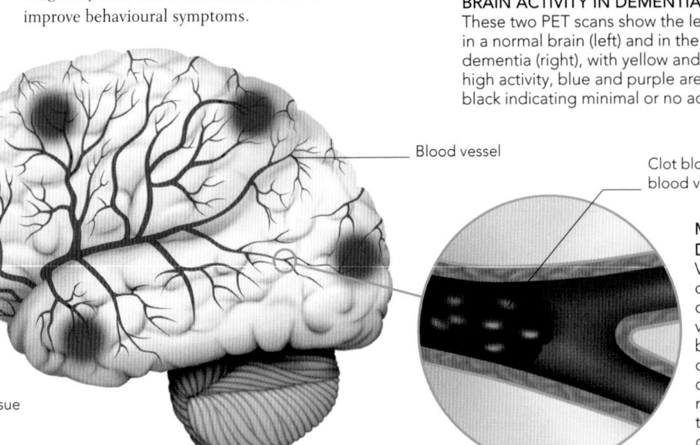

MULTI-INFARCT DEMENTIA
Vascular dementia can occur due to a series of blockages of blood vessels that supply the brain, usually due to clots. Each clot prevents oxygenated blood from reaching a small area of the brain, causing tissue death (infarct) in the affected area.

ALZHEIMER'S DISEASE

THE MOST COMMON CAUSE OF DEMENTIA, THIS IS A PROGRESSIVE DEGENERATIVE CONDITION IN WHICH PLAQUES CAUSE DAMAGE TO THE BRAIN.

Alzheimer's disease is rare before the age of 60, but increasingly common thereafter. Most cases occur without an identifiable cause. Mutations in several genes are associated with this disorder, however, and the genetic component is especially strong in the relatively rare cases of early onset disease (symptoms occurring before 60). In late-onset Alzheimer's disease, mutations in genes responsible for the production of a blood protein called apoliprotein E are implicated. These genes result in a protein (beta amyloid) being deposited in the brain as plaques, which leads to the death of neurons. Alzheimer's disease is also associated with reduced levels in the brain of the neurotransmitter acetylcholine. Additionally, it is thought that the disruption of the mechanism that controls the inflow of calcium ions into neurons may be involved, leading to excessive calcium in the neurons, which prevents them from receiving impulses from other brain neurons. Symptoms may vary from one person to another, but typically Alzheimer's progresses through three stages (see panel, left). Alzheimer's disease is usually diagnosed from the symptoms, although brain scans, blood tests, and neuropsychological tests are also carried out.

STAGES OF ALZHEIMER'S DISEASE

The symptoms and progression of Alzheimer's disease vary from person to person. However, the symptoms become increasingly severe as the disease progresses and larger areas of the brain are damaged, although in some cases there may be periods in which the person seems to improve. Generally, there are three broad stages in the development of Alzheimer's disease.

STAGE	SYMPTOMS
Stage 1	The person becomes increasingly forgetful, and these memory problems may cause anxiety and depression. However, memory deterioration is a normal feature of ageing and is not in itself evidence of Alzheimer's.
Stage 2	Severe memory loss, particularly for recent events, along with confusion about time and/or place; diminished concentration; aphasia (inability to find the right word); and anxiety, unstable moods, and personality changes.
Stage 3	In the third stage, confusion becomes very severe and there may be psychotic symptoms, such as delusions or hallucinations. There may also be abnormal reflexes and incontinence.

Treatment

Treatment for this disorder is aimed at slowing down the degeneration, but it does not completely halt decline, and eventually complete nursing care is needed. Acetylcholinesterase inhibitors may slow progress of Alzheimer's disease in the early and middle stages, and memantine in the later stages.

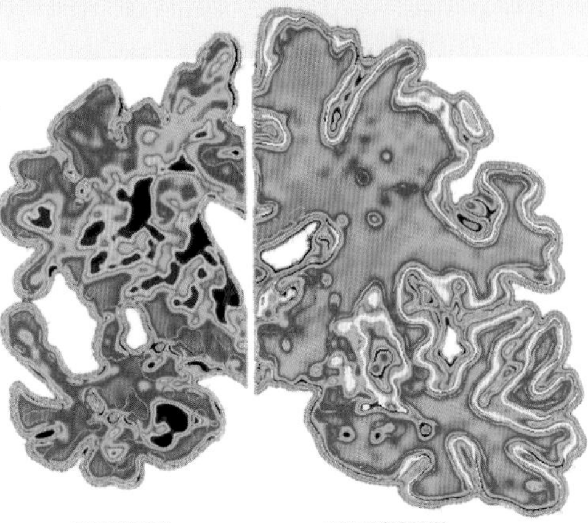

ANATOMICAL CHANGES
These two vertical sections through the brain show the loss of brain tissue and increased surface folding in Alzheimer's disease (left) compared to a healthy brain (right).

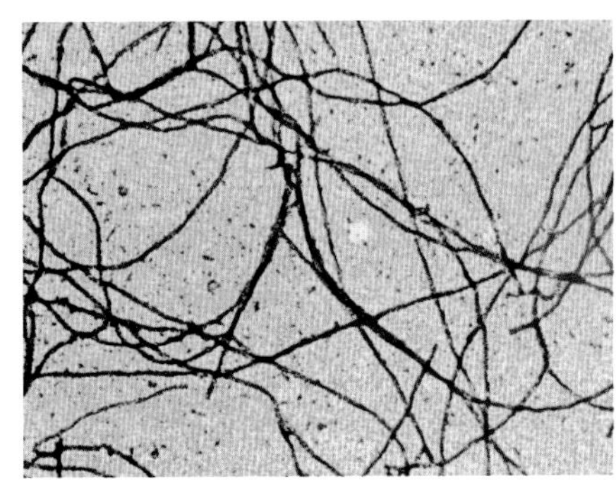

PROTEIN FILAMENTS
Alzheimer's disease is often associated with the formation of tangled masses of protein filaments (shown in purified form in this micrograph), which may develop to form plaques.

CREUTZFELDT–JAKOB DISEASE

DEMENTIA CAN BE CAUSED BY AN ABNORMAL PRION PROTEIN THAT ACCUMULATES IN THE BRAIN AND CAUSES WIDESPREAD DESTRUCTION OF BRAIN TISSUE.

Prions are proteins that occur naturally in the brain, but their function is unknown. These proteins may become abnormally distorted, forming clusters in the brain and destroying brain tissue. This tissue destruction leaves holes in the brain, giving it a sponge-like appearance, and results in various neurological dysfunctions, dementia, and finally death. There are four main types of Creutzfeldt–Jakob disease: sporadic CJD; familial CJD; iatrogenic CJD; and variant CJD, which is caused by infection with bovine spongiform encephalopathy (BSE).

Initial symptoms include memory lapses, mood changes, and apathy. These may be followed by clumsiness, confusion, unsteadiness, and speech problems. Towards the final stages there may be uncontrollable muscle spasms, stiffness of the limbs, impaired vision, incontinence, progressive dementia, seizures, and paralysis. Eventually, CJD is fatal.

VARIANT CJD AND BSE

Creutzfeldt–Jakob disease, previously an obscure illness, came to public prominence in the 1990s when a few people developed a form of the disease – known as variant CJD (vCJD) – after eating meat from cattle infected with bovine spongiform encephalopathy (BSE), commonly known as "mad cow disease". Initially it was thought that BSE was not transmissible to humans but this proved to be wrong, and stringent measures were introduced to prevent infected meat from entering the human food supply. As a result, the number of deaths in the UK from vCJD declined from a peak of 28 in 2000 to 1 in 2008.

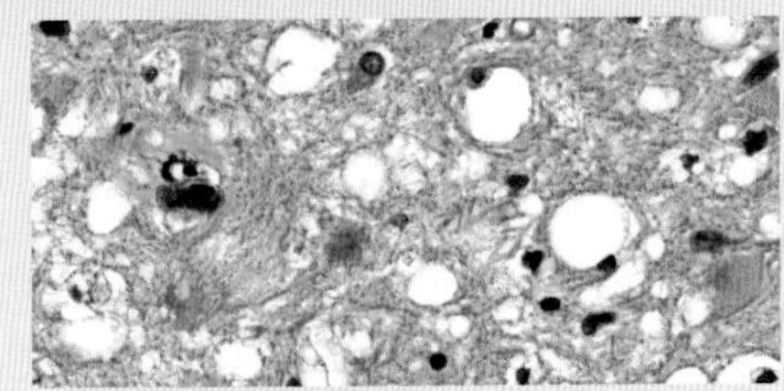

BRAIN TISSUE IN CJD
This micrograph of brain cortex tissue from a person with variant CJD shows the characteristic sponge-like appearance that is caused by the loss of neurons.

TYPES OF CJD

There are four main types of Creutzfeldt–Jakob disease (CJD). They are differentiated principally by the cause of the disease, although there are also other differences between them, such as the typical age of onset and the general length of illness.

TYPE OF CJD	CHARACTERISTICS
Sporadic CJD	Also known as classic or spontaneous CJD, this is the most common form of the disease. It mainly affects people over 50, and usually progresses rapidly (over a period of months).
Familial CJD	This is an inherited form of CJD, caused by a genetic mutation. It first appears between the ages of 20 and 60 and typically has a long course, generally between 2 and 10 years.
Iatrogenic CJD	This rare form of CJD is due to contamination with blood, tissue, or other substances from an infected person as a result of a medical procedure, such as brain surgery or certain hormone treatments.
Variant CJD (vCJD)	This type of CJD is acquired by eating meat contaminated with BSE. Typically, the disease lasts about a year before causing death. This type is rare, as there are measures to prevent infected meat from entering the food supply.

BRAIN SURGERY

SURGERY ON THE BRAIN IS A SPECIALIZED FIELD OF NEUROSURGERY IN WHICH OPERATIONS ON THE BRAIN OR MENINGES ARE CARRIED OUT THROUGH AN OPENING MADE IN THE SKULL (A CRANIOTOMY) OR, MORE RARELY, VIA THE NOSE AND NASAL CAVITY.

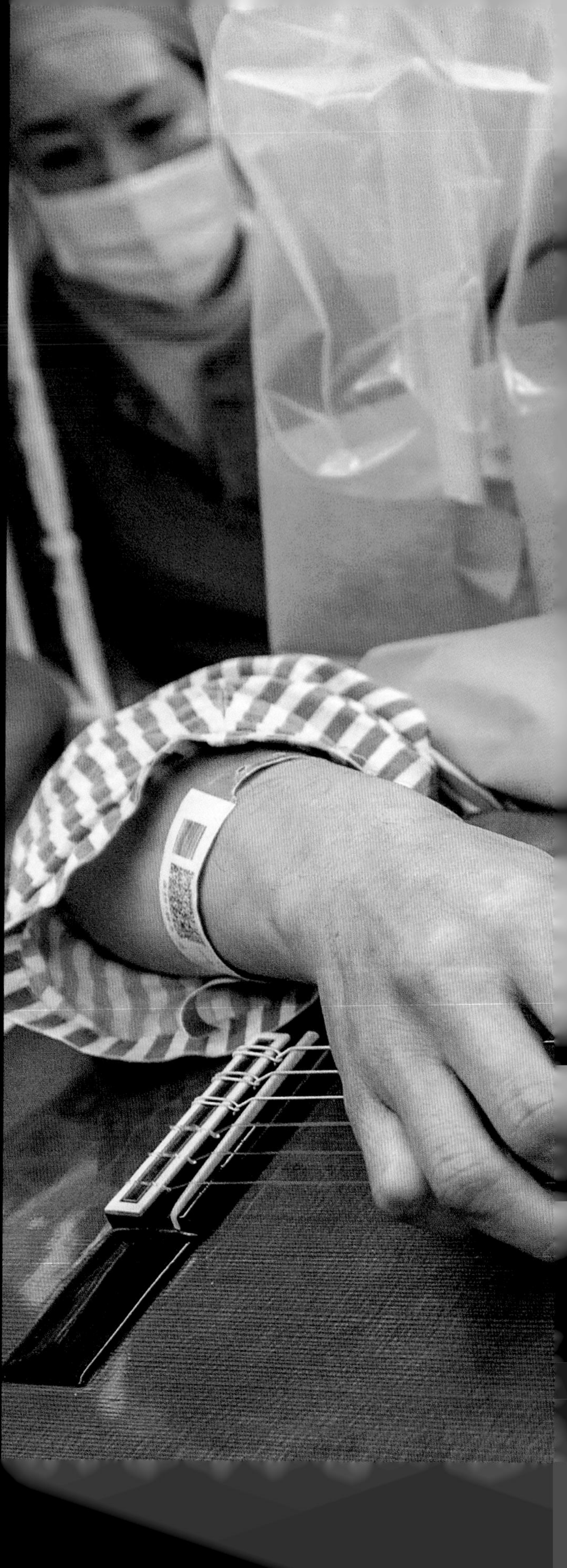

USES OF BRAIN SURGERY

Surgery may be used to treat various disorders. These include tumours of the brain or the meninges; raised pressure inside the skull due to a haemorrhage, haematoma, or hydrocephalus; traumatic brain injury, for example due to a head wound; blood vessel abnormalities, such as aneurysms; and brain abscesses. Less commonly, surgery may be used to treat severe cases of epilepsy that have not responded to medication, and to obtain biopsy samples. A highly experimental form of brain surgery known as deep brain stimulation, which involves placing electrodes inside the brain, has been used to treat a few patients with movement disorders such as Parkinson's disease (see p.234) and Tourette's syndrome (see p.243).

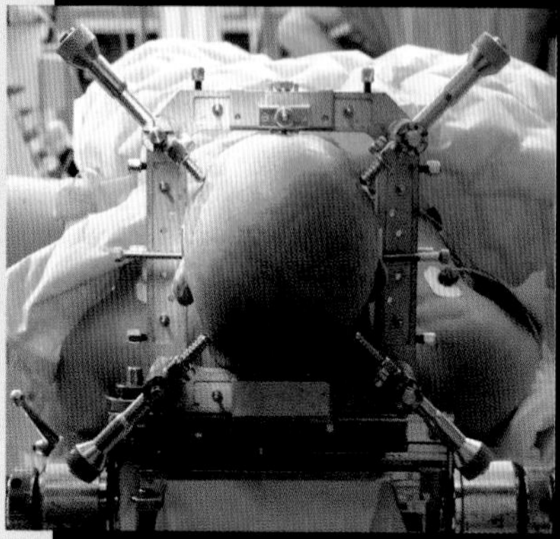

STEREOTACTIC BRAIN SURGERY
A patient about to undergo deep brain stimulation first has a frame fixed to the scalp. The frame helps the surgeon navigate to the precise site in the brain where electrodes are to be implanted.

TRANSNASAL SURGERY

A minimally invasive procedure, transnasal surgery involves inserting an endoscope (viewing tube) through the nose to reach the base of the brain. The endoscope enables the surgeon to view the operation site, and instruments can be passed along it to perform surgical procedures. The main use of this type of brain surgery is to remove tumours of the pituitary gland or of the meninges at the base of the brain. It leaves no external scar, usually requires only a short hospital stay, and tends to cause less pain afterwards than traditional surgery.

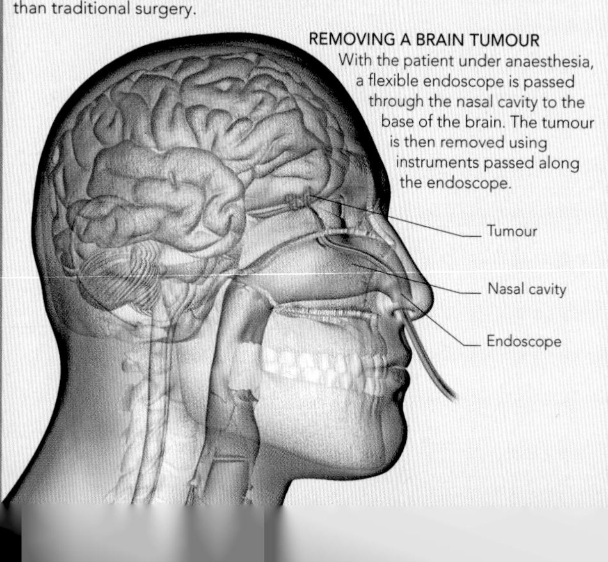

REMOVING A BRAIN TUMOUR
With the patient under anaesthesia, a flexible endoscope is passed through the nasal cavity to the base of the brain. The tumour is then removed using instruments passed along the endoscope.

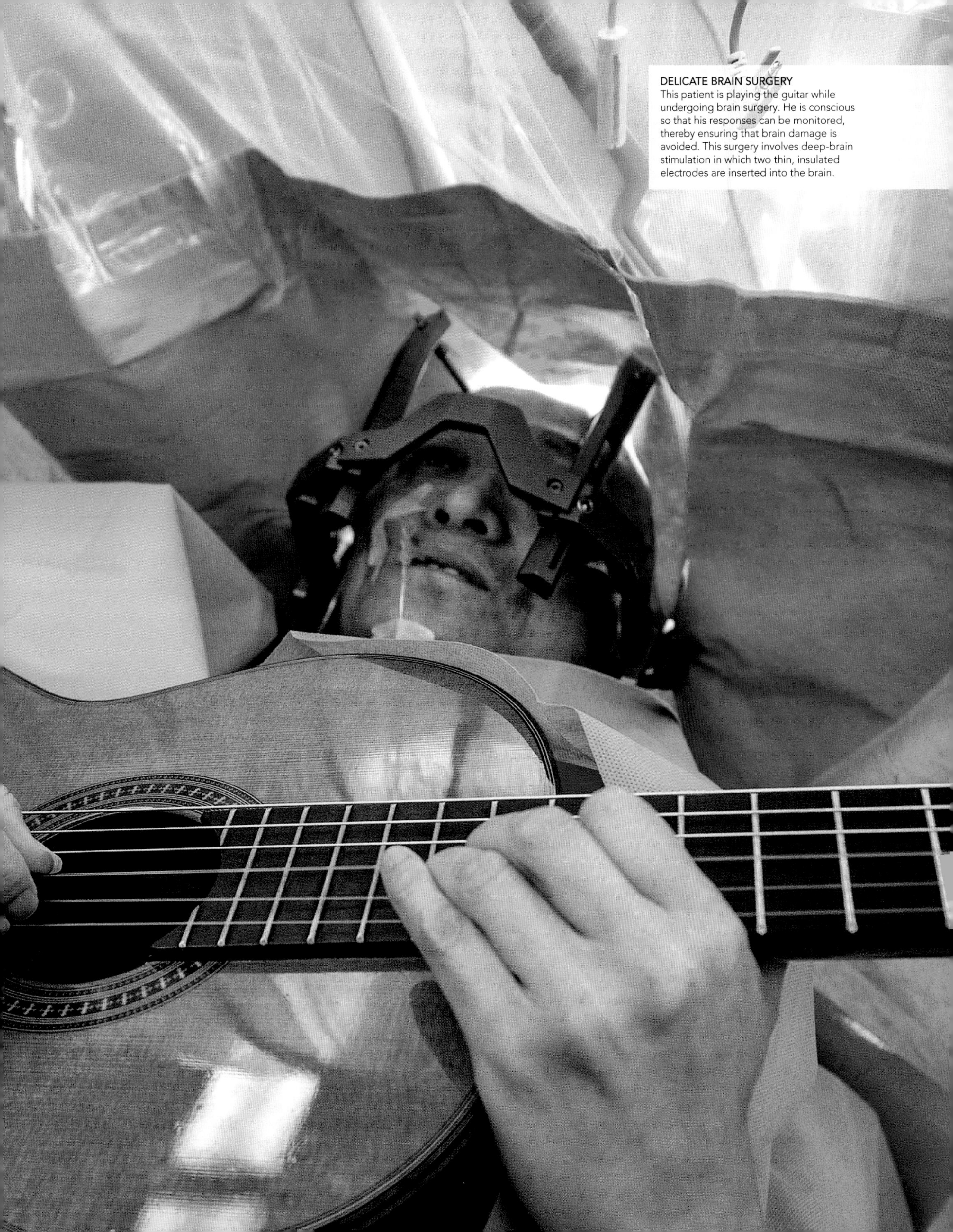

DELICATE BRAIN SURGERY
This patient is playing the guitar while undergoing brain surgery. He is conscious so that his responses can be monitored, thereby ensuring that brain damage is avoided. This surgery involves deep-brain stimulation in which two thin, insulated electrodes are inserted into the brain.

PARKINSON'S DISEASE

THIS IS A PROGRESSIVE BRAIN DISORDER THAT CAUSES TREMORS, MUSCLE RIGIDITY, PROBLEMS WITH MOVEMENT, AND DIFFICULTY KEEPING BALANCE.

Parkinson's disease is caused by degeneration of cells in the substantia nigra nuclei of the midbrain. These cells produce dopamine, a neurotransmitter that helps to control muscles and movement. Damage to the cells reduces dopamine production, leading to the characteristic motor symptoms of Parkinson's disease.

In most cases, the underlying cause is not known, although in a very few cases, specific genetic mutations have been linked to Parkinson's disease.

Symptoms usually develop gradually (over months or years), typically beginning with a tremor in a hand, arm, or leg that is worse when at rest. As the disease progresses, it becomes difficult to initiate voluntary movements; walking becomes a shuffling motion – it may be difficult to take the first step, and the normal arm swing when walking may be reduced or lost; muscles become rigid; handwriting becomes small and illegible; posture becomes stooped; and there may be loss of facial expression.

In the late stages, there may be problems speaking, swallowing may be difficult, and depression may occur. The intellect is usually unaffected, although dopamine depletion may cause symptoms of dementia.

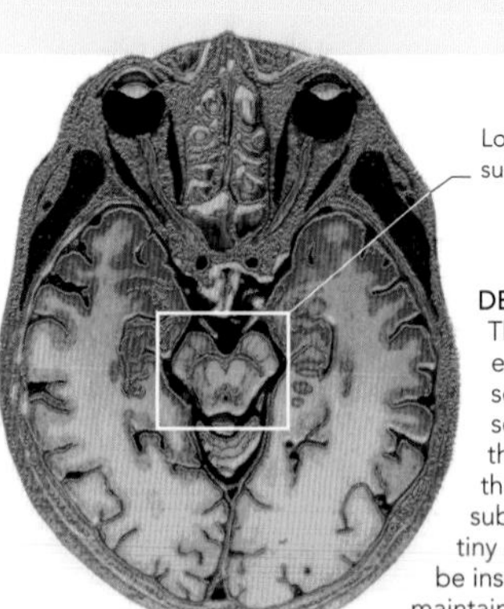

DEEP IN THE BRAIN
This colour-enhanced MRI scan of a horizontal section through the head shows the location of the substantia nigra. A tiny electrode may be inserted here to maintain neuronal activity.

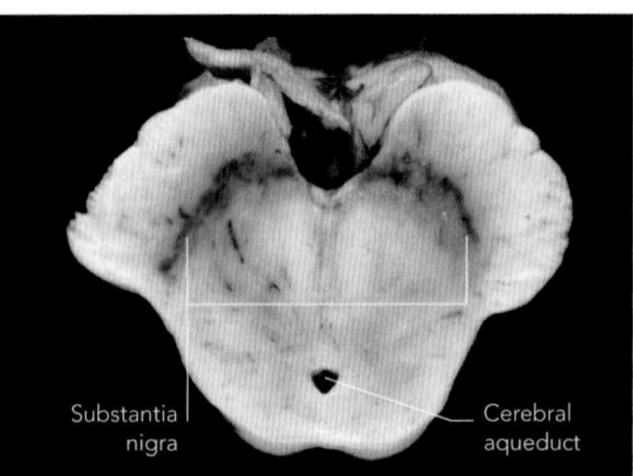

HEALTHY BRAIN
This section of brain tissue shows the substantia nigra in a healthy brain, with the dark pigmented areas of the substantia nigra clearly visible.

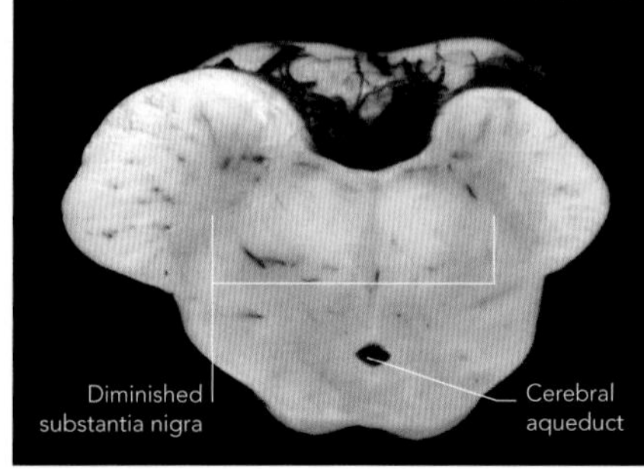

DISEASED BRAIN
In this section of brain tissue of a person with Parkinson's disease, the pigmented neurons in the substantia nigra are significantly reduced.

PARKINSONISM

The term "parkinsonism" refers to any condition that causes the movement abnormalities that occur in Parkinson's disease resulting from the reduced production of dopamine (for example, tremors, muscle stiffness, and slow movements). Parkinson's disease is the most common cause of parkinsonism, but not everybody with parkinsonism has Parkinson's disease. Other causes include stroke, encephalitis, meningitis, head injury, prolonged exposure to herbicides and pesticides, other degenerative nerve diseases, and certain drugs, such as some antipsychotic drugs.

HUNTINGTON'S DISEASE

HUNTINGTON'S IS A RARE, INHERITED DISEASE IN WHICH NEURONS IN THE BRAIN DEGENERATE, LEADING TO JERKY, UNCONTROLLED MOVEMENTS AND DEMENTIA.

The underlying cause of Huntington's disease is a single abnormal gene that occurs when a group of DNA base pairs is repeated many times. The faulty gene generates an abnormal version of Huntingtin protein, which then builds up in nerve cells and leads to the degeneration of neurons in the basal ganglia and cerebral cortex.

Effects

Symptoms usually start to appear between the ages of 35 and 50, although they may sometimes start in childhood. Early symptoms include chorea (jerky, rapid, uncontrollable movements), clumsiness, and involuntary facial grimaces and twitches. Other symptoms then develop, including speech problems; difficulty swallowing; depression; apathy; and dementia, which usually takes the form of lack of concentration, memory problems, and personality and mood changes (including aggressive or antisocial behaviour). The disease usually progresses slowly, eventually causing death some 10–30 years after symptoms first appear.

A diagnosis of Huntington's disease is made from the symptoms, with brain scans, and also genetic (to test for the abnormal gene) and neuropsychological testing.

There is no cure for Huntington's disease, and drug treatment is aimed at reducing the symptoms. Keeping physically and mentally active is also advised.

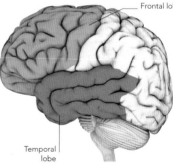

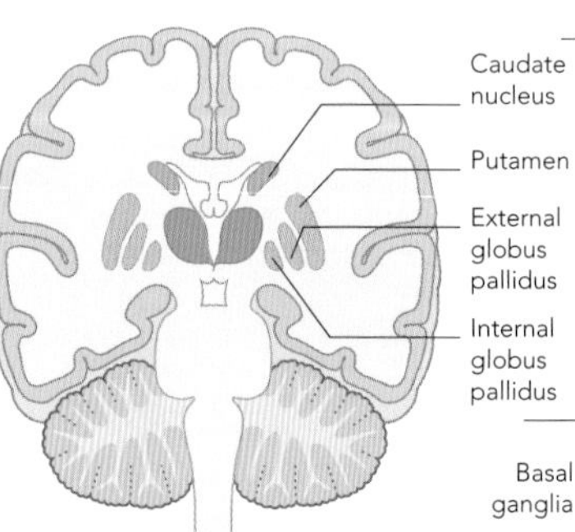

Frontal lobe

Temporal lobe

AFFECTED AREAS
Huntington's disease causes degeneration of neurons in the basal ganglia (primarily in the caudate nuclei, putamen, and globus pallidus). It is also associated with degeneration in the frontal and temporal lobes.

AFFECTED PARENT
UNAFFECTED PARENT
Huntington's gene
Normal gene
AFFECTED CHILDREN
UNAFFECTED CHILDREN

INHERITANCE PATTERN
Huntington's disease is inherited in an autosomal dominant fashion, which means that if one parent has a copy of the gene, each child has a 1 in 2 chance of inheriting the faulty gene and therefore of developing the disease in adulthood.

A C T G T T C A G C A G C A G

3 CAG REPEATS

GENETIC DEFECT
The genetic abnormality that causes Huntington's disease is a sequence of DNA on chromosome 4 in which a group of base pairs (CAG) is repeated numerous times. Whether or not a person develops the disease depends on the number of CAG repeats (see table, right).

HUNTINGTON'S DISEASE AND CAG REPEATS

NUMBER OF REPEATS	EFFECTS
0–15	No adverse effect; Huntingtin protein functions normally.
16–39	Huntington's disease may or may not develop.
40–59	Huntingtin abnormal; Huntington's disease will eventually develop.
60 or more	Huntingtin abnormal; Huntington's disease will develop early.

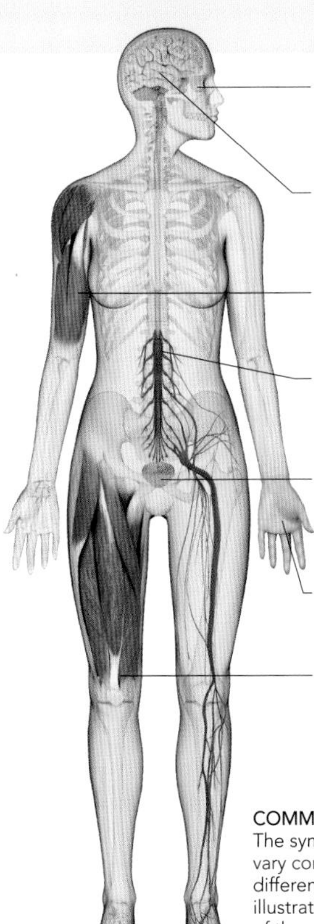
Vision
Blurred and/or double vision; loss of centre of visual field
Co-ordination
Impaired co-ordination; loss of balance
Muscle strength
Weakness in limbs; paralysis
Motor control
Plaques on motor nerve tracts may affect movement
Bladder
Urinary incontinence due to loss of sphincter control
Sensation
Numbness, tingling, and/or pain
Movement
A feeling of muscle weakness, poor co-ordination, and unsteadiness can make walking difficult

COMMON EFFECTS OF MS
The symptoms of MS vary considerably among different people. The illustration shows some of the more common symptoms of the condition.

MULTIPLE SCLEROSIS

A PROGRESSIVE DISEASE, MULTIPLE SCLEROSIS CAUSES THE DESTRUCTION OF THE MYELIN SHEATHS THAT SURROUND NEURONS IN THE BRAIN AND SPINAL CORD.

Multiple sclerosis (MS) is thought to be an autoimmune disease in which the body's immune system destroys the cells that produce the myelin sheaths that surround and insulate neurons. Eventually hardened (sclerosed) plaques of scar tissue form over the demyelinated areas and the neurons themselves degenerate. The effect of these changes is to impair or block nerve impulses. The reason for this autoimmune reaction is not known, although there may be genetic, environmental, and/or infectious factors involved.

The course and symptoms of MS vary among individuals. In addition to common symptoms (see illustration, left), there may also be mental changes, such as poor memory, anxiety, and depression. The most common type is relapsing-remitting MS, in which attacks (relapses) of gradually worsening symptoms are followed by periods of remission. In progressive MS, symptoms worsen without remission. In most cases, relapsing-remitting MS may develop into progressive MS.

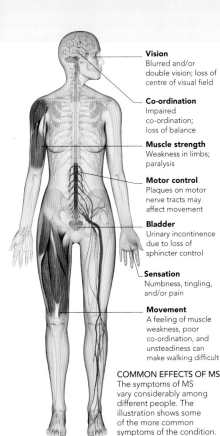

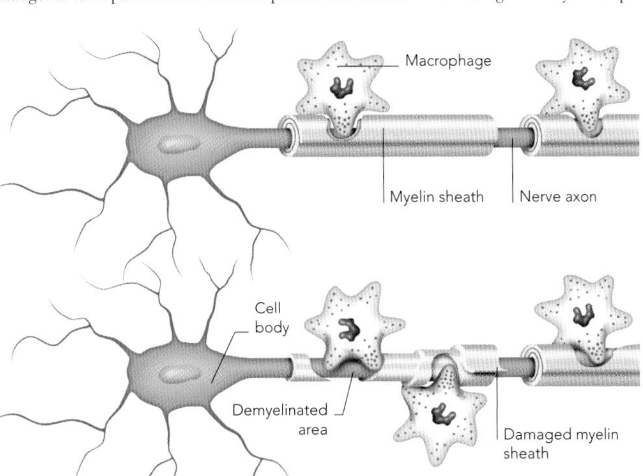
Macrophage
Myelin sheath
Nerve axon
Cell body
Demyelinated area
Damaged myelin sheath

EARLY STAGE
In the early stages of MS, the fatty myelin sheaths that surround the nerve axons are damaged. Macrophages, a type of white blood cell, remove the damaged areas, leading to demyelinated patches along the axons and impairing nerve conduction.

LATE STAGE
As the disorder progresses, there is an increasing amount of damage to the myelin sheaths and more nerves become affected, leading to a worsening of symptoms. Hardened (sclerosed) patches form over the demyelinated areas and eventually the nerve degenerates.

MOTOR NEURON DISEASE

IN THIS GROUP OF DISORDERS, PROGRESSIVE DEGENERATION OF MOTOR NEURONS LEADS TO INCREASING WEAKNESS AND WASTING OF MUSCLES.

In most cases, the cause of motor neuron disease (MND) is not known. However, genetic factors are thought to be important in affecting a person's susceptibility to the condition. Some rare types of MND are inherited. Motor neuron disease can affect the upper motor neurons (those originating in the motor cortex or brainstem) and/or the lower motor neurons (those in the spinal cord and brainstem that connect the central nervous system to the muscles). Damage to the upper motor neurons is indicated by spasticity, muscle weakness, and exaggerated reflexes. Damage to the lower motor neurons produces a weakening of muscles, paralysis, and atrophy of the skeletal muscles.

In addition to muscular symptoms, some people also experience personality changes and depression, but intellect, vision, and hearing remain unaffected. There are many types of motor neuron disease, the most common of which are amyotrophic lateral sclerosis (ALS, or Lou Gehrig's disease) and progressive bulbar atrophy. Both these types affect both the upper and lower motor neurons.

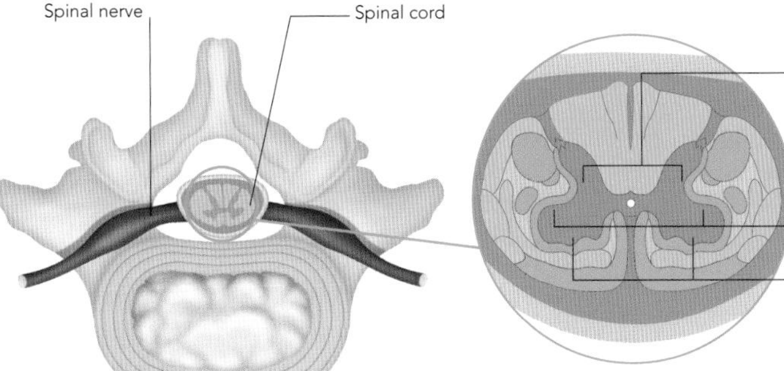
Spinal nerve
Spinal cord
Dorsal (back) horns
Neurons in these horns receive sensory information from around the body
Lateral (side) horns
Neurons here convey signals to and from the internal organs. These horns are not found at all levels of the spinal cord
Ventral (front) horns
Neurons here send motor nerve fibres to skeletal muscles, causing them to contract

NERVE TRACTS OF THE SPINAL CORD
Nerve fibres in the spinal cord are grouped into bundles, or tracts, depending on the type and direction of nerve impulses they convey. MND may affect the lower motor neurons, in the ventral horns of the spinal cord.

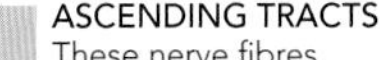

ASCENDING TRACTS
These nerve fibres convey sensory signals from the body to the brain.

DESCENDING TRACTS
These convey motor signals from the brain to the skeletal muscles of the torso and limbs.

Mouth and throat
Difficulty swallowing, speaking, and chewing

Neck
Muscles in the neck become weak, causing the head to fall forwards

Chest and diaphragm
Difficulty breathing as muscles involved in breathing become weak

Leg and arm muscles
Weakness and stiffness in the legs, arms, and hands; muscles may occasionally cramp or spasm; eventually, inability to walk

AFFECTED AREAS
The effects of MND depend on the specific form of the disease, and there is also some variation among different individuals. In almost all cases, the disease is progressive and ultimately fatal. The principal effects of the main types of the condition are shown here.

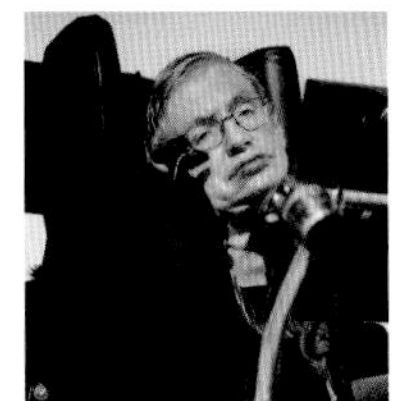

STEPHEN HAWKING
Renowned theoretical physicist and cosmologist Stephen Hawking died in 2018, aged 76. Few people with motor neuron disease have survived to such an age. Hawking retained his brilliant mind and worked practically until the end of his life.

PARALYSIS

PARTIAL OR COMPLETE LOSS OF CONTROLLED MOVEMENT DUE TO IMPAIRED MUSCLE FUNCTION MAY BE THE RESULT OF A NERVE OR MUSCLE DISORDER.

Paralysis can affect areas ranging from a single small muscle to most of the major muscles of the body. It is classified by the areas of body affected. Hemiplegia is paralysis of one half of the body. Paraplegia is the paralysis of both legs and sometimes part of the trunk. Quadriplegia is paralysis of all four limbs and the trunk. Paralysis may also be classified as "flaccid" (causing floppiness) or "spastic" (causing rigidity).

Paralysis can be caused by any injury or disorder that affects the motor cortex or the motor nerve pathways that run from the motor cortex via the spinal cord and peripheral nerves to the muscles. It may also result from a muscle disorder or myasthenia gravis (a disorder affecting the junction between nerves and muscles). The affected area sometimes feels numb.

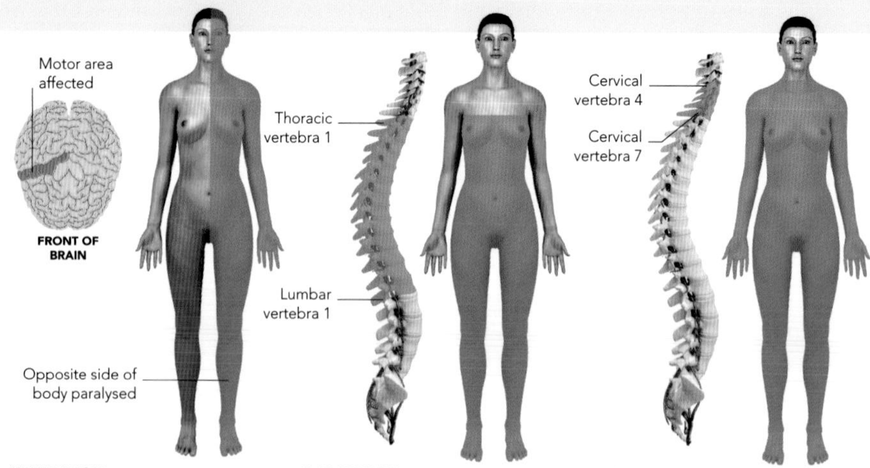

HEMIPLEGIA
Paralysis of one half of the body may be caused by damage to the motor area of the brain on the opposite side.

PARAPLEGIA
Both legs and possibly part of the trunk may be paralysed as a result of damage to the middle or lower spinal cord.

QUADRIPLEGIA
Damage to motor nerves in the lower neck causes quadriplegia. Damage higher in the neck is usually fatal.

DOWN'S SYNDROME

ALSO KNOWN AS TRISOMY 21, DOWN'S SYNDROME IS A CHROMOSOMAL ABNORMALITY THAT AFFECTS BOTH MENTAL AND PHYSICAL DEVELOPMENT.

One of the most common chromosomal abnormalities, Down's syndrome is usually the result of an extra copy of chromosome 21; affected people therefore have 47 chromosomes in all of their body cells, rather than 46. It may also result when part of chromosome 21 breaks off and attaches to another chromosome, a process called translocation, so that cells have the normal number of chromosomes but chromosome 21 is abnormally sized. Very rarely, Down's syndrome may be the result of mosaicism, in which some body cells have 47 chromosomes and some have 46. Exactly how these abnormalities produce the characteristic mental and physical features of Down's is not known.

In most cases there is no identifiable reason for the chromosomal abnormality, although maternal age is a risk factor – after the early 30s, the risk of having a child with Down's increases significantly. Paternal age can also be a risk factor, if the father is over 50. Parents who already have a child with Down's or who have abnormalities of their own chromosome 21 have a higher risk of having a baby with Down's syndrome.

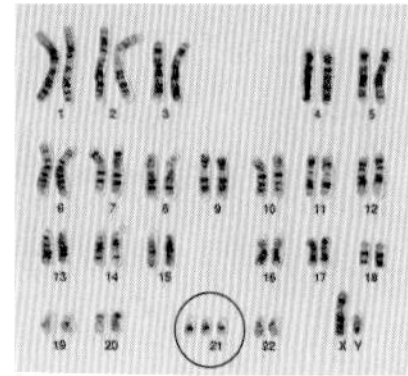

NORMAL CHROMOSOME COMPLEMENT
This karyotype (a photograph of the full set of chromosomes) shows the chromosome complement of a normal male, comprising a total of 46 chromosomes: 22 pairs of autosomes plus one pair of sex chromosomes (X and Y).

TRISOMY 21
This karyotype shows the chromosome complement of a male with Down's syndrome. There are three chromosome 21s (hence the term "trisomy 21") instead of the normal two, resulting in the characteristic symptoms of Down's syndrome.

Symptoms

There is considerable variation in the severity of symptoms, but typically they include slow motor and language development, and learning difficulties. Physical symptoms may include a small face with upward-sloping eyes; a flattened back of the head; a short neck; a large tongue; small hands with a single horizontal crease on the palm; and short stature.

There is also increased risk of various disorders, such as heart disease (often associated with congenital heart problems), hearing problems, underactivity of the thyroid gland, narrowing of the intestines, leukaemia, and respiratory-tract and ear infections. Adults are at increased risk of eye problems such as cataracts. In older people there is a heightened risk of Alzheimer's disease. People with Down's syndrome have lower than normal life expectancy, but some survive into old age.

Tests

Pregnant women with a higher than normal risk of producing a child with Down's syndrome may be offered amniocentesis – a diagnostic test that can detect chromosome abnormalities and other genetic disorders. It involves inserting a needle through the mother's abdomen into the uterus and withdrawing a small amount of amniotic fluid. The fluid is then sent to a laboratory for analysis; reports usually take a few days. Amniocentesis is usually performed between 14 and 20 weeks' gestation.

Although it is thought a safe procedure, it carries a small risk of miscarriage – roughly one in 300. Miscarriages can occur because of infection in the uterus, waters breaking, or labour being induced prematurely. In very rare cases, the needle may come into contact with the baby. Great precautions are taken by using ultrasound to guide the needle away from the baby. The mother may experience a sharp pain when the needle enters the skin and again when it enters the uterus. She may also experience cramps after the procedure, or minor fluid leakage from the site. Having amniocentesis provides parents with the chance to pursue interventions – such as fetal surgery for spina bifida – and to plan, if necessary, for having a child with special needs. It also gives women the opportunity to opt for an abortion if they do not want to carry the child to term.

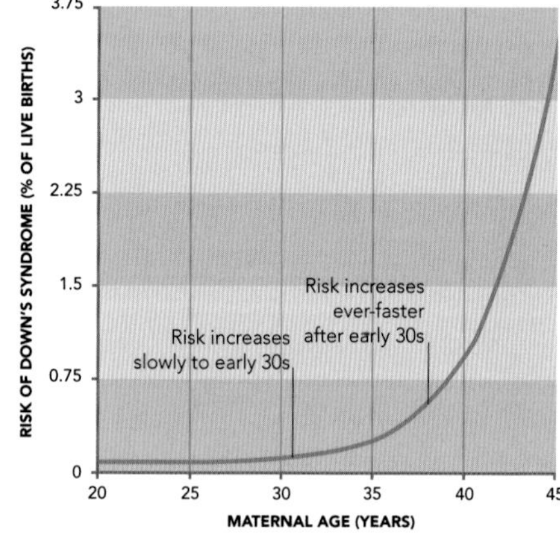

MATERNAL AGE AND DOWN'S SYNDROME
The risk of having a child with Down's syndrome is related to the mother's age – increasing slowly up to the early 30s, and then at an ever-faster rate with increasing maternal age.

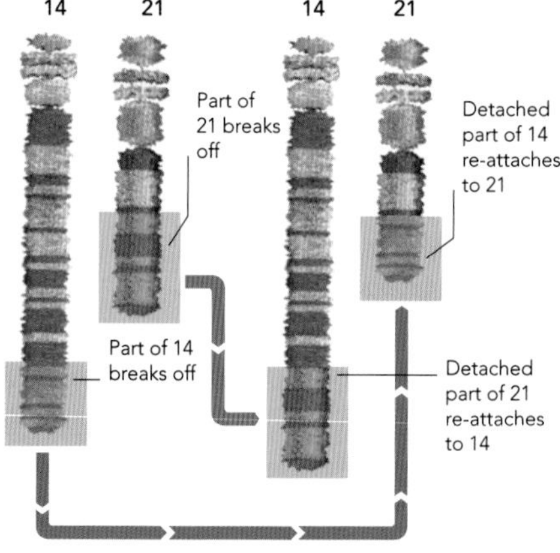

BALANCED TRANSLOCATION
Down's syndrome may be caused by a translocation, in which part of chromosome 21 breaks off and re-attaches to another chromosome. A balanced translocation occurs when part of the other chromosome in turn moves to chromosome 21.

TYPES OF CEREBRAL PALSY	
Cerebral palsy can be classified into four main types, primarily on the basis of the type of movement abnormality, although there may also be other symptoms.	
TYPE	**CHARACTERISTICS**
Spastic cerebral palsy	Exaggerated reflexes; stiff, difficult movement due to tight, stiff, and weak muscles.
Athetoid cerebral palsy	Involuntary writhing movements, especially in the face, arms, and trunk; difficulty maintaining posture.
Ataxic cerebral palsy	Problems maintaining balance; shaky movements of the hands and feet; and speech difficulties.
Mixed cerebral palsy	A combination of symptoms from the other types; often tight muscle tone and involuntary movements.

CEREBRAL PALSY

CEREBRAL PALSY REFERS TO A GROUP OF DISORDERS THAT AFFECT MOVEMENT AND POSTURE DUE TO BRAIN DAMAGE OR THE FAILURE OF THE BRAIN TO DEVELOP PROPERLY.

There are many possible causes of cerebral palsy, and often the cause is not identified. Usually, the brain damage occurs before or around birth. Possible causes include extreme prematurity; lack of oxygen to the fetus before or during birth (hypoxia); hydrocephalus (see below); infections transmitted from the mother to the fetus; or haemolytic disease, which is caused by a blood incompatibility between the mother and the fetus. After birth, infections such as encephalitis and meningitis, head injury, or a brain haemorrhage may cause cerebral palsy.

In addition to movement and posture abnormalities and the difficulties that these can cause (such as difficulty walking, talking, and eating), cerebral palsy may also give rise to various other problems, such as vision and hearing impairment and epilepsy. It may also sometimes cause learning difficulties. The severity of symptoms varies widely among different people, from slight clumsiness to severe disability.

There is no cure for cerebral palsy, but treatment includes physiotherapy, occupational therapy, and speech therapy. Drugs may be used to control muscle spasms and increase joint mobility. Surgery may help correct any deformities that have developed as a result of abnormal muscle development. Cerebral palsy is not progressive.

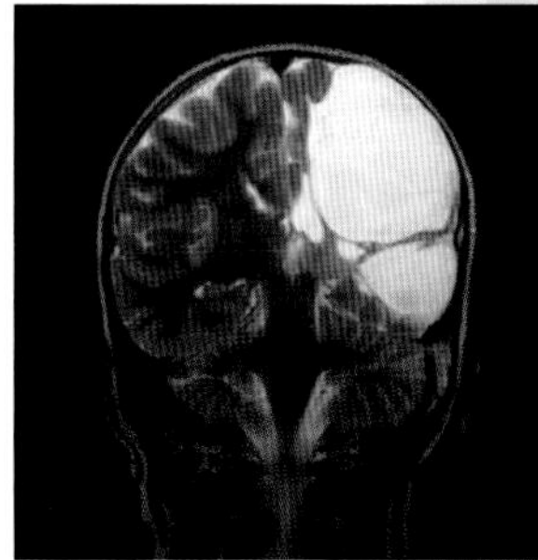

BRAIN DAMAGE
This MRI scan shows the head of a child with cerebral palsy. The abnormal brain tissue (in the left side of the brain, but seen on the right of this image) has resulted in paralysis of the right side of the body.

HYDROCEPHALUS

COMMONLY KNOWN AS WATER ON THE BRAIN, HYDROCEPHALUS IS AN EXCESSIVE BUILD-UP OF CEREBROSPINAL FLUID WITHIN THE SKULL.

Hydrocephalus occurs either because excess cerebrospinal fluid is produced or because the fluid does not drain away normally. The fluid accumulates in the skull and compresses the brain, which may lead to brain damage.

This condition can be present at birth, often in association with other abnormalities, such as a neural-tube defect. The main symptom is an abnormally large head that continues to grow rapidly. Without treatment, severe brain damage may occur, which may lead to cerebral palsy or other physical or mental disabilities, or may even be fatal.

Hydrocephalus may occur later in life, as a result of a head injury, brain haemorrhage, infection, or a brain tumour. It usually clears up once the cause is treated.

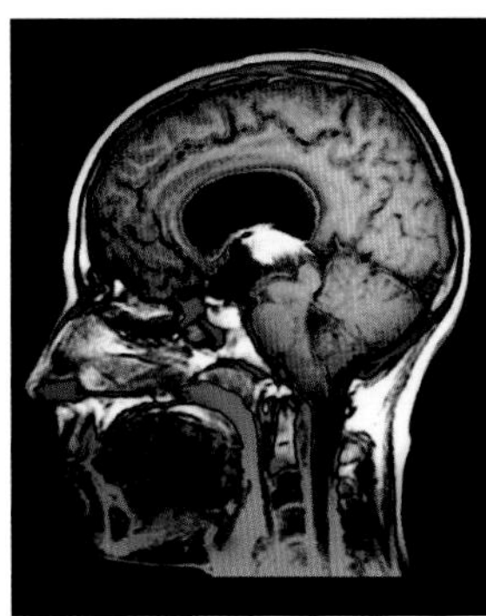

ENLARGED VENTRICLES
In this MRI scan through the centre of the head, the ventricles (black areas in the middle of the brain) are enlarged due to hydrocephalus. This abnormal accumulation of cerebrospinal fluid has compressed the brain.

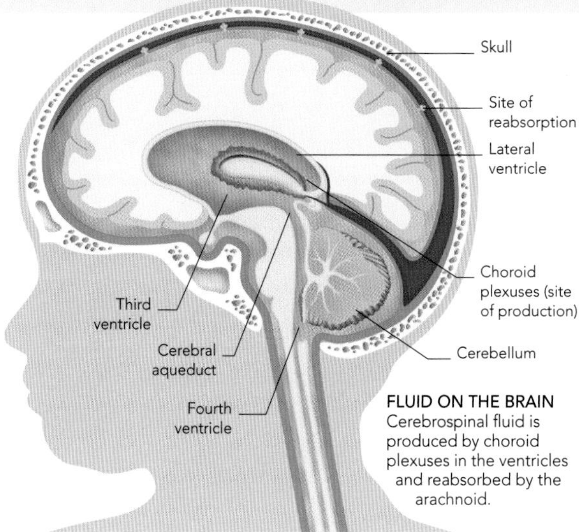

FLUID ON THE BRAIN
Cerebrospinal fluid is produced by choroid plexuses in the ventricles and reabsorbed by the arachnoid.

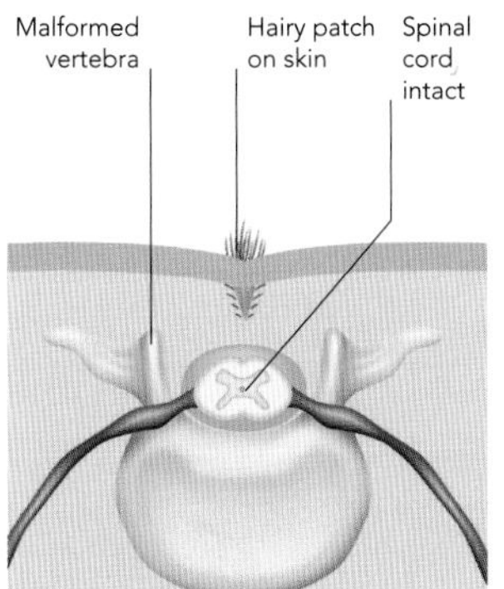

SPINA BIFIDA OCCULTA
In spina bifida occulta, the only defect is malformation of one or more vertebrae; the spinal cord is undamaged. There may be a hair tuft, dimpling, or a fatty lump at the base of the spine.

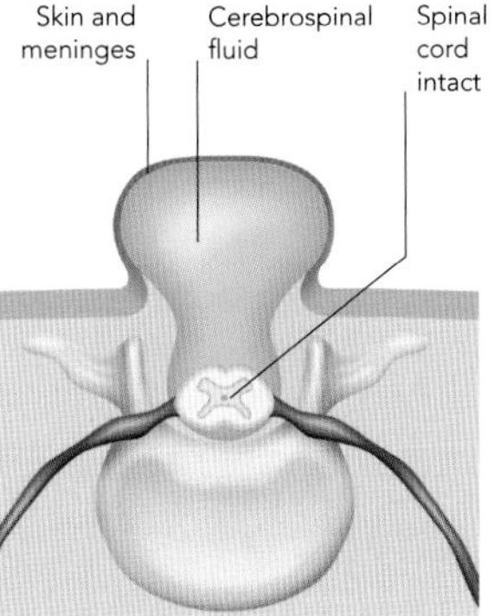

MENINGOCELE
In meningocele, the meninges protrude through the malformed vertebra, forming a sac filled with cerebrospinal fluid, which is called a meningocele. With this type of defect the spinal cord is not damaged.

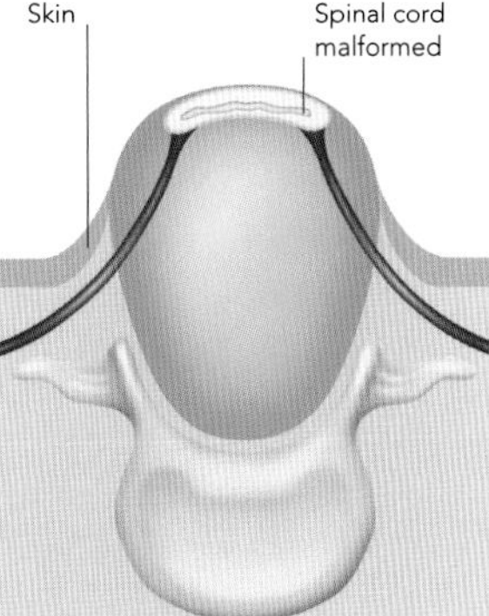

MYELOMENINGOCELE
This is the most severe form of spina bifida, in which the spinal cord is malformed and, contained within a sac of cerebrospinal fluid, protrudes through a defect in the skin.

NEURAL-TUBE DEFECTS

A NUMBER OF DEVELOPMENTAL ABNORMALITIES OF THE BRAIN OR SPINAL CORD CAN OCCUR WHEN THE NEURAL TUBE DOES NOT FORM PROPERLY.

The neural tube is the region along the back of an embryo that develops into the brain, spinal cord, and meninges. The cause of neural-tube defects is unknown, but they tend to run in families and have been associated with certain anticonvulsant drugs during pregnancy. A lack of folic acid during early pregnancy is also associated with the defects.

The most common types are anencephaly and spina bifida. In anencephaly there is a complete lack of a brain, which is always fatal. In spina bifida the vertebrae do not close completely around the spinal cord. In the most severe form of spina bifida, called myelomeningocele, the spinal cord is malformed and there may be paralysis of the legs and loss of bladder control.

NARCOLEPSY

THIS IS A NEUROLOGICAL DISORDER CHARACTERIZED BY CHRONIC DROWSINESS AND RECURRENT, SUDDEN EPISODES OF SLEEP THROUGHOUT THE DAYTIME.

This condition is thought to be due to abnormally low levels of proteins called hypocretins (also known as orexins) in the brain. Hypocretins are produced by cells in the hypothalamus and help regulate sleep and wakefulness. In people with narcolepsy, these cells are damaged. The underlying cause of the damage is not known, but it may be due to an autoimmune response, possibly triggered by an infection. A genetic factor may be involved, as the condition tends to run in families.

The main symptoms are overwhelming drowsiness and an uncontrollable urge to sleep – people with narcolepsy may fall asleep without warning at any time and place. Other common symptoms include a sudden loss of muscle tone (cataplexy) while awake and hallucinations at the start or end of sleep.

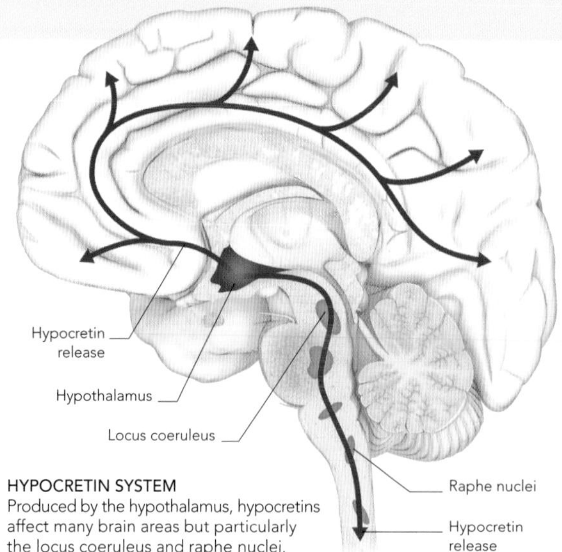

HYPOCRETIN SYSTEM
Produced by the hypothalamus, hypocretins affect many brain areas but particularly the locus coeruleus and raphe nuclei.

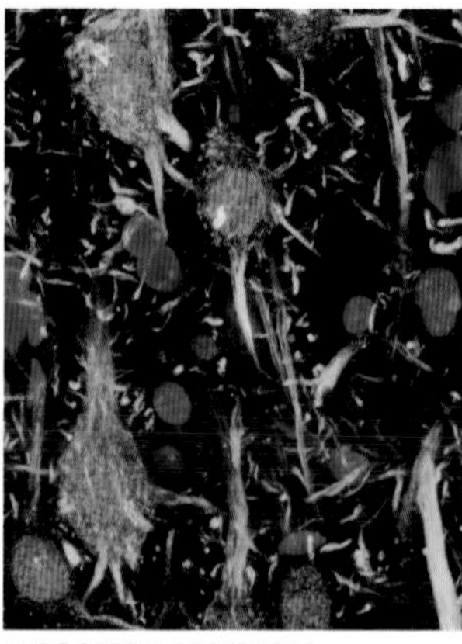

HYPOCRETIN RECEPTORS
This light micrograph of brain tissue shows a large number of neurons with hypocretin receptors (coloured red).

COMA

A STATE OF UNCONSCIOUSNESS IN WHICH THERE IS A LACK OF RESPONSIVENESS TO INTERNAL AND EXTERNAL STIMULI IS CALLED A COMA.

Coma results from damage or disturbance to parts of the brain involved in maintaining consciousness or conscious activity, especially the limbic system and the brainstem. A wide range of problems can cause a coma, including head injury; lack of blood supply to the brain, as may occur after a heart attack or stroke; infections, such as encephalitis and meningitis; toxins, such as carbon monoxide or drug overdoses; and prolonged high or low blood-sugar levels, as can occur in diabetes mellitus.

Symptoms

There are varying degrees of coma. In less severe forms, the person may respond to certain stimuli and spontaneously make small movements. In the condition known as a persistent vegetative state there may be sleep–wake cycles, movements of the eyes and limbs, and even speech, although the person does not appear to respond to any stimuli. In a deep coma, the person does not respond to any stimuli nor make any movements, although automatic responses such as blinking and breathing may be maintained. In severe cases, in which the lower brainstem is damaged, vital functions such as breathing are impaired or lost and life support is necessary. Total and irreversible loss of brainstem function is classed as brain death.

Coma is diagnosed when a person remains persistently unconscious and unresponsive to stimuli. It is an emergency and requires immediate treatment.

1 **Conscious** Normal responses to stimuli such as sound, light, pain, and orientation (prompt response to questions about name, date, time, and/or location).

2 **Confused** The person is aware but bewildered and disorientated (does not respond promptly to questions about name, date, time, and/or location).

3 **Delirious** The person is disorientated, restless, or agitated, and shows a marked impairment of attention; there may be hallucinations or delusions.

4 **Obtunded** The person is sleepy, shows a marked lack of interest in the surroundings, and responds very slowly to stimuli.

5 **Stuporous** A sleep-like state with little or no spontaneous activity; typically, a person responds only to painful stimuli (by moving away) or by grimacing.

6 **Comatose** The person cannot be woken and does not respond to any stimuli, even painful ones; there is no gag reflex, and the pupils may not respond to light.

LEVELS OF CONSCIOUSNESS
There are various systems used to classify levels of consciousness, one of which is outlined here. The depth of a coma may also be assessed using a scale, most commonly the Glasgow Coma Scale.

BRAIN DEATH

Brain death is the irreversible cessation of functions of the brain and particularly the brainstem. The brainstem is responsible for maintaining vital functions such as breathing and heartbeat. If there is no activity in the brainstem and it is damaged so severely and irreversibly that these vital functions cannot be carried out independently without a life-support machine, a person may be diagnosed as brain dead. To confirm the diagnosis, a series of tests are carried out by two experienced senior doctors. These tests include checking responses to stimuli, checking functions controlled by the brainstem, and testing the ability to breathe without life support. Only if both doctors are in agreement that brainstem and brain functions have been irreversibly lost is the diagnosis of brain death confirmed.

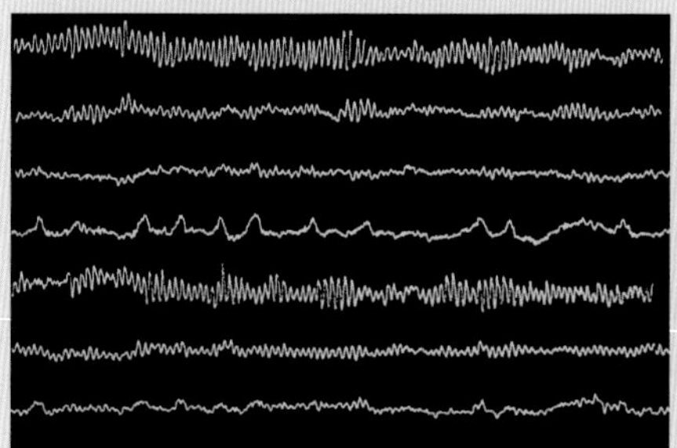

NORMAL EEG
Brain activity can be assessed by electroencephalography (EEG), in which electrodes are attached to the scalp and connected to a machine that records the levels of electrical activity in the brain.

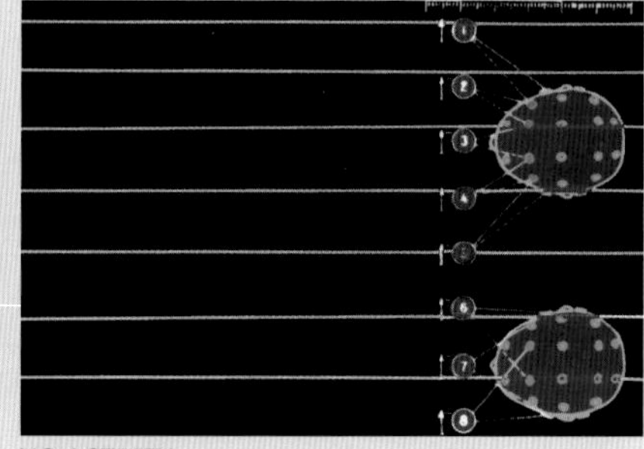

NO ACTIVITY
Electroencephalography can be used to help diagnose brain death. If the EEG lines are flat, as in the recording above, it indicates that there is no activity in the brain, which is one of the criteria used to diagnose brain death.

DEPRESSION

DEPRESSION IS CHARACTERIZED BY PERSISTENT FEELINGS OF INTENSE SADNESS, HOPELESSNESS, AND LOSS OF INTEREST IN LIFE THAT INTERFERE WITH EVERYDAY LIFE.

In many cases, depression occurs without an obvious cause. A number of factors may trigger it, such as a physical illness; hormonal disorders or the hormonal changes during pregnancy (antenatal depression) or after childbirth (postnatal depression); or distressing life events, such as a bereavement. It may also occur as a side effect of certain drugs, such as oral contraceptives. Depression is more common in women, it tends to run in families, and various genetic mutations are associated with this disorder.

Various biological abnormalities have been found in the brains of depressed people, such as decreased levels of the neurotransmitter serotonin, raised levels of the enzyme monoamine oxidase, loss of cells from the hippocampus (an area of the brain involved in mood and memory), and abnormal patterns of neural activity in the amygdala and parts of the prefrontal cortex. However, the mechanisms by which such biological abnormalities may lead to depression are not known.

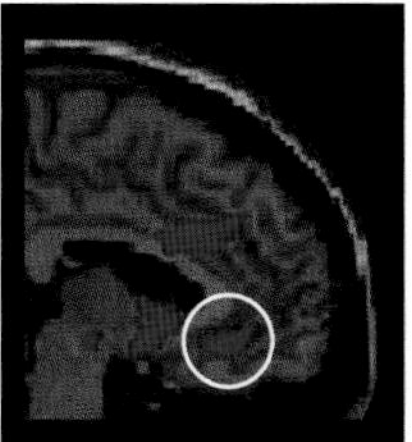

BEFORE TREATMENT

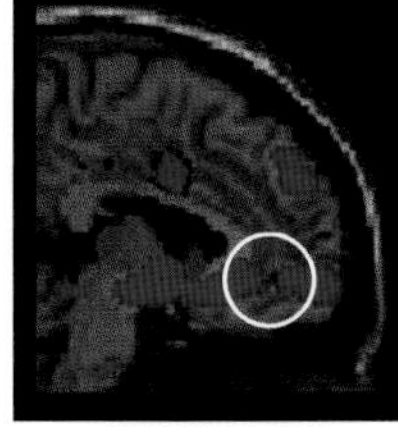

AFTER TREATMENT

DEEP BRAIN STIMULATION
In the PET scan on the left, a patient suffering from depression shows overactivity in the cingulate cortex (circled). After six months of deep brain stimulation, activity in this area (shown in the scan to the right) decreased and symptoms had improved.

SEASONAL AFFECTIVE DISORDER

Commonly known as SAD, seasonal affective disorder is a type of depression in which mood changes occur according to the season. The cause is not known, although it is thought that changes in daylight levels may cause alterations in brain chemistry that affect mood. Typically, the onset of winter brings depression, tiredness, lack of energy, cravings for sugary and starchy food, weight gain, anxiety and irritability, and avoidance of social activities. The symptoms then spontaneously clear up with the coming of spring. SAD can usually be treated with daily light therapy (sitting in front of a special light box that produces bright light similar to daylight) or antidepressants.

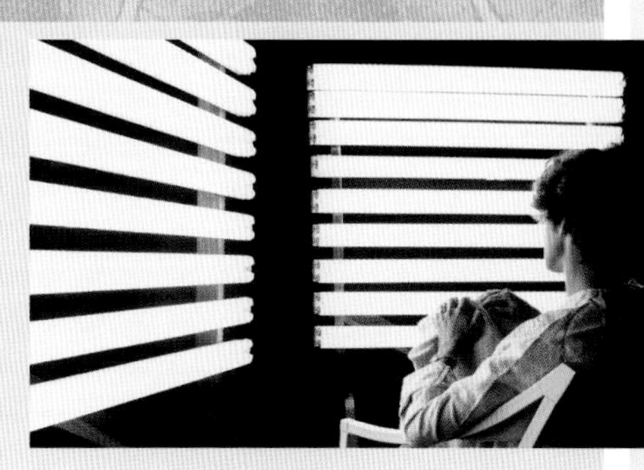

Symptoms and treatment

There is considerable variation among different people in the symptoms and in their severity. Most people experience several of the following: feeling unhappy most of the time; loss of interest and enjoyment in life; difficulty coping and making decisions; impaired concentration; persistent tiredness; agitation; changes in appetite and weight; disrupted sleeping patterns; loss of interest in sex; loss of self-confidence; irritability; and thoughts of, or attempts at, suicide. In some people, episodes of depression alternate with periods of extreme highs (manic episodes); this is known as bipolar disorder (see below).

Usually depression is treated with a talking therapy, antidepressant drugs, or both. Experimental treatment using deep brain stimulation (where implanted electrodes stimulate areas of the brain) is also being studied.

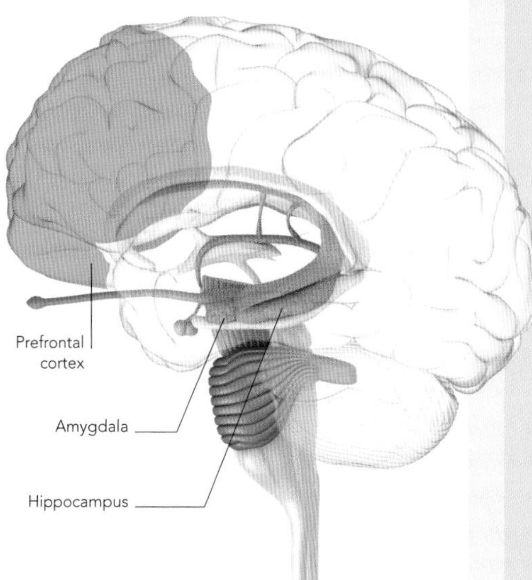

BRAIN AREAS
The biological basis of depression is not fully understood but several areas of the brain are thought to be involved, including the prefrontal cortex, hippocampus, and amygdala.

BIPOLAR DISORDER

BIPOLAR DISORDER IS A MOOD DISORDER CHARACTERIZED BY MOOD SWINGS BETWEEN DEPRESSION AND MANIA.

The exact cause of bipolar disorder (sometimes called manic–depressive illness) is not known, although it is believed that it results from a combination of biochemical, genetic, and environmental factors. The levels of certain neurotransmitters in the brain, such as norepinephrine, serotonin, and dopamine, may play a role. Bipolar disorder tends to run in families and has a strong genetic component. However, environmental factors, such as a major life event, may act as triggers.

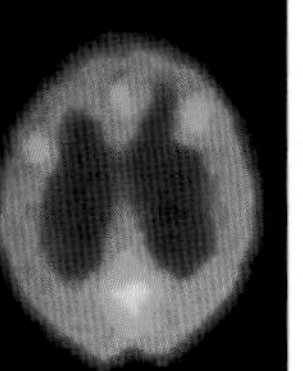

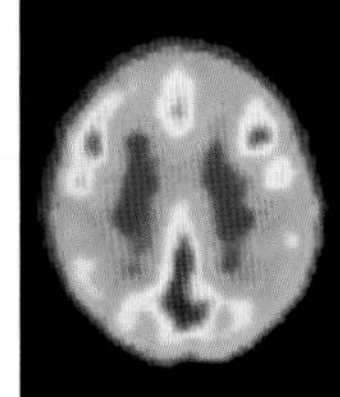

BRAIN ACTIVITY IN BIPOLAR DISORDER
These PET scans show brain activity during normal periods (left) and increased levels of activity during a manic phase (right).

Symptoms

Typically, symptoms of depression and mania alternate, with each episode lasting for an unpredictable period. Between mood swings, a person's mood and behaviour are often normal. Symptoms of a depressive episode may include feelings of hopelessness, disturbed sleep, changes in appetite and weight, tiredness, a loss of interest in life, and a loss of self-confidence; there may also be suicide attempts. Symptoms of a manic episode may include extreme optimism, increased energy levels, drive and activity, inflated self-esteem, racing thoughts, and risk-taking behaviour.

CREATIVITY AND BIPOLAR DISORDER

Biographical studies suggest that bipolar disorder may be more common among accomplished artists than in the general population, and some artists seem to be able to utilize periods of mania as a spur to creativity. For example, the musical output of the German composer Robert Schumann (1810–56) – illustrated on the graph below – shows a link between his bouts of mania and the number of compositions he produced. He was most productive during manic phases and least productive when depressed. However, the quality of his work was not affected by his moods.

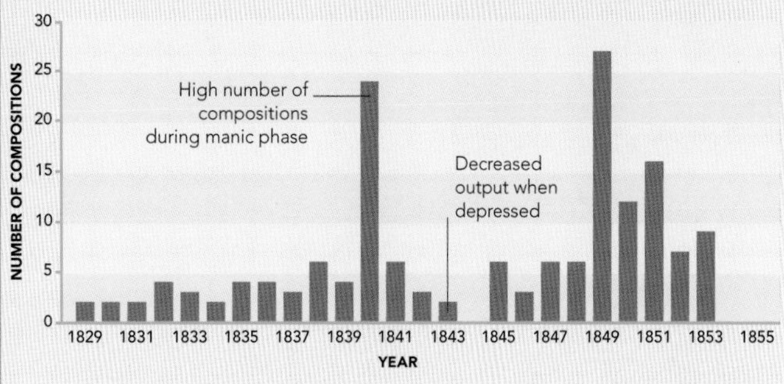

ANXIETY DISORDERS

THIS IS A GROUP OF DISORDERS IN WHICH FEELINGS OF ANXIETY AND/OR PANIC OCCUR FREQUENTLY ENOUGH TO CAUSE PROBLEMS IN COPING WITH EVERYDAY LIFE.

Temporary feelings of nervousness, apprehension, and even panic in stressful situations are normal and appropriate. However, when these anxiety reactions occur frequently in ordinary situations and disrupt normal activities, it is considered to be a disorder. In a few cases there may be an identifiable physical cause for persistent anxiety, such as a thyroid disorder or substance abuse, and sometimes generalized anxiety may develop after a stressful life event, such as a bereavement. In most cases the cause is not known, although a family history of an anxiety disorder increases the risk of developing one. The brain mechanisms underlying anxiety disorders are also unknown, although disruption of neurotransmitters in the frontal lobes or limbic system may be involved.

Whatever the underlying cause, the effect is to disrupt the body's normal control of its stress response – the "fight or flight" response. With anxiety disorders either the stress response fails to turn off or the stress response becomes activated at inappropriate times.

There are several forms of anxiety disorder. The most common is generalized anxiety disorder, which is characterized by excessive, inappropriate worrying that lasts for at least six months. Another form of anxiety disorder is panic disorder, in which there are sudden, unexpected attacks of intense anxiety or fear.

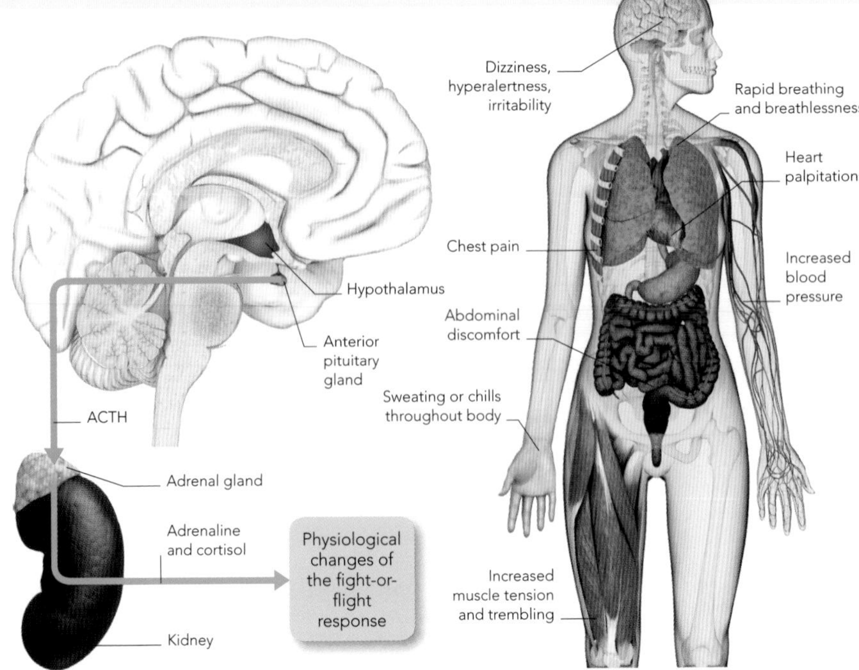

STRESS RESPONSE
In response to stress, the hypothalamus stimulates the pituitary gland to produce adrenocorticotropic hormone (ACTH). ACTH stimulates production of adrenaline and cortisol by the adrenal glands, and these hormones produce the fight-or-flight response.

PHYSICAL EFFECTS OF ANXIETY
Activation of the body's flight-or-fight stress response produces widespread effects on the body. Normally, this response turns off when the stress disappears, but in anxiety disorders the stress response may be oversensitive or may fail to turn off.

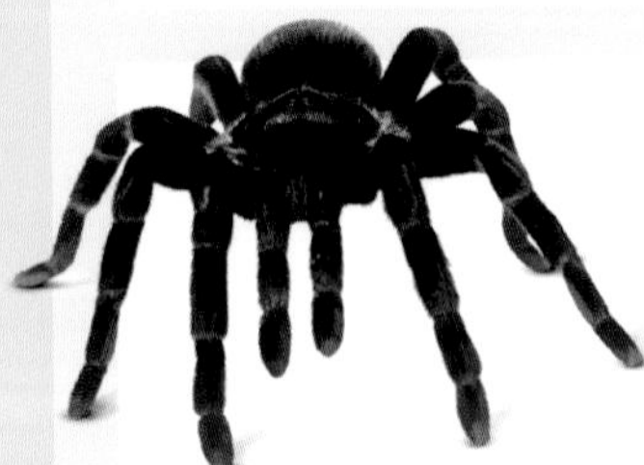

FEAR OF SPIDERS
Arachnophobia is one of the most common phobias. Sufferers may experience anxiety about encountering a spider even when it is extremely unlikely.

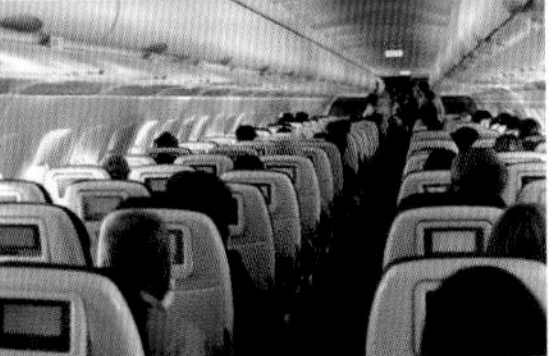

AVIOPHOBIA
Fear of flying may occur by itself or as a manifestation of other phobias, such as acrophobia (fear of heights) or claustrophobia.

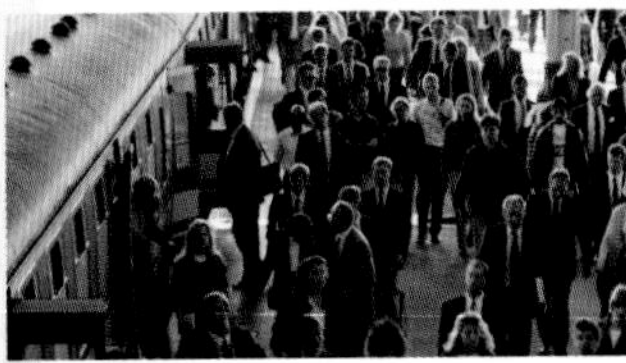

FEAR OF CROWDS
Enochlophobia may be associated with other fears, such as fear of catching a disease or being trampled.

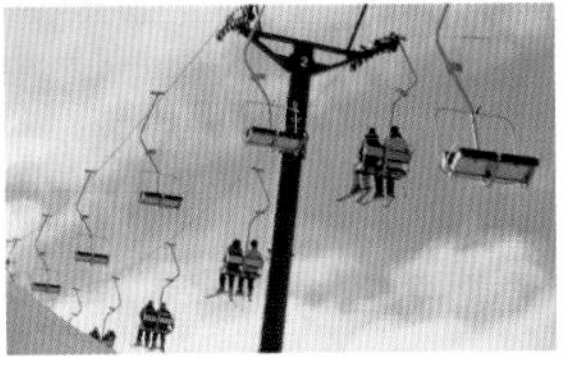

ACROPHOBIA
Fear of heights is a generalized fear of being in a high place, even an enclosed space such as a high floor in a building.

PHOBIAS

A PHOBIA IS CONSIDERED TO BE A DISORDER WHEN PERSISTENT, IRRATIONAL FEARS OF PARTICULAR THINGS, ACTIVITIES, OR SITUATIONS DISRUPT EVERYDAY LIFE.

There are many different forms of phobia, but they can be categorized into two broad types: simple and complex. Simple phobias are fears of specific objects or situations, for example, spiders (arachnophobia) or enclosed spaces (claustrophobia). Complex phobias are more pervasive and involve several anxieties. For example, agoraphobia may involve fear of crowds and public places or of travelling in planes, buses or other forms of public transport; it also includes anxiety about being unable to escape to a safe place, usually home. Social phobia (also known as social anxiety disorder) is another complex phobia in which there is intense anxiety in social or performance situations (such as public speaking) because of fear of public embarrassment or humiliation.

Causes and effects

The causes of phobias are not known for certain, Some phobias tend to run in families, which may be a result of children learning a specific fear from their parents. In other cases, a phobia may develop in response to a traumatic event or situation.

The main symptom of a phobia is an intense, uncontrollable anxiety when confronted by the feared object or situation. Merely anticipating an encounter with the feared object or situation can cause anxiety. In severe cases there may be symptoms of a panic attack, such as sweating, palpitations, breathing difficulty, and trembling, when the object or situation is actually encountered. There is also usually a strong desire to avoid the feared object or situation, often to the extent of taking extreme measures. These effects can severely limit normal everyday activities and sometimes a person with a phobia may try using drugs or alcohol in an attempt to reduce the anxiety.

COMMON PHOBIAS

NAME	DESCRIPTION
Astraphobia	Fear of thunder and lightning
Carcinophobia	Fear of cancer
Claustrophobia	Fear of enclosed spaces
Cynophobia	Fear of dogs
Mysophobia	Fear of contamination by germs
Necrophobia	Fear of death or dead things
Nosophobia	Fear of developing a specific disease
Nyctophobia	Fear of the dark
Ophidiophobia	Fear of snakes
Trypanophobia	Fear of injections or medical needles

POST-TRAUMATIC STRESS DISORDER

A SEVERE ANXIETY RESPONSE CAN DEVELOP AFTER A PERSON IS INVOLVED IN OR WITNESSES A DISTRESSING OR LIFE-THREATENING EVENT, SUCH AS A TERRORIST ATROCITY, NATURAL DISASTER, RAPE OR PHYSICAL VIOLENCE, SERIOUS PHYSICAL INJURY, OR MILITARY COMBAT.

The external cause of post-traumatic stress disorder (PTSD) is the experience of trauma. In the brain itself, various abnormalities in areas involved in memory, the stress response, and the processing of emotions have been identified. The amygdala (involved in memory and emotion processing) is overactivated in response to memories of traumatic events whereas the prefrontal cortex is under-responsive to fearful stimuli, which may result in its failure to inhibit the amygdala and thereby inhibit traumatic memories. The thalamus may also be involved; some people have a genetic constitution that is associated with an enlarged thalamus, which may in turn lead to an exaggerated response to fearful memories and an increased susceptibility to PTSD.

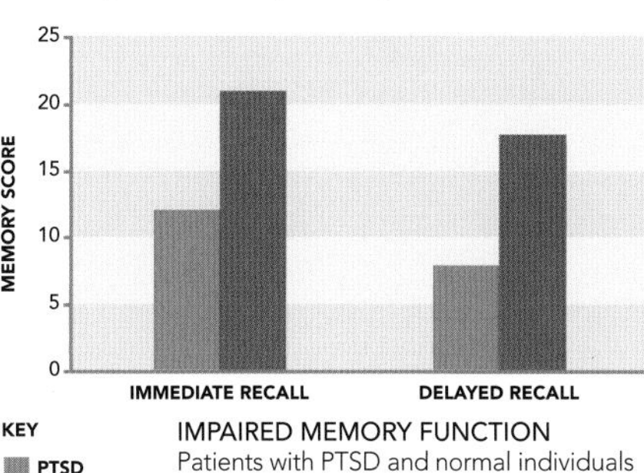

KEY
PTSD PATIENTS
CONTROLS

IMPAIRED MEMORY FUNCTION
Patients with PTSD and normal individuals (controls) were read a paragraph and asked to recall it immediately and after a delay. PTSD patients scored lower on both tests.

Symptoms and treatment

The symptoms of PTSD may develop immediately after a traumatic event or may not appear for months. They may include flashbacks or nightmares that trigger the same intense fear originally felt; emotional numbness; loss of enjoyment in usually pleasurable activities; memory problems; hypervigilance and an exaggerated startle response; sleeping problems; and irritability.

SHELL SHOCK

Stress reaction to the trauma of combat – shell shock – came to be widely recognized during World War I. Today, the term "shell shock" is categorized as "combat stress reaction" and refers to a collection of short-lived physical and mental symptoms, such as exhaustion and hypervigilance. If symptoms persist long-term, the condition is usually categorized as PTSD.

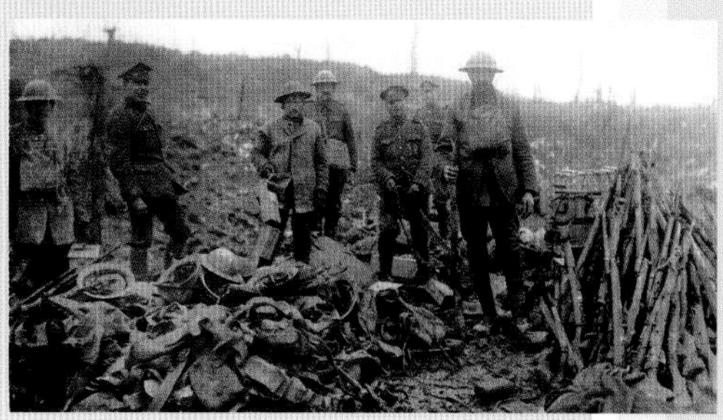

OBSESSIVE–COMPULSIVE DISORDER

COMMONLY KNOWN AS OCD, OBSESSIVE–COMPULSIVE DISORDER IS CHARACTERIZED BY RECURRENT THOUGHTS THAT CAUSE ANXIETY AND/OR OVERWHELMING URGES TO PERFORM REPETITIVE ACTS OR RITUALS IN AN ATTEMPT TO RELIEVE ANXIETY.

The exact cause of OCD is not known, but it is generally thought to be due to a combination of factors and may have different causes in different people. OCD tends to run in families, so there may be a genetic link in some cases. It has also been associated with childhood infection with streptococcus bacteria. Brain imaging studies have found evidence of abnormal physiological connections in the communication loop between the orbitofrontal cortex, caudate nucleus, and thalamus involving the neurotransmitter serotonin. In addition, personality type may be a factor, as perfectionists appear to be more susceptible to developing OCD.

Symptoms

Symptoms typically appear during the teenage or early adult years and may consist of obsessions, compulsions, or both. Obsessions are thoughts, feelings, or images that recur involuntarily and provoke anxiety. For example, there may be an excessive fear of dirt that may be so powerful that the person fears leaving home in case he or she becomes contaminated. Compulsions are actions that a person feels compelled to carry out repeatedly in an effort to ward off anxiety, such as repeatedly checking things such as locks or doors. The person may recognize that the obsessions and/or compulsions are unreasonable but cannot control them.

Diagnosis and outlook

To be diagnosed with OCD, the symptoms must cause anxiety, must be present on most days for at least two weeks, and must interfere significantly with everyday life. With treatment most people recover, although symptoms may recur under stress. Deep brain stimulation, in which tiny electrodes are inserted into the brain to modulate the activity, is a promising new treatment for this condition.

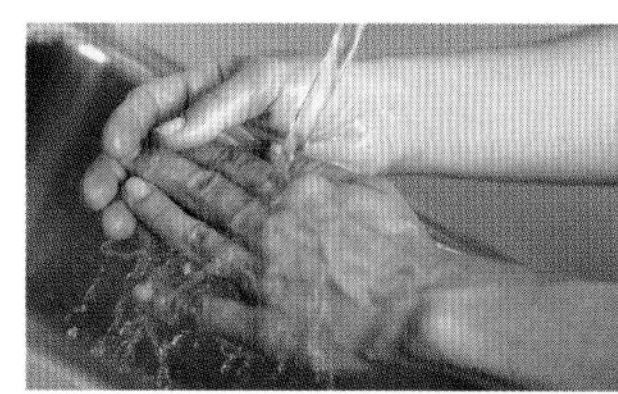

COMPULSIVE BEHAVIOUR
Compulsions, such as constant handwashing, are actions that a person feels compelled to carry out repeatedly.

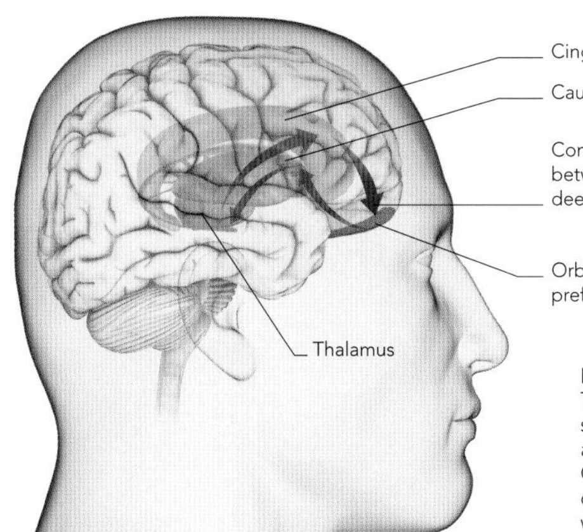

BRAIN CIRCUIT IN OCD
This disorder may be associated with abnormalities in the communication circuit between the orbital prefrontal cortex and deeper brain structures.

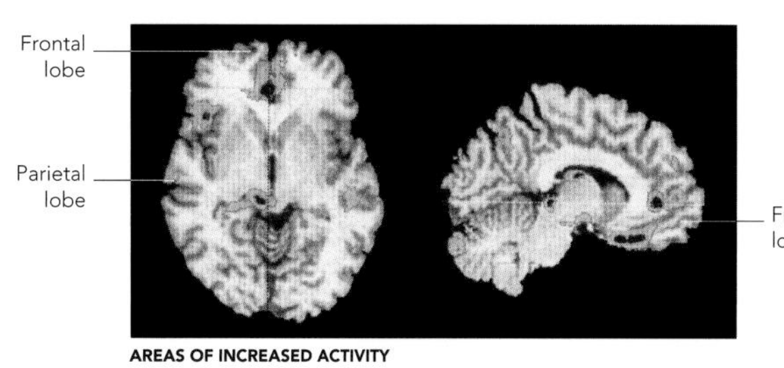

BRAIN ACTIVITY IN OCD
These coloured PET scans show patterns of brain activity associated with OCD. In the top pair, the colours show areas in which activity is increased when OCD symptoms get stronger. The bottom scans show areas of decreased activity when symptoms strengthen.

BODY DYSMORPHIC DISORDER

BODY DYSMORPHIC DISORDER (BDD) IS A MENTAL HEALTH PROBLEM IN WHICH A PERSON IS EXCESSIVELY CONCERNED ABOUT A PERCEIVED DEFECT IN HIS OR HER APPEARANCE AND THIS PREOCCUPATION WITH BODY IMAGE CAUSES SIGNIFICANT DISTRESS.

The cause of body dysmorphic disorder is unclear, although it is thought to be due to a combination of several factors, possibly including low levels of serotonin. It may occur in combination with other disorders, such as eating disorders, obsessive-compulsive disorder, and generalized anxiety disorder, although it is not clear whether there is a causative relationship with such disorders.

Many people are dissatisfied with some aspect of their appearance, but people with BDD are obsessed with one or more perceived flaws. Typical signs of BDD include refusing to be in photographs; trying to hide the "flaw" with clothing or make-up; constantly checking one's appearance in mirrors; frequently comparing one's appearance with that of others; often seeking reassurance about one's appearance; frequently touching the perceived flaw; and picking the skin to make it smooth. In addition, a person may feel anxious and self-conscious around other people because of the perceived flaw and may avoid social situations in which it might be noticed. In some cases, medical and surgical treatment may be sought to correct the perceived flaw.

Diagnosis

Body dysmorphic disorder is diagnosed by psychiatric evaluation. To be diagnosed with this disorder, preoccupations with appearance must cause considerable distress and interfere with everyday life.

Right hemisphere

Active area in left hemisphere

PROCESSING FACES IN BDD
Studies of BDD patients have revealed that they tend to use the left side of the brain, which normally processes complex detail, for processing pictures of faces. Normal people usually use their right hemisphere, unless they are examining a face closely.

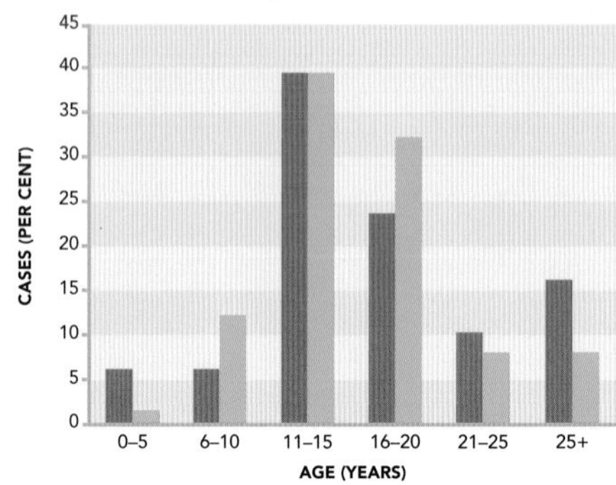

AGE OF ONSET
Body dysmorphic disorder most commonly first appears during puberty or early adulthood. The peak age of onset is 11–15 years for both males and females, with about 40 per cent of cases starting in this age group.

SOMATIZATION DISORDER

IN THIS CHRONIC PSYCHOLOGICAL PROBLEM, A PERSON COMPLAINS OF PHYSICAL SYMPTOMS FOR WHICH NO UNDERLYING PHYSICAL CAUSE IS FOUND.

A person with this disorder typically experiences several physical symptoms that persist for years. The symptoms are not generated intentionally and are often severe enough to interfere with everyday life, but no physical cause for them can be identified.

The symptoms may affect any part of the body, but complaints involving the digestive, nervous, and reproductive systems are the most common. If symptoms involve the voluntary central nervous system, such as paralysis, the condition is sometimes classed as conversion disorder (formerly known as hysteria).

The cause of somatization disorder is not known. In some cases it may be associated with other disorders such as anxiety and depression, but it is not clear whether these are causes or effects of the disorder.

HYSTERIA

The term "hysteria" originates from the Greek word *hysterikos*, which referred to a medical disorder caused by disturbances of the uterus. The Austrian psychoanalyst Sigmund Freud (see p.189) suggested that hysteria was an attempt by the subconscious to protect the patient from stress. The term is no longer generally used in psychiatry, although it is still in everyday use to refer to a state of uncontrollable emotional excess.

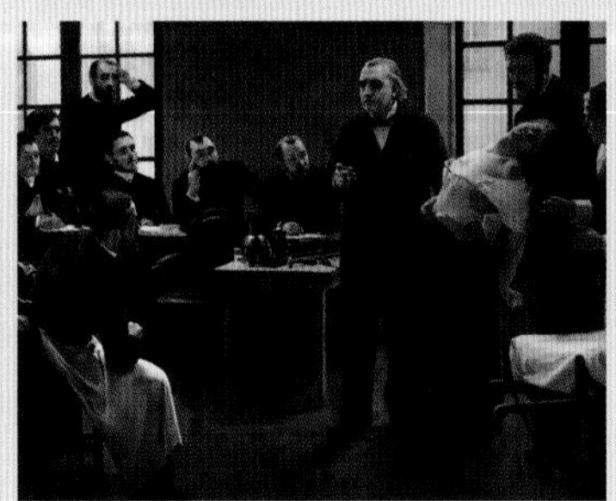

DEMONSTRATION OF HYSTERIA
Hysteria was believed to be an inherited neurological disorder by the French neurologist Jean-Martin Charcot (1825–93), who used hypnosis to induce hysteria in patients and then studied the results.

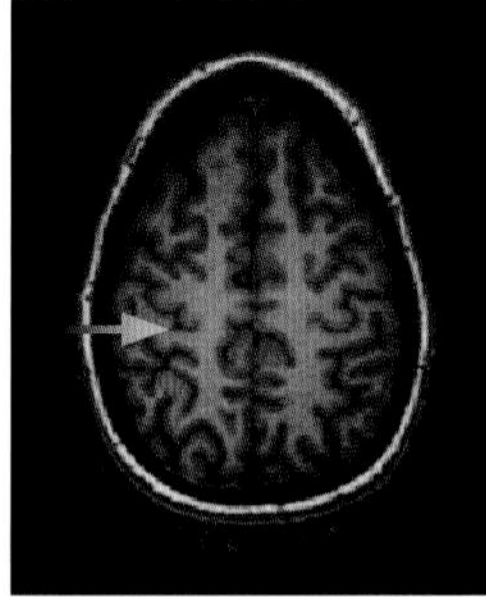

LEFT HAND STIMULATED

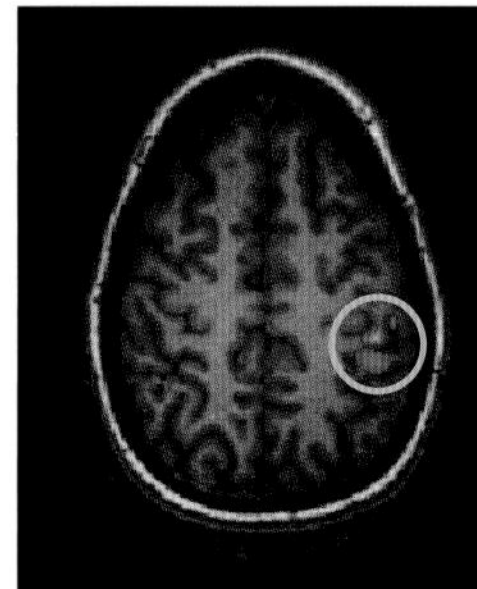

RIGHT HAND STIMULATED

BRAIN ACTIVITY
Unusual patterns of brain activity may be detected in some cases of somatization disorder. These MRI scans show the brain of a person who experiences a loss of sensation in the left hand (the right side of the brain appears on the left in the images). The scans reveal an absence of brain activity (shown by the arrow) in the right somatosensory cortex when the left hand is stimulated. There is normal brain activity (circle) when the unaffected right hand is stimulated.

HYPOCHONDRIA

THIS DISORDER IS CHARACTERIZED BY EXCESSIVE AND UNREALISTIC ANXIETY ABOUT HAVING A SERIOUS ILLNESS.

In hypochondria (also known as hypochondriases) trivial symptoms assume unrealistic significance. The symptoms are real, such as a cough or headache, but people with hypochondria are genuinely worried that they indicate a serious disease, such as lung cancer or a brain tumour. In mild forms, the person may simply worry constantly. In more severe cases, hypochondria can seriously disrupt everyday life, with the person making frequent visits to the doctor to have tests. Even when the test results prove negative, people may remain convinced that they have a serious illness and often seek other medical opinions. In addition, the person may believe they have a particular disease after hearing about it; for example, after hearing about Alzheimer's disease, an instance of momentary forgetfulness might lead the person to believe they have that disease. Many people with hypochondria also have other mental health disorders, such as depression, obsessive–compulsive disorder, phobia, or generalized anxiety disorder.

MUNCHAUSEN'S SYNDROME

SOMETIMES ALSO KNOWN AS HOSPITAL ADDICTION SYNDROME, MUNCHAUSEN'S SYNDROME IS A RARE PSYCHIATRIC CONDITION IN WHICH A PERSON REPEATEDLY SEEKS MEDICAL ATTENTION FOR FAKED OR SELF-INDUCED SYMPTOMS OF ILLNESS.

People with Munchausen's syndrome are aware that they are fabricating symptoms, unlike those with hypochondria, who truly believe they are ill. They do not fake illness in order to receive tangible benefits (such as financial gain). Instead, the motive seems to be to obtain investigation, treatment, and attention from medical personnel. People with the syndrome often have a good medical knowledge and create plausible symptoms and explanations for their faked illness, which makes diagnosis of Munchausen's syndrome very difficult. As well as lying about symptoms, they may try to manipulate test results – for example, by adding blood to a urine sample – and may even inflict symptoms on themselves; they may injure themselves or ingest poisons, for instance. Typically, they attend many different hospitals, often repeatedly presenting the same symptoms. In a related condition, known as Munchausen's by proxy or fabricated and induced illness (FII), people may invent or induce symptoms in somebody else. This usually involves a parent faking or inducing symptoms in their child.

Diagnosis is difficult and involves carrying out various tests to exclude an underlying illness. If a genuine underlying cause is not found, a diagnosis is made from a psychiatric assessment.

FEIGNING DISEASE

Many people feign illness at some point in their lives, but in the majority of cases it is simply an occasional occurrence – to avoid going to work or school, for example. However, in some people fabricating illness is a pathological problem. This chart summarizes the ways in which feigning illness can be classified.

Non-pathological
This form of feigning typically involves using minor symptoms as a means of avoidance or of getting attention. The feigning tends to occur only sporadically and for no tangible gain.

Pathological
Pathological disease feigning, unlike the non-pathological form, tends to occur repeatedly and usually involves the feigner obtaining a significant tangible gain, such as a financial reward.

Malingering
This is the intentional use of false or exaggerated symptoms to obtain a significant gain, such as financial compensation or sympathy. It is not a disorder itself, but it may indicate a mental problem.

Factitious disorders
These involve intentional disease forgery to obtain emotional gain, such as sympathy, attention, and nurturing. Extreme forms of factitious disorders include Munchausen's syndrome.

TOURETTE'S SYNDROME

TOURETTE'S SYNDROME IS A NEUROLOGICAL DISORDER THAT IS CHARACTERIZED BY SUDDEN, REPETITIVE, INVOLUNTARY MOVEMENTS (CALLED MOTOR TICS) AND NOISES OR WORDS (CALLED VOCAL TICS).

In most cases, Tourette's syndrome runs in families and genetic factors may be involved, although the relevant genes and the mode of inheritance have not been identified. In some cases, known as sporadic Tourette's syndrome, there is no apparent inherited link. Various brain abnormalities have been implicated, including malfunctioning of the basal ganglia, thalamus, and frontal cortex, and abnormalities in the neurotransmitters serotonin, dopamine, and norepinephrine, although their causative relationship to Tourette's has not been established. Environmental factors may also play a role in the development of Tourette's syndrome.

Symptoms and effects

The characteristic symptoms of Tourette's syndrome are motor tics, such as blinking, facial twitches, shoulder shrugging, and head jerking, and vocal tics, such as grunting or repeating words. The involuntary utterances of swear words (coprolalia) is a well-known feature, but is comparatively rare. Other mental health problems, such as depression or anxiety disorders, may also develop. Typically, the symptoms first appear during childhood and get worse during the teenage years but then improve. However, in some cases the condition gets progressively worse and lasts throughout adulthood.

Diagnosis

For a positive diagnosis of Tourette's, both motor and vocal tics must be present and they must not be due to another medical condition, medications, or other substances. They must occur several times a day on most days or intermittently for more than a year.

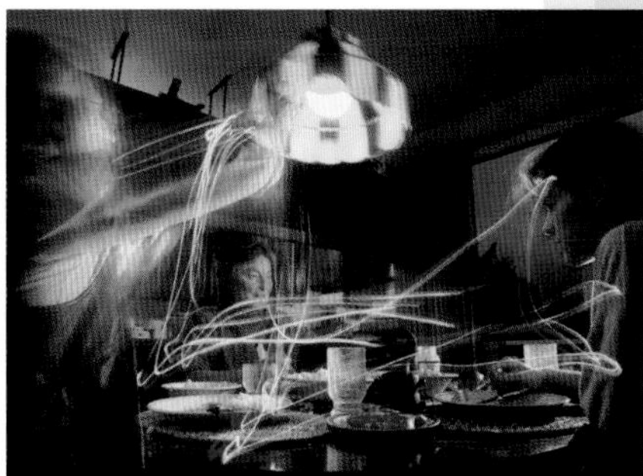

TOURETTE'S MOTOR TICS
This long-exposure photograph illustrates the repetitive movements characteristic of Tourette's syndrome. A Tourette's sufferer, on the left, has had lights attached to his fingers to show his hand movements.

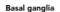

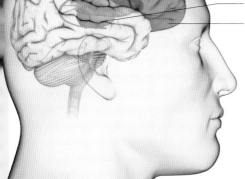

Basal ganglia
Responsible for implementing movement routines

Thalamus
Filters and relays nerve impulses to the cortex

Frontal cortex
Plays a key role in sequencing actions

IMPLICATED BRAIN AREAS
Brain studies of people with Tourette's have found abnormalities in certain areas of the brain, including the basal ganglia, thalamus, and frontal cortex, but it is not clear if these are a cause or effect of the disorder.

EXPERIMENTAL TREATMENT

Most people with Tourette's learn to live with it and do not require treatment. In severe cases, it is usually treated primarily with medication to help control the tics, although talking therapy may also be useful, particularly if there are other problems such as anxiety or obsessions. In a few, very severe, debilitating cases that have not responded to other treatments, deep-brain stimulation has been used. However, this procedure is still highly experimental and it is not yet clear whether the benefits outweigh the risks.

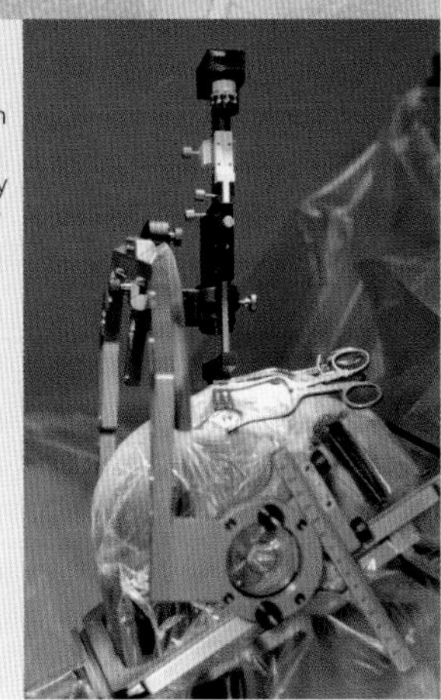

DEEP BRAIN STIMULATION
This procedure involves surgically implanting a device known as a brain pacemaker into the brain (as shown here). The pacemaker sends electrical impulses to specific areas of the brain, thereby controlling their activity.

SCHIZOPHRENIA

A SERIOUS MENTAL HEALTH DISORDER, SCHIZOPHRENIA IS CHARACTERIZED BY DISTORTIONS IN THINKING, PERCEPTIONS OF REALITY, EXPRESSION OF EMOTIONS, SOCIAL RELATIONSHIPS, AND BEHAVIOUR.

Contrary to popular belief, schizophrenia is not a "split personality", but rather a form of psychosis in which a person is not able to distinguish what is real from what is imagined.

The cause of schizophrenia is not known, although it is believed to result from a combination of genetic and environmental factors. Schizophrenia runs in families, and a person who has a close family member with the disorder is at increased risk of developing it. However, it is believed that genetic susceptibility alone is insufficient to cause schizophrenia and environmental factors are also necessary. Among the environmental factors that may be involved are exposure to infection or malnutrition before birth, stressful life events, and the use of marijuana. Excess dopamine levels may also be involved as all antipsychotic drugs block dopamine, and drugs that release dopamine can trigger schizophrenia. Various brain abnormalities have been identified in people with schizophrenia, including unusually low levels of glutamate receptors and a reduction of grey matter in certain brain regions, notably the hippocampus, frontal lobes, and temporal lobes. However, the significance of these abnormalities in schizophrenia has not been established.

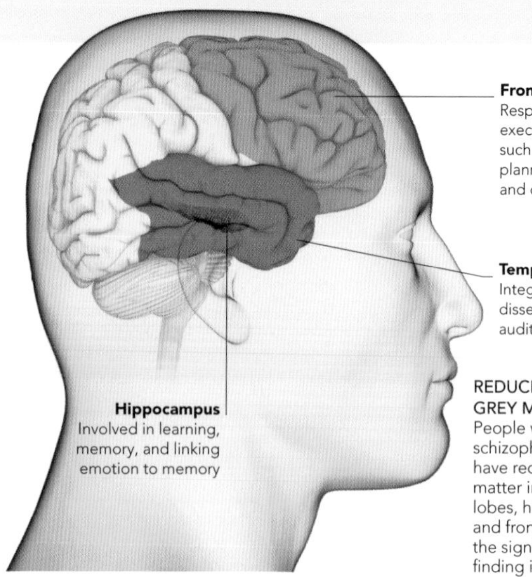
Frontal lobe
Responsible for executive functions, such as attention, planning, motivation, and decision-making
Temporal lobe
Integrates and disseminates auditory information
Hippocampus
Involved in learning, memory, and linking emotion to memory

REDUCED GREY MATTER
People with schizophrenia typically have reduced grey matter in the temporal lobes, hippocampus, and frontal lobes, but the significance of this finding is not clear.

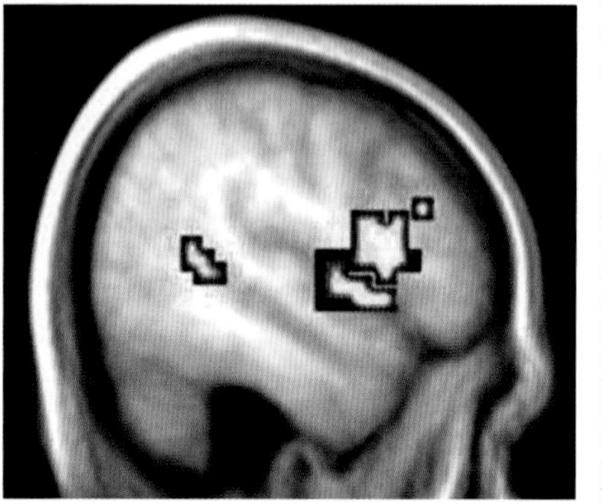

HEARING VOICES
During auditory hallucinations, fMRI scans show activity mainly in right-hemisphere language areas, rather than in the left-hemisphere areas typically active in speech production. This may explain why the speech produced by the "voices" is simple and derogatory and why the patient mistakenly attributes them to an external source.

Symptoms and treatment

Schizophrenia can take various forms (see panel, left). The symptoms typically develop during late adolescence or early adulthood in men, and some 4–5 years later in women. Different individuals may have different patterns of symptoms, and with varying degrees of severity. However, in general they may include delusions; hallucinations, especially auditory ones; jumbled, incoherent speech (so-called "word salad"); lack of emotions or inappropriate emotions, such as amusement at bad news; disorganized thoughts; clumsiness; involuntary or repetitive movements; social isolation; neglect of personal health and hygiene; and unresponsive (catatonic) behaviour.

Schizophrenia is diagnosed from the symptoms, but various tests are also usually performed to exclude other possible causes of abnormal behaviour. Treatment is with medication, such as antipsychotic drugs, and talking therapy. About 1 in 5 people make a full recovery, but for the remainder schizophrenia is lifelong.

TYPES OF SCHIZOPHRENIA

TYPE	DESCRIPTION
Paranoid schizophrenia	Delusions (particularly about being persecuted) and hallucinations are present, but thinking, speech, and emotions are often relatively normal.
Disorganized schizophrenia	Thinking and speech are confused and disordered, and emotions may be flat or inappropriate; behaviour is disorganized and often disrupts everyday activities, such as cooking or washing.
Catatonic schizophrenia	Lack of responsiveness to the surroundings and immobility are typical features; in some cases, the person may exhibit strange postures or purposeless movements, or repeat overheard words.
Undifferentiated schizophrenia	Some of the symptoms of paranoid, disorganized, or catatonic schizophrenia are present, but the pattern of symptoms does not clearly fall into any of the types above.
Residual schizophrenia	Symptoms of schizophrenia are present, but these are now significantly less severe than when the schizophrenia was originally diagnosed.

LOSS OF TISSUE
These MRI scans of a pair of twins show that the ventricles (indicated by arrows) are enlarged – suggesting loss of brain tissue – in the twin on the right, who is schizophrenic. The twin on the left is not affected.

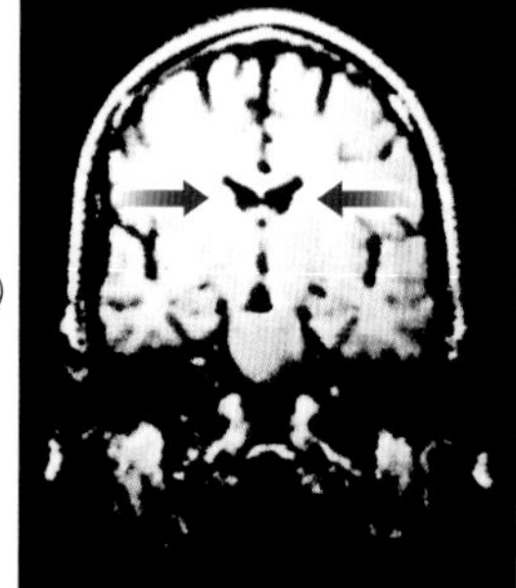

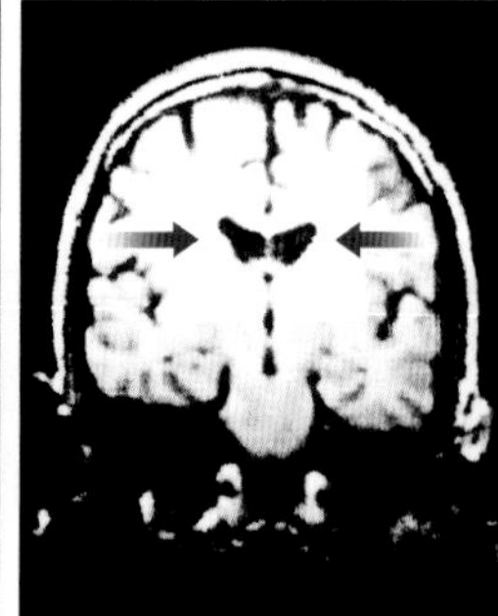

DELUSIONAL DISORDER

THIS DISORDER IS A TYPE OF PSYCHOSIS CHARACTERIZED BY THE PRESENCE OF PERSISTENT, IRRATIONAL BELIEFS THAT ARE NOT CAUSED BY ANOTHER MENTAL DISORDER.

In delusional disorder, the delusions are "non-bizarre" (involving things that are within the realms of possibility). Apart from the delusion and behaviour related to it, someone with the disorder often functions normally, although they can become so preoccupied with the delusion that everyday life is disrupted. The cause of delusional disorder is not known, but it is more common in people with family members who have the disorder or schizophrenia. Socially isolated people tend to be more susceptible, and in some cases it may also be triggered by stress.

There are several types of delusional disorder: jealous (the delusion that their partner is unfaithful); persecutory (a belief that somebody is hounding or trying to harm them); erotomanic (somebody – often a celebrity – is in love with them); grandiose (an inflated sense of worth, power, talent, or knowledge); somatic (the delusion that they have a physical defect or medical problem); and mixed (two or more of the other delusional types).

DE CLERAMBAULT'S SYNDROME
Also called erotomania, de Clerambault's syndrome is a rare delusional disorder in which the sufferer believes that another person is in love with him or her. This disorder is a central theme in British novelist Ian McEwan's *Enduring Love*.

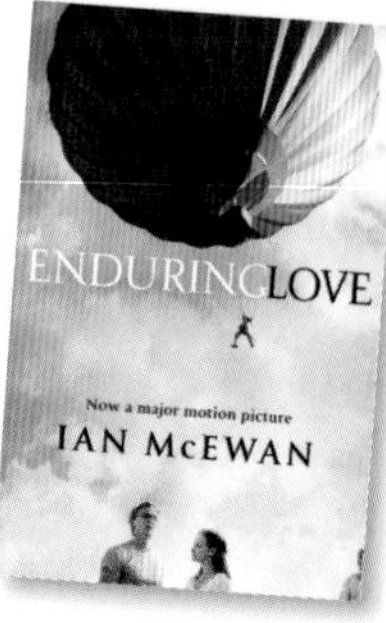
ENDURING LOVE
IAN McEWAN

ADDICTIONS

AN ADDICTION IS A STATE OF BEING SO DEPENDENT ON SOMETHING THAT IT BECOMES DIFFICULT OR IMPOSSIBLE TO DO WITHOUT IT FOR ANY SIGNIFICANT PERIOD.

It is possible to become addicted to anything, but whatever the addiction is, the person cannot control it. An addiction may be to a substance or to an activity.

It is believed that addictive substances or activities affect the brain so that it reacts in the same way that it responds to pleasurable experiences, by increasing the release of the neurotransmitter dopamine. It is not known why some people seem to be more likely to become addicted than others, although it is thought that genetic susceptibility and environmental factors probably play a role. For example, children who grow up in a family where there is drug or alcohol abuse are more likely to become addicted.

Although some symptoms are specific to the addictive substance or activity, there are several general symptoms that occur in all addictions. These include the development of tolerance – the need for increasing amounts to produce the desired effect; unpleasant physical and/or psychological withdrawal symptoms when the substance or activity is stopped; and continuing to use the substance or engage in the activity even though it may be detrimental to physical or mental health, or relationships.

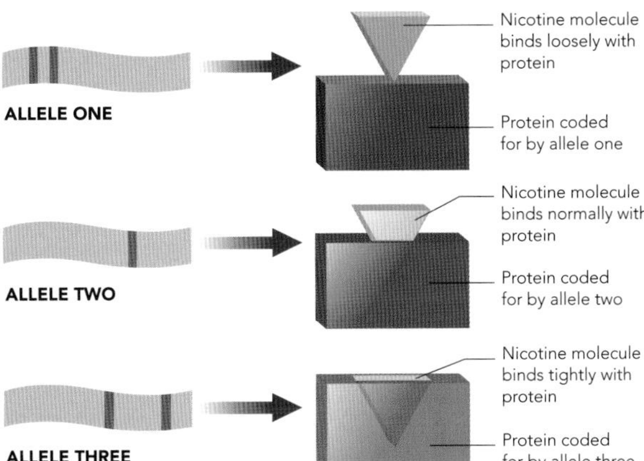

GENES AND NICOTINE ADDICTION

Research indicates that there may be a genetic factor involved in some addictions. In people who carry one version (allele) of a particular gene, the allele may code for a protein that binds only loosely with nicotine. In people who carry other alleles, the proteins they code for may bind normally or tightly to nicotine. The tightness of binding alters the effects nicotine has on the body, which may, in turn, affect the susceptibility to nicotine addiction.

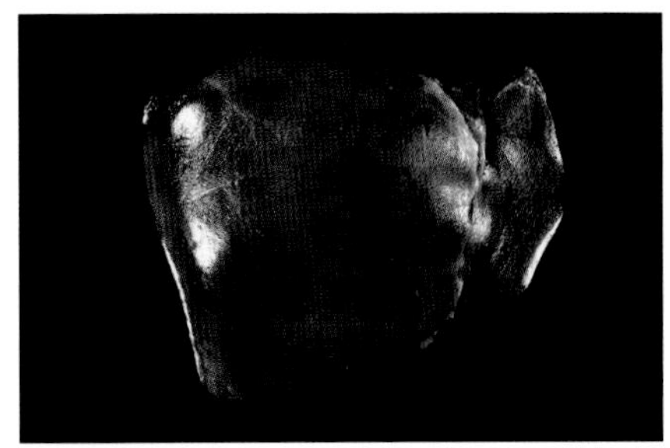

HEALTHY LIVER
A normal, healthy liver is dark red in colour, has a smooth outer surface without lumps or scar tissue, and is also free of areas of discoloration.

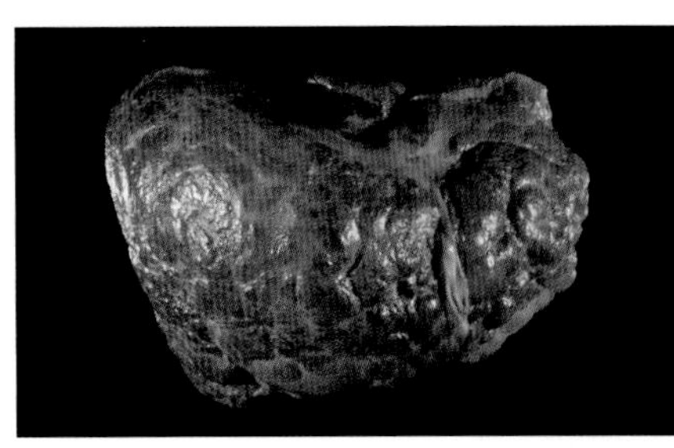

CIRRHOTIC LIVER
This liver shows advanced cirrhosis, with large areas of scar tissue, a lumpy surface, and general discoloration. Cirrhosis is one of the possible complications of alcohol addiction.

PERSONALITY DISORDERS

THIS IS A GROUP OF DISORDERS IN WHICH A PERSON'S HABITUAL BEHAVIOUR AND THOUGHT PATTERNS CAUSE RECURRENT PROBLEMS IN THEIR EVERYDAY LIFE.

The cause of personality disorders is not known but they are thought to be due to a combination of genetic and environmental influences. Factors that may increase the risk of developing a personality disorder include a family history of such a disorder or another mental illness; abuse during childhood; a dysfunctional family life during childhood; and having conduct disorder (see p.248) in childhood.

There are many types of personality disorders (see panel, below), but in general they are all characterized by an inflexible way of thinking and behaving, irrespective of the situation. Symptoms tend to develop in adolescence or early adulthood and may vary in severity. Often a person with a personality disorder is not aware that their behaviour and thought patterns are inappropriate, but they may be aware of problems with personal, social, or work relationships, and these problems may cause them distress. Specific symptoms depend on the type of personality disorder a person has.

TYPES OF PERSONALITY DISORDERS

Personality disorders are classified into three broad groups, known as clusters, according to the behavioural symptoms and types of thinking exhibited.

Cluster A The disorders that comprise this group are characterized by odd or eccentric behaviour and/or thinking.

Paranoid People with paranoid personality disorder are suspicious and distrustful of others, may believe others are trying to harm them, and tend to be hostile and emotionally detached.

Schizoid Those with this disorder are uninterested in social relationships, introverted and solitary, and have a limited range of emotional expression; often they seem unable to recognize normal social cues.

Schizotypal People with this type are socially and emotionally detached and exhibit peculiarities of behaviour and thinking, such as "magical" thinking (believing their thoughts can influence others).

Cluster B These are characterized by dramatic, erratic, or overemotional thinking and behaviour.

Antisocial Previously called sociopaths, people with this personality disorder persistently disregard the feelings, rights, and safety of others; they may also persistently lie, steal, or behave aggressively.

Borderline Borderline types have problems with self-identity and fear being alone, yet often have volatile relationships; they engage in impulsive or risky behaviour; and tend to have unstable moods.

Histrionic Histrionic types are highly emotional and constantly seek attention; they tend to be very sensitive to the opinions of others and overly concerned with their physical appearance.

Narcissistic Narcissistic types believe that they are superior to others, but still constantly seek approval; they tend to exaggerate their achievements and exhibit marked lack of empathy.

Cluster C The personality disorders that comprise this group are distinguished by habitual patterns of anxious, fearful, or inhibited thinking or behaviour.

Avoidant People with avoidant personality disorder feel inadequate and are oversensitive to criticism or rejection; they are timid and extremely shy in social situations, which may lead to social isolation.

Dependent People with this type of personality disorder are extremely dependent on, and submissive towards, others; they feel unable to cope with everyday life alone and often feel an urgent need to be in a relationship.

Obsessive-compulsive Those with this personality disorder conform rigidly to rules and moral codes, are inflexible, and often want to be in control; also tend to be perfectionists. This is not the same as OCD (see p.241), which is an anxiety disorder.

EATING DISORDERS

AN EATING DISORDER IS A CONDITION IN WHICH THERE ARE EXTREME PREOCCUPATIONS WITH FOOD AND/OR WEIGHT AND DISTURBANCES IN EATING BEHAVIOUR.

The causes of eating disorders are not clear, although a combination of biological, genetic, psychological, and social factors are thought to be involved. The effects of social and peer pressure to be thin may be a contributory factor. Anxiety about body image, low self-esteem, and depression, may also be involved.

Types of eating disorders

Eating disorders are most common in adolescent girls and young women, but also affect older women and males. The most common types are anorexia nervosa, bulimia nervosa, and binge-eating disorder.

Anorexia nervosa is characterized by self-starvation and excessive weight loss. Its main features are an intense fear of being fat or gaining weight; a resistance to maintaining normal weight; and the denial of the seriousness of low body weight. It can be fatal.

Bulimia nervosa is characterized by binge eating and then repeated compensatory actions to prevent weight gain, such as self-induced vomiting, laxative or diuretic use, excessive exercise, or fasting. It can result in life-threatening heart abnormalities due to an imbalance of electrolytes.

Binge-eating disorder is similar to bulimia nervosa but without the compensatory actions to counter the binges, which can lead to obesity.

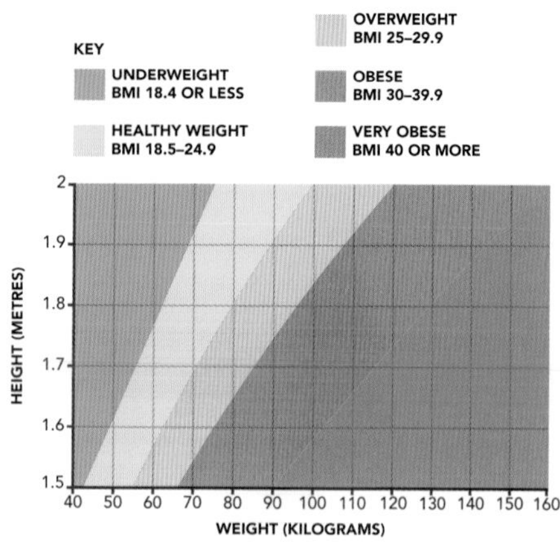

BODY MASS INDEX
Body mass index (BMI) is a figure that indicates whether wa person is within a healthy weight range. Adults with anorexia nervosa have a BMI of 17.5 or less.

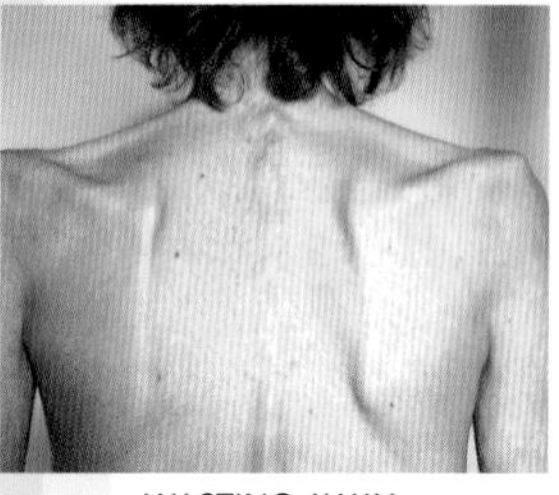

WASTING AWAY
The extreme weight loss associated with anorexia nervosa leads to wasting of body tissues, as is evident in this person with this disorder.

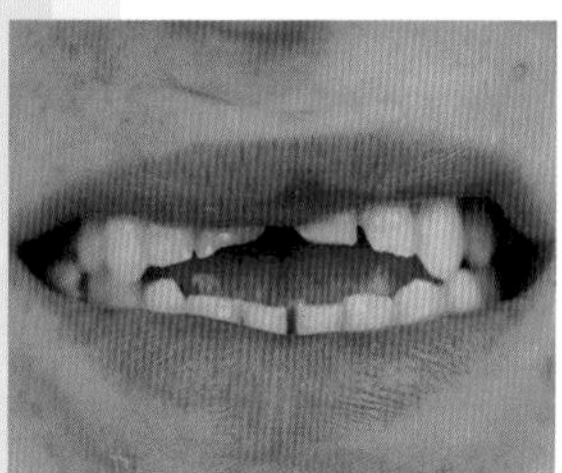

DENTAL EROSION
Repeated self-induced vomiting in bulimia nervosa can lead to erosion of tooth enamel by stomach acid, and this may lead to loss of teeth.

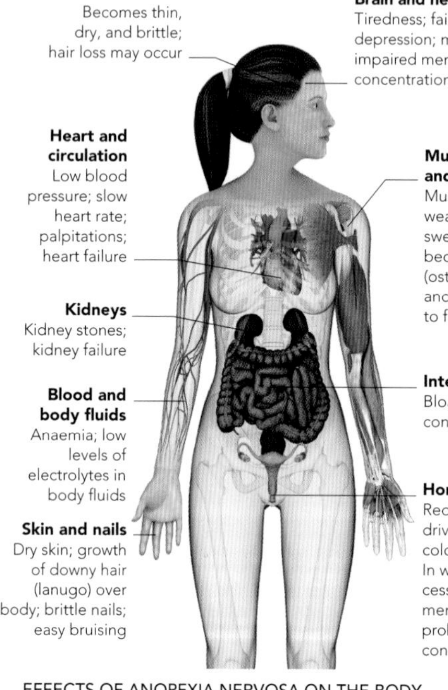

EFFECTS OF ANOREXIA NERVOSA ON THE BODY
The most obvious effect of anorexia nervosa is extreme weight loss. However, it can also have a number of other effects on the body and may even be fatal.

Brain and nervous system
Dizziness; depression; low self-esteem; often a realization that eating behaviour is abnormal

Heart and circulation
Low blood pressure; slow and/or irregular heart rate; heart-muscle disorders; heart failure

Stomach
Pain; bloating; delayed emptying; ulceration; stomach rupture

Skin
Dry skin

Muscles
Weakness

Mouth and teeth
Swollen, sore cheeks; gum disease; sensitive teeth; tooth erosion and decay; tooth loss

Throat and oesophagus
Sore, irritated throat; inflammation of oesophagus; oesophageal rupture

Blood and body fluids
Anaemia; low levels of electrolytes in body fluids; dehydration

Intestines
Irregular bowel movements; bloating; abdominal cramps; constipation; diarrhoea

Hormones
Irregular or absent menstrual periods

EFFECTS OF BULIMIA NERVOSA ON THE BODY
Bulimia nervosa tends to have less obvious outward effects than anorexia nervosa as the person is often of normal weight. However, repeated bingeing and purging can have widespread physical effects.

ATTENTION DEFICIT HYPERACTIVITY DISORDER

COMMONLY KNOWN AS ADHD, ATTENTION DEFICIT HYPERACTIVITY DISORDER IS ONE OF THE MOST COMMON BEHAVIOURAL DISORDERS OF CHILDHOOD.

ADHD is characterized by persistent difficulty in paying attention and/or hyperactivity. It is most common in children, but it may persist into adulthood. ADHD tends to run in families and in most cases genetic inheritance, probably involving many genes, is thought to be the most probable underlying cause. However, this genetic predisposition interacts with various other factors, such as exposure to certain toxins (such as nicotine and alcohol) before birth, brain damage before birth or in the early years of life, and food allergies. There is no evidence that parenting problems cause ADHD, but they may influence its severity and a child's coping strategies. Some brain abnormalities have been found in children with ADHD, including low dopamine levels. Drugs that increase dopamine levels in the brain, such as Ritalin, may lessen symptoms. Symptoms usually appear during early childhood and may become worse when the child starts school. Due to the various ADHD-related problems, there may also be difficulty in making friends, low self-esteem, anxiety, or depression.

TYPES OF ADHD
Attention deficit hyperactivity disorder can be categorized into three broad types, according to the predominant type of behaviour exhibited.

Inattentive Symptoms include a short attention span; poor concentration; difficulty with carrying out instructions; and changing activities often.

Hyperactive/impulsive Characterized by fidgeting; excessive activity; acting without thinking; excessive talking; and repeatedly interrupting a speaker.

Combined Symptoms include those of both other types, such as a short attention span, overactivity, and acting without thinking.

DEVELOPMENTAL DELAY

DEVELOPMENTAL DELAY IS A TERM USED WHEN A BABY OR YOUNG CHILD HAS NOT ACQUIRED THE SKILLS AND ABILITIES NORMALLY ACHIEVED BY A PARTICULAR AGE.

In the few first years of life there are important stages – developmental milestones – when a child is normally expected to have acquired certain basic physical, mental, social, and langugae skills. Child development is assessed in several areas, including physical and motor development; vision, hearing, speech, and mental development; and social and emotional development.

Generalized or specific delay

Delays can vary in severity and may affect one or more areas of development. Generalized delay affects most areas of development and may be due to various factors, such as severe visual or hearing impairment; brain damage; learning difficulties; Down's syndrome; severe, prolonged disease, such as heart disease, muscle disease, or a nutritional disorder; or a lack of physical, emotional, or mental stimulation.

Developmental delay may also occur in specific areas only. Delay in movement and walking is quite common, and often a child catches up. However, there may be a serious underlying cause such as muscular dystrophy, cerebral palsy, or a neural-tube defect (as per p.237). Delay in speech and language development may have various causes, including lack of stimulation, hearing problems, or more rarely, autism. Generalized difficulty with muscle control that affects speaking, which may be due to cerebral palsy, for example, can also cause delay in this area.

WALKING UNAIDED
Being able to walk without help is one of the key developmental milestones. Typically, children manage this when between about 10 and 19 months old.

Diagnosis and treatment

Often delays are first noticed by parents, but a delay may also be detected during routine developmental checks. If a problem is suspected, a full developmental assessment is done, and the child may be referred to a specialist. Treatment depends on the severity and type of delay. It may include physical aids, such as glasses or hearing aids, therapies such as speech therapy, and possibly special educational help.

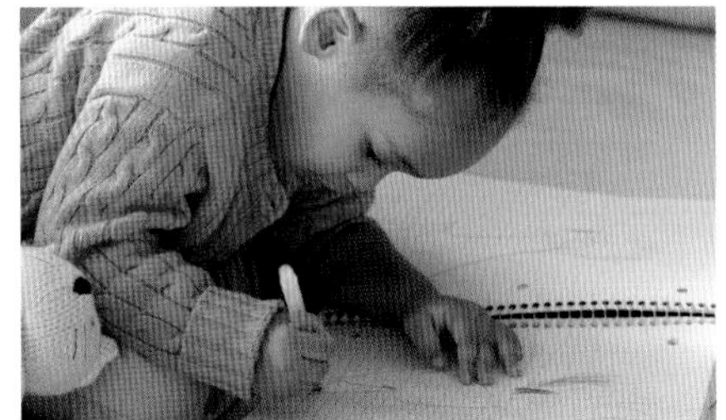

SCRIBBLING AND DRAWING
Normally, a child likes to scribble from about one year old, and by the age of about three most children are able to draw a reasonably straight line.

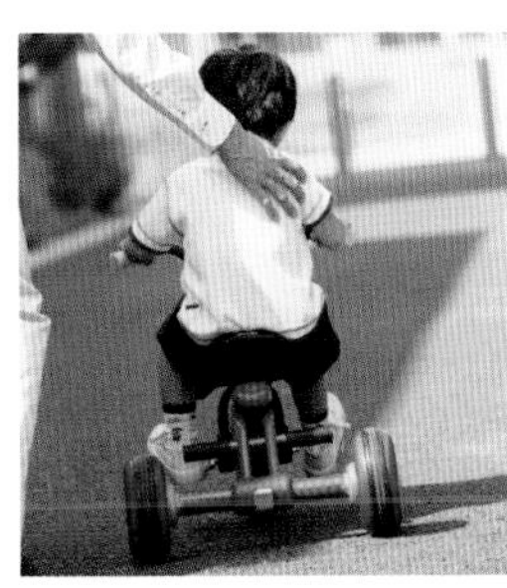

RIDING A TRICYCLE
The ability to pedal a tricycle is an indicator of motor-skill and physical development. Normally, this ability develops between about two and three years of age.

DEVELOPMENTAL MILESTONES

AGE (YEARS): 0, 1, 2, 3, 4, 5

PHYSICAL AND MOTOR SKILLS

Babies are born able to perform basic reflex actions such as grasping. By a process of trial and error, they gradually acquire other physical skills and develop motor co-ordination. Initially, babies master control of their body posture and head, then go on to develop physical skills, such as crawling, standing, and walking.

- Can lift head to 45°
- Can walk without help
- Can hop on one leg
- Can bear weight on legs
- Can roll over
- Can walk upstairs without help
- Can stand by hoisting up own weight
- Can balance on one foot for a second
- Can sit unsupported
- Can pedal a tricycle
- Can crawl
- Can kick a ball
- Can catch a bounced ball

VISION AND MANUAL DEXTERITY

A newborn baby can only see clearly up to about a metre away. Vision gradually improves, and after about six months objects several metres away are clear. With the improvement in vision, and also with the continuing maturation of the motor system, dexterity and hand–eye co-ordination develop.

- Holds hands together
- Can copy a circle
- Likes to scribble
- Plays with feet
- Can draw a straight line
- Can copy a square
- Reaches out for a rattle
- Can pick up a small object
- Can grasp object between finger and thumb
- Can draw a rudimentary likeness of a person

SOCIAL SKILLS AND LANGUAGE

Within a few weeks of birth, a baby turns towards sounds, and also starts to squeal and smile spontaneously. As the baby hears language, he or she starts to associate words with objects, and may start to say "dada" and "mama" to the parents as early as about nine months of age. Social skills improve rapidly as the ability to communicate develops.

- Can drink from a cup
- Stays dry at night
- Smiles spontaneously
- Stays dry in the day
- Says "dada" and "mama" to parents
- Knows first and last names
- Squeals
- Can put two words together
- Can dress without help
- Starts to learn single words
- Can talk in full sentences

AGE (MONTHS): 0, 2, 4, 6, 8, 10, 12, 14, 16, 18, 20, 22, 24, 26, 28, 30, 32, 34, 36, 38, 40, 42, 44, 46, 48, 50, 52, 54, 56, 58, 60

LEARNING DISABILITY

LEARNING DISABILITY REFERS TO PROBLEMS IN UNDERSTANDING, REMEMBERING, USING, OR RESPONDING TO INFORMATION.

There are differences in opinion about what the term "learning disability" encompasses but, in general, it applies to conditions in which there is developmental delay. Confusingly, learning difficulty may also refer to a specific difficulty, for example, in reading or writing.

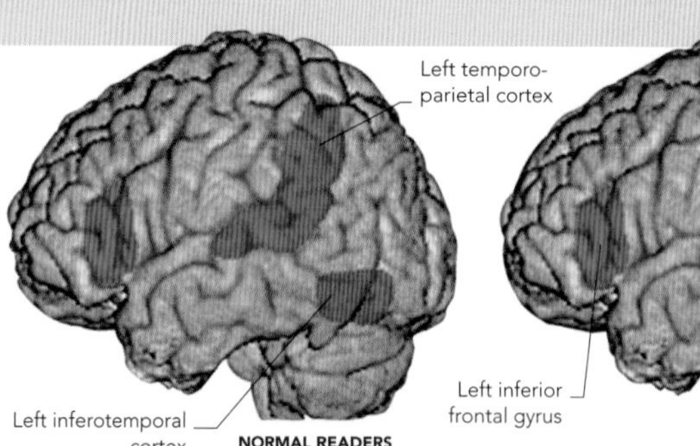

DYSLEXIC BRAIN
These two images show the areas of the brain that are active while reading in normal people (far left) and those with dyslexia (left). Only the left inferior frontal gyrus is active in those with dyslexia, whereas in normal readers other areas are also active.

Types

Learning disabilities are commonly categorized as generalized or specific. Generalized learning disability affects all or almost all intellectual functions, leading to developmental delay. In addition to below-average intelligence, there may also be behavioural problems and, in severe cases, physical developmental problems as well, impairing motor skills and co-ordination.

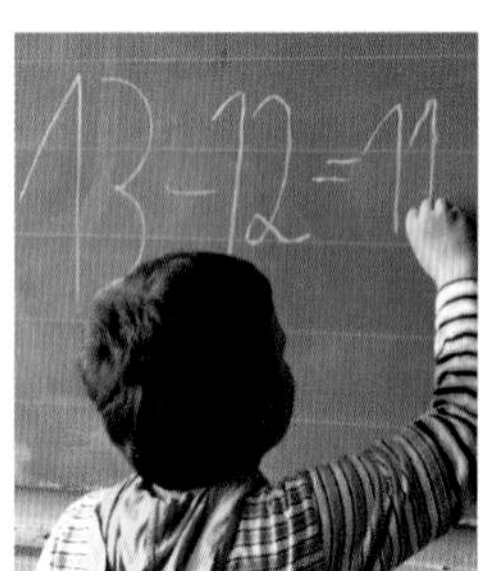

DYSCALCULIA
Difficulty with mathematics – dyscalculia – is the numerical counterpart of dyslexia. It usually first becomes apparent in the early school years when a child has problems with learning number facts and calculations such as addition and subtraction.

Specific learning disabilities (see table, below) affect only one or a few areas of mental functioning and, in many cases, intelligence is not impaired.

People with learning disability may also have various associated conditions, such as ADHD (see p.246), autistic disorder (see opposite page), or epilepsy (see p.226).

Causes

Learning disability can have a wide range of causes, including genetic abnormalities, such as Williams syndrome, or chromosomal abnormalities, such as Down's syndrome (see p.236) and fragile X syndrome (see below). Other factors include problems with brain development before or during birth, possibly due to exposure to toxins such as alcohol or drugs in the uterus, lack of oxygen, or premature or prolonged labour; and a head injury, malnutrition, or exposure to environmental toxins (such as lead) at a young age.

If a learning disability is suspected, a developmental assessment will be carried out. Hearing, vision, and other medical and genetic tests will also be done to check for underlying physical causes of the learning difficulties.

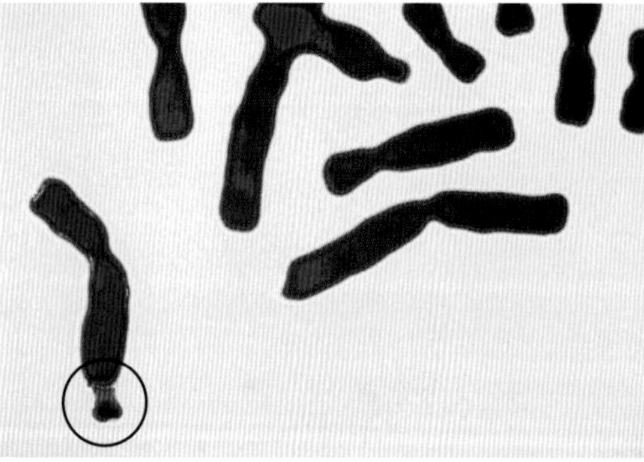

FRAGILE X SYNDROME
This syndrome is a major cause of severe learning disability in boys. It is caused by a constriction near the end of an X chromosome (circled), making it prone to break.

COMMON SPECIFIC LEARNING DISABILITIES

TYPE	DESCRIPTION
Dyslexia	Impaired ability to learn to read and/or write. As well as poor reading and spelling, there may also be difficulty with sequences, such as date order, and problems with organizing thoughts.
Dyscalculia	Difficulty performing mathematical calculations and trouble with learning mathematical concepts, such as quantity and place value, and with organizing numbers.
Amusia	Commonly called tone deafness, the inability in a person with normal hearing to recognize musical notes, rhythms, or tunes or to reproduce them.
Dyspraxia	The inability to make skilled movements with accuracy. It can cause difficulty with establishing spatial relationships, such as positioning objects accurately.
Specific language impairment	Difficulties with understanding and/or expressing oral language in a child with no physical impediment to hearing or speaking and no generalized developmental delay.

CONDUCT DISORDER

CONDUCT DISORDER IS A BEHAVIOURAL DISORDER IN WHICH A CHILD OR ADOLESCENT REPEATEDLY AND PERSISTENTLY BEHAVES IN A WAY THAT IS ANTISOCIAL.

Various factors put a child at increased risk of conduct disorder, including genetic factors, an unstable and/or violent family life, lack of supervision, abuse, and bullying. Learning disabilities (see above), attention deficit hyperactivity disorder (see p.246), and mental health problems such as depression also increase the risk. Children with conduct disorder also tend to have abnormal responses to reward and punishment.

Symptoms and effects

Symptoms vary from individual to individual, but they include aggressive behaviour, physical cruelty, theft or persistent lying, deliberate destruction of property, and violations of rules, such as playing truant from school. In some cases, a child may also engage in alcohol or drug abuse. Many children act in an antisocial or disruptive way from time to time, but in a child with conduct disorder the behaviour occurs repeatedly over a period of several months or longer. As a result of such behaviour, a child may find it difficult to make friends, have low self-esteem, and do poorly at school.

A diagnosis is usually based on a psychiatric assessment of the child's behaviour patterns. Treatment of conduct disorder, through talking therapies such as cognitive-behavioural therapy, can be difficult, but early treatment is more likely to be effective. It is important that parents are involved in the treatment.

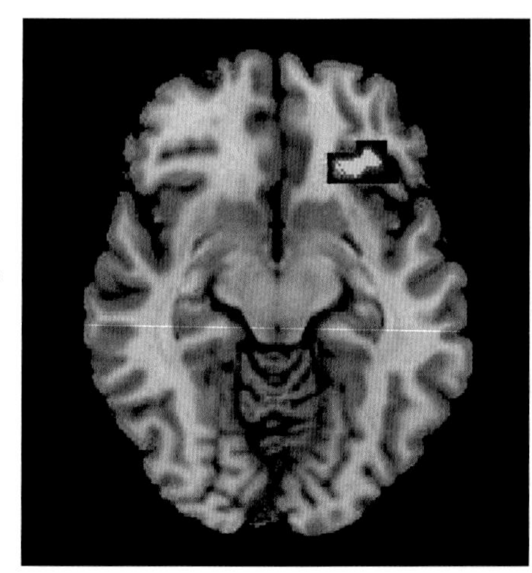

REDUCED BRAIN ACTIVITY
Children with conduct disorder tend to show reduced activity in the right orbitofrontal cortex (orange in this fMRI scan) when rewarded for a task. This supports the idea that this disorder arises from abnormal responses to the rewards and punishments that normally shape behaviour.

AUTISM SPECTRUM DISORDERS

THIS IS A GROUP OF DEVELOPMENTAL DISORDERS CHARACTERIZED BY PROBLEMS WITH COMMUNICATION, SOCIAL RELATIONSHIPS, AND REPETITIVE BEHAVIOUR.

There are several types of autism spectrum disorders, but the main ones are autistic disorder (sometimes referred to as "classic" autism) and high-functioning autism.

Autistic disorder usually appears in early childhood, before the age of about three years. It produces problems in three main developmental areas: impaired social skills, impaired communication, and restricted behaviour. Typically, a child fails to respond to their name or to other speech directed at them; avoids eye contact; resists physical contact; starts talking late and speaks with an abnormal tone or rhythm; shows abnormal response to social cues, such as faces and voices; performs repetitive movements, such as rocking; develops specific routines and becomes disturbed when they are changed; and may be unusually sensitive to sound, light, and touch, but sometimes ignore sensory signals. About half of all children with autistic disorder have learning difficulties and some children develop seizures. However, some children with autism have a high ability in one area, such as rote memory or precocious reading, and, rarely a child may have an exceptional ability in a specific area (called savant syndrome), such as mathematics. Children with high-functioning autism tend to have similar symptoms, but in a less severe form. Many children are of average or above average intelligence and develop speech and language skills at the normal time. However, they have very narrow interests, find it difficult to interact socially with their peers, and are usually inflexible in their behaviour and routines.

There is no cure for autism spectrum disorders, and treatment is based on supportive education to help a child reach his or her potential.

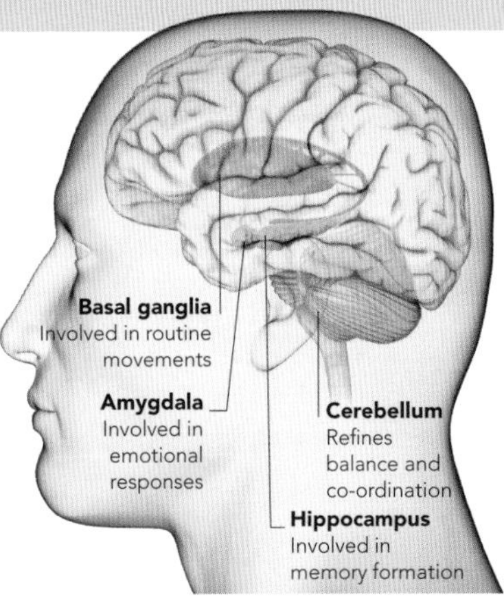

AFFECTED AREAS OF THE BRAIN
Autism has been associated with abnormalities in many brain regions (including those shown here), but their causal connection to autism is not yet clear.

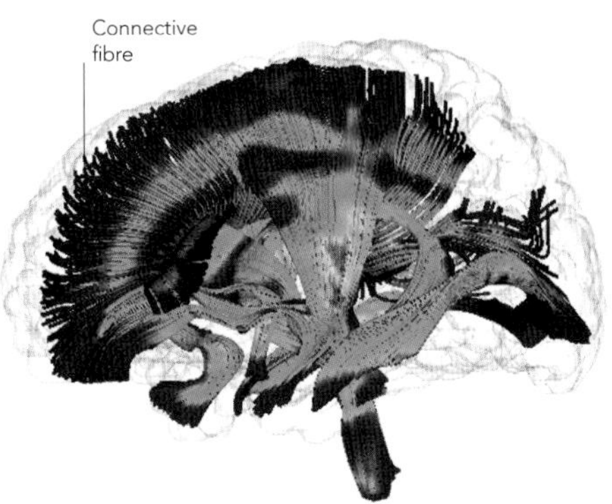

ORGANIZED CONNECTIONS
This diffusion tensor scan shows the clear, organized tracts of connective tissue in a healthy six-month-old brain. These fibres are disorganized in a person that goes on to develop autism.

RARE AUTISM SPECTRUM DISORDERS	
TYPE	**DESCRIPTION**
Rett syndrome	This autism spectrum disorder affects females almost exclusively, and is caused by a mutation in a single gene. Typically, there is a period of normal development but then autism-like symptoms begin to appear, usually between about six and 18 months of age. The child's development then regresses: she shies away from social contact and no longer responds to her parents. The child stops talking, if she had been talking before, loses co-ordination of her feet, has repeated writhing movements of her hands, and has inappropriate outbursts of crying or laughter.
Childhood disintegrative disorder	This very rare form of autism spectrum disorder primarily affects males. As with Rett syndrome, there is a period of normal development followed by the onset of autism-like symptoms and regression. Symptoms typically appear between the ages of three and four years, although they may sometimes appear as early as two years. There are extensive and severe losses of previously acquired social, language, and motor skills, and there may also be loss of bladder and bowel control, repetitive, stereotyped behaviour patterns, seizures, and severe intellectual impairment.

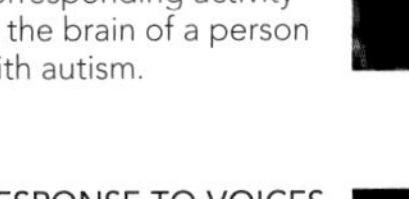

RESPONSE TO FACES
In these two MRI scans the yellow and red colours show areas of brain activity when looking at faces. In a normal person, there is activity in the fusiform gyrus of the temporal lobe (circled) but no corresponding activity in the brain of a person with autism.

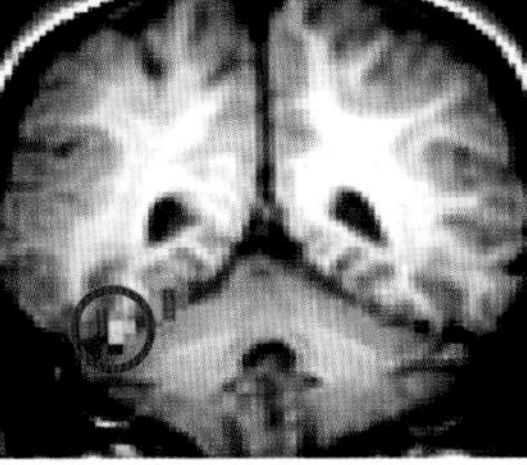

NORMAL BRAIN

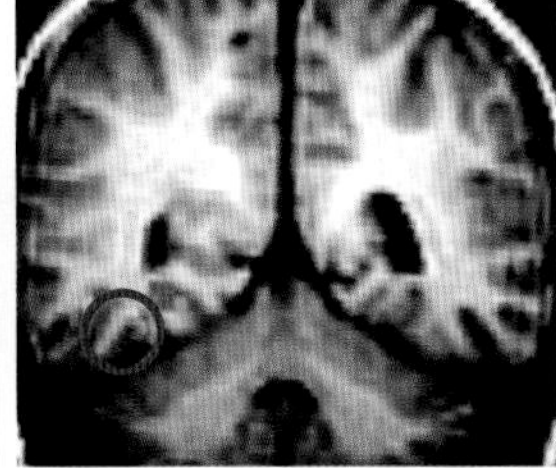

AUTISTIC BRAIN

RESPONSE TO VOICES
These two images show brain activity when normal people and those with autism listened to human voices. In the normal people, the superior temporal sulcus was active (the yellow and red area) whereas there was no activity in that area in those with autism.

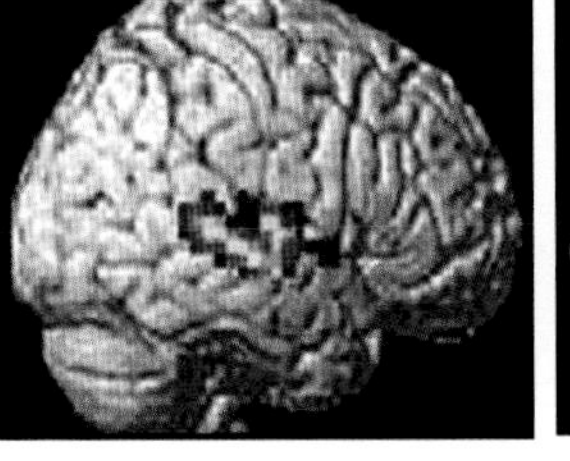

NORMAL BRAIN

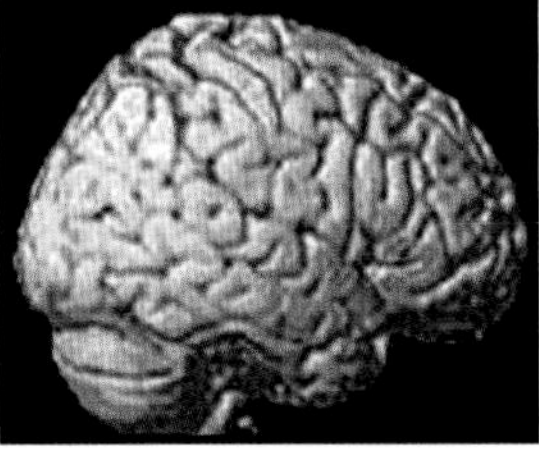

AUTISTIC BRAIN

TEMPLE GRANDIN

One of the best-known writers on autism, Temple Grandin is herself a high-functioning autist who has graphically described what it is like to have autism. Born in 1947 in the US, she was diagnosed with autism at the age of three. After a supportive early education, she attended ordinary schools, where she was often teased and picked on for being different. Nevertheless, she graduated from college and became a prominent researcher in animal science and welfare as well as an advocate for people with autism. In the field of animal welfare, she considers her autism, hypersensitivity to stimuli, and unusual visual thought processes to be a positive advantage, giving her a unique insight into the stresses livestock are vulnerable to. As a result of her early childhood experiences, Grandin is an advocate of early intervention and a supportive educational regime in autism, to help direct children with autism in productive directions. Even though autism affects every aspect of her life, Temple Grandin has said that she would not support a cure for all autism spectrum disorders.

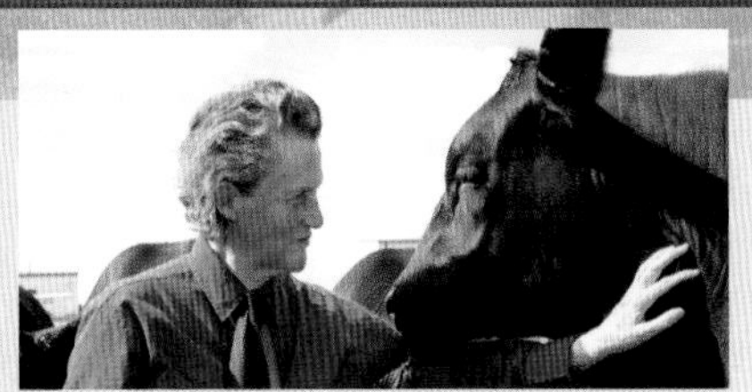

UNIQUE INSIGHT
Temple Grandin became famous for her ability to understand animals' minds and use her insights to improve their lives. Today she helps people on the autism spectrum to be more comfortable in the world.

GLOSSARY

A

acalculia The inability to perform numerical calculations due to neurological injury; see also *dyscalculia*.

acetylcholine A neurotransmitter that plays an important role both in learning and memory, and in sending messages from motor nerves to visceral muscles.

action potential A brief pulse of electrical current, generated by a neuron, which may be transmitted to neighbouring cells.

adrenaline and noradrenaline Hormones and neurotransmitters secreted by the adrenal gland; also referred to as epinephrine and norepinephrine.

afferent Travelling towards or entering; see also *efferent*.

agonist A molecule that binds to a receptor and stimulates the cell to fire; see also *antagonist*. An agonist is often a chemical that mimics the effect of a naturally occuring neurotransmitter.

agraphia The inability to write due to neurological injury.

alexia The inability to read due to neurological injury; also known as word blindness.

amnesia A general term for memory deficit.

amygdala A nucleus in the limbic area of the temporal lobe that is crucial to emotion.

androgens The sex steroid hormones (including testosterone), responsible for male sexual maturation and associated with stereotypically masculine behavioural traits.

angular gyrus A ridge of the neocortex in the parietal lobe, next to the temporal and occipital lobe. It is concerned with the position of the body in space and linking sound and meaning.

anomia The inability to name objects.

anosmia The inability to smell.

anosognosia The failure, due to neurological injury, to be aware of a deficit in oneself, such as paralysis or blindness.

ANS See *autonomic nervous system*.

antagonist A molecule that blocks or prevents activation of a receptor.

anterior The front, or towards the front.

anterograde amnesia The loss of memory of things that occur after a brain injury, especially after concussion.

apraxia A partial or total inability to perform co-ordinated movements, including speech.

arachnoid membrane The middle of the three meninges (layers of tissue that cover the brain).

arcuate fasciculus The nerve-fibre tract that connects Broca's and Wernicke's areas.

ascending reticular formation A part of the reticular formation, responsible for the arousal and sleep–wake cycle.

association areas The regions of the brain that combine different types of information to produce a "whole" experience.

astrocyte A type of support cell that provides brain cells with nutrients and insulation.

ataxia A symptom of neurological disorder in which the sufferer experiences difficulty with balance and co-ordinated movement.

athetosis A condition in which muscles make slow, involuntary, writhing movements, seen in some forms of epilepsy.

attention deficit hyperactivity disorder (ADHD) A syndrome of learning and behavioural problems characterized by a short attention span and often by inappropriately energetic or frenzied activity. It usually occurs first in early childhood.

auditory cortex The region of the brain responsible for receiving and processing information relating to sound.

autonomic nervous system (ANS) A component of the peripheral nervous system, responsible for regulating the activity of internal organs. It includes both the sympathetic and parasympathetic nervous systems.

axon The fibre-like extension of a neuron that carries electrical signals to other cells. Most neurons have only one axon.

B

basal ganglia A bundle of nuclei in the base of the forebrain, including the striatum and globus pallidus. It is mainly concerned with selecting and mediating movements.

bilateral On both sides of the body; for example, both brain hemispheres.

bipolar disorder An illness that is characterized by dramatic mood swings.

blindsight The ability to respond to visual stimuli in spite of being blind due to damage to the visual cortex.

blood–brain barrier A network of tightly packed cells surrounding the brain, which prevents toxic molecules from entering.

bottom-up Usually refers to relatively "raw" information flowing from the primary sensory areas of the brain rather than from areas involved in thinking, imagining, or creating expectations.

brainstem The lower part of the brain that becomes the spinal cord.

brainwaves The regular oscillations (firings) of neurons. Different rates of firing indicates different mental states; see also *electroencephalograph* (EEG).

Broca's area A frontal-lobe brain region, concerned with articulating speech.

Brodmann areas The microscopically distinct cortical areas that were mapped out by neurologist Korbinian Brodmann (1868–1918).

C

Capgras' delusion A rare syndrome in which people believe that a close friend or spouse has been replaced by a double. It is thought to be caused by damage to nerve pathways concerned with emotional recognition.

caudal Towards the tail end; see also *posterior*.

caudate nucleus A part of the striatum.

cell body The central structure of a neuron; also referred to as the soma.

central fissure Also called the central sulcus. A long, deep fissure that runs across the brain, dividing the parietal and frontal lobes.

central nervous system (CNS) The brain and spinal cord.

cerebellum The "small brain" behind the cerebrum that helps regulate posture, balance, and co-ordination.

cerebral cortex The outer, wrinkled "grey" part of the cerebral hemispheres.

cerebral hemispheres The two halves of the brain.

cerebrospinal fluid (CSF) The fluid found in the brain's ventricles, which brings nutrients to, and removes waste from, the brain.

cerebrum The major part of the brain, excluding the cerebellum and brainstem.

cerebellar penducles The short, stalk-like extensions of the cerebellum, which connect it to the brainstem.

cholinergic system The nerve pathways that are activated by the neurotransmitter acetylcholine.

cingulate cortex The area of cortex that makes up the sides of the longitudinal fissure. It is closely connected to the underlying limbic system as well as to cortical areas of the brain, and is important in combining "top-down" and "bottom-up" information to guide actions.

circadian rhythm A cycle of behaviour or physiological change lasting about 24 hours.

cochlea The spiral-shaped bony canal in the inner ear, containing the hair cells that transduce sound.

cognition Conscious and unconscious brain processes, such as perceiving, thinking, learning, and remembering information.

commisserectomy The surgical severing of the corpus callosum.

computed tomography (CT) A scanning technique that uses weak levels of X-ray to produce images of the brain and body.

concussion A brain trauma, usually caused by a blow to the head and resulting in temporary loss of consciousness.

cone A colour-sensitive receptor cell in the retina, used primarily for daytime vision.

contralateral On the other side of the body or brain. Damage to the brain often leads to problems on the contralateral side of the body; see also *ipsilateral*.

coronal A vertical "slice" through the brain, running parallel to the shoulders.

corpus callosum The thick band of nerve tissue that connects the left and right hemipsheres of the brain and carries information between them.

cortex See *cerebral cortex*.

Cotard's syndrome A rare disorder in which a patient asserts that they are dead, often claiming to smell rotting flesh or feel worms crawling over their skin.

cranial fossa The various bowl-shaped cavities in the skull. The posterior cranial fossa houses the brainstem and cerebellum.

cranial nerves The 12 pairs of nerves that arise from the brainstem. These include the olfactory nerve, which conveys information about smell to the brain, and the optic nerve, which carries data about vision.

cranium The skull.

D

decussation The crossing of nerve fibres, as in the optic chiasm.

delusion A false belief that is not easily eradicated by exposure to evidence that reveals its falsity.

dementia A loss of brain function due to degeneration through age or cumulative damage to the brain.

dendrite A branch that extends from a neuron's cell body and receives signals from other neurons.

dentate gyrus The part of the hippocampus containing nerve cells that receive input from the entorhinal cortex.

depression A common illness characterized by intense and chronically low mood and energy levels.

diencephalon A part of the brain that includes the thalamus and the area that surrounds it.

dopamine A neurotransmitter that produces motivation and strong feelings of pleasurable anticipation.

dorsal At or towards the (upper) back.

dorsal horn The back part (in cross section) of the spinal cord, where nerve fibres, especially pain-carrying fibres, merge with the spinal cord to travel upwards towards the brain.

dorsal route The pathway in the visual system that connects the visual cortex to the parietal lobe, also referred to as the "where" or "how" pathway; see also *ventral route*.

dorsolateral prefrontal cortex The area of the frontal lobe concerned with planning, organization, and various other executive functions of cognition.

dura mater The top of the three layers of tissue separating the brain from the skull; see also *meninges*.

dyscalculia A condition associated with difficulty in learning simple arithmetical operations in the absence of any other intellectual problems.

dyslexia A condition associated with difficulty in learning to read and write in the absence of any other intellectual problems.

E

EEG See *electroencephalograph*.

efferent Leading away from; see also *afferent*.

electroencephalograph (EEG) A graphic record of the electrical activity of the brain, made by attaching electrodes to the scalp that pick up the underlying brainwaves.

encephalin A type of endorphin.

encephalitis Inflammation of the brain.

endorphins A group of chemicals produced by the brain, which produce effects similar to those of opium.

entorhinal cortex The main route for information entering the hippocampus.

epilepsy An illness characterized by repeated seizures.

epinephrine See *adrenaline and noradrenaline*.

event-related potential (ERP) The neural activity generated in response to a given stimulus recorded by EEG.

excitatory neurotransmitter A type of neurotransmitter that encourages neurons to fire; see also *inhibitory neurotransmitter*.

explicit memory The memories that can be consciously retrieved and reported.

F

fissure A deep cleft, or sulcus, on the surface of the brain.

fMRI See *functional magnetic resonance imaging*.

forebrain A major part of the brain, including the cerebrum, thalamus, and hypothalamus.

fornix An arching band of nerve tissue that carries signals around the limbic system from the hippocampus at one end, to the mammillary bodies at the other.

fovea The central part of the retina, composed of densely packed cones. It is the area of the retina that has the highest visual acuity.

frontal lobe The area at the front of the brain, responsible for thinking, making judgements, planning, decision-making and conscious emotion.

functional imaging A range of techniques that allow neural activity to be measured and shown as visual images.

functional magnetic resonance imaging (fMRI) A brain-imaging technique in which magnetic resonance imaging is used to measure the changes in blood properties associated with neural activity; see also *magentic resonance imaging*.

fusiform gyrus A long cortical bulge on the underside of the temporal lobe, important for object and face recognition; see also *ventral route*.

G

gamma-aminobutyric acid (GABA) The major inhibitory neurotransmitter in the brain.

ganglion A cluster of interactive nuclei. The term also refers to light-sensitive cells in the retina.

Geschwind's territory A region of the brain concerned with language.

glial cells Also referred to as glia, the brain cells that support neurons by performing a variety of "housekeeping" functions in the brain. They may also mediate signals between neurons.

globus pallidus A part of the basal ganglia involved in movement control; see also *basal ganglia*.

glutamate The most common excitatory neurotransmitter in the brain.

grand mal See *seizure*.

grey matter The darker tissues of the brain, made up of densely packed cell bodies, as seen in the cortex.

gustatory cortex The area of the brain responsible for processing taste.

gyrus (*pl.* gyri) The bulges of tissue on the surface of the brain.

H

hallucination A false perception that occurs in the absence of any sensory stimuli.

hemiplegia A condition in which there is paralysis of one half of the body.

hemisphere One of the two halves of the brain.

hindbrain The back part of brain, adjoining the spine, which includes the cerebellum, pons, and medulla.

hippocampus A part of the limbic system lying on the inside of each temporal lobe. It is crucial for spatial navigation and encoding and retrieving long-term memories.

hormones The chemical messengers secreted by endocrine glands to regulate the activity of target cells. They play a role in sexual development, metabolism, growth, and many other physiological processes.

hypothalamus A cluster of nuclei that controls many bodily functions, including feeding, drinking, and the release of many hormones.

I

illusion A false perception or distortion of the senses often caused by unconscious brain processes.

implicit memory The memories that cannot be retrieved consciously, but are activated as part of particular skills or actions, or in the form of an emotion linked to an event that cannot be made conscious. Implicit memories underlie the learning of physical skills such as playing a ball game or tying a shoelace; see also *procedural memory*.

inferior Below or underneath.

inferior colliculi The principal midbrain nuclei of the auditory pathway.

inhibitory neurotransmitter A type of neurotransmitter that stops neurons firing; see also *excitatory neurotransmitter*.

insula Also referred to as the insular cortex, the brain region that lies in a deep recess between the temporal and frontal lobes.

intelligence quotient (IQ) A score based on a range of tests that represents the relative intelligence of a person.

interneuron A "bridging" neuron connecting afferent and efferent neurons.

ipsilateral On the same side of the body to that in which a condition occurs; see also *contralateral*.

IQ See *intelligence quotient*.

K

Korsakoff's syndrome A brain disease associated with chronic alcoholism. Symptoms include delirium, insomnia, hallucinations, and a lasting amnesia.

L

lateral On or to the side.

lateral geniculate nucleus (LGN) A nucleus in the thalamus that acts as a relay in the visual pathway.

lesion An area of injury or cell death.

limbic system A set of brain structures lying along the inner border of the cortex, crucial for emotion, memory, and mediating consciousness.

lobe One of four main areas of the brain that are delineated by function (occipital, temporal, parietal, and frontal).

longitudinal fissure Also called the longitudinal sulcus, the deep groove that marks the division of the two cerebral hemispheres.

long-term memory The final phase of memory, in which information storage may last from hours to a lifetime.

long-term potentiation (LTP) A change in a neuron that increases the likelihood of it firing in unison with one that it has fired with before.

M

magnetic resonance imaging (MRI) A brain-imaging technique that provides high-resolution pictures of brain structures.

magnetoencephalography (MEG) A non-invasive functional brain-imaging technique that is sensitive to rapid changes in brain activity. Recording devices (SQUIDS) measure small magnetic fluctuations associated with neural activity in the cortex and present these in visual form.

magnocellular The pathways from large retinal ganglion cells to cortical visual areas. They are sensitive to movement.

mamillary bodies The small limbic-system nuclei that are concerned with emotion and memory.

medial In the middle.

medulla Also known as the medulla oblongata or myencephalon. A part of the brainstem situated between the pons and the spinal cord. It is responsible for maintaining vital bodily processes, such as breathing and heart rate.

melatonin A hormone that helps to regulate the sleep–wake cycle. It is produced by the pineal gland.

meninges The three layers of protective tissue between the brain and the skull.

mesencephalon Also referred to as the "midbrain", the area of the brain between the forebrain and the brainstem, involved in eye movement, body movement, and hearing. It includes the basal ganglia.

midbrain See *mesencephalon*.

mind The thoughts, feelings, beliefs, intentions, and so on, that arise from the processes of the brain.

motor cortex The region of the brain containing neurons that send signals, directly or indirectly, to the muscles. It stretches around the brain like an alice band.

motor neuron A neuron that infiltrates muscle and causes it to contract or stretch.

MRI See *magnetic resonance imaging*.

myelencephalon See *medulla*.

myelin The fatty material that surrounds and insulates the axons of some neurons.

N

narcolepsy An illness characterized by uncontrolled bouts of sleeping.

near-infrared spectroscopy (NIRS) A functional imaging technique that shows varying levels of oxygen use in the brain (a marker of neural activity) by measuring the reflection of near-infrared light from cerebral tissues.

neocortex The wrinkled outer layer of the brain; also referred to as the cerebral cortex.

nervous system The nerve cells that connect to the brain and extend throughout the entire body. They are grouped into the central nervous system (CNS) and the peripheral nervous system (PNS).

neurogenesis The generation of new neurons in the brain.

neuron Also referred to as a nerve cell, a brain cell that signals to others by generating and passing on electrical signals.

neurotransmitter A chemical secreted by neurons that carries signals between them across synapses.

nociceptive Responding to painful or noxious stimuli.

norepinephrine An excitatory neurotransmitter, also known as noradrenaline; see also *adrenaline*.

nucleus A bound cluster or group of nerve cells with specialist functions.

nucleus accumbens A limbic-system nucleus that processes information related to motivation and reward.

occipital lobe The back part of the cerebrum, mainly dedicated to visual processing.

olfactory nerve/system The nerve/body system that responds to smell molecules.

opium A drug derived from poppy seeds that produces intense euphoria, pain relief, and relaxation.

optic chiasm The point of decussation (crossing) of the optic nerves from each eye; see also *decussation*.

optic nerve A bundle of nerve fibres carrying signals from retinal ganglion cells into the main part of the brain for processing.

oscillations The rhythmic firings of neurons.

oxytocin A neurotransmitter involved in social bonding.

P

parasympathetic nervous system A branch of the autonomic nervous system, concerned with the conservation of the body's energy. It inhibits the sympathetic nervous system.

parietal lobe The top-back subdivision of the cerebral cortex, mainly concerned with spatial computation, body orientation, and attention.

Parkinson's disease An illness characterized by tremors and slowness of action; it is thought to be caused by degeneration of dopamine-producing cells.

parvocellular The nerve pathways from small areas of the retina to cortical visual areas. They are sensitive to colour and form.

peptides The chains of amino acids that can function as neurotransmitters or hormones.

peripheral nervous system (PNS) The part of the nervous system that includes all nerves and neurons outside the brain and spinal cord.

PET See *positron emission tomography*.

phantom limb An absent limb (usually amputated) that the person continues to experience as part of their body.

pia matter The innermost layer of the meninges; a thin, elastic tissue that covers the surface of the brain.

pineal gland A pea-sized gland located near the thalamus that produces melatonin, which regulates the sleep-wake cycle.

pituitary gland A hypothalamic nucleus that produces hormones, including oxytocin.

plasticity The capacity of the brain to change its structure and function.

pons A part of the hindbrain lying in front of the cerebellum.

positron emission tomography (PET) A functional imaging technique for measuring brain function in living subjects by detecting the location and concentration of small amounts of radioactive chemicals associated with specific neural activity.

posterior Towards the back or tail end. Also referred to as "caudal".

postsynaptic neuron A neuron that receives messages from another; see also *presynaptic neuron*.

prefrontal cortex The region of the brain in the forward-most part of the frontal cortex, involved in planning and other higher-level cognition.

premotor cortex A part of the frontal cortex concerned with planning movements.

presynaptic neuron A neuron that releases a neurotransmitter to carry signals across a synapse to another neuron; see also *postsynaptic neuron*.

primary cortex A region of the brain that first receives sensory information from organs, such as the primary visual cortex.

procedural memory A form of implicit memory relating to learned movements, for example, riding a bicycle.

proprioception Sensory information relating to balance and the position of the body in space.

prosopagnosia The inability to recognize faces.

psychasthenia A condition in which the sufferer experiences heightened sensitivity to negative stimuli, resulting in chronic anxiety.

psychedelic A drug that distorts perception, thought, and feeling.

psychoactive Changing brain function, usually referring to drugs.

psychosis A condition in which a person loses touch with reality.

psychotherapy The treatment of a mental disorder using psychological rather than medical methods.

putamen A part of the striatum, which itself is part of the basal ganglia, that is mainly concerned with regulating movement and procedural learning.

pyramidal neuron An excitatory neuron with a distinctive triangular body, found in the cortex, hippocampus, and amygdala.

Q

qualia The conscious, subjective sensations that arise from stimulation of sense organs, such as pain, warmth, or seeing a colour.

R

raphe nuclei The brainstem nuclei that mainly release serotonin and have wide-ranging effects on mental function.

rapid eye movement (REM) A phase of sleep characterized by rapid eye movements and vivid dreams.

reflex An involuntary movement, controlled by neurons in the spinal cord.

reticular formation A complex area in the brainstem containing various nuclei that affect arousal, sensation, motor function, and vegetative functions such as heartbeat and breathing.

retina The part of the eye containing light-sensitive cells, which send electrical signals to the visual area of the brain for processing into visual imagery.

re-uptake The process by which excess neurotransmitters are removed from the synapse by being carried by transporter cells back into the axon terminals that first released them.

rhombencephalon See *hindbrain*.

rod A sensory neuron located in the outer edge of the retina. It is sensitive to low-intensity light and is specialized for night vision.

rostral Towards or at the front side of the body; see also *anterior*.

S

sagittal A vertical plane passing through the brain from front to back. The mid-sagittal, or median, plane splits the brain into left and right hemispheres.

schizophrenia An illness characterized by intermittent psychosis.

seizure A disruption of normal neural activity. Grand mal seizures involve widespread synchronous neural firing, which produces unconsciousness.

serotonin A neurotransmitter that regulates many functions, including mood, appetite, and sensory perception.

short-term memory A phase of memory in which a limited amount of information may be held for several seconds to minutes; see also *working memory*.

single photon emission computed tomography (SPECT) An imaging process that measures the emission of single photons of a given energy from radioactive tracers in the brain, giving a measure of neural activity.

somatosensory cortex An area of the brain concerned with receiving and processing information about bodily sensations, such as pain and touch.

SPECT See *single photon emission computed tomography*.

SQUIDS See *magnetoencephalography*.

striate cortex An area of the visual cortex characterized (in cross section) by visually distinct strips of cells.

striatum A structure in the basal ganglia composed of the caudate and the putamen.

sulcus (*pl.* sulci) A valley or groove in the brain surface (the opposite of gyrus).

superior Towards or at the top.

superior colliculi Paired structures of nuclei of the midbrain that play a part in relaying visual information.

supplementary motor cortex An area in the front of the motor cortex involved in planning actions that are under internal control, such as actions done from memory rather than guided by current sensations.

survival value The benefit to an individual's chances of surviving and reproducing that is conferred by a particular physical or behavioural characteristic.

sympathetic nervous system A part of the autonomic nervous system that speeds up heart rate, among other things, in response to stimulation; see also *parasympathetic nervous system*.

synaesthaesia The experience of having two or more senses "blended" in response to a stimulus – for example, a shape might be tasted as well as seen, or a sound may be seen as well as heard.

synapse A gap between two neurons that is bridged by neurotransmitters.

T

tegmentum The lower-back part of the midbrain.

telencephalon The largest part of the brain; see also *cerebrum* and *forebrain*.

temporal lobe A division of the cerebral cortex at the side of the head, concerned with hearing, language, and memory.

thalamus Large paired masses of grey matter lying between the brainstem and the cerebrum, the key relay station for sensory information flowing into the brain.

TMS see *transcranial magnetic stimulation*.

top-down A phrase used to distinguish "processed" information or knowledge that is used to interpret "raw" sensory data.

transcranial magnetic stimulation (TMS) A method by which electrical activity in the brain is influenced by a magnetic field, usually generated by a wand held on the scalp.

U

unilateral On one side of the body; see also *bilateral*.

V

V1 The primary visual cortex – other visual areas are often referred to as V2, V3, V4, and so on.

ventral Towards the lower, front surface (such as the abdomen of an animal).

ventral route The pathway in the visual system that connects the visual cortex to the temporal lobe, concerned with the recognition of objects and faces.

ventral tegmental area (VTA) A group of dopamine-containing neurons that make up a key part of the brain's reward system.

ventricle A cavity within the brain containing cerebrospinal fluid.

ventromedial prefrontal cortex A part of the prefrontal cortex, associated with emotions and judgement.

visual cortex The surface of the occipital lobe in which visual information is processed.

W

Wernicke's area The major language area, in the temporal lobe, concerned with comprehension. In most people, it is situated in the left hemisphere, near the junction with the parietal lobe.

white matter A type of brain tissue that is made up of densely packed axons that carry signals to other neurons. It is distinguished from cell bodies by the lighter colour. White matter generally lies beneath the grey matter that forms the cortex.

working memory A process by which information is held "in mind" as active neural traffic until it is forgotten, or encoded in long-term memory.

INDEX

Page numbers in **bold** indicate extended treatments of a topic.

M

N

ACKNOWLEDGMENTS

For the third edition, DK would like to thank Dharini Ganesh for editorial assistance, Pooja Pipil and Garima Agarwal for design assistance, Helen Peters for compiling the index, and Jamie Ambrose for proof-reading.

The publisher would like to thank the following for their kind permission to reproduce their photographs:

(Key: a-above; b-below/bottom; c-centre; f-far; l-left; r-right; t-top)

Edward H. Adelson: 87cr; **Alamy Images:** Alan Dawson Photography 146bl, Alan Graf / Image Source Salsa 173br, allOver photography 45tr, Bubbles Photolibrary 186cr, Mary Evans Picture Library 174br, Photo by M. Flynn / © Salvador Dali, Gala-Salvador Dali Foundation, DACS, London 2009 191t, Paul Hakimata 200tl, Barrie Harwood 202cr, Hipix 10bc, Kirsty McLaren 130c, Mira 44bc, 115cr, Robin Nelson 179c, Old Visuals 92cra, Photogenix 122tl, Pictorial Press 200-201, Stephanie Pilick / dpa picture alliance archive 181b, Simon Reddy 116t, Supapixx 153tr, Tetra Images 123tl, vario images GmbH & Co. KG 190cr; ZUMA Press, Inc. 135br; **Arionauro Cartuns:** 171cr; **Helen Dr Jason J.S. Barton:** 85cr; **George Bartzokis, M.D, UCLA Neuropsychiatric Hospital and Semel Institute:** 214cl; **Dr Theodore W Berger, University of Southern California:** 161tl; **Blackwell Publishing:** European Journal of Neuroscience Vol 25, Issue 3, pp863-871, Renate Wehrle et al, Functional microstates within human REM sleep: first evidence from fMRI of a thalamocortical network specific for phasic REM periods. © 2007 John Wiley & Sons / Image courtesy Renate Wehrle 189fcr; **© EPFL / Blue Brain Project:** 74cb, 75c, Thierry Parel 75cr; **The Bridgeman Art Library:** Archives Charmet 8ftl, 10cl, Bibliothèque de l'Institut de France 7tl, The Detroit Institute of Arts, USA / Founders Society purchase with Mr & Mrs Bert L. Smokler & Mr & Mrs Lawrence A. Fleischman funds 189bc, Maas Gallery, London 134c, Peabody Essex Museum, Salem, Massachusetts, USA 172bl, Royal Library, Windsor 174tr; **Vergleichende Lokalisationslehre der Grosshirnrinde, Dr K Brodmann:** 1909, publ: Verlag von Johann Ambrosius Barth, Leipzig 67bc; **Dr Peter Brugger:** 173cr; **Caltech Brain Imaging Center:** J. Michael Tyszka & Lynn K. Paul 204ca; **Center for Brain Training (www.centerforbrain.com):** 222bl; **Copyright Clearance Center - Rightslink:** Brain 2008 131(12):3169-3177; doi:10.1093 / brain / awn251, Iris E. C. Sommer et al, Auditory verbal hallucinations predominantly activate the right inferior frontal area. Reprinted by permission of Oxford University Press 193cra, Brain Lang 80: 296-313, 2002, Murray Grossman et al, Sentence processing strategies in healthy seniors with poor comprehension: an fMRI study (c) 2002 with permission from Elsevier 215tl, Brain Vol 125, No 8, 1808-1814, Aug 2002, Sterling C. Johnson et al, Neural correlates of self-reflection (c) 2002. Reprinted with permission of Oxford University Press 192bl, Brain, Vol. 122, No. 2, 209-217, Feb 1999, Noam Sobel et al, Blind smell: brain activation induced by an undetected air-borne chemical © 1999 by permission of Oxford University Press 98bl, Current Biology, Vol. 13, December 16, 2003, Nouchine Hadjikhani and Beatrice de Gelder, Seeing Fearful Body Expressions Activates the Fusiform Cortex and Amygdala, 2201-2205, Fig. 1, © 2003, with permission from Elsevier Science Ltd. 144br, Int J Dev Neurosci. 2005 Apr-May;23(2-3):125-41, Robert Schultz, Developmental deficits in social perception in autism: the role of the amygdala and fusiform face area © 2005, with permission from Elsevier 249cr, International Journal of Psychophysiology, V63, No 2 Feb 2007 p214-220, Michael J Wright & Robin C. Jackson, Brain regions concerned with perceptual skills in tennis, An fMRI study (c) 2007 with permission from Elsevier 121, Journal of Neurophysiology 96: 2830-2839, 2006; doi:10.1152 / jn.00628.2006, Arthur Wingfield & Murray Grossman, Language and the Aging Brain: Patterns of Neural Compensation Revealed by Functional Brain Imaging © 2006 The American Physiological Society 215, Journal of Neurophysiology Vol 82 No 3 Sept 1999 1610-1614, 128cl, Journal of Neuroscience, Aug 27, 2008 Vol 28 p8655-8657, Duerden & Laverdure-Dupont, Practice makes cortex, (c) The Society of Neuroscience 157tr, Journal of Neuroscience, May 28, 2008, 28(22):5623-5630. Todd A. Hare et al, Dissociating the Role of the Orbitofrontal Cortex and the Striatum in the Computation of Goal Values and Prediction Errors © 2008. Printed with permission from The Society for Neuroscience 169t, Journal of Neuroscience, Nov 7, 2007, 12190-12197; Hongkeun Kim, Trusting our memories: Dissociating the Neural Correlates of Confidence in Veridical versus Illusory Memories, © 2007, Society for Neuroscience 164c, Michael S Beauchamp & Tony Ro; Adapted with permission from Figure 1, Neural Substrates of Sound-Touch Synesthesia after a Thalamic Lesion; Journal of Neuroscience 2008 28:13696-13702 78bl, The Journal of Neuroscience, December 7, 2005 • 25(49):11489 –11493, Peter Kirsch et al, Oxytocin Modulates Neural Circuitry for Social Cognition and Fear in Humans 127tc, Reprinted from The Lancet, Volume 359, Issue 9305, Page 473, 9 February 2002, Half a Brain, Johannes Borgstein & Caroline Grootendorst, © 2002, with permission from Elsevier 205tr, Nature 373, 607-609 (Feb 16, 1995), Bennett A. Shaywitz et al Yale, Sex differences in the functional organization of the brain for language. Reprinted by permission from Macmillan Publishers Ltd 198cl, Nature 415, 1026-1029 (28 Feb 2002), Antoni Rodriguez-Fornells et al Brain potential and functional MRI evidence for how to handle two languages with one brain © 2002. Reprinted by permission of Macmillan Publishers Ltd 149tr, Nature 419, 269-270 (Sept 19, 2002), Olaf Blanke et al, Neuropsychology: Stimulating illusory own-body perceptions (c) 2002. Reprinted by permission from Macmillan Publishers Ltd 173cr, Nature Neuroscience 7, 801-802 (18 July 2004) | doi:10.1038 / nn1291, Hélène Gervais et al, Abnormal cortical voice processing in autism © 2004 Reprinted by permission from Macmillan Publishers Ltd / image courtesy Mônica Zilbovicius 249crb, Nature Neuroscience Vol 10, 1 Jan 2007 p119 Figure 3, Yee Joon Kim et al, Attention induces synchronization-based response in steady-state visual evoked potentials © 2007. Reprinted by permission from Macmillan Publishers Ltd. 183tr, Nature Reviews Neuroscience 4, 37-48, Jan 2003 | doi:10.1038 / nrn1009; Arthur W. Toga & Paul M Thompson, Mapping brain asymmetry © 2003. Reprinted by permission from Macmillan Publishers Ltd / image courtesy Dr Arthur W. Toga, Laboratory of Neuro Imaging at UCLA 57cr, Nature Reviews Neuroscience 7, 406-413 (May 2006) | doi:10.1038 / nrn1907, Usha Goswami, Neuroscience and education: from research to practice? © 2006. Reprinted by permission from Macmillan Publishers Ltd / courtesy Dr Guinevere Eden, Georgetown University, Washinton DC 248t, redrawn by DK courtesy Nature Reviews Neuroscience 3, 201-215 (March 2002), Maurizio Corbetta & Gordon L. Shulman, Control of goal-directed and stimulus-driven attention in the brain © 2002 Reprinted by permission from Macmillan Publishers Ltd. 183cb, NeuroImage 15: 302-317, 2002 Murray Grossman et al, Age-related changes in working memory during sentence comprehension: an fMRI study (c) 2002 with permission from Elsevier 215ftl, Neuron 6 March 2013, 77(5): 980-991, fig 6; Charles E. Schroeder et al, "Mechanisms Underlying Selective Neuronal Tracking of Attended Speech at a Cocktail Party" © 2013 with permission from Elsevier (http: // dx.doi.org / 10.1016 / j.neuron.2012.12.037) 92tr, Neuron Vol 42 Issue 4, 27 May 2004, p687-695, Jay A. Gottfried et al, Remembrance of Odors Past: Human Olfactory Cortex in Cross-Modal Recognition Memory; with permission from Elsevier 162tr, Neuron, Vol 42, Issue 2, 335-346, Apr 22, 2004, Christian Keysers et al, A Touching Sight (c) 2004 with permission from Elsevier 122bl, Neuron, vol 45 issue 5, 651-660, 3 March 2005, Helen S. Mayberg et al Deep Brain Stimulation for Treatment-Resistant Depression (c) 2005 with permission from Elsevier Science & Technology Journals 239cl, Neuron, Vol 49, Issue 6, 16 Mar 2006, p917-927, Nicholas B Turke-Browne, Do-Joon Yi & Marvin M. Chun, Linking Implicit and Explicit Memory: Common Encoding Factors and Shared Representations © 2006 with permission from Elsevier 159crb, Psychiatric Times Vol XXII No 7, May 31, 2005, Dean Keith Simonton, PhD, Are Genius and Madness Related: Contemporary Answers to an Ancient Question, (c) 2005 CMPMedica, reproduced with permission of CMPMedica 170br, Science 2010: 329 (5997): 1358-1361 "Prediction of Individual Brain Maturity Using fMRI", fig. 2, Nico U.F. Dosenbach et al (c) 2010 The American Association for the Advancement of Science - Reprinted with permission from AAAS 210cr, Science Feb 20, 2004; © 2004 The American Association for the Advancement of Science, T. Singer, B. Seymour, J. O'Doherty, H. Kaube, R.J. Dolan, C.D. Frith, Empathy for Pain involves the affective but not sensory components of pain 138br, Science, 13 July 2007, Vol 317. No. 5835, pp.215-219, fig 2, Brendan E. Depue et al, Prefrontal regions orchestrate suppression of emotional memories via a two-phase process. Reprinted with permission from AAAS 158cl, Science, Oct 10, 2003, Vol 302, No 5643 p290-292, Naomi I. Eisenberger et al, Does Rejection Hurt? An fMRI Study of Social Exclusion © 2003 The American Association for the Advancement of Science 139tl, Science, Vol 264, Issue 5162, 1102-1105 (c) 1994 by American Association for the Advancement of Science / H. Damasio, T. Grabowski, R. Frank, A.M. Galaburda & A.R. Damasio, "The return of Phineas Gage: clues about the brain from the skull of a famous patient" / Dept of Image Analysis Facility, University of Iowa 141cr, Trends in Cognitive Sciences, Vol 11 Issue 4, Apr 2007 p158-167 Naotsugu Tsuchiya & Ralph Adolphs, Emotion & consciousness © 2007 Elsevier Ltd / image: Ralph Adolphs 128tr; **Corbis:** Alinari Archives 6tl, Steve Allen 39bc, The Art Archive 8tl, 8cb, Bettmann 6tc, 6tr, 7tc, 8tc, 8bl, 8bc, 9ca, 9br, 11tr, 75br, 136cl, 136c, 136fcl, 173cra, 187br, 204-205, 205cra, Blend Images 215c, Bloomimage 186bl, Keith Brofsky 144tr, Fabio Cardoso 157c, Peter Carlsson / Etsa 96br, Christophe Boisvieux 118bl, Gianni Dagli Orti 85bl, Kevin Dodge 140l, Ecoscene / Angela Hampton 39cr, EPA 186tl, 190t, 248cla, ER Productions 222cr, Fancy / Veer 159tc, Peter M. Fisher 179tr, Robert Garvey 134tl, Rune Hellestad 196cl, Hulton Collection 99cr, Hutchings Stock Photography 104c, Image 100 157bl, Tracy Kahn 168c, Ed Kashi 151tr, Helen King 183cr, 183cr (Man using computer), Elisa Lazo de Valdez 180tl, Walter Lockwood 182cra, Tim McGuire 39t, MedicalRF.com 9tr, Mediscan 199cr, Moodboard 38br, 123tr, 157br, 182cr, Greg Newton 186fbr, Tim Pannell 186br, PoodlesRock 7tr, Premium Stock 157cr, Louie Psihoyos 99bl, Radius Images 185b, Redlink 182tr, Reuters 196-197, Lynda Richardson 159cl, Chuck Savage 138bc, 198tr, Ken Seet 135t, Sunset Boulevard 57t, Sygma 84br, 180bc, Tim Tadder 38tr, 39bl, William Taufic 172tl, 184c, 189br, TempSport 118-119, Thinkstock 38c, Visuals Unlimited 213tr, Franco Vogt 193c, Zefa 101br, 182ftr, 186bc, 192r, 214cr; **Luc De Nil, PhD:** & Kroll, R. (2000). Nieuwe inzichten in de rol van de hersenen tijdens het stotteren van volwassenen aan de hand van recent onderzoek met Positron Emission Tomography (PET). Signaal 32, 13-20. 149cr; **Dr Jean Decety:** Neuropsychologia, Vol 46, Issue 11, Sep 2008, 2607-2614, Jean Decety, Kalina J. Michalska & Yoko Akitsuki, Who caused the pain? An fMRI investigation of empathy and intentionality in children. © 2008 with permission from Elsevier. 140tr; **Dr José Delgado** : 10bl; **Brendan E. Depue:** 164b; **DACS (Design And Artists Copyright Society):** 191; **Dorling Kindersley:** Bethany Dawn 138clb, Colin Keates / Courtesy of the Natural History Museum, London 49cr; **Dreamstime.com:** Sean Pavone 175cl; Photoeuphoria 152tl; **Henrik Ehrsson et al:** Neural substrate of body size: illusory feeling of shrinking of the waist; PLoS Biol 3(12): e412, 2005 174cr; **© 2012 The M.C. Escher Company - Holland. All rights reserved. www.mcescher.com:** 175br; **Henrik Ehrsson et al:** Staffan Larsson 193bl; **Explore-At-Bristol:** 87c; **eyevine:** 11cl; **Dr Anthony Feinstein, Professor of Psychiatry, University of Toronto:** 242crb; **Professor John Gabrieli:** Stanford Report, Tuesday February 25, 2003, Remediation training improves reading ability of dyslexic children 153clb; **Getty Images:** AFP 145t, 202bl, The Asahi Shimbun 216bl, Assembly 187t, John W. Banagan 240fbl, Blend Images 247t, The Bridgeman Art Library / National Portrait Gallery, London 205cla, Maren Caruso 100cr, Pratik Chorge / Hindustan Times 216r, Comstock Images 134tr, Digital Vision 144tc, ElementalImaging 116-117, 153cr, 170bl, 185cr, Gazimal 182crb, Tim Graham 162br, Louis Grandadam 153cr, Hulton Archive 11bl, 93cr, 129b, 160-161 (girls icecream), 162-163t, 190b, 201tr, 202br, 205c, 222tl, 222tr, 242bl, International Rescue 105, Lifestock 144cb, Tanya Little 184br, Don Mason 135cb, Victoria Pearson 215tr, Peter Ginter 243t, Hulton Archive /Stringer 199fcl, Photo and Co 127cra, Photodisc 215cr, 241cr, Popperfoto 241tr, Louie Psihoyos 239tr, Purestock 215tc, Juergen Richter 175tr, Charlie Schuck 162bl, Chad Slattery 131, Henrik Sorensen 189bl, Sozaijiten / Datacraft 247cr, Tom Stoddart 119br, David Sutherland 191b, Time & Life Pictures 8crb, VCG 217bl, Bruno Vincent 235bc; WireImage 240clb, Elis Years 240bl; **Jordan Grafman PhD:** 141tl; **Dr Hunter Hoffman, U.W.:** 109t, 109c, 109cr; **Courtesy of the Laboratory of Neuro Imaging at UCLA and Martinos Center for Biomedical Imaging at MGH, Consortium of the Human Connectome Project - www.humanconnectomeproject.org ; Courtesy of the Laboratory of Neuro Imaging at UCLA and Martinos Center for Biomedical Imaging at MGH, Consortium of the Human Connectome Project - www.humanconnectomeproject.org ; Courtesy of the Laboratory of Neuro Imaging at UCLA and Martinos Center for Biomedical Imaging at MGH, Consortium of the Human Connectome Project - www. humanconnectomeproject.org ; :** 74r; **Imprint Academic:** The Volitional Brain: Towards a neuroscience of free will, Ed Benjamin Libet, Anthony Freeman & Keith Sutherland © 1999 / Cover illustration by Nicholas Gilbert Scott, Cover design by J.K.B. Sutherland 11cr; **Photographic Unit, The Institute of Psychiatry, London:** 247cl; **iStockphoto.com:** 175c, Jens Carsten Rosemann 85t, Kiyoshi Takahase Segundo 181cr; **Frances Kelly :** Lorna Selfe 174tc; **Pilyoung Kim et al:** Fig. 1 from "The Plasticity of Human Maternal Brain: Longitudinal Changes in Brain Anatomy During the Early Postpartum Period", Behavioural Neuroscience 2010, Vol 124, No. 5 695-700 (c) 2010 American Psychological Association DOI: 10.1037 / a0020884 213bl; **© 2008 Little et al. This is an open-access article distributed under the terms of the Creative Commons Attribution License, which permits unrestricted use, distribution, and reproduction in any medium, provided the original author and source are credited (see http:// creativecommons.org/licenses/by/2.5/).; :** Little AC, Jones BC, Waitt C, Tiddeman BP, Feinberg DR, et al. (2008) Symmetry Is Related to Sexual Dimorphism in Faces: Data Across Culture and Species. PLoS ONE 3(5): e2106. doi:10.1371 / journal.pone.0002106 134bl; **Ian Loxley / TORRO / The Cloud Appreciation Society:** 172-173t; **Library of Congress, Washington, D.C.:** Official White House photo by Pete Souza. 199cl, Orren Jack Turner, Princeton, N.J. 199c; **Mairéad MacSweeney:** Brain. 2002 Jul;125(Pt 7):1583-93, B Woll, R Campbell, PK McGuire, AS David, SC Williams, J Suckling, GA Calvert, MJ Brammer; Neural systems underlying British Sign Language & audio-visual English processing in native users © 2002. Reprinted by permission of Oxford University Press 78cl; **Rogier B. Mars:** Rogier B. Mars, Franz-Xaver Neubert, MaryAnn P. Noonan, Jerome Sallet, Ivan Toni and Matthew F. S. Rushworth, On the relationship between the 'default mode network"and the 'social brain'; Front. Hum. Neurosci., 21 June 2012 | doi: 10.3389 / fnhum.2012.00189 184bl; **Mediscan:** 246tl; **Pierre Metivier:** 178tc; **Massachusetts Institute of Technology (MIT):** Ben Deen / Rebecca Saxe / Department of Brain and Cognitive Sciences and the McGovern Institute, MIT / Nat Comm 8, Article number: 13995 (2017) 209bc; **MIT Press Journals:** Journal of Cognitive Neuroscience Nov 2006, Vol 18, No 11, p1789-1798, Angela Bartolo et al, Humor Comprehension and Appreciation: A FMRI study, © 2006 Massachusetts Institute of Technology 171crb, Journal of Cognitive Neuroscience, Fall 1997, V9; No 5 p664-686, D. Bavelier et al, Sentence reading: a functional MRI study at 4 Tesla, © 1997 Massachusetts Institute of Technology 146br; **The National Gallery, London:** Applied Vision Research Unit / Professor Alastair Gale, Dr David Wooding, Dr Mark Mugglestone & Kevin Purdy with support of Derby University / Telling Time exhibition at National Gallery 86-87; **The Natural History Museum, London:** 103cr; **Neuramatix (www.neuramatix. com):** 75bl;-**Oregon Brain Aging Study, Portland VAMC and Oregon Health & Science University:** 214-215b; **Oxford University Press:** 78; **Professor Eraldo Paulesu:** 153cla; **Pearson Asset Library:** Pearson Education Ltd / Jules Selmes 122br; **Pearson Group:** © 1991 Pearson Assessment. Reproduced with permission. 85br; **Jack Pettigrew, FRS:** 87br; **(c) Philips:** Philips Design concept dress 'Bubelle' 129cl, 129c; **Photolibrary:** David M. Dennis 8t; **PLoS Biology:** Cantlon JF, Brannon EM, Carter EJ, Pelphrey KA (2006) Functional Imaging of Numerical Processing in Adults and 4-y-Old Children. PLoS Biol 4(5): e125 doi:10.1371 / journal.pbio.0040125 169b, Gross L (2006) Evolution of Neonatal Imitation. PLoS Biol 4(9): e311, Sept 5, 2006 doi:10.1371 / journal.pbio.0040311. © 2006 Public Library of Science 11br; **PNAS, Proceedings of the National Academy of Sciences:** Based on Fig. 4 from https: // doi.org / 10.1073 / pnas.0903627106 147bc, Based on Fig. 3.from https: // doi.org / 10.1073 / pnas.0402680101 Copyright (2004) National Academy of Sciences, U.S.A. 210-211b, 103, 15623-15628, Oct 17 2006, Jordan Grafman et al, Human fronto–mesolimbic networks guide decisions about charitable donation © 2006 National Academy of Sciences, USA 141tc, June 16, 2008 (DOI: 10.1073 / pnas.0801566105) Ivanka Savic & Per Lindström, PET and MRI show differences in cerebral asymmetry and functional connectivity between homo- and heterosexual subjects © 2008 National Academy of Sciences, USA 198bl, March 19, 2002 V99, No 6 4115-4120, Jeremy R. Gray et al, Integration of emotion & cognition in the lateral prefrontal cortex © 2002 National Academy of Sciences, USA 169c, Vol 105 no. 39 15106-15111, Sept 30, 2008, Jean-Claude Dreher et al, Age-related changes in midbrain dopaminergic regulation of the human reward system, © 2008 National Academy of Sciences, USA 130bl; **Press Association Images:** 182b, **Public Health Image Library:** Sherif Zaki, MD, PhD; Wun-Ju Shieh, MD, PhD, MPH 231b; **Marcus E. Raichle, Department of Radiology, Washington University School of Medicine, St. Louis, Missouri:** 148bl; **The Random House Group Ltd:** Vintage Books, Ian McEwan, Enduring Love, 2004 244br; **Courtesy of the Rehabilitation Institute of Chicago:** 218-219b; **M. Reisert:** University Medical Center Freiburg; based on the algorithm in M. Reisert et al, Global fiber reconstruction becomes practical, NeuroImage Volume 54, Issue 2, 15 January 2011 pages 955-962 (http: / / www.ncbi. nlm.nih.gov / pubmed / 20854913) 204cl; **Courtesy of Professor Katya Rubia:** based on data published in the American Journal of Psychiatry, 2009; 166: 83-94 248b; **Kosha Ruparel & Daniel Langleben, University of Pennsylvania:** 217cra; Rex by Shutterstock: Imaginechina 232-233; **Science Photo Library:** 12c, 14, 16, 17, 18, 19, 20, 21, 22, 23, 24, 25, 26, 27, 28, 29, 30, 31, 32, 33, 34, 35, 51r, 113cl, 125r, 126cl, 174cl, 215cl, 228tr, 238bc, AJ Photo / Hop American 193cla, Anatomical Travelogue 177r, Tom Barrick, Chris Clark, SGHMS 13tr, 75cla, Dr Lewis Baxter 239bl, David Becker 81tl, Tim Beddow 244cl, Juergen Berger 218bl, Biophoto Associates 68bc, Dr Goran Bredberg 90br, BSIP VEM 238br, BSIP, Asteier-Chru, Lille 232cl, BSIP, Ducloux 96cl, BSIP, SEEMME 12br, Oscar Burriel 188cr, 187bc, Scott Camazine 12bc, CNRI 230l, 245tr, 245cr, Custom Medical Stock Photo 248cl, Thomas Deerinck, Ncmir 59, 68fbl, 126bc, 155r, Steven Needell 141crb, 141br, Department of Nuclear Medicine, Charing Cross Hospital 224bl, Eye of Science 71c, 197bc, 218bc, Don Fawcett 111r, 119tl, Simon Fraser 146tr, 237t, Simon Fraser / Royal Victoria Infirmary, Newcastle Upon Tyne 9tc, 207r, Dr David Furness, Keele University 69bl, GJLP 7bl, Pascal Goetgheluck 104br, Steve Gschmeissner 58l, 61cr, 68bl, 96t, 107bl, C.J. Guerin, PhD, MRC Toxicology Unit 57br, 60l, 63cr, 65cr, 238t, Dr M O Habert, Pitie-Salpetriere, ISM 181cl, Prof J J Hauw 234cl, Innerspace Imaging 9bl, 9-241 (sidebar), ISM 46, Nancy Kedersha 4-5, 8-256 (sidebar), 36-37, 50-51, 76-77, 110-111, 124-125, 132-133, 142-143, 154-155, 166-167, 176-177, 194-195, 206-207, 220-221, Nancy Kedersha / UCLA 68cl, James King-Holmes 91c, 109b, Mehau Kulyk 223cl, 227tr, Living Art Enterprises, LCC 12bl, 44br, 126br, Dr Kari Lounatmaa 227tl, 228tc, Dr John Mazziotta Et Al / Neurology 12tr, 93cl, Duncan Shaw 100tl, Medi-mation 232b, MIT AI Lab / Surgical Planning Lab / Brigham & Women's Hospital 10br, Hank Morgan 12cr, 181fcl, 189cl, 189cr, 189fcl, John Greim 112cr, Paul Parker 81br, Prof. P. Motta / Dept. of Anatomy / University 'La Sapienza', Rome 81bl, 91tr, National Institutes of Health 230r, National Library of Medicine 9cr, Susumu Nishinaga 94br, David Parker 77r, Alfred Pasieka 61cl, 80t, 133r, 135bc, 167r, 231t, 234t, Pasieka 170cla, Alain Pol, ISM 47, Dr Huntington Potter 231cr, C. Pouedras 5br, Philippe Psaila 7br, 107tl, John Reader 100tr, Jean-Claude Revy ISM 12cl, Sovereign, ISM 6bl, 6bc, 6br, 13cra, 13c, 37r, 62l, 64t, 208t, Dr Linda Stannard 228tl, Andrew Syred 195r, Sheila Terry 102l, 153cb, Alexander Tsiaras 7bc, 13br, US National Library of Medicine 10tr, Wellcome Dept. of Cognitive Neurology 57bl, 127cr, 143r, 241br, Professor Tony Wright 91bc, Dr John Zajicek 71cr, 221r, Zephyr 13cr, 57bc, 119crb, 218tl, 225cra, 225cb, 227br, 228cl, 229bl, 237c; **seeingwithsound.com:** Peter B L Meijer 89br; **Roger Shepard:** Adapted from L'egs-istential Quandry, 1974, pen and ink; Published in artist's book, Mind Sights, 1990 W.H. Freeman 175bc; **Society for Neuroscience:** Fig. 8 / Nemrodov et al., "The Neural Dynamics of Facial Identity Processing: Insights from EEG-Based Pattern Analysis and Image Reconstruction" 217tc; **Stephen Wiltshire Gallery, London:** Stephen Wiltshire, Aerial view of Houses of Parliament and Westminster Abbey, 23 June 2008 164-165; **© 2009 Michael J Tarr:** 83cra; **Taylor & Francis Books (UK):** Riddoch MJ, Humphreys GW. Birmingham Object Recognition Battery (BORB). Lawrence Erlbaum Associates, 1993 85crb; **The Art Archive:** Musée Condé Chantilly / Gianni Dagli OrtiAA 11tl; **Thanks to Flickr user Reigh LeBlanc for the use of this image:** 69bc; **TopFoto.co.uk:** 173bl, Imageworks 83bl; **Peter Turkeltaub, MD, PhD:** 152cr; **UCLA Health:** 203t; **Dept of Neurology, University Hospital of Geneva :** paper, ref: Seeck et al (1998) Electroeneph 226t; **University of California, Los Angeles:** 242tl; **Dr Katy Vincent, University of Oxford:** 108c; **Image: Tor Wager:** from H. Kober et al, NeuroImage 2008 Aug 15;42(2): 998-1031, Functional grouping and cortical-subcortical interactions in emotion: a meta-analysis of neuroimaging studies, fig. 7 (http: // www.ncbi.nlm.nih.gov / pubmed / 18579414) 127cla; **Wellcome Images:** 222cra, Wellcome Photo Library 91br, Wessex Reg. Genetics Centre 236bl, 236bc; **Susan Whitfield-Gabrieli, McGovern Institute for Brain Research at MIT:** 185cl; **Wikimedia Commons:** Thomasbg 243br, Van Gogh, Starry Night, MoMA, New York 170-171t; **Wikipedia:** 10c, Histologie du Systeme Nerveux de l'Homme et des Vertebretes, Vols 1 & 2, A. Maloine. Paris 1911 9c, Sternberg, Robert J. (1986). "A triangular theory of love", Psychological Review 93 (2): 119–135, doi:10.1037 / 0033-295X.93.2.119 134ca; **John Wiley & Sons Ltd:** Chris Frith, Making up the Mind – How the brain creates our mental world, 2007 Blackwell Publishing © 2007 John Wiley & Sons Ltd / image courtesy Chiara Portas 13bc, Psychological Science, Vol 19 Issue 1, p12-17, Trey Hedden et al, Cultural Influences on Neural Substrates of Attentional Control, © 2009 Association of Psychological Science 199br, **David Williams, University of Rochester:** 81tr; **Dr Daniel R. Winberger:** 244cb; **Adapted with permission of S.F. Witelson:** Reprinted from The Lancet, Vol 353 Issue 9170, p2150, (19 June 1999), Sandra F. Witelson et al, The exceptional brain of Albert Einstein, (c) 1999 with permission from Elsevier & S.F. Witelson 205br; **Rosalie Winard / Temple Grandin:** 249br, **Jason Wolff, PhD, UNC:** 249tr; **Professor Michael J Wright:** International Journal of Psychophysiology, V63, No 2 Feb 2007 p214-220, Michael J. Wright & Robin C. Jackson, Brain regions concerned with perceptual skills in tennis, An fMRI study © 2007 with permission from Elsevier 121t; **Professor Semir Zeki:** 128br

Front & Back Endpapers: **Science Photo Library:** Innerspace Imaging

All other images © Dorling Kindersley

For further information see: **www.dkimages.com**

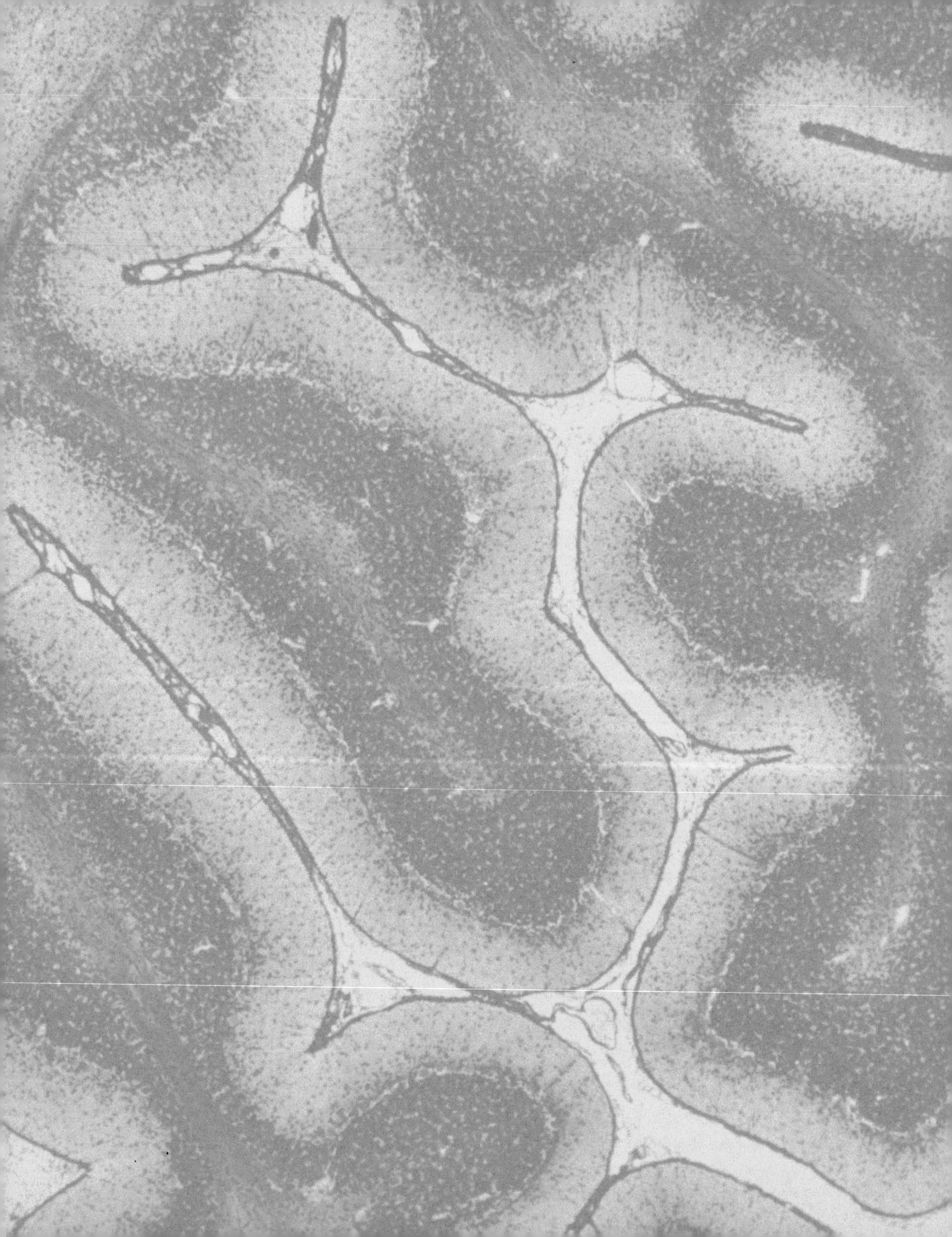